Springer Series in Statistics

Advisors:
P. Bickel, P. Diggle. S. Fienbnerg, K. Krickeberg,
I. Olkin, N. Wermuth, S. Zeger

Springer
New York
Berlin
Heidelberg
Hong Kong
London
Milan
Paris
Tokyo

Springer Series in Statistics

Andersen/Borgan/Gill/Keiding: Statistical Models Based on Counting Processes.
Atkinson/Riani: Robust Diagnostic Regression Analysis.
Berger: Statistical Decision Theory and Bayesian Analysis, 2nd edition.
Borg/Groenen: Modern Multidimensional Scaling: Theory and Applications
Brockwell/Davis: Time Series: Theory and Methods, 2nd edition.
Chan/Tong: Chaos: A Statistical Perspective.
Chen/Shao/Ibrahim: Monte Carlo Methods in Bayesian Computation.
David/Edwards: Annotated Readings in the History of Statistics.
Devroye/Lugosi: Combinatorial Methods in Density Estimation.
Efromovich: Nonparametric Curve Estimation: Methods, Theory, and Applications.
Eggermont/LaRiccia: Maximum Penalized Likelihood Estimation, Volume I: Density Estimation.
Fahrmeir/Tutz: Multivariate Statistical Modelling Based on Generalized Linear Models, 2nd edition.
Farebrother: Fitting Linear Relationships: A History of the Calculus of Observations 1750-1900.
Federer: Statistical Design and Analysis for Intercropping Experiments, Volume I: Two Crops.
Federer: Statistical Design and Analysis for Intercropping Experiments, Volume II: Three or More Crops.
Ghosh/Ramamoorthi: Bayesian Nonparametrics.
Glaz/Naus/Wallenstein: Scan Statistics.
Good: Permutation Tests: A Practical Guide to Resampling Methods for Testing Hypotheses, 2nd edition.
Gouriéroux: ARCH Models and Financial Applications.
Gu: Smoothing Spline ANOVA Models.
Györfi/Kohler/Krzyżak/ Walk: A Distribution-Free Theory of Nonparametric Regression.
Haberman: Advanced Statistics, Volume I: Description of Populations.
Hall: The Bootstrap and Edgeworth Expansion.
Härdle: Smoothing Techniques: With Implementation in S.
Harrell: Regression Modeling Strategies: With Applications to Linear Models, Logistic Regression, and Survival Analysis
Hart: Nonparametric Smoothing and Lack-of-Fit Tests.
Hastie/Tibshirani/Friedman: The Elements of Statistical Learning: Data Mining, Inference, and Prediction
Hedayat/Sloane/Stufken: Orthogonal Arrays: Theory and Applications.
Heyde: Quasi-Likelihood and its Application: A General Approach to Optimal Parameter Estimation.
Huet/Bouvier/Gruet/Jolivet: Statistical Tools for Nonlinear Regression: A Practical Guide with S-PLUS Examples.
Ibrahim/Chen/Sinha: Bayesian Survival Analysis.
Jolliffe: Principal Component Analysis.
Kolen/Brennan: Test Equating: Methods and Practices.

(continued after index)

Mark J. van der Laan
James M. Robins

Unified Methods for Censored Longitudinal Data and Causality

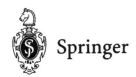

Mark J. van der Laan
Department of Biostatistics
University of California
Berkeley, CA 94720
USA
laan@stat.berkeley.edu

James M. Robins
Department of Epidemiology
Harvard School of Public Health
Boston, MA 02115
USA
robins@hsph.harvard.edu

Library of Congress Cataloging-in-Publication Data
Laan, M.J. van der.
    Unified methods for censored longitudinal data and causality / Mark J. van der Laan,
James M. Robins.
      p. cm. — (Springer series in statistics)
    Includes bibliographical references and indexes.
    ISBN 0-387-95556-9 (alk. paper)
    1. Nonparametric statistics. 2. Longitudinal method. 3. Estimation theory.
I. Robins, James M. II. Title. III. Series.
QA278.8.L33 2002
519.5′4—dc21   2002030239

ISBN 0-387-95556-9   Printed on acid-free paper.

© 2003 Springer-Verlag New York, Inc.
All rights reserved. This work may not be translated or copied in whole or in part without the written permission of the publisher (Springer-Verlag New York, Inc., 175 Fifth Avenue, New York, NY 10010, USA), except for brief excerpts in connection with reviews or scholarly analysis. Use in connection with any form of information storage and retrieval, electronic adaptation, computer software, or by similar or dissimilar methodology now known or hereafter developed is forbidden. The use in this publication of trade names, trademarks, service marks, and similar terms, even if they are not identified as such, is not to be taken as an expression of opinion as to whether or not they are subject to proprietary rights.

Printed in the United States of America.

9 8 7 6 5 4 3 2 1   SPIN 10887878

www.springer-ny.com

Springer-Verlag   New York   Berlin   Heidelberg
A member of BertelsmannSpringer Science+Business Media GmbH

Preface

This project started out with a joint publication with Richard Gill (Gill, van der Laan, Robins, 2000, technical report) on locally efficient estimation in censored data models. Therefore we are particularly grateful to Richard for his contributions. The writing of the book began during Mark van der Laan's sabbatical at the Department of Statistics, University of Auckland, New Zealand, which involved discussions with Alastair Scott and Chris Wild. We owe thanks to Alastair and Chris for their interest, stimulus, and helpful remarks.

An earlier version of this book has been used in a course in the Biostatistics Department at University of California, Berkeley, directed at Ph.D students in biostatistics and statistics. We thank these students for their helpful comments that led to an improved presentation. In spite of the difficulty of the materials, the students were highly motivated to master it and successfully applied the methodology to important practical problems. Collaborations with current and previous Ph.D students on research topics in censored data and causal inference have helped in writing this book. We, therefore, owe thanks to Van der Laan's students Alan Brookhart, Jennifer Bryan, Sunduz Keles, Alan Hubbard, Romain Neugebauer, Maja Pavlic, Katherine Pollard, Chris Quale, Tanya Henneman, Annette Molinaor, and Zhuo Yu and Robins's students Nuala McGrath, Jon Page, and Eric Tchetgen. In addition, collaborations with other researchers have been an important stimulus. In particular, we would like to thank Miguel Hernan, Babette Brumback, Andrea Rotnitzky, Steve Mark, Marshall Joffee, Niels Keiding, Whitney Newey, Jacqueline Witteman, Steve Cole, Sander Greenland, Ya'acov Ritov, Chris Andrews, Larry Wasserman, Alan Hubbard, Nick Jewell, Susan Murphy, Dan Scharfstein and Aad van der Vaart. The enthusiasm of epidemiologists John Colford, Bill Satariano, and Ira Tager for statistical methods suitable for addressing causal questions of interest in their studies on AIDS, air pollution, drinking water, and effect of excercise on survival, has been particularly stimulating.

As always, efforts such as writing a book are a product of the community one works in. Therefore it is difficult to mention everybody who has contributed in one way or another to this book. Mark van der Laan would like to give special thanks to Martine since writing this book would have been hard without her wonderful support, and to Laura, Lars, and Robin as well for not having lost track of the important things in life. Mark van der Laan also thanks Nick Jewell for his continuous intellectual interest and moral support during the writing of this book, and Bonnie Hutchings for being an incredible asset to our Department. James Robins would like to specially thank Andrea Rotnitzky for being both intellectual soulmate and supportive friend, Susanna Kaysen for her extended hospitality at Casa Kaysen, and Valérie Ventura for just about everything.

Mark van der Laan has been supported in his research efforts over the period of work on this book (1994-2002) by a FIRST award (GM53722) grant from the National Institute of General Medical Sciences and a NIAID grant (1-R01-AI46182-01), National Institute of Health. James Robins has been supported by an NIAID grant.

Mark J. van der Laan

James M. Robins

Contents

Preface			v
Notation			1
1	**Introduction**		**8**
	1.1	Motivation, Bibliographic History, and an Overview of the book.	8
	1.2	Tour through the General Estimation Problem.	16
		1.2.1 Estimation in a high-dimensional full data model	17
		1.2.2 The curse of dimensionality in the full data model	21
		1.2.3 Coarsening at random	23
		1.2.4 The curse of dimensionality revisited	27
		1.2.5 The observed data model	40
		1.2.6 General method for construction of locally efficient estimators	40
		1.2.7 Comparison with maximum likelihood estimation	45
	1.3	Example: Causal Effect of Air Pollution on Short-Term Asthma Response	48
	1.4	Estimating Functions	55
		1.4.1 Orthogonal complement of a nuisance tangent space	55
		1.4.2 Review of efficiency theory	61
		1.4.3 Estimating functions.	62
		1.4.4 Orthogonal complement of a nuisance tangent space in an observed data model	64

	1.4.5	Basic useful results to compute projections	68
1.5	Robustness of Estimating Functions		69
	1.5.1	Robustness of estimating functions against misspecification of linear convex nuisance parameters. . .	69
	1.5.2	Double robustness of observed data estimating functions.	77
	1.5.3	Understanding double robustness for a general semiparametric model	79
1.6	Doubly robust estimation in censored data models. . . .		81
1.7	Using Cross-Validation to Select Nuisance Parameter Models		93
	1.7.1	A semiparametric model selection criterian	94
	1.7.2	Forward/backward selection of a nuisance parameter model based on cross-validation with respect to the parameter of interest.	97
	1.7.3	Data analysis example: Estimating the causal relationship between boiled water use and diarrhea in HIV-positive men	99

2 General Methodology　102

2.1	The General Model and Overview		102
2.2	Full Data Estimating Functions.		103
	2.2.1	Orthogonal complement of the nuisance tangent space in the multivariate generalized linear regression model (MGLM)	105
	2.2.2	Orthogonal complement of the nuisance tangent space in the multiplicative intensity model	107
	2.2.3	Linking the orthogonal complement of the nuisance tangent space to estimating functions	111
2.3	Mapping into Observed Data Estimating Functions . . .		114
	2.3.1	Initial mappings and reparametrizing the full data estimating functions	114
	2.3.2	Initial mapping indexed by censoring and protected nuisance parameter	124
	2.3.3	Extending a mapping for a restricted censoring model to a complete censoring model	125
	2.3.4	Inverse weighting a mapping developed for a restricted censoring model	126
	2.3.5	Beating a given RAL estimator	128
	2.3.6	Orthogonalizing an initial mapping w.r.t. G: Double robustness	131
	2.3.7	Ignoring information on the censoring mechanism improves efficiency	135
2.4	Optimal Mapping into Observed Data Estimating Functions		137

			Contents	ix

		2.4.1	The corresponding estimating equation	139
		2.4.2	Discussion of ingredients of a one-step estimator .	141
	2.5	Guaranteed Improvement Relative to an Initial Estimating Function		142
	2.6	Construction of Confidence Intervals		144
	2.7	Asymptotics of the One-Step Estimator		145
		2.7.1	Asymptotics assuming consistent estimation of the censoring mechanism	146
		2.7.2	Proof of Theorem 2.4	150
		2.7.3	Asymptotics assuming that either the censoring mechanism or the full data distribution is estimated consistently	151
		2.7.4	Proof of Theorem 2.5	152
	2.8	The Optimal Index		153
		2.8.1	Finding the optimal estimating function among a given class of estimating functions	159
	2.9	Estimation of the Optimal Index		166
		2.9.1	Reparametrizing the representations of the optimal full data function	167
		2.9.2	Estimation of the optimal full data structure estimating function	169
	2.10	Locally Efficient Estimation with Score-Operator Representation		170
3	**Monotone Censored Data**			**172**
	3.1	Data Structure and Model		172
		3.1.1	Cause-specific censoring	175
	3.2	Examples		176
		3.2.1	Right-censored data on a survival time	176
		3.2.2	Right-censored data on quality-adjusted survival time	177
		3.2.3	Right-censored data on a survival time with reporting delay	179
		3.2.4	Univariately right-censored multivariate failure time data	181
	3.3	Inverse Probability Censoring Weighted (IPCW) Estimators		183
		3.3.1	Identifiability condition	183
		3.3.2	Estimation of a marginal multiplicative intensity model	184
		3.3.3	Extension to proportional rate models.	191
		3.3.4	Projecting on the tangent space of the Cox proportional hazards model of the censoring mechanism	192
	3.4	Optimal Mapping into Estimating Functions		195

- 3.5 Estimation of Q 196
  - 3.5.1 Regression approach: Assuming that the censoring mechanism is correctly specified 197
  - 3.5.2 Maximum likelihood estimation according to a multiplicative intensity model: Doubly robust .. 198
  - 3.5.3 Maximum likelihood estimation for discrete models: Doubly robust 200
  - 3.5.4 Regression approach: Doubly robust 201
- 3.6 Estimation of the Optimal Index 204
  - 3.6.1 The multivariate generalized regression model .. 205
  - 3.6.2 The multivariate generalized regression model when covariates are always observed 206
- 3.7 Multivariate failure time regression model 208
- 3.8 Simulation and data analysis for the nonparametric full data model 211
- 3.9 Rigorous Analysis of a Bivariate Survival Estimate ... 217
  - 3.9.1 Proof of Theorem 3.2 221
- 3.10 Prediction of Survival 224
  - 3.10.1 General methodology 225
  - 3.10.2 Prediction of survival with Regression Trees ... 230

4 Cross-Sectional Data and Right-Censored Data Combined   232
- 4.1 Model and General Data Structure 232
- 4.2 Cause Specific Monitoring Schemes 234
  - 4.2.1 Overview 235
- 4.3 The Optimal Mapping into Observed Data Estimating Functions 236
  - 4.3.1 Identifiability condition 239
  - 4.3.2 Estimation of a parameter on which we have current status data 241
  - 4.3.3 Estimation of a parameter on which we have right-censored data 243
  - 4.3.4 Estimation of a joint-distribution parameter on which we have current status data and right-censored data 244
- 4.4 Estimation of the Optimal Index in the MGLM 245
- 4.5 Example: Current Status Data with Time-Dependent Covariates 246
  - 4.5.1 Regression with current status data 248
  - 4.5.2 Previous work and comparison with our results . 250
  - 4.5.3 An initial estimator 251
  - 4.5.4 The locally efficient one-step estimator 252
  - 4.5.5 Implementation issues 253
  - 4.5.6 Construction of confidence intervals 255

		Contents	xi

		4.5.7	A doubly robust estimator	256
		4.5.8	Data-adaptive selection of the location parameter	257
		4.5.9	Simulations	257
		4.5.10	Example 1: No unmodeled covariate	258
		4.5.11	Example 2: Unmodeled covariate	258
		4.5.12	Data Analysis: California Partners' Study	260
	4.6	Example: Current Status Data on a Process Until Death		262

5 Multivariate Right-Censored Multivariate Data — 266

	5.1	General Data Structure	266
		5.1.1 Modeling the censoring mechanism	268
		5.1.2 Overview	270
	5.2	Mapping into Observed Data Estimating Functions	271
		5.2.1 The initial mapping into observed estimating data functions	271
		5.2.2 Generalized Dabrowska estimator of the survival function in the nonparametric full data model	273
		5.2.3 Simulation study of the generalized Dabrowka estimator.	275
		5.2.4 The proposed mapping into observed data estimating functions	276
		5.2.5 Choosing the full data estimating function in MGLM	282
	5.3	Bivariate Right-Censored Failure Time Data	282
		5.3.1 Introduction	282
		5.3.2 Locally efficient estimation with bivariate right-censored data	286
		5.3.3 Implementation of the locally efficient estimator	290
		5.3.4 Inversion of the information operator	292
		5.3.5 Asymptotic performance and confidence intervals	293
		5.3.6 Asymptotics	294
		5.3.7 Simulation methods and results for the nonparametric full data model	299
		5.3.8 Data analysis: Twin age at appendectomy	302

6 Unified Approach for Causal Inference and Censored Data — 311

	6.1	General Model and Method of Estimation	311
	6.2	Causal Inference with Marginal Structural Models	318
		6.2.1 Closed Form Formula for the Inverse of the Nonparametric Information Operator in Causal Inference Models.	324
	6.3	Double Robustness in Point Treatment MSM	326
	6.4	Marginal Structural Model with Right-Censoring	329

	6.4.1	Doubly robust estimators in marginal structural models with right-censoring	334
	6.4.2	Data Analysis: SPARCS	338
	6.4.3	A simulation for estimators of a treatment-specific survival function	343
6.5	Structural Nested Model with Right-Censoring		347
	6.5.1	The orthogonal complement of a nuisance tangent space in a structural nested model without censoring	353
	6.5.2	A class of estimating functions for the marginal structural nested model	357
	6.5.3	Analyzing dynamic treatment regimes	359
	6.5.4	Simulation for dynamic regimes in point treatment studies	360
6.6	Right-Censoring with Missingness.		362
6.7	Interval Censored Data		366
	6.7.1	Interval censoring and right-censoring combined .	368

References   **371**

Author index   **388**

Subject index   **394**

Example index   **397**

Notation

CAN: consistent and asymptotically normal.
RAL: regular and asymptotically linear.
SRA: sequential randomization assumption.
CAR: coarsening at random.
i.i.d.: identically and independently distributed.
MGLM: multivariate generalized linear regression model.
$\max_{\mathbf{x} \in S}^{-1} \mathbf{f}(\mathbf{x})$: this denotes the argument at which the function $f : S \to \mathbb{R}$ is maximal.
$\min_{\mathbf{x} \in S}^{-1} \mathbf{f}(\mathbf{x})$: this denotes the argument at which the function $f : S \to \mathbb{R}$ is minimal.
$\mathbf{P_1 \equiv P_2}$ for two probability measures P_1, P_2: this means that P_1 is absolutely continuous w.r.t. P_2 (which we denote with $P_1 \ll P_2$) and P_2 is absolutely continuous w.r.t. P_1 ($P_2 \ll P_1$). In other words, dP_1/dP_2 and dP_2/dP_1 exist.
$\mathbf{dG_1/dG} < \infty$: same as $G_1 \ll G$, but where G_1, G refer to the conditional distributions of Y, given X.
$\mathbf{Y} = \mathbf{\Phi}(\mathbf{X}, \mathbf{C})$: denotes observed data on a subject (or more general, the experimental unit), which is a function of a full data structure X and censoring variable C. It is always assumed that we observe n i.i.d. $Y_1, \ldots, Y_n$ copies of Y.
$\mathcal{X}$: outcome space of X.
$\mathcal{Y}$: outcome space of Y.
$\bar{\mathbf{X}}(\mathbf{t}) = (\mathbf{X}(\mathbf{s}) : \mathbf{s} \le \mathbf{t})$: full data process up to point t.
$\mathbf{X} \equiv \bar{\mathbf{X}}(\mathbf{T})$: time-dependent full data process up to a possibly random endpoint T.

2 Notation

F_X: the probability distribution of the full data X.
G: the conditional probability distribution of C, given X, also called the censoring mechanism, treatment mechanism, or action mechanism, depending on what C stands for. When we define CAR, we do this in terms of the conditional distribution of Y, given X, which is determined by G, and, by CAR, it is the identifiable part of G. In this book we frequently denote the conditional distribution of Y, given X, with G as well.
$P_{F_X, G}$: the distribution of the observed data Y, which only depends on G through the conditional distribution of Y, given X.
$\mathcal{G}$: a model for the censoring mechanism G (i.e., it is known that $G \in \mathcal{G}$).
$\mathcal{G}(\text{CAR})$: all conditional distributions G of C, given X, satisfying coarsening at random (CAR).
$\mathcal{M}^F$: a model for F_X (i.e., the full data model).
$\mathcal{M} = \{P_{F_X,G} : F_X \in \mathcal{M}^{F,w}, G \in \mathcal{G}(\text{CAR})\} \cup \{P_{F_X,G} : F_X \in \mathcal{M}^F, G \in \mathcal{G}\}$, the observed data model allowing that either the working model $\mathcal{M}^{F,w}$ for F_X or the censoring model $\mathcal{G}$ for G is misspecified, but not both.
$\mathcal{M}(\mathcal{G}) = \{P_{F_X,G} : F_X \in \mathcal{M}^F, G \in \mathcal{G}\}$: the observed data model when assuming a correctly specified model $\mathcal{G}$ for G.
$\mathcal{M}(\mathbf{G}) = \{P_{F_X,G} : F_X \in \mathcal{M}^F\}$: the observed data model if the censoring mechanism G is known.
$\mathcal{M}(\mathbf{CAR}) = \{P_{F_X,G} : F_X \in \mathcal{M}^F, G \in \mathcal{G}(\text{CAR})\}$: the observed data model if the censoring mechanism is only known to satisfy CAR.
$\mu = \mu(\mathbf{F_X}) \in \mathbb{R}^k$: the Euclidean parameter of F_X of interest.
$\mathbf{Z} = \mathbf{g}(\mathbf{X}^* \mid \alpha) + \epsilon$: a multivariate generalized regression model (a particular choice of full data model), where Z is a p-variate outcome, X^* is a vector of covariates, $g(X^* \mid \alpha)$ is a p-dimensional vector whose components are regression curves parametrized with a regression parameter $\alpha \in \mathbb{R}^k$, ϵ is a p-variate residual satisfying $E(K(\epsilon_j) \mid X^*) = 0$, $j = 1, \ldots, p$, for a given monotone nondecreasing function K.
$K(\cdot)$: monotone function specifying the location parameter (e.g., mean, median, truncated mean, smooth median) of the conditional distribution of Z, given X^*, modeled by $g(X^* \mid \alpha)$. For example, 1) $K(\epsilon) = \epsilon$, 2) $K(\epsilon) = I(\epsilon > 0) - (1 - p)$, 3) $K(\epsilon) = \epsilon$ on $[-\tau, \tau]$ and $K(\epsilon) = \tau$ for $\epsilon > \tau$, $K(\epsilon) = -\tau$ for $\epsilon < -\tau$ correspond with mean regression, pth quantile regression (e.g., $p = 0.5$ gives median regression), and truncated mean regression, respectively.
$N(t)$: a counting process being a part of the full data X.
$\lambda(t)dt = E(dN(t) \mid \bar{Z}(t-)) = Y(t)\lambda_0(t)\exp(\beta W(t))dt$: a multiplicative intensity model (a particular full data model), where $\bar{Z}(t)$ is a given function of $\bar{X}(t)$ including the past $\bar{N}(t)$ of the counting process N, $Y(t)$ is an indicator function of $\bar{Z}(t-)$ (indicator that $N(\cdot)$ is at risk of jumping at time t), and $W(t)$ is a vector of covariates extracted from $\bar{Z}(t-)$. We also consider the case where $\bar{Z}(t-)$ does not include the past of N. In this case, we refer to these models as proportional rate models. We also consider discrete multiplicative intensity models, where $\lambda(t) = Y(t)\Lambda_0(dt)\exp(beta W(t))$ is

now a conditional probability.
$\bar{F} = 1 - F$.
$<S_1, \ldots, S_k>$: linear span of k elements (typically scores in $L_0^2(F_X)$ or $L_0^2(P_{F_X,G})$) in a Hilbert space.
$<\vec{S}> \equiv <S_1, \ldots, S_k>$: linear span of the k components of $\vec{S}$.
$\langle f, g \rangle$: inner product defined in a Hilbert Space.
$\langle f, (g_1, \ldots, g_k) \rangle \equiv (\langle f, g_1 \rangle, \ldots, \langle f, g_k \rangle)$.
$H_1 \oplus H_2 = \{h_1 + h_2 : h_j \in H_j, j = 1, 2\}$: the sum space spanned by two orthogonal sub-Hilbert spaces H_1, H_2 of a certain Hilbert space.
$H_1 + H_2 = \{h_1 + h_2 : h_j \in H_j, j = 1, 2\}$: the sum space spanned by two sub-Hilbert spaces H_1, H_2 of a certain Hilbert space.
$\Pi(\cdot \mid H)$: the projection operator onto a subspace H of a certain Hilbert space.
$L_0^2(F_X)$: Hilbert space of functions $h(X)$ with $E_{F_X} h(X) = 0$ with inner product $\langle h, g \rangle_{F_X} = E_{F_X} h(X) g(X)$ and corresponding norm $\| h \|_{F_X} = \sqrt{E_{F_X} h^2(X)}$.
$T^F(F_X) \subset L_0^2(F_X)$: the tangent space at F_X in the full data model $\mathcal{M}^F$. This is the closure of the linear space spanned by scores of a given class of one-dimensional submodels $\epsilon \to F_\epsilon$ that cross F_X at $\epsilon = 0$.
$T^F_{nuis}(F_X) \subset L_0^2(F_X)$: the nuisance tangent space at F_X in the full data model $\mathcal{M}^F$. This is the closure of the linear space spanned by scores of a given class of one-dimensional submodels $\epsilon \to F_\epsilon$ that cross F_X at $\epsilon = 0$ and satisfy $d/d\epsilon \mu(F_\epsilon)|_{\epsilon=0} = 0$.
$T^{F,\perp}_{nuis}(F_X) \subset L_0^2(F_X)$: the orthogonal complement of the nuisance tangent space $T^F_{nuis}(F_X)$ in model $\mathcal{M}^F$, where μ is the parameter of interest. The class of full data estimating functions $D_h(\cdot \mid \mu, \rho)$, $h \in \mathcal{H}^F$, is chosen so that $T^{F,\perp}_{nuis}(F_X) \supset \{D_h(X \mid \mu(F_X), \rho(F_X)) : h \in \mathcal{H}^F\}$, where the right hand side is chosen as rich as possible so that we might even have equality.
D_h, defined in full data model $\mathcal{M}^F$: full data estimating function $D_h : \mathcal{X} \times \{(\mu(F_X), \rho(F_X)) : F_X \in \mathcal{M}^F\} \to \mathbb{R}$ for parameter μ with nuisance parameter ρ. Here $h \in \mathcal{H}^F$ indexes different possible choices of full data estimating functions.
$\mathcal{H}^F$: index set providing a rich class of full data estimating functions satisfying:
$$D_h(X \mid \mu(F_X), \rho(F_X)) \in T^{F,\perp}_{nuis}(F_X) \text{ for all } h \in \mathcal{H}^F.$$
$D_h, h \in \mathcal{H}^{F,k}$: for $h = (h_1, \ldots, h_k) \in \mathcal{H}^{Fk}$,
$$D_{h_1,\ldots,h_k}(X \mid \mu, \rho) = (D_{h_1}(X \mid \mu, \rho), \ldots, D_{h_k}(X \mid \mu, \rho)).$$
A full data structure estimating function D_h, $h \in \mathcal{H}^{Fk}$, defines an estimating equation for μ: given an estimate of ρ, one can estimate μ with the solution of the k-dimensional equation $0 = \sum_{i=1}^n D_h(X_i \mid \mu, \rho_n)$.
$D_h(X \mid \mu, \rho)$: full data estimating function D_h evaluated at X, μ, ρ. Sometimes, $D_h(X \mid \mu, \rho)$ is used to denote the actual estimating function,

4   Notation

just to make its arguments explicit.

$\mathcal{D}(\mu,\rho) = \{D_h(X \mid \mu,\rho) : h \in \mathcal{H}^F\}$: all possible full data functions obtained by varying h, but fixing μ, ρ.

$\mathcal{D} = \{D_h(X \mid \mu(F_X), \rho(F_X)) : F_X \in \mathcal{M}^F, h \in \mathcal{H}^F\}$: all possibly full data structure estimating functions obtained by varying h and F_X.

$\mathbf{S_{eff}^{*F}}(\cdot \mid \mathbf{F_X})$: the canonical gradient (also called efficient influence curve) of the pathwise derivative of the parameter $\mu(F_X)$ in the full data model $\mathcal{M}^F$.

$\mathbf{T_{nuis}^{F,\perp,*}}(\mathbf{F_X})$: the set of all gradients of the pathwise derivative at F_X of the parameter $\mu(F_X)$ in the full data model $\mathcal{M}^F$ whose components span $T_{nuis}^{F,\perp}(F_X)$.

$\mathbf{D_{h_{eff}}}(\cdot \mid \mu(\mathbf{F_X}), \rho(\mathbf{F_X})) = S_{eff}^{*F}(\cdot \mid F_X)$: that is, h_{eff} indexes the optimal estimating function in the *full data structure model*. Here $h_{eff} = h_{eff}(F_X)$ depends on F_X. Off course, one still obtains an optimal estimating function by putting a $k \times k$ fixed matrix in front of S_{eff}^{*F}.

$\mathcal{F}(\mathbf{t})$: a predictable observed subject-specific history up to time t, typically representing all observed data up to time point t on a subject.

$\mathbf{A}$: a time-dependent possibly multivariate process $A(t) = (A_1(t), \ldots, A_k(t))$ whose components describe specific censoring (e.g., treatment) actions at time t. Here A represents the censoring variable C for the observed data structure. Typically, $A_j(t)$, $j = 1, \ldots, k$, are counting processes.

$\mathcal{A}$: the support of the marginal distribution of A.

$\alpha(\mathbf{t}) = E(dA(t) \mid \mathcal{F}(t))$: the intensity (possibly discrete, $\alpha(t) = P(dA(t) = 1 \mid \mathcal{F}(t))$ at given grid points) of counting process $A(t)$ w.r.t. the history $\mathcal{F}(t)$.

$\mathbf{Y} = (\mathbf{A}, \mathbf{X_A})$: a particular type of observed censored data, where for the full data we have $X = (X_a : a \in \mathcal{A})$, and A tells us what component of X we observe. For example, $A(t)$ can be the indicator $I(C \leq t)$ of being right-censored by a dropout time C. If the full data model is a causal model and there is no censoring, then $A(t)$ is the treatment that the subject receives at time t. If the observed data structure includes both treatment assignment and censoring, then $A(t)$ is the multivariate process describing the treatment actions and censoring actions assigned to the subject at time t.

$\mathbf{L_0^2(P_{F_X,G})}$: Hilbert space of functions $V(Y)$ with $E_{P_{F_X,G}} V(Y) = 0$ with inner-product $\langle h, g \rangle_{P_{F_X,G}} = E_{P_{F_X,G}} h(Y) g(Y)$ and corresponding norm $\parallel h \parallel_{P_{F_X,G}} = \sqrt{E_{P_{F_X,G}} h^2(Y)}$.

$\mathbf{T(P_{F_X,G})} \subset L_0^2(P_{F_X,G})$, $\mathbf{T_{nuis}(P_{F_X,G})} \subset L_0^2(P_{F_X,G})$, $\mathbf{T_{nuis}^\perp(P_{F_X,G})} \subset L_0^2(P_{F_X,G})$ are the observed data tangent space, observed data nuisance tangent space, and the orthogonal complement of the observed data nuisance tangent space at $P_{F_X,G}$, respectively, in model $\mathcal{M}(CAR)$ (or, if made explicit in $\mathcal{M}(\mathcal{G})$), where μ is the parameter of interest.

$\mathbf{T_{CAR}(P_{F_X,G})} = \{V(Y) : E_G(V(Y) \mid X) = 0\} \subset L_0^2(P_{F_X,G})$: the nuisance

tangent space of G in model $\mathcal{M}(CAR)$.
$\mathbf{T_2}(\mathbf{P_{F_X,G}}) \subset T_{CAR}(P_{F_X,G})$ or $\mathbf{T_G}(\mathbf{P_{F_X,G}}) \subset T_{CAR}(P_{F_X,G})$: the nuisance tangent space of G in the observed data model $\mathcal{M}(\mathcal{G})$.
$D \to \mathbf{IC_0}(\mathbf{Y} \mid \mathbf{Q_0}, \mathbf{G}, \mathbf{D})$, $D \to \mathbf{IC}(\mathbf{Y} \mid \mathbf{F_X}, \mathbf{G}, \mathbf{D})$, $D \to \mathbf{IC}(\mathbf{Y} \mid \mathbf{Q}, \mathbf{G}, \mathbf{D})$: mapping from a full data function into an observed data function indexed by nuisance parameters $Q_0(F_X,G), G$, F_X, G or $Q(F_X,G), G$. $IC_0(Y \mid Q_0, G, D)$ stands for an initial mapping and $IC(Y \mid F_X, G, D)$ and $IC(Y \mid Q(F_X,G), G, D)$ for the optimal mapping orthogonalized w.r.t. T_{CAR} or a mapping orthogonalized w.r.t. a subspace of T_{CAR}. In many cases, it is not convenient to parametrize IC in terms of F_X, G, but instead parametrize it by a parameter $Q = Q(F_X,G)$ and G. We note that the dependence of these functions on F_X and G is only through the F_X-part of the density of Y and the conditional distribution of Y, given X, respectively.

The mapping IC_0 satisfies for each $P_{F_X,G} \in \mathcal{M}(\mathcal{G})$: for a non empty set of full data functions $\mathcal{D}(\rho_1(F_X), G)$, we have

$$E_G(IC_0(Y \mid Q, G, D) \mid X) = D(X) \quad F_X\text{-a.e. for all } Q \in \mathcal{Q}_0. \qquad (1)$$

For IC, we have the additional property at each $P_{F_X,G} \in \mathcal{M}(CAR)$:

$$IC(Y \mid Q(F_X,G), G, D) = IC_0(Y \mid Q_0(F_X,G), G, D) \\ - \Pi_{F_X,G}(IC_0(Y \mid Q_0(F_X,G), G, D) \mid T_{CAR}),$$

or the projection term can be a projection on a subspace of T_{CAR}. Here $\Pi(\cdot \mid T_{CAR})$ denotes the projection operator in the Hilbert space $L_0^2(P_{F_X,G})$ with inner product $\langle f, g \rangle_{P_{F_X,G}} = E_{P_{F_X,G}} f(Y)g(Y)$.

$\mathcal{D}(\rho_1(\mathbf{F_X}), \mathbf{G})$: the set of full data functions in $\mathcal{D}$ for which (1) holds. Thus, these are the full data structure functions that are mapped by IC_0 into unbiased observed data estimating functions. By making the appropriate assumption on the censoring mechanism, one will have that $\mathcal{D}(\rho_1(F_X), G) = \mathcal{D}$, but one can also decide to make this membership requirement $D_h(\cdot \mid \mu(F_X), \rho(F_X)) \in \mathcal{D}(\rho_1(F_X), G)$ a nuisance parameter of the full data structure estimating function: see next entry.

$\mathbf{D_h}(\cdot \mid \mu(\mathbf{F_X}), \rho(\mathbf{F_X}, \mathbf{G}))$, $h \in \mathcal{H}^F$: these are full data structure estimating functions satisfying $D_h(\cdot \mid \mu(F_X), \rho(F_X, G)) \in \mathcal{D}(\rho_1(F_X), G))$ for all $h \in \mathcal{H}^F$. Formally, they are defined in terms of initially defined full data estimating functions D_h as

$$D_h^r(\cdot \mid \mu, \rho, \rho_1, G) \equiv D_{\Pi(h \mid \mathcal{H}^F(\mu,\rho,\rho_1,G))}(\cdot \mid \mu, \rho),$$

where $\mathcal{H}^F(\mu, \rho, \rho_1, G) \subset \mathcal{H}^F$ are the indexes that guarantee that $E_G(IC_0(Y \mid Q_0, G, D_h(\cdot \mid \mu, \rho)) \mid X) = D_h(X \mid \mu, \rho)$ F_X-a.e and $\Pi(\mid \mathcal{H}^F(\mu, \rho, \rho_1, G))$ is a mapping from $\mathcal{H}^F$ into $\mathcal{H}^F(\mu, \rho, \rho_1, G)$ that is the identity mapping on $\mathcal{H}^F(\mu, \rho, \rho_1, G)$. Thus, if $D_h(\cdot \mid \mu(F_X), \rho(F_X)) \in \mathcal{D}(\rho_1(F_X), G)$ for all $P_{F_X,G} \in \mathcal{M}(\mathcal{G})$, then $D_h^r = D_h$. For notational convenience, we denote $D_h^r(\cdot \mid \mu, \rho, \rho_1, G)$ with $D_h(\cdot \mid \mu, \rho)$ again, but where ρ

now includes the old ρ, ρ_1, and G.

$IC(Y \mid Q, G, D_h(\cdot \mid \mu, \rho))$: an observed data estimating function for μ with nuisance parameters $Q(F_X, G), G$, and ρ, which is obtained by applying the mapping $D \to IC(Y \mid Q, G, D)$ to the particular full data estimating function D_h. If $h = (h_1, \ldots, h_k) \in \mathcal{H}^{Fk}$, then $IC(Y \mid Q, G, D_h(\cdot \mid \mu, \rho))$ denotes

$$(IC(Y \mid Q, G, D_{h_1}(\cdot \mid \mu, \rho)), \ldots, IC(Y \mid Q, G, D_{h_k}(\cdot \mid \mu, \rho))).$$

$\mathbf{S}^*_{\mathbf{eff}}(\mathbf{Y} \mid \mathbf{F_X}, \mathbf{G})$: the canonical gradient (also called the efficient influence curve) of the pathwise derivative of the parameter μ in the observed data model $\mathcal{M}$.

$IC(Y \mid F_X, G, D_{h_{opt}}(\cdot \mid \mu(F_X), \rho(F_X, G))) = S^*_{eff}(Y \mid F_X, G)$: that is, h_{opt} indexes the choice of full data estimating function that results in the optimal observed data estimating function for μ in the *observed data model* $\mathcal{M}, \mathcal{M}(\mathcal{G})$, and $\mathcal{M}(CAR)$. Here $h_{opt} = h_{opt}(F_X, G)$ depends on F_X and G.

$\mathbf{h_{ind, F_X}} : L^2_0(F_X) \to \mathcal{H}^F$: We call it the *index mapping* since it maps a full data function into an index h defining the projection onto $T^{F, \perp}_{nuis}(F_X)$. It is defined by

$$D_{h_{ind, F_X}(D)}(X \mid \mu(F_X), \rho(F_X)) = \Pi(D \mid T^{F, \perp}_{nuis}(F_X)).$$

$\mathbf{A_{F_X}} : L^2_0(F_X) \to L^2_0(P_{F_X, G}) : A_{F_X}(h)(Y) = E_{F_X}(h(X) \mid Y)$: the nonparametric score operator that maps a score of a one-dimensional fluctuation F_ϵ at F_X into the score of the corresponding one-dimensional fluctuation $P_{F_\epsilon, G}$ at $P_{F_X, G}$.

$\mathbf{A_G} : L^2_0(P_{F_X, G}) \to L^2_0(F_X): A_G(V)(X) = E_G(V(Y) \mid X)$: the adjoint of the nonparametric score operator A_{F_X}.

$\mathbf{I_{F_X, G}} = A_G^\top A_{F_X} : L^2_0(F_X) \to L^2_0(F_X): \mathbf{I}_{F_X, G}(h)(X) = E_G(E_{F_X}(h(X) \mid Y) \mid X)$: the nonparametric information operator. If we write $\mathbf{I}^{-1}_{F_X, G}(h)$, then it is implicitly assumed that $I_{F_X, G}$ is 1-1 and h lies in the range of $I_{F_X, G}$.

$\mathbf{IC(Y \mid F_X, G, D)} \equiv A_{F_X} \mathbf{I}^-_{F_X, G}(D)$ is an optimal mapping (assuming that the generalized inverse is defined) from full data estimating functions into the observed data estimating function. For any $IC_0(Y \mid F_X, G, D)$ satisfying $E(IC_0(Y \mid F_X, G, D) \mid X) = D(X)$ F_X-a.e., the optimal mapping can be more generally defined by $IC(Y \mid F_X, G, D) = IC_0(Y \mid F_X, G, D) - \Pi(IC_0(Y \mid F_X, G, D) \mid T_{CAR}(P_{F_X, G}))$.

$\mathbf{I}^*_{\mathbf{F_X, G}} = \Pi(\mathbf{I}_{F_X, G} \mid T^F(F_X))$: the information operator. If we write $I^{*-1}_{F_X, G}(h)$, then it is implicitly assumed that $\mathbf{I}^*_{F_X, G}$ is 1-1 and h lies in the range of $I^*_{F_X, G}$.

The projection operator can be expressed as a sum of a projection on a finite space and the projection on $T^{F, \perp}_{nuis}$ since $T^F(F_X) = \langle S_{eff}(\cdot \mid F_X)\rangle \oplus T^F_{nuis}(F_X)$.

$S^*_{eff}(Y \mid F_X, G) = A_{F_X} \mathbf{I}^{*-}_{F_X, G}(S^{*F}_{eff}(\cdot \mid F_X))$: that is, the efficient influence curve can be expressed in terms of the inverse of the information operator, assuming that the inverse is defined.

R(B): the range of a previously defined linear operator **B**.
N(B): the null space of a previously defined linear operator **B**.
$\overline{\mathbf{H}}$ for a set of elements in a Hilbert space $L_0^2(P_{FX,G})$ is defined as the closure of its linear span.
Pf $\equiv \int f(y) dP(y)$.
$\mathcal{L}(\mathcal{X})$: all real-valued functions of X that are uniformly bounded on a set that contains the true X with probability one.
$\mathcal{H}$: some index set indexing observed data estimating functions.
$\mathbf{c}(\mu) = d/d\mu EIC(Y \mid Q, G, D_h(\cdot \mid \mu, \rho))$ $(h = (h_1, \ldots, h_k))$: the derivative matrix of the expected value of the observed data estimating function.

1
Introduction

1.1 Motivation, Bibliographic History, and an Overview of the book.

In most empirical studies, the full (equivalently, complete) data X on certain subjects are censored (equivalently, missing or coarsened). That is, the data X that one would wish to collect are incompletely observed for a (possibly improper) subset of the study subjects; instead, only a random function (equivalently, a random coarsening) Y of X is observed. Furthermore, over the past decades, data from epidemiological, biostatistical, and econometric studies have become increasingly high-dimensional as longitudinal designs that collect data on many time-varying covariate processes at frequent intervals have become commonplace. Scientific interest, however, often focuses on a low-dimensional functional μ of the distribution F_X of the full data – say, as an example, the medians of the treatment-arm specific distributions of time to tumor recurrence in a cancer clinical trial in which recurrence times are right censored by lost -to-follow-up. In such a trial, X is often high dimesional because the study protocol specifies comprehensive laboratory and clinical measurements be taken monthly. In such settings, the use of non-or semiparametric models for F_X that do not model the components of F_X that are of little scientific interest have become commonplace, so as to insure that misspecification of the functional form of a parametric model for the entire distribution F_X does not induce biased estimates of μ. The methodology described in this book was developed to meet the analytic challenges posed by high dimensional censored data in which a low-dimensional functional μ of the distribution F_X is the parameter of scientific interest.

We provide a general estimating function methodology for locally semiparametric efficient (LSE) estimation of smooth parameters (i.e., parameters estimable at rate $\sqrt{n}$) μ of large non- or semiparametric models for the law F_X of very high dimensional data X based on the observed data Y, when the data are coarsened at random (CAR). The data are said to be CAR if the coarsening mechanism (i.e., the conditional density g of the conditional distribution $G(\cdot \mid X)$ of the observed data Y given the full data X) is only a function of the observed data Y (Heitjan and Rubin, 1991, Jacobsen and Keiding, 1995, and Gill, van der Laan, and Robins, 1997), in which case we refer to the coarsening mechanism $G(\cdot \mid X)$ as a CAR mechanism.

When the data are CAR, the likelihood for Y factors into a part that depends only on the distribution of X and a part that equals the CAR mechanism g. As a consequence, all methods of estimation that obey the likelihood principle (including Bayesian methods with F_X and g apriori independent, and the methods of parametric maximum likelihood, nonparametric maximum likelihood and maximum regularized likelihood) must ignore the CAR mechanism g and thus provide the same inference regardless of whether g is completely known, completely unknown, or known to lie in a (variation independent) parametric or semiparametric model. Because of a historical preference for methods that obey the likelihood principle, a CAR mechanism is referred to as ignorable (Rubin, 1976). However Robins and Ritov (1997) showed that, with high dimensional coarsened at random data, any method of estimation must perform poorly in realistic-sized samples if the CAR mechanism is completely unknown. It follows that, even when the CAR mechanism is completely known or known to follow a lower dimensional model, methods that obey the likelihood principle and thus ignore the coarsening mechanism may perform poorly in realistic-sized samples; in contrast, our generalized estimating functions depend on the CAR mechanism (or a model-based estimate thereof) and thus violate the likelihood principle, yet yield estimators that perform well in the moderate-sized samples occurring in practice. Thus the slogan "With high dimensional censored data, one cannot ignore an ignorable coarsening mechanism."

The general estimating function approach to estimation of parameters of a full-data model based on censored data with known or correctly modelled CAR mechanism was originally introduced by Robins and Rotnitzky (1992), drawing on advances in the efficiency theory of semiparametric models due to Bickel, Klaassen, Ritov, and Wellner (1993), Newey (1990), van der Vaart (1988, 1991), among others. Robins and Rotnitzky restricted their investigation to data structures for which the full data X has a positive probability of being completely observed. As one example, Robins and Rotnitzky (1992) considered the data strucuture in which $X = \{T, (X(t); 0 \leq t \leq T)\}$ is a high-dimensional multivariate time-dependent covariate process $X(t)$ observed till death T that is subject to right censoring by lost to follow-up. In this setting CAR is equivalent to the assumption that the conditonal cause-specific hazard of censoring at each t depends on X only through the past $\{X(u); 0 \leq u \leq t\}$. Robins and Rotnitzky (1992) used their methodology to construct locally efficient estimators of the marginal survival function of T and of regression parameters in the Cox-proportional hazards model and accelerated failure time model for the law of T given baseline covariates Z. The authors showed that their locally efficient general estimating function methodology allowed them to both (i) correct for any bias due to informative censoring attributable to the covariate process $X(t)$ and (ii) to recover information from the censored observations by nonparametrically exploiting the correlation between the process $X(t)$ observed up to the censoring time and the unobserved failure time T. Additional papers by these authors and colleagues considered multivariate regression models for repeated measure outcomes and median regression models for failure time outcomes subject to right censoring and/or missing regressors. (Robins, 1993a, 1996, Robins and Rotnitzky, 1992, 1995b, 1996, Robins, Rotnitzky and Zhao, 1994, 1995, Rotnitzky and Robins, 1995a,b, Robins, Hsieh, Newey, 1995, among various other references) . Robins, Rotnitzky and Zhao (1995), Robins and Rotnitzky (1995), Robins and Wang (1998), and Robins and Gill (1997) considered CAR data with non monotone missing data patterns.

The Robins-Rotnitzky locally efficient estimating function methodology has recently been used to solve a number of interesting statistical problems. Pavlic, van der Laan and Buttler (2001) estimated the parameters of a multiplicative intensity model and of a proportional rate model in the presence of informative censoring attributable to time-dependent covariates that were not included as regressors in the models. Quale, van der Laan and Robins (2001) constructed locally efficient estimators of a multivariate survival function when failure times are subject to failure-time-specific censoring times which required iteratively solving an integral equation that did not admit a closed form solution. In this same setting, but including time-dependent covariate processes in the observed data structure, Keles, van der Laan, and Robins (2002) proposed closed form estimators that are easier to compute and almost as efficient as the Quale et al. iterative estimator. Van der Laan, Hubbard, and Robins (2002) constructed locally efficient closed-form estimators of a a multivariate survival function when the survival times are subject to a commom censoring time. Van der Laan, Hubbard (1998, 1999), building on Hu, Tsiatis (1996), and Zhao and Tsiatis (1997) constructed locally efficient estimators of (i) a survival function from right censored data subject to reporting delays and (ii) the quality-adjusted survival time distribution from right-censored data. Strawderman (2000) and Bang and Tsiatis (2002), respectively, used the Robins-Rotnitzky methodology to estimate the mean of an increasing stochastic process parameters and the parameters of a median regression model for medical costs from right censored data. Datta, Satten and Datta (2000) used the methodology to estimate a three state illness-death model from right censored data.

The Robins and Rotnitzky (1992) methodology was later extended to censored data structures in which the full data on a subject are never observed. Van der Laan and Hubbard (1997), Van der Laan and Robins (1998), Andrews, Van der Laan and Robins (2000), and van der Laan (2000) considered estimation of the marginal survival function of T and of regression parameters of an accelerated failure time model for the law of T given baseline covariates Z from current status and/or interval censored data structures wherein the failure time variable T is never exactly observed but the intensity function for monitoring whether failure T has occured by time t depends on the observed history $\{X(u); 0 \leq u \leq t\}$ of a multivariate covariate process.

Robins (1993b, 1998b, 1999) extended the methodology of Robins and Rotnitzky (1992) to estimate the parameters of longitudinal counterfactual causal models under a sequential randomization assumption (SRA) by exploiting the fact that counterfactual causal inference is formally a missing data problem (Rubin, 1978). The full data structure X is the set of counterfactual treatment-specific responses indexed by the set of potential treatments. The observed data structure Y consists of the actual treatment received and its corresponding treatment-specific response. Because only one of the potential treatments is actually received, X is never fully observed. The SRA is the assumption that the conditional probability of receiving a particular treatment at time t may depend on past treatment and response history but does not further depend on the unobserved counterfactual responses. Robins, Rotnitzky, and Scharfstein (1999) showed that, under fairly general conditions, the SRA is equivalent to CAR and extended the Robins and Rotnitzky (1992) general estimating function technology to this causal inference missing data problem. Because many readers may be less familiar with the causal inference literature than with the censored or missing data literature we provide some useful references. Rubin (1978), Rosenbaum (1984, 1987, 1988), Rosenbaum and Rubin (1983, 1984, 1985) and Robins, Mark, Newey (1992) consider causal inference for time-independent treatments. Robins (1989a,b, 1992, 1994, 1998a,b,c, 1999) introduces structural nested and marginal structural models for the causal effect of time-dependent treatments from longitudinal (panel) data and provides a locally efficient estimating function methodology . Hubbard, van der Laan, Robins (1999) develop closed form locally efficient estimators of treatment specific survival functions right-censored data. Mark, Robins (1993), Robins, Greenland (1994), Hernan, Brumback, Robins (2000), Henneman and van der Laan (2002), Bryan, Yu and van der Laan (2002), Yu and van der Laan (2002) apply this methodology to (re)analyze a number of interesting data sets .

In this book, we review the aforementioned developments and further generalize the general estimating function methodology to cover any CAR data structure. Our principle concern will be with the estimation of causal and non-causal parameters in longitudinal studies in which data are available on all time dependent covariates that predict both (i) subsequent response and (ii) subsequent treatment and/or censoring, so that the data are CAR.

As discussed above, we can use our general estimating function methodology to obtain $n^{1/2}-$ consistent estimators $\widehat{\mu}$ of a smooth parameters μ of a very large non- or semiparametric model for the law F_X of a high-dimensional X from CAR data Y, provided either that the CAR mechanism G is known or that we can correctly specify a lower dimension model for G. Now, in observational studies in which data are missing by happenstance and subjects self-select treatment, even if we are willing to assume the data are CAR, nonetheless the density g of Y given X will not be known; further, we cannot be certain the lower dimensional model we assume for g is correct. Thus we cannot be assured that our estimator $\widehat{\mu}$ is consistent. Because of this uncertainty, we might choose to specify a lower dimensional (say a fully parametric) working submodel $f(X; \mu, \eta)$ of our large non- or semiparametric model for F_X and then estimate the finite dimensional parameters (μ, η) based on the data Y by parametric maximum likelihood. The difficulty with this approach is that, if the parametric submodel $f(X; \mu, \eta)$ is misspecified, the parametric MLE of μ will be inconsistent. However, because of the curse of dimensionality, we cannot obtain estimators with reasonable finite sample performance if we do not place additional modelling restrictions on either the CAR mechanism G or on our large non- or semiparametric model for F_X. Hence, the best that can be hoped for is to find a doubly robust estimator. An estimator is doubly robust (equivalently, doubly protected) if it is consistent asymptotically normal (CAN) under the assumption of CAR when either (but not necessarily both) a lower dimensional model for G or a lower dimensional model for F_X is correct. A doubly robust estimator is locally semiparametric efficient (LSE) if it is the asymptotically most efficient doubly robust estimator of μ when both the lower dimensional models for G and F_X happen to be correct.

It turns out that, as discussed by Scharfstein, Rotnitzky, and Robins (1999), Neugebauer, van der Laan (2002), and later in this chapter, with a little care, we can guarantee that the aforementioned LSE estimator of μ in the semiparametric model that assumes a correct lower dimensional model for g is actually a LSE doubly robust estimator. Specifically the aforementioned LSE estimator of μ based on our general estimating function methodology actually depends not only on an estimate of g but also on an estimate of the law F_X. Further, because of the curse of dimensionality, it is necessary that F_X be estimated using a lower dimensional working submodel. If the model for g is correct, our LSE estimator is CAN for μ regardless of whether our working submodel for F_X is correct. However, if this submodel is correct, our estimator of μ attains the efficiency bound for the semiparametric model that assumes a correct lower dimensional model for G.

Now, if we take care that our estimate of F_X under the lower dimensional submodel is the MLE and thus depends only on the F_X part of the likelihood, then the estimator of μ considered in the previous paragraph is actually a LSE doubly robust estimator; in particular, it is CAN for μ even if the model for g is incorrect, provided the lower dimensional (say, parametric) submodel for F_X is correct. Even more surprisingly, Scharfstein, Rotnitzky, and Robins (1999) and Neugebauer, and van der Laan (2002) show that, when the lower dimensional (say, parametric) model for F_X happens to be correct, this doubly robust estimator of μ, like the parametric MLE, may be CAN, even when μ is not identified under the observed data model in which the true density g of Y given X is completely known. Non-identifiability of μ in this latter model occurs when the support set for Y at each value of X under the known density g is very small. See Section 1.6 for details. Thus, in CAR models, it is best to (i) simultaneously model the coarsening (i.e., censoring and/or treatment) mechanism and the law of the full data with lower dimensional models, (ii) estimate them both by maximum likelihood separately from the two parts of the likelihood, and (iii) finally obtain a LSE doubly robust estimator with our general estimating function methodology (see e.g., Scharfstein, Rotnitzky, and Robins, 1999, and Robins, 2000). Yu, and van der Laan (2002) implement this strategy and provide explicit algorithmic and computational suggestions: See Section 1.6. This strategy, however, is not always computationally feasible; in that case, alternative approaches to doubly robust estimation are available as developed in Robins (2000) and Tchetgen and Robins (2002). See Sections 3.5 and 6.4.

Certain semiparametric models in addition to CAR censored data models also admit doubly robust estimators. As far as we are aware, Brillinger (1983) was the first to call attention to and provide examples of DR-like estimators. Other examples are given by Ruud (1983, 1986), Duan and Li (1987, 1991), Newey (1990), Robins, Mark and Newey (1992), Ritov and Robins (1997), and Lipsitz and Ibrahim (1999). Scharfstein, Rotnitzky, Robins (1999), Robins (2000), and Neugebauer, van der Laan (2002) went beyond individual examples to provide a broad theory of double robustness in missing data and counterfactual causal inference models in which the data was CAR. Robins, Rotnitzky, and Van der Laan (2000) extended the results in Scharfstein, Rotnitzky, Robins (1999), and Robins (2000) to cover DR estimation in any model in which locally variation-independent (possibly infinite-dimensional) parameters κ and γ index the law of the observed data, the likelihood factorized as $L(\kappa, \gamma) = L_1(\kappa) L_2(\gamma)$, and the smooth finite-dimensional parameter $\mu(\kappa, \gamma) = \mu(\kappa)$ only depended on κ. All of the above mentioned examples are special cases of the general results in Robins, Rotnitzky, van der Laan (2000). Robins and Rotnitzky (2001), in the most comprehensive investigation of double robustness to date, provide a summary of known results concerning the existence and construction of doubly robust estimators, including results for missing data models with data that are not CAR.

One could wonder about the actual advantage of using doubly robust estimators as, in practice, all models including the lower dimensional models for both G and F_X are misspecified. Thus, even a doubly robust estimator of μ may be considerably biased. In our opinion, however, a doubly robust estimator has the following advantage that argues for its routine use: if either the lower dimensional model for F_X or for G is nearly correct, then the bias of doubly robust estimator of μ will be small. Thus, a doubly robust estimator gives the analyst two chances, instead of only one, to obtain a nearly unbiased estimator of μ. Furthermore informal but sensitive goodness of fit tests can be based on doubly robust estimators. See Robins and Rotnitzky (2001) for details. Yu, van der Laan (2002) demonstrate in a simulation study that the maximum likelihood estimator is much less robust than doubly robust estimators to model misspecification.

Van der Vaart, van der Laan (2001), van der Laan, Yu (2001), and Robins and Rotnitzky (2001) show that our general estimating function methodolgy can also be used to obtain doubly robust estimators of non-smooth parameters (such as the density of a continuous random variable) in both CAR censored data models and in certain other semiparametric models by approximating the non-smooth parameter by a smooth parameter, applying the locally efficient estimating function methodology to estimate the smooth parameter, and allowing the approximation to improve at an appropriate rate with increasing sample size. In van der Vaart, van der Laan (2001) this approach is used to estimate a survival function based on current status data in the prescence of a time-dependent surrogate processes. In this monograph, however, we largely restrict attention to the estimation of smooth parameters.

In this book we assume that the data are CAR. This assumption will in general be correct only when data have been obtained on all time-independent and time-dependent covariates that predict both (i) subsequent outcomes and (ii) subsequent treatment and/or censoring. In certain settings CAR may not hold even approximately. For example subjects often refrain from answering specific questions in surveys of religious, financial or sexual practices, but their reasons for nonresponse (censoring) are unavailable to the data analyst. Thus methods for the analysis of non-CAR coarsened data are also important. In a series of papers, Robins, Rotnitzky and Scharfstein have developed a general estimating function sensitivity analysis methodology for locally semiparametric efficient (LSE) estimation of smooth parameters (i.e., parameters estimable at rate $\sqrt{n}$) μ of large non- or semi- parametric models for the law F_X of very high dimensional data X based on the observed data Y, when the data are not coarsened at random. For further information, the interested reader may consult Rotnitzky, Robins (1997), Rotnitzky, Robins, and Scharfstein

1.1. Motivation, Bibliographic History, and an Overview of the book. 15

(1998) Scharfstein, Rotnitzky, and Robins (1999), and Robins, Rotnitzky, Scharfstein (1999).

Robins (1987), Robins and Rotnitzky (1992), Robins, Rotnitzky, and Zhao (1995), Robins (1997), Pearl (1995), and Pearl and Robins (1995) provide conditions under which CAR is violated but causal effects can still be nonparametrically identfied by the G-computation functional algorithm of Robins (1986). Furthermore the induced model for the obervable data Y under these conditions is the same as under CAR, so the theory and methodology developed in this book for CAR models still applies. See Subsection 3.3.2 and Section 6.2 for examples. Pearl (1995,2000) describes additional assumptions characterized in terms of missing arrows on "causal" directed acyclic graphs under which causal effects are nonparametrically identified by a functionals of the observed data distribution other than the G-computation algorithm functional. Though these additional identification results are quite interesting, the application of these latter results to complex longitudinal studies with high dimensional time-dependent data structures as considered in this book has been limited because their use requires detailed knowledge of the underlying causal structure, which rarely exists.

The book is organized as follows. Chapter 1 provides an overview of the mathematical tools that lie at the foundation of our methodology. Specifically we review the modern theory of semiparametric models based on tangent spaces and Hilbert space projections on these spaces. We then use this theory to derive our estimating function methodology and prove that these estimating functions are doubly robust. Next we apply our general estimating function methodology to several important examples. Chapter 2 is more technical and provides a rather complete treatment of our locally efficient estimating function methodology and its associated asymptotic theory. Although the theory and methods developed in this chapter are illustrated with concrete examples, nonetheless Chapter 2 is the most difficult in the book . The remaining chapters 3-6, however, cover specific data structures and models and are sufficiently self-contained that they can be read before chapter 2, although occassionally one will be referred back to a result in chapter 2. Chapter 3 treats right-censored data. Chapter 4 treats current status data and a combination of current status data and right-censored data. Chapter 5 treats multivariate right-censored data. Finally, Chapter 6 provides a general methodology for estimation of causal and non-causal parameters from longitudinal data, complicated by right censoring of some responses and interval censoring of other responses. Most of the methods discussed in chapters 3-6 have been implemented with Splus or C-software by Ph.D students in Biostatistics and Statistics. Examples of these data analyses and simulations are provided toward the end of each chapter.

With the help of students and colleagues, we have applied our locally efficient, doubly robust, estimating function methodology to a large variety of realistic and difficult data structures and models commonly encountered in biostatistical and epidemiologic practice. It is our belief that a reader who has mastered the techniques described in this book will be ready to attack the many possible variations of the examples covered in the book.

1.2 Tour through the General Estimation Problem.

In both observational and experimantal studies, the full (equivalently, complete) data structure X that one would wish to collect is often incompletely observed on some, possibly all, subjects. In such cases, we say that the study data is subject to censoring or missingness. As an example, in a study of a cohort of HIV infected subjects, the full data X on a subject might consist of the time from seroconversion to the development of AIDS, the time from seroconversion to death, and the time-dependent covariate processes encoding a subjects CD4 lymphocyte count, viral load, and antiviral treatment history from seroconversion to death. Due to the finite duration of the study, to limitations of funds and resources, and/or to the logistical impossibility of performing hourly or even daily laboratory tests, X is only partially observed. We denote a unit or subject's full data structure with random variable X which may be incompletely observed. Rather we observe the random variable

$$Y = \Phi(X, C) \text{ for a known many-to-one-mapping } \Phi, \qquad (1.1)$$

where Φ is a known function and C is the censoring or missingness variable that determines what part of X is observed. The following examples should help clarify the notation.

Example 1.1 (Repeated measures data with missing covariate)
Let Z be a p-dimensional vector of outcomes and let E be a vector of accurately measured exposures based on blood tests. Let V be a vector of variables that one wants to adjust for in a regression model (such as confounding factors for the causal effect of E on Z). Our goal is to estimate the regression parameters $\alpha = (\alpha_1, \ldots, \alpha_k)$ in a model for the conditional mean of Z, given $X^* = (E, V)$,

$$Z = g(X^* \mid \alpha) + \epsilon, \ E(\epsilon \mid X^*) = 0, \qquad (1.2)$$

where ϵ is a p-dimensional vector of residuals and $g(X^* \mid \alpha) = (g_1(X^* \mid \alpha), \ldots, g_p(X^* \mid \alpha))$ is a known function and α is an unknown parameter to be estimated.

Let E^* be a vector of poorly measured surrogates for E obtained on each subject from questionnaire responses. In general one would not wish to adjust for these surrogates E^* in the regression model (1.2) because of the possibility of differential misclassification (i.e., the possibility that E^* and Z may be conditionally dependent given E and V). However if it is

1.2. Tour through the General Estimation Problem.

very expensive to measure E it may be feasible to obtain data on E only on a subset of the study subjects. In that case, data on on E^* may be useful either to explain informative missingness and/or to recover information from the censored observations (i.e., from the observations lacking data on E) Let Δ be the indicator that E is observed; Then $C = \Delta$ and $Y = \Phi(X, C) = (C, CX + (1-C)W)$, where $W = (Z, V, E^*)$.

Example 1.2 (Repeated measures data with right-censoring) Consider a longitudinal study in which each subject is supposed to be monitored at time points $0, \ldots, p$, but some subjects drop out before they reach the endpoint p. Let $X = \{X(t) : t = 0, \ldots, p\}$ represent the full data structure on a subject, where $X(t)$ is typically a multivariate vector. Let $\bar{X}(t) = (X(0), \ldots, X(t))$ denote the history through time t. We assume that the measurements $X(t)$ can be divided in outcomes $Z(t)$, covariates $X^*(t)$ that one wants to adjust for in a regression model, and extraneous covariates $V^*(t)$. Let $Z = (Z(0), \ldots, Z(p))$, $X^* = (X^*(0), \ldots, X^*(p))$, and $V^* = (V^*(0), \ldots, V^*(p))$. Consider a regression model

$$Z = g(X^* \mid \alpha) + \epsilon, \quad E(\epsilon \mid X^*) = 0, \tag{1.3}$$

where $g(X^* \mid \alpha) = (g_0(X^* \mid \alpha), \ldots, g_p(X^* \mid \alpha))$ and $g_j(X^* \mid \alpha)$ only depends on the history $(X^*(0), \ldots, X^*(j))$ of X^* up to point j, $j = 0, \ldots, p$. For example, if X^* is univariate, we might have

$$g_t(X^* \mid \alpha) = \alpha_0 + \alpha_1 t + \alpha_2 X^*(0) + \alpha_3 (X^*(t) - X^*(0)). \tag{1.4}$$

For other longitudinal data models, we refer to Diggle, Liang and Zeger (1994). Our goal is to estimate the regression parameters $\alpha = (\alpha_1, \ldots, \alpha_k)$.

Let C be the discrete drop-out time with values in $\{0, \ldots, p\}$. The observed data structure is given by $Y = \Phi(X, C) = (C, \bar{X}(C)) = (X(0), \ldots, X(C))$. In other words, if $C = j$, then the subject was followed up to (and including) visit j. □

We assume throughout that we have n study units (or subjects) and observe n identically and independently distributed observations (copies) $Y_1, \ldots, Y_n$ of the random variable Y. We will suppose that the full data structure distribution F_X of X is known to be an element of a specified full data structure model $\mathcal{M}^F$ and that there is a Euclidean parameter $\mu = \mu(F_X) \in \mathbb{R}^k$ of interest. For instance, in both Examples 1.1 and 1.2, μ is the regression parameter.

1.2.1 Estimation in a high-dimensional full data model

Our estimating function methodology for estimating the k-dimensional parameter μ based on the observed data $Y_1, \ldots, Y_n$ requires that we can find a class of k-dimensional estimating functions whose components, when evaluated at any $F_X \in \mathcal{M}^F$, are elements of the orthogonal complement $T_{nuis}^{F,\perp}(F_X)$ of the nuisance tangent space $T_{nuis}^F(F_X)$ in model $\mathcal{M}^F$ at F_X.

To formalize this, recall that an unbiased estimating function $D(X \mid \mu)$ that does not depend on any nuisance parameters is a k-dimensional vector function of the data X and the parameter $\mu \in R^k$ that has mean zero under all F_X in $\mathcal{M}^F$; that is, $E_{F_X} D(X \mid \mu(F_X)) = 0$. More generally, an estimating function $D(X \mid \mu, \rho)$ can also depend on a parameter ρ whose domain is the set $\mathcal{R} = \{\rho(F_X); F_X \in \mathcal{M}^F\}$ of possible values of a nuisance parameter $\rho(F_X)$. In this case, $D(X \mid \mu, \rho)$ is unbiased if

$$E_{F_X} D(X \mid \mu(F_X), \rho(F_X)) = 0 \text{ for all } F_X \in \mathcal{M}^F. \quad (1.5)$$

An estimating function $D(X \mid \mu, \rho)$ of the dimension of μ yields an estimating equation $0 = \sum_{i=1}^n D(X_i \mid \mu, \rho_n)$ for μ by replacing the parameter ρ by an estimate ρ_n and setting its empirical mean equal to zero. We can let the estimate $\rho_n(\mu)$ of $\rho(F_X)$ depend on μ; when it does, we obtain the estimating equation $0 = \sum_{i=1}^n D(X_i \mid \mu, \rho_n(\mu))$. To simplify the asymptotics of an estimator defined by a solution of an estimating equation, it is beneficial to have that the nuisance parameter ρ be locally variation-independent of μ. We have that μ and ρ are globally variation independent if each element of in $\{\mu(F_X); F_X \in M^F\} \times R$ is equal to $(\mu(F_X), \rho(F_X))$ for some $F_X \in M^F$. Similarly μ and ρ are locally variation independent if for each $F_X \in M^F$ there is a neighborhood $N(F_X) \subset M^F$ (in a natural topology) such that μ and ρ are variation independent in the local model $N(F_X)$. When μ and ρ are not variation independent we will, when possible, reparametrize the estimating function as $D^r(X \mid \mu, \rho_1) \equiv D(X \mid \mu, \rho(\mu))$, where ρ_1 and μ are now globally or locally variation independent. Although in many models it may not be possible to define a reparamaterization that yields global variation independence, one can essentially always find a reparameterization that leads to local variation independence. It is only local variation independences that is required to simplify the asymptotics of our estimators. For notational convenience, we denote the reparametrized estimating function with $D(X \mid \mu, \rho)$ again. That is, throughout the book, unless stated otherwise, one can take the parameters μ and ρ to be locally variation independent.

Let $(L_0^2(F_X), \langle f, g \rangle_{F_X} = E_{F_X} f(X)g(X))$ be the Hilbert space of mean zero one-dimensional random variables with finite variance and covariance inner product. Informally, the nuisance tangent space $T_{nuis}^F(F_X)$ at F_X is the subspace of $(L_0^2(F_X), \langle f, g \rangle_{F_X} = E_{F_X} f(X)g(X))$ defined as the closed linear span of all nuisance scores obtained by taking standard scores of one-dimensional parametric submodels that do not fluctuate the parameter of interest μ (see, e.g., Bickel, Klaassen, Ritov and Wellner, 1993). More formally, let $\{\epsilon \to F_{\epsilon, g} : g\}$ be a class of one-dimensional submodels indexed by g with parameter ϵ through F_X at $\epsilon = 0$, and let $T^F(F_X) \subset L_0^2(F_X)$ be the closure of the linear span of the corresponding scores $s(g)$ at $\epsilon = 0$. The nuisance tangent space is defined by $\{s(g) \in T^F(F_X) : \frac{d}{d\epsilon} \mu(F_{\epsilon,g})|_{\epsilon=0} = 0\}$; that is, these are the scores of the 1-d models that do not vary the parameter of interest μ to first order. We illustrate these concepts in the two regression model examples.

Example 1.3 (Repeated measures data with missing covariate; continuation of example 1.1) In this example, the full data structure model for $X = (Z, E, V, E^*)$ is characterized by the sole restriction (1.2). The parameter of interest is μ, and all other components of the distribution F_X represent the nuisance parameter η. The nonparametric maximum likelihood estimator of (α, η) suffers from the curse of dimensionality so that an estimating function approach to construct estimators is useful again. Lemma 2.1 in Chapter 2 proves that the orthogonal complement of the nuisance tangent space at (α, η) is given by

$$T_{nuis}^{F,\perp}(\alpha, \eta) = \{h(X^*)\epsilon(\alpha) \in L_0^2(F_X) : h(X^*) \, 1 \times p\}.$$

We will now explain the sense in which the orthogonal complement of the nuisance tangent space indeed generates all estimating functions of interest based on the full data structure X. The representation of the orthogonal complement $(\alpha, \eta) \to T_{nuis}^{F,\perp}(\alpha, \eta)$ of the nuisance tangent space as a function of (α, η) implies the following class of estimating equations for α: For any given $k \times p$ matrix function h of X^*, we could estimate α with the solution α_n of the k-dimensional estimating equation

$$0 = \frac{1}{n} \sum_{i=1}^{n} h(X_i^*)\epsilon_i(\alpha). \tag{1.6}$$

We will refer to h as an index of the estimating function. In other words, given a univariate class of estimating functions $(D_h : h \in \mathcal{H}^F)$ with h $1 \times p$ such that $(D_h(\cdot \mid \mu(F_X), \rho(F_X)) : h \in \mathcal{H}^F) \in T_{nuis}^{F,\perp}(F_X)$, we obtain a class of k-dimensional estimating functions $(D_h : h \in \mathcal{H}^{Fk})$ by defining for $h \in \mathcal{H}^{Fk}$, $D_h = (D_{h_1}, \ldots, D_{h_k})$. Recall that an estimator α_n is called asymptotically linear with influence curve $IC(X)$ if $\alpha_n - \alpha$ can be approximated by an empirical mean of $IC(X)$:

$$\alpha_n - \alpha = \frac{1}{n} \sum_{i=1}^{n} IC(X_i) + o_P(1/\sqrt{n}).$$

Under standard regularity conditions (in particular, on h), the estimator α_n solving (1.6) is asymptotically linear with influence curve

$$IC_h(X) \equiv E\left\{h(X^*)\frac{d}{d\alpha^\top}g(X^* \mid \alpha)\right\}^{-1} h(X^*)\epsilon(\alpha), \tag{1.7}$$

where $\frac{d}{d\alpha^\top}g(X^* \mid \alpha)$ is a $p \times k$ matrix and we implicitly assumed that the determinant of the $k \times k$ matrix $E\left\{h(X^*)\frac{d}{d\alpha}g(X^* \mid \alpha)\right\}$ is non zero. Thus, the influence curve at F_X is a standardized version of the estimating function itself. A well-known and important fundamental result (see e.g.,

Bickel, Klaassen, Ritov and Wellner, 1993) is that any regular asymptotically linear (RAL) estimator of μ at the full data distribution $F_{\alpha,\eta}$ has an influence curve whose components are contained in the orthogonal complement $T_{nuis}^{F,\perp}(\alpha,\eta)$ of the nuisance tangent space. We recall that an estimator μ_n of μ is regular at F_X if, for each 1-dimensional regular submodel F_ϵ with parameter ϵ and $F_{\epsilon=0} = F_X$, $\sqrt{n}(\mu_n - \mu(F_{\epsilon_n = 1/\sqrt{n}}))$ converges under (i.e., when sampling from) F_{ϵ_n} to a common limit distribution Z (independent of the choice of submodel). This proves that, given any regular asymptotically linear estimator of α, we can find a candidate estimating equation of the type (1.6) so that its solution is asymptotically equivalent with the estimator under appropriate regularity conditions (typically the same as needed for the given estimator). In this sense, the mapping from (α,η) to the orthogonal complement of the nuisance tangent space $T_{nuis}^{F,\perp}(\alpha,\eta)$ actually identifies *all* estimating functions for α of interest, which is a fundamental result used throughout this book.

By the multivariate central limit theorem, we have that $\sqrt{n}(\alpha_n - \alpha)$ converges in distribution to a normal limit distribution with mean vector zero and covariance matrix $\Sigma = E\{IC_h(X)IC_h(X)^\top\}$. The efficient score $h_{opt}(X^*)\epsilon(\alpha)$ for μ is defined to be the vector of the projections of the components of the score for μ onto the orthogonal complement $T_{nuis}^{F,\perp}$ of the nuisance tangent space. The inverse of the covariance matrix of the efficient score is referred to as the semiparametric variance bound (SVB) for the model; the asymptotic covariance matrix of every regular estimator is at least as large (in the positive definite-sense) as the SVB (Bickel, Klaassen, Ritov and Wellner, 1993). The optimal estimating function is obtained by choosing $h = h_{opt}$ so that $h_{opt}(X^*)\epsilon(\alpha)$ equals the actual efficient score. Lemma 2.1 in Chapter 2 proves that this efficient score is defined by the index

$$h_{opt}(X^*) = \frac{d}{d\alpha}g(X^* \mid \alpha)_{k \times p}^\top E(\epsilon(\alpha)\epsilon(\alpha)^\top \mid X^*)_{p \times p}^{-1}, \qquad (1.8)$$

a result first proved by Chamberlain (1987). Note that this optimal index h_{opt} depends on the full data distribution F_X and is thus unknown. This suggests estimating α with the solution α_n of the estimating equation

$$0 = \frac{1}{n}\sum_{i=1}^{n} h_n(X_i^*)\epsilon_i(\alpha)$$

indexed by h_n, where h_n is an estimator of h_{opt}. Estimation of h_{opt} requires an initial estimate of α and an estimate of the $p \times p$ covariance matrix $E(\epsilon(\alpha)\epsilon(\alpha)^\top \mid X^*)$. One can obtain an initial consistent estimator $\alpha_{n,0}$ of α by solving the estimating function according to a simple choice h independent of the true parameters (e.g., $h(X^*) = d/d\alpha g(X^* \mid \alpha_0)$) at a guessed α_0). In order to construct a globally efficient estimator of α, one needs a globally consistent estimate of h_{opt}; that is, one needs a consistent estimator of the conditional covariance matrix $E(\epsilon(\alpha_{n,0})\epsilon(\alpha_{n,0})^\top \mid X^*)$ at each full data distribution in the full data model. If X^* is multidimensional, then a nonparametric estimate of the covariance matrix will require a multivariate smooth and will usually result in an estimator of α with poor performance in finite samples. As a consequence, globally efficient estimators of α are not attractive estimators in practice. However, we can obtain a so called locally consistent estimate h_n of h_{opt} by estimating the covariance matrix $E(\epsilon(\alpha_{n,0})\epsilon(\alpha_{n,0})^\top \mid X^*)$ of the estimated error term according to a lower-dimensional guessed (e.g, a multivariate normal) model. If the guessed (equivalently, working) model for the covariance matrix is correct, then the estimator α_n is an asymptotically efficient estimator of α. Furthermore, α_n remains consistent and asymptotically normal as long as h_n converges to *some* h. We say that α_n is a locally efficient estimator since it is efficient at a guessed submodel and is consistent and asymptotically normal over the whole full data structure model. The asymptotic covariance matrix of μ_n can be estimated consistently with $1/n \sum_i \widehat{IC}_{h_n}(X_i)\widehat{IC}_{h_n}(X_i)^\top$, where $\widehat{IC}_{h_n}$ estimates the influence curve (1.7). □

Example 1.4 (Repeated measures data with right-censoring; continuation of Example 1.2) Before considering the observed data structure, it is necessary to understand the estimation problem for the case where we observe n i.i.d. observations of the full data structure X. But this is is equivalent to the full data model in the previous example. Thus, for any given matrix function h of X^*, we could estimate α with the solution α_n of

$$0 = \frac{1}{n}\sum_{i=1}^n h(X_i^*)\epsilon_i(\alpha).$$

The optimal estimating function is obtained by choosing $h = h_{opt}$, where $h_{opt}(X^*) = \{\frac{d}{d\alpha}g(X^* \mid \alpha)^\top\} E(\epsilon(\alpha)\epsilon(\alpha)^\top \mid X^*)^{-1}$. Given an estimator h_n of h_{opt}, involving an estimate of the covariance matrix $E(\epsilon(\alpha)\epsilon(\alpha)^\top \mid X^*)$ of the error term computed under a guessed lower-dimensional model, one estimates α by the solution of the corresponding estimating function

$$0 = \frac{1}{n}\sum_{i=1}^n h_n(X_i^*)\epsilon_i(\alpha).$$

If the guessed model for the covariance matrix is correct, then this procedure yields a fully efficient estimator of α, and otherwise the estimator is still consistent and asymptotically normal. □

1.2.2 The curse of dimensionality in the full data model

In this subsection, we discuss the curse of dimensionality using our multivariate regression full data structure model as an illustration.

Example 1.5 The curse of dimensionality; continuation of Example 1.2 Suppose that X^* has many continuous components and we assume that $E(\epsilon(\mu)\epsilon(\mu)^\top \mid X^*)$ is unrestricted except for being a continuous function of the continuous components of X^*. To simplify the notation, we assume μ is one-dimensional. It is possible to use multivariate smoothing to construct a globally efficient RAL estimator $\mu_{n,globeff}$ of μ under the standard asymptotic theory of Bickel, Klaassen, Ritov and Wellner (1993) by using a smooth to obtain a globally consistent estimator of $E(\epsilon(\mu)\epsilon(\mu)^\top \mid X^*)$; that is, the estimator will have asymptotic variance equal to the semiparametric variance bound $I^{-1}(\mu, \eta)$ (i.e., the inverse of the variance of the efficient score) at each law (μ, η) allowed by the model. However, in finite samples and regardless of the choice of smoothing parameter (e.g., bandwidth), the actual coverage rate of the Wald interval $\mu_{n,globeff} \pm z_{\alpha/2} I^{-1/2}(\mu, \eta)/\sqrt{n}$ based on $\mu_{n,globeff}$ and the semiparametric variance bound $I^{-1}(\mu, \eta)$ will be considerably less than its nominal $(1-\alpha)$ level at laws (μ, η) at which $E(\epsilon(\mu)\epsilon(\mu)^\top \mid X^*)$ is a very wiggly function of X^*. Here $z_{\alpha/2}$ is the upper $\alpha/2$ quantile of a standard normal. This is because (i) if a large bandwidth is used, the estimate of $E(\epsilon(\mu)\epsilon(\mu)^\top \mid X^*)$ will be biased so that h_{opt} and its estimate will differ greatly but (ii) if a small bandwidth is used, the second-order $o_P(1/\sqrt{n})$ terms in the asymptotic linearity expansion $\mu_{n,globeff} - \mu = \frac{1}{n}\sum_{i=1}^n IC(Y_i) + o_P(1/\sqrt{n})$, where $IC(Y)$ denotes the influence curve of $\mu_{n,globeff}$, will be large, adding variability. Thus, standard asymptotics is a poor guide to finite sample performance in high-dimensional models when X^* has many continuous components. Robins and Ritov (1997) proposed an alternative curse of dimensionality appropriate (CODA) asymptotics that serves as a much better guide.

Under CODA asymptotics, an estimator $\mu_{n,globeff}$ of a one-dimensional parameter μ is defined to be globally CODA-efficient if $\mu_{n,globeff} \pm z_{\alpha/2} I^{-1/2}(\mu, \eta)/\sqrt{n}$ (or equivalently $\mu_{n,globeff} \pm z_{\alpha/2} \widetilde{I}^{-1/2}(\mu, \eta)/\sqrt{n}$, where $\widetilde{I}$ is a uniformly consistent estimator of I) is an asymptotic $(1-\alpha)$ confidence interval for μ uniformly over all laws (μ, η) allowed by the model. An estimator $\mu_{n,loceff}$ is locally CODA-efficient at a working submodel if (i) $\mu_{n,loceff} \pm z_{\alpha/2} I^{-1/2}(\mu, \eta)/\sqrt{n}$ is an asymptotic $(1-\alpha)$ confidence interval for μ uniformly over all laws (μ, η) in the submodel and (ii) $\mu_{n,loceff} \pm z_{\alpha/2}\sigma_n$ is an asymptotic $(1-\alpha)$ confidence interval for μ uniformly over all laws (μ, η), where σ_n is the nonparametric bootstrap estimator of the standard error of $\mu_{n,loceff}$ (or any other robust estimator of its asymptotic standard error). Given (ii), condition (i) is implied by $\sqrt{n}\sigma_n$ converging to $I^{-1/2}$ uniformly over (μ, η) in the working submodel. These definitions extend to a vector parameter μ by requiring that they hold for each one-dimensional linear combination μ of the components. Arguments similar to those in Robins and Ritov (1997) show that in the model with $E(\epsilon(\mu)\epsilon(\mu)^\top \mid X^*)$ unrestricted, except by continuity and a bound on its matrix norm, no globally efficient CODA estimators exist (owing to undercoverage under certain laws (μ, η) depending on the sample size n), but the locally efficient RAL estimator of the previous paragraph is locally CODA-efficient as well. Further, in moderate-sized samples, the nominal $1 - \alpha$ Wald interval confidence interval $\mu_{n,loceff} \pm z_{\alpha/2}\sigma_n$ for μ based on the locally efficient estimator above and its estimated variance will cover at near its nominal rate under all laws allowed by the model, with length near $2z_{\alpha/2}I^{-1/2}(\mu, \eta)/\sqrt{n}$ at laws in the working submodel. Thus, CODA asymptotics is much more reliable than standard asymptotics as a guide to finite sample performance.

Now $\mu_{n,globeff}$ can be made globally CODA-efficient if we impose the additional assumption that $E(\epsilon(\mu)\epsilon(\mu)^\top \mid X^*)$ is locally smooth (i.e., has bounded derivatives to a sufficiently high order) in the continuous components of X^*. However, when X^* is high-dimensional, even when local smoothness is known to be correct, the asymptotics based on the larger model that only assumes continuity of the conditional covariance provides a more relevant and appropriate guide to moderate sample performance. For example, with moderate-sized samples, for any estimator $\mu_{n,globeff}$, there will exist laws (μ, η) satisfying the local smoothness assumption such that the coverage of $\mu_{n,globeff} \pm z_{\alpha/2}I^{-1/2}(\mu, \eta)/\sqrt{n}$ will be considerably less than its nominal $(1 - \alpha)$. This is due to the curse of dimensionality: in high-dimensional models with moderate sample sizes, local smoothness assumptions, even when true, are not useful, since essentially no two units will have X^*-vectors close enough to one another to allow the "borrowing of information" necessary for smoothing. Thus, in high-dimensional models, we suggest using a CODA asymptotics that does not impose smoothness, even when smoothness is known to hold. □

1.2.3 Coarsening at random

The distribution of Y is indexed by the distribution F_X of the full data structure X and the conditional distribution $G(\cdot \mid X)$ of the censoring variable C, given X. Because, for a given X, the outcome of C determines what we observe about X, we refer to the conditional distribution $G(\cdot \mid X)$ as the censoring or coarsening mechanism. If the censoring variable C is allowed to depend on unobserved components of X, then μ is typically not identifiable from the distribution of Y without additional strong untestable assumptions. When the censoring distribution only depends on the observed components of X, we say that the censoring mechanism satisfies *coarsening at random* (CAR).

In this book we will assume that the censoring mechanism G satisfies CAR. Formally, CAR is a restriction on the conditional distribution $G_{Y|X}$ of Y, given X (which implies that it is also a restriction on G). If Y includes the censoring variable C itself as a component, then the conditional distribution $G_{Y|X}$ of Y, given X, can be replaced by G itself in the definition of

CAR. If Y does not include the censoring variable C, then the definition of CAR on $G_{Y|X}$ is weaker than the same definition applied to G.

Let $\mathcal{X}$ and $\mathcal{C}$ be the sample spaces of X and C, respectively. We first formally define CAR in the case where X is a discrete random variable. Let $C(y) = \{x^* \in \mathcal{X}; \Phi(x^*, c^*) = y \text{ for some } c^* \in \mathcal{C}\}$ be the subset of the support $\mathcal{X}$ of X whose elements x are consistent with the observation y. If X is discrete, then CAR is the assumption

$$P(Y = y \mid X = x) = P(Y = y \mid X = x') \text{ for any } (x, x') \in C(y). \quad (1.9)$$

If, as in the previous examples, observing Y implies observing C so that C is always observed, then CAR can also be written

$$P(C = c \mid X = x) = P(C = c \mid X = x') = h(y) \text{ for any } (x, x') \in C(y) \quad (1.10)$$

for some function $h(\cdot)$ of $y = \Phi(c, x)$. If C is not always observed, this last assumption is more restrictive than CAR. Assumption (1.9) is also equivalent to

$$P(Y = y \mid X = x) = P(Y = y \mid X \in C(y)) \text{ for all } x \in C(y), \quad (1.11)$$

or equivalently the density $P(Y = y \mid X = x)$ is only a function of y. In other words, there is no $x \in C(y)$ that makes the observation $Y = y$ more likely. Therefore, under CAR, observing $Y = y$ is not more informative than observing that X falls in the *fixed given* set $C(y)$. As a consequence, under CAR, we have the following factorization of the density of the observed data structure:

$$\begin{aligned} P(Y = y) &= P(X \in C(y)) P(Y = y \mid X = x) \\ &= P(X \in C(y)) P(Y = y \mid X \in C(y)). \quad (1.12) \end{aligned}$$

Coarsening at random was originally formulated for discrete data by Heitjan and Rubin (1991).

A generalization to continuous data is provided in Jacobsen and Keiding (1995), whose definition is further generalized in Gill, van der Laan, and Robins (1997). A general definition of CAR in terms of the conditional distribution of the observed data Y, given the full data structure X, is given in Gill, van der Laan and Robins (1997): for each x, x'

$$P_{Y|X=x}(dy) = P_{Y|X=x'}(dy) \text{ on } \{y : x \in C(y)\} \cap \{y : x' \in C(y)\}. \quad (1.13)$$

Given this general definition of CAR, it is now also possible to define coarsening at random in terms of densities: for every $x \in C(y)$, we have that, for a dominating measure ν of G that satisfies (1.13) itself,

$$g_{Y|X}(y \mid x) \equiv \frac{dP(y \mid X = x)}{d\nu(y \mid X = x)} = h(y) \text{ for some measurable function } h. \quad (1.14)$$

Thus the density $g_{Y|X}(y \mid x)$ of $G_{Y|X}$ does not depend on the location of $x \in C(y)$. Therefore, the heuristic interpretation of CAR is that, given the full data structure $X = x$, the censoring action determining the observed data $Y = y$ is only based on the observed part $C(y)$ of x. As mentioned above, if observing Y implies observing C, then (1.14) translates into $g(c \mid x) = h(y)$ for some function h of $y = \Phi(c, x)$.

In this book, we can actually replace (1.13) by the minimally weaker condition that

$$g_{Y|X}(Y \mid X) = h(Y) \text{ with probability } 1 \qquad (1.15)$$

for some $h(\cdot)$. Again, if observing Y implies observing C so that C is always observed, then this last equation is equivalent to

$$g(C \mid X) = h(Y) \text{ with probability } 1 \qquad (1.16)$$

for some function $h(\cdot)$.

Example 1.6 (Repeated measures data with missing covariate; continuation of Example 1.1) In this example, C is the always observed variable Δ. Thus, CAR is the assumption that $p_G(\Delta|X) = h(Y) = h(\Delta, W, \Delta E)$. Thus $pr_G(\Delta = 0|X)$ is a function only of W so that

$$pr_G(\Delta = 1|X) = pr_G(\Delta = 1|W) \equiv \Pi_G(W) \equiv \Pi(W) \qquad (1.17)$$

does not depend on E. □

Example 1.7 (Repeated measures data with right-censoring; continuation of Example 1.2) In this example, the conditional distribution of the always observed variable C, given X, is a multinomial distribution with the probability of $C = j$, $j = 0, \ldots, p$, being a function of X. It is easy to show that CAR is the assumption that the probability that a subject drops out at time j given the subject is yet to drop out (i.e., is at risk at j) is only a function of the past up to and including point j,

$$\begin{aligned}\lambda_C(j \mid X) &\equiv P(C = j \mid X, C \geq j) = P(C = j \mid C \geq j, \bar{X}(j)) \quad (1.18)\\ &\equiv \lambda_C(j \mid \bar{X}(j)),\end{aligned}$$

where $\lambda_C(j \mid \cdot)$ is the discrete conditional hazard of C at j given the information $\cdot$. □

Example 1.8 (Right-censored data) Let T be a univariate failure time variable of interest, W be a 25-d covariate vector (e.g., 25 biomarkers/gene expressions for survival), and C be a censoring variable. Suppose that we have the full data $X = (T, W)$ and the observed data $Y = (\tilde{T} = \min(T, C), \Delta = I(\tilde{T} = T), W)$. Let $G(\cdot \mid X)$ be the conditional distribution of C, given X, and let $g(\cdot \mid X)$ be its density w.r.t. a dominating measure that satisfies CAR as defined by (1.13) itself such as the Lebesgue measure or counting measure on a given set of points. CAR is then equivalent to

$$g(C \mid X) = g(C \mid W) \text{ on } C < T. \qquad (1.19)$$

Except when the conditional law of C, given $C > T$, is a point mass, the assumption $g(C \mid X) = h(Y)$ is strictly stronger than CAR because the additional non identifiable restriction $g(c_1 \mid X) = g(c_2 \mid X)$ for $c_1 > c_2 > T$ will hold. If we redefine the variable C to be infinity when $T < C$, then C is always observed, the conditional law of C given $C > T$ is a point mass at ∞, and CAR becomes $g(C \mid X) = h(Y)$. Whether or not C has been redefined, CAR is equivalent to the assumption that the cause-specific conditional hazard of C given X only depends on W; that is,

$$\lambda_C(t \mid X) \equiv \lambda_C(t \mid W), \ 0 < t < \infty, \qquad (1.20)$$

where $\lambda_C(t \mid \cdot) = \lim_{h \to 0} P(t+h < C \leq t \mid X, C \geq t, T \geq t)/h$ for C a continuous random variable. □

Coarsening at random implies factorization of the density of Y at y in F_X and G parts as in (1.12): for example, if $F_X(C(y)) > 0$, then $p_{F_X,G}(y) = F_X(C(y))h(y)$, with $h(y) = g_{Y|X}(y \mid x)$. Under mild regularity conditions, Gill, van der Laan and Robins (1997) show that even when $F_X(C(y)) = 0$, the density $p_{F_X,G}(y)$ (w.r.t. a dominating measure satisfying CAR itself) factors as a product $p_{F_X}(y)h(y)$, where $h(y) = g_{Y|X}(y \mid X)$ and $p_{F_X}(y)$ only depends on the measure F_X. Thus, the maximum likelihood estimator (MLE) of F_X based on $Y_1,\ldots,Y_n$ ignores the censoring mechanism G by simply interpreting $Y_i = y_i$ as $X_i \in C(y_i)$, $i = 1,\ldots,n$. The MLE of F_X can typically be computed with the EM-algorithm (e.g., Dempster, Laird and Rubin, 1977) either by assuming a nonparametric full data model and maximizing an unrestricted multinomial likelihood defined over given support points or assuming a parametric full data model and maximizing the parametric log-likelihood (Little and Rubin, 1987). The G part of the likelihood of $Y = y$ is the conditional density of $Y = y$, given X, which by CAR indeed only depends on y.

Let $\mathcal{G}(CAR)$ be the set of all conditional distributions G satisfying CAR (i.e., satisfying (1.13) or (1.14) w.r.t. a particular dominating measure μ satisfying CAR itself). Consider the observed data model $\mathcal{M}(CAR) = \{P_{F_X,G} : F_X \in \mathcal{M}^F, G \in \mathcal{G}(CAR)\}$ defined by the assumptions $G \in \mathcal{G}(CAR)$ and $F_X \in \mathcal{M}^F$. Let $T(P_{F_X,G}) \subset L_0^2(P_{F_X,G})$ be the closure of the linear span of all scores of one-dimensional submodels $\epsilon \to P_{F_\epsilon,G_\epsilon}$ with parameter ϵ through $P_{F_X,G}$ at $\epsilon = 0$. Here $L_0^2(P_{F_X,G}) = \{h(Y) : E_{P_{F_X,G}} h^2(Y) < \infty, E_{P_{F_X,G}} h(Y) = 0\}$ is the Hilbert space endowed with inner product $\langle h, g \rangle_{P_{F_X,G}} = E_{P_{F_X,G}} h(Y)g(Y)$. The sub-Hilbert space $T(P_{F_X,G})$ is called the observed data tangent space. It is shown in Gill, van der Laan and Robins (1997) that if F_X is completely unspecified (i.e., the full data structure model $\mathcal{M}^F$ is nonparametric), then the observed data model $\mathcal{M}(CAR)$ for the distribution of Y characterized by the sole restriction CAR (1.13) is locally saturated in the sense that $T(P_{F_X,G}) = L_0^2(P_{F_X,G})$. An important consequence of this result is that in this nonparametric CAR model all *regular* asymptotically linear estimators of the parameter μ are asymptotically equivalent and efficient. Because of its importance, we will give here the proof of this local saturation result.

Lemma 1.1 *Consider the model*

$$\mathcal{M}(CAR) = \{P_{F_X,G} : F_X \text{ unrestricted}, G \in \mathcal{G}(CAR)\}$$

for the observed data structure $Y = \Phi(C, X)$. *The tangent space* $T(P_{F_X,G})$ *equals* $L_0^2(P_{F_X,G})$.

Proof. By CAR, we have that the density $p(y)$ of $P_{F_X,G}$ w.r.t. a dominating measure factorizes (Gill, van der Laan and Robins, 1997): $p(y) = p_{F_X}(y)h(y)$ with $h(y) = g_{Y|X}(y \mid X)$. As one-dimensional submodels through F_X (at parameter value $\epsilon = 0$), we take $dF_{X,\epsilon}(x) = (1 + \epsilon s(x))dF_X(x)$, $s \in L_0^2(F_X)$. As one-dimensional submodels through G, we take $dG_\epsilon(y \mid x) = (1 + \epsilon v(y))dG(y \mid x)$, $v \in \{V(Y) \in L_0^2(P_{F_X,G}) : E(V(Y) \mid X) = 0\}$. A general result is that the score of the one-dimensional model $P_{F_{X,\epsilon},G}$ equals $E_{F_X}(s(X) \mid Y)$ (Gill, 1989). As a consequence, the collection of all scores of the corresponding one-dimensional submodels $P_{F_{X,\epsilon},G_\epsilon}$ through $P_{F_X,G}$ (obtained by varying s, v over all possible functions) is given by

$$S(P_{F_X,G}) \equiv \{E_{F_X}(s(X) \mid Y) : s \in L_0^2(F_X)\} \oplus \{V(Y) : E_G(V(Y) \mid X) = 0\}. \tag{1.21}$$

Let the nonparametric score operator $A_{F_X} : L_0^2(F_X) \to L_0^2(P_{F_X,G})$ be defined by $A_{F_X}(s)(Y) = E(s(X) \mid Y)$. The adjoint of A_{F_X} is given by $A_G^\top : L_0^2(P_{F_X,G}) \to L_0^2(F_X)$, $A_G^\top(V)(X) = E(V(Y) \mid X)$. This proves that the closure $T(P_{F_X,G})$ of $S(P_{F_X,G})$ equals the closure of the range of A_{F_X} plus the null space of its adjoint: $T(P_{F_X,G}) = \overline{R(A_{F_X})} \oplus N(A_G^\top)$. A general Hilbert space result is that for any Hilbert space operator $A : H_1 \to H_2$ with adjoint $A^\top : H_2 \to H_1$, $\overline{R(A)} + N(A^\top) = H_2$. This proves the lemma. $\square$

Gill, van der Laan and Robins (1997) also prove that if the distribution of $Y = \Phi(C, X)$ has a finite support set, then the hypothesis that G satisfies CAR cannot be rejected; that is, the model $\mathcal{M}(CAR) = \{P_{F_X,G} : F_X \text{ unrestricted}, G \in \mathcal{G}(CAR)\}$ is a nonparametric model for the law of Y. It follows that the observing data $(Y_1, ..., Y_n)$ can never lead one to reject the hypothesis that the law of Y lies in the model $\mathcal{M}(CAR)$, regardless of the support of Y.

In many of the specific data structures covered in this book, it will be possible to provide an easy-to-interpret definition of CAR. If the censoring is multivariate in nature, CAR is typically a very complicated and hard-to-understand assumption, but we will always be able to define large easy-to-interpret submodels of CAR.

1.2.4 *The curse of dimensionality revisited*

When X is high-dimensional, the existence of locally CODA-efficient estimators with good moderate sample performance in the full data model $\mathcal{M}^F$

(based on observing $X_1, \ldots, X_n$) does not imply their existence in the observed data model $\mathcal{M}(CAR) = \{P_{F_X,G} : F_X \in \mathcal{M}^F, G \in \mathcal{G}(CAR)\}$ (based on observing $Y_1, \ldots, Y_n$), thereby creating the need for further modeling assumptions on G or F_X; that is, when X is high-dimensional and the sample size is moderate, there may be no estimator of μ that has, under all laws allowed by model $\mathcal{M}(CAR)$, an approximately normal sampling distribution centered near μ with variance small enough to be of substantive interest. Further, if we adopt a CODA asymptotics that imposes no smoothness, then there will generally exist (i) no uniformly consistent estimator of μ, (ii) no estimator of μ that attains a pointwise (i.e., non-uniform) rate of convergence of n^α under all laws allowed by the model for any $\alpha > 0$; and (iii) no "valid" $1 - \alpha$ interval estimator for μ exists. By valid we mean that, under all laws, the coverage is at least $(1 - \alpha)$ at each sample size n and the length goes to zero in probability with increasing sample size. This reflects the fact that, in order to construct a uniformly consistent estimator of μ under model $\mathcal{M}(CAR)$, it is necessary to use multivariate nonparametric smoothing techniques to estimate conditional means or densities given a high-dimensional covariate, which would require impractically large samples when X is high-dimensional.

Practical estimators (say, $\mu_n = \Phi(P_n)$ for some ϕ) are typically reasonably smooth functionals of the empirical distribution P_n so that its first-order linear approximation (i.e., the functional derivative $d\Phi(P_n - P)$ applied to $(P_n - P)$, which is the empirical mean in (1.22) of its influence function; see Gill, 1989) is representative of its finite sample behavior. Informally, one might coin in the phrase "an estimator suffers from the curse of dimensionality" if it is a highly non smooth functional of the empirical distribution P_n so that the second-order terms in (1.22) heavily influence its finite sample behavior. Variance of an estimator and smoothness of the estimator as a functional of the empirical distribution P_n (measured by the size of its second order terms) are typically tradeoffs, so that it is no surprise that in many models the unregularized nonparametric maximum likelihood estimator suffers from the curse of dimensionality (i.e., large second order terms) while many practical good estimators are available (as in our full data repeated measures examples above). The following examples illustrate this type of failure of maximum likelihood estimation nicely.

Example 1.9 (Right censored data; continuation of Example 1.8)
Let $\mu = F_T(t) = P(T \leq t)$ be the parameter of interest. If censoring is absent, then we would estimate μ with the empirical cumulative distribution function of $T_1, \ldots, T_n$. If censoring is independent (i.e., $g(c \mid W) = g(c)$), then we could estimate μ with the Kaplan–Meier estimator (Kaplan and Meier, 1958; Wellner, 1982; Gill, 1983), which is inefficient since it ignores the covariates W. In general, the Kaplan-Meier estimator is an inconsistent estimator under the sole assumption (1.19). The F_X part of the likelihood

of Y under CAR is given by
$$L(Y \mid F_X) = dF_{T|W}(\tilde{T} \mid W)^\Delta (1 - F_{T|W}(\tilde{T} \mid W))^{1-\Delta} dF_W(W).$$
Let $L(Y_1, \ldots, Y_n \mid F_X) = \prod_{i=1}^n L(Y_i \mid F_X)$ be the likelihood of an i.i.d. sample $Y_1, \ldots, Y_n$. The maximum likelihood estimator of $F_{T|W=W_i}$ is given by the Kaplan–Meier estimator based on the subsample $\{Y_j : W_j = W_i\}$, $i = 1, \ldots, n$. The maximum likelihood estimator of F_W is the empirical distribution function that puts mass $1/n$ on each observation W_i, $i = 1, \ldots, n$. If W is continuous, then each subsample only consists of one observation so that, if $\Delta_i = 1$, then the Kaplan-Meier estimator of $F_{T|W=W_i}$ puts mass 1 on $\tilde{T}_i$, and if $\Delta_i = 0$, then it puts mass zero on $[0, \tilde{T}_i]$ and is undefined on $(\tilde{T}_i, \infty)$. It follows that the MLE results in an inconsistent estimator of $F_T(t)$. Thus, if W is continuous, then the curse of dimensionality causes the MLE to be inconsistent.

Suppose that each of the 25 components of W is discrete with 20 possible outcomes. Then, the outcome space of W has 20^{25} values w_j. In that case, the maximum likelihood estimator of $F_{T|W}(\cdot \mid w_j)$ is *asymptotically* consistent and normally distributed so that the NPMLE of $F_T(t)$ is also asymptotically consistent and normally distributed. However, one needs on the order of 20^{25} observations to have Kaplan–Meier estimator of $F_{T|W}(\cdot \mid W = w_j)$ be well defined with high probability. Therefore, one needs a sample size on the order of 20^{25} observations in order for the MLE of $F_T(t)$ to have a reasonable practical performance. In this case, we conclude that the curse of dimensionality does not cause inconsistency of the MLE but causes a miserable finite sample performance for any practical sample size. □

Example 1.10 (Repeated measures data with missing covariate; continuation of Example 1.1) Under CAR, the F_X part of the likelihood of the observed data $Y_1, \ldots, Y_n$ is given by
$$L(Y_1, \ldots, Y_n \mid F_X) = \prod_{i=1}^n dF_X(X_i)^{\Delta_i} dF_W(W_i)^{1-\Delta_i}.$$

This F_X-part of the likelihood of the observed data $Y_1, \ldots, Y_n$ can be parametrized by α and a nuisance parameter η that includes the unspecified conditional error distribution of ϵ, given X^*, the unspecified conditional distribution of extraneous surrogates E^* given Z, X^*, and the unspecified marginal distribution of X^*. A maximum likelihood estimator of α is defined as the maximizer of the profile likelihood for α (i.e., the likelihood with the nuisance parameter replaced by $\widehat{\eta}(\alpha)$, where $\widehat{\eta}(\alpha)$ is the maximum likelihood estimator w.r.t. η for given α). Thus $\widehat{\eta}(\alpha)$ involves maximizing a likelihood w.r.t. the high dimensional nuisance parameter η. As a consequence, the maximum likelihood estimator $\widehat{\eta}(\alpha)$, or any approximation or regularization of this maximum likelihood estimator, such as a penalized or sieve maximum likelihood estimator, is either extremely variable in moderate sized samples if not oversmoothed, but may be biased if oversmoothed. Thus $\hat\eta(\alpha)$ is only acceptable for large sample sizes. Obviously, this implies that the maximum likelihood estimator of α or any approximation thereof also suffers heavily from this curse of dimensionality. □

Example 1.11 (Repeated measures data with right-censoring; continuation of Example 1.2) Under CAR, the F_X part of the likelihood of the observed data $Y_1, \ldots, Y_n$ is given by

$$L(Y_1, \ldots, Y_n \mid F_X) = \prod_{i=1}^{n} dF_X(\bar X_i(c))\big|_{c=C_i},$$

where $dF_X(\bar X(c))$ represents the density of the sample path $\bar X(c)$ under F_X w.r.t. some dominating measure (discrete or continuous). Again, we note that the full data model only specifies a mean of one of the components of F_X so that maximum likelihood estimation will perform miserably at finite sample sizes and may even be inconsistent. □

The fact that the maximum likelihood estimator, or more generally any globally efficient estimator, has a bad practical performance does not exclude the presence of other inefficient but practical estimators. In fact, in the *full data* multivariate generalized regression models (repeated measures) of Examples 1.1 and 1.2, we have already seen that no globally efficient practical estimators of μ exist, but nice locally efficient estimators are available. However, Lemma 1.1 teaches us that if F_X is completely unspecified, then all *regular* asymptotically linear estimators of the parameter μ in the observed data model $\mathcal{M}(CAR)$ are asymptotically equivalent and efficient. Thus, in this nonparametric coarsening at random model for Y, one has no other choice than to construct globally efficient estimators, such as the nonparametric maximum likelihood estimator. From a practical point of view, the lesson is that if the maximum likelihood estimator of F_X in the observed data model $\mathcal{M}(CAR)$ based on $Y_1, \ldots, Y_n$ has a bad practical performance, then there will not exist regular asymptotically linear estimators with good practical performance in $\mathcal{M}(CAR)$.

To further understand the difficulty in estimating μ in model $\mathcal{M}(CAR)$, recall that the observed data nuisance tangent space $T_{nuis}(P_{F_X,G})$ for the parameter of interest μ is the closure of the linear span of all scores of one-dimensional submodels $\epsilon \to P_{F_\epsilon, G_\epsilon}$ for which $d/d\epsilon\,\mu(P_{F_\epsilon,G_\epsilon})|_{\epsilon=0} = 0$. The observed nuisance tangent space is a sub-Hilbert space of $L_0^2(P_{F_X,G}) = \{h(Y): E_{P_{F_X,G}} h^2(Y) < \infty, E_{P_{F_X,G}} h(Y) = 0\}$ endowed with inner product $\langle h, g\rangle_{P_{F_X,G}} = E_{P_{F_X,G}}[h(Y)g(Y)]$. We also recall that an estimator μ_n is called asymptotically linear at $P_{F_X,G}$ with influence curve $IC(Y)$ if

$$\mu_n - \mu = \frac{1}{n}\sum_{i=1}^{n} IC(Y_i) + o_P(1/\sqrt{n}) \qquad (1.22)$$

and that the components of the influence function $IC(Y)$ of any regular asymptotically linear estimators of μ must lie in the orthocomplement $T_{nuis}^{\perp}(P_{F_X,G})$ of the observed data nuisance tangent space $T_{nuis}(P_{F_X,G})$. Our next goal is to try to understand why in the models of the previous examples it is not possible to obtain an estimator μ_n satisfying the expansion above for any element $IC(Y)$ in the orthogonal complement $T_{nuis}^{\perp}$ in the absence of smoothness assumptions. To do so, we must first determine the form of $T_{nuis}^{\perp}$.

Consider a full data structure model $\mathcal{M}^F$ and associated observed data model $\mathcal{M}(CAR)$ in which G is assumed to satisfy CAR but is otherwise unrestricted (i.e., $G \in \mathcal{G}(CAR)$). Our general representation theorem (Theorem 1.3) at the end of this chapter, first established in Robins and Rotnitzky (1992), represents the orthogonal complement $T_{nuis}^{\perp} = T_{nuis}^{\perp}(P_{F_X,G})$ of the nuisance tangent space T_{nuis} in the observed data model $\mathcal{M}(CAR)$ at $P_{F_X,G}$ as the range of a mapping $D \to IC_0(D) - \Pi(IC_0(D) \mid T_{CAR})$, where the initial mapping $D \to IC_0(D)$ satisfies $E(IC_0(D)(Y) \mid X) = D(X)$ F_X-a.e., applied to the orthogonal complement $T_{nuis}^{F,\perp}(F_X)$ of the nuisance tangent space in the full data model $\mathcal{M}^F$. The mapping is defined as an initial mapping (typically an inverse probability of censoring weighted mapping) minus a projection of this initial mapping on the tangent space $T_{CAR} = T_{CAR}(P_{F_X,G})$ for G in model $\mathcal{M}(CAR)$ at $P_{F_X,G}$. $T_{CAR}(P_{F_X,G})$ consists of all functions of the observed data that have mean zero given the full data, namely

$$T_{CAR}(P_{F_X,G}) = \{V(Y) \in L_0^2(P_{F_X,G}) : E_G(V(Y) \mid X) = 0\} \qquad (1.23)$$

To understand why this space should be T_{CAR}, note that any parametric submodel $f(Y|X;\omega) = m(Y;\omega)$ of $\mathcal{G}(CAR)$ with true value $\omega = 0$ must have a score $\partial \log m(Y;\omega)/\partial \omega$ at $\omega = 0$ that is a function only of Y and has conditional mean zero, given X. By choosing $f(Y|X;\omega) = (1 + \omega V(Y))g(Y \mid X)$ for bounded $V(Y)$ satisfying $E_G(V(Y) \mid X) = 0$ and then taking the closure in $L_0^2(P_{F_X,G})$, we obtain the set $T_{CAR}(P_{F_X,G})$. Note that $T_{CAR}(P_{F_X,G})$ depends on F_X as well as on G because whether $V(Y)$ has a finite variance (and thus belongs to $L_0^2(P_{F_X,G})$) depends on F_X.

Below, using this general representation of $T_{nuis}^{\perp}(P_{F_X,G})$, we will determine the orthogonal complement of the nuisance tangent space (or equivalently all influence curves/functions of regular asymptotically linear estimators) in model $\mathcal{M}(CAR)$ for our examples. Subsequently, we will note that any function of Y and the empirical distribution P_n (say $IC_{FC}(Y \mid P_n)$) for which $IC_{FC}(Y \mid P)$ would equal an influence function $IC(Y \mid P)$ at P for each $P \in \mathcal{M}(CAR)$ is a highly non smooth function of the empirical distribution P_n, because $IC(Y \mid P)$ depends on conditional expectations given high dimensional continuous covariates. Such a function $IC_{FC}(Y \mid P_n)$ is said to be Fisher consistent for $IC(Y \mid P)$. Clearly $IC_{FC}(\cdot \mid P_n)$ will fail to be consistent in $L_2(P_{F_X,G})$ for the function

$IC(\cdot \mid P)$. Klaassen (1987) shows that a necessary condition for construction of a regular asymptotically linear estimator of μ with a given influence function is that one can estimate this influence function consistently. Therefore one is forced to consider non-Fisher consistent estimators $IC_n(Y)$ of $IC(Y \mid P)$ which use regularization (smoothing) to estimate the conditional expectations in $IC(Y \mid P)$. However, in the absence of smoothness assumptions on these conditional expectations, the bias of any regularized estimator will imply that $\int IC_n(Y)dP(Y)$ will not be $o_P(n^{-1/2})$ at all laws allowed by the model. However, Klaassen (1987) shows that a necessary condition for construction of a RAL estimator of μ is that this integral be $o_p(n^{-1/2})$.

Therefore, our argument shows that without smoothness assumptions (as in CODA theory) in these examples there will not exist any regular asymptotically linear estimators in model $\mathcal{M}(CAR)$. For a formal theory of the curse of dimensionality, we refer to Robins and Ritov (1997).

Example 1.12 (Right-censored data with time-independent covariates; continuation of Example 1.9) In the nonparametric full data model, the orthogonal complement of the nuisance tangent space of $\mu = F_T(t)$ is spanned by $D(T \mid \mu) \equiv I(T \leq t) - \mu$. By the general result in Gill, van der Laan and Robins (1997), we have that the orthogonal complement of the nuisance tangent space in model $\mathcal{M}(CAR)$ is also spanned by one function $IC(Y \mid F_X, G, \mu)$ of the data Y, which is thus the one-dimensional space spanned by the efficient influence function. Thus, a necessary condition to construct a regular asymptotically linear estimator in model $\mathcal{M}(CAR)$ is that one can estimate this function $IC(Y \mid F_X, G, \mu)$ consistently in $L_2(P)$ and that the estimator has bias of $o_P(n^{-1/2})$.

Let $\Delta(t) = I(C > \min(T, t))$. Our general representation theorem (Theorem 1.3) at the end of this chapter, first established in Robins and Rotnitzky (1992), represents the orthogonal complement of the nuisance tangent space in the observed data model $\mathcal{M}(CAR)$ as the range of a specified mapping applied to the orthogonal complement of the nuisance tangent space in the full data model $\mathcal{M}^F$. The mapping is defined as the projection of an inverse probability of censoring weighted mapping

$$D \to IC_0(Y \mid G, D) \equiv \frac{D(T \mid \mu)\Delta(t)}{\bar{G}(\min(T,t) \mid W)}$$

onto the orthogonal complement of the tangent space $T_{CAR}(P_{F_X,G}) = \{h(Y) \in L_0^2(P_{F_X,G}) : E_G(h(Y) \mid X) = 0\}$ of G in model $\mathcal{M}(CAR)$. The projection onto T_{CAR},

$$\Pi(IC_0 \mid T_{CAR}) = \int_0^{\tilde{T}} H(u, W) dM_G(u),$$

where

$$H(u, W) = \left\{ E(IC_0(Y) \mid C = u, W, T \geq u) - E(IC_0(Y) \mid W, \tilde{T} \geq u) \right\}$$

1.2. Tour through the General Estimation Problem.   33

and $dM_G(u) = I(\tilde{T} \in du, \Delta = 0) - I(\tilde{T} \geq u)\Lambda_C(du \mid W)$, is provided in Theorem 1.1 later in this section. Applying it to $D(T \mid \mu) \equiv I(T \leq t) - \mu$ and splitting up the integrals as $\int_0^{\tilde{T}} = \int_0^{\min(t,\tilde{T})} + \int_{\min(t,\tilde{T})}^{\tilde{T}}$ yields (after cancellation of $\int_{\min(t,\tilde{T})}^{\tilde{T}}$)

$$IC(Y) = \frac{D(T \mid \mu)\Delta(t)}{\bar{G}(\min(T,t) \mid W)}$$
$$+ \int_0^{\min(t,\tilde{T})} E\left(\frac{D(T \mid \mu)\Delta(t)}{\bar{G}(\min(T,t) \mid W)} \mid W, \tilde{T} \geq u\right) dM_G(u),$$

where

$$E\left(\frac{D(T \mid \mu)\Delta(t)}{\bar{G}(\min(T,t) \mid W)} \mid W, \tilde{T} \geq u\right) = \frac{F(t \mid W, \tilde{T} \geq u) - F(t)}{\bar{G}(u \mid W)}.$$

Thus estimation of this efficient influence function $IC(Y)$ requires estimation of $G(\cdot \mid W)$ and $F(t \mid W, \tilde{T} \geq u)$. Since W is 25-dimensional, globally consistent estimation of each of these nuisance parameters requires a 25-dimensional smoothing procedure. Such a smoothing procedure will only be consistent under additional smoothness assumptions, and besides it will not have a decent performance in finite samples. This shows that no *practical* regular asymptotically linear estimators of the marginal failure time distribution $F_T(t)$ exist in model $\mathcal{M}(CAR)$ even were smoothness assumptions imposed. □

Example 1.13 (Repeated measures data with missing covariate; continuation of Example 1.1) In the previous coverage of this example, we explained that in the full data world, globally efficient estimators are not practical, but good locally efficient estimators exist. Locally efficient estimators exist because the orthogonal complement of the nuisance tangent space in the full data model, which identifies all estimating functions, was given by functions $h(X^*)\epsilon(\alpha)$ that thus do not depend on nuisance parameters. In the observed data model $\mathcal{M}(CAR)$, defined by the restrictions (1.2) and (1.17), we will see that it is impossible to construct any practical estimators at all.

In order to show this, we need to find the orthogonal complement of the nuisance tangent space in the model $\mathcal{M}(CAR)$ and show that each of these elements depends on nuisance parameters that cannot be well estimated at reasonable sample sizes. Note that in the observed data model $\mathcal{M}(CAR)$, the nuisance parameter consists of the full data nuisance parameter η and the censoring mechanism $\Pi(W)$.

To begin with, consider the inverse of probability of censoring weighted estimating functions

$$\left\{h(X^*)\epsilon(\alpha)\frac{\Delta}{\Pi(W)} : h\right\}. \tag{1.24}$$

34   1. Introduction

Thus, given an estimator of the nuisance parameter Π, one could use as estimating equation for α

$$0 = \frac{1}{n}\sum_{i=1}^n h(X_i^*)\epsilon_i(\alpha)\frac{\Delta_i}{\Pi_n(W_i)}.$$

However, under the sole restriction CAR (1.17), estimation of $\Pi(W)$ requires nonparametrically fitting a multivariate regression of the same dimension as W. As a consequence, these Horvitz–Thompson types of estimating functions do not result in practical estimators over the whole model $\mathcal{M}(CAR)$. Now (1.24) is a subset of the orthogonal complement of the nuisance tangent space of η in the observed data model with Π known. However, under CAR, the tangent space $T_{CAR}(P_{F_X,G})$ of G when only assuming (1.17) is also contained in the orthogonal complement of the nuisance tangent space of η in the observed data model with Π known. In fact, our representation theorem (Theorem 1.3) shows that adding the tangent space $T_{CAR}(P_{F_X,G})$ to (1.24) yields the complete orthogonal complement of the nuisance tangent space of η in the model with Π known. The tangent space $T_{CAR}(P_{F_X,G})$ of the conditional distribution G of Δ, given W, consists of all functions of (Δ, W) with conditional mean zero, given W. One can represent this tangent space as

$$T_{CAR}(P_{F_X,G}) = \left\{(\Delta - \Pi(W))\frac{\phi(W)}{\Pi(W)} : \phi\right\}.$$

Thus, the complete orthogonal complement of the nuisance tangent space of η in the observed data model with Π known is given by

$$\left\{h(X^*)\epsilon(\alpha)\frac{\Delta}{\Pi(W)} - (\Delta - \Pi(W))\frac{\phi(W)}{\Pi(W)} : h, \phi\right\}. \quad (1.25)$$

Thus, in the observed data model with Π known, we have access to a rich class (1.25) of estimating functions for α *without* a nuisance parameter; namely, any choice of ϕ, h provides an estimating function.

The orthogonal complement of the nuisance parameter (η, G) in $\mathcal{M}(CAR)$ is the subspace of (1.25) consisting of the functions in (1.25) that are *also* orthogonal to G. Thus, this space is given by

$$\left\{h(X^*)\epsilon(\alpha)\frac{\Delta}{\Pi(W)} - (\Delta - \Pi(W))\frac{\phi_{opt,h}(W)}{\Pi(W)} : h, \phi\right\},$$

where $\phi_{opt,h}$ is chosen so that $(\Delta - \Pi(W))\frac{\phi_{opt,h}(W)}{\Pi(W)}$ equals the projection of $h(X^*)\epsilon(\alpha)\frac{\Delta}{\Pi(W)}$ onto $T_{CAR}(P_{F_X,G})$. It is not hard to show that the projection of a function of the data onto $T_{CAR}(P_{F_X,G})$ in Hilbert space $L_0^2(P_{F_X,G})$ is obtained by first taking the conditional expectation, given W, Δ, and subtracting from this object its conditional mean, given W.

1.2. Tour through the General Estimation Problem. 35

Thus

$$\phi_{opt,h}(W) = E\left\{h(X^*)\epsilon(\alpha)\frac{\Delta}{\Pi(W)} \mid W\right\}.$$

We conclude that the orthogonal complement of the nuisance parameter (η, G) in the model $\mathcal{M}(CAR)$ is given by

$$\left\{h(X^*)\epsilon(\alpha)\frac{\Delta}{\Pi(W)} - (\Delta - \Pi(W))\frac{E\left\{h(X^*)\epsilon(\alpha)\frac{\Delta}{\Pi(W)} \mid W\right\}}{\Pi(W)} : h\right\}. \tag{1.26}$$

Each of the elements, indexed by h, in this orthogonal complement of the nuisance tangent space implies an estimating function for α (and a corresponding influence curve) with nuisance parameters being Π and the full data parameter

$$Q_X(W) \equiv E_{F_X}\left\{h(X^*)\epsilon(\alpha) \mid W\right\} = E_{F_X}\left\{h(X^*)\epsilon(\alpha)\frac{\Delta}{\Pi(W)} \mid W\right\}.$$

Nonparametric estimation of both nuisance parameters $\Pi(W)$ and $Q_X(W)$ requires a multivariate smoothing procedure of the same dimension as W. Thus, without additional assumptions on the full data model and censoring mechanism Π, none of these nuisance parameters can be reasonably well estimated with finite sample sizes. $\square$

Example 1.14 (Repeated measures data with right-censoring; continuation of Example 1.2) In the previous coverage of this example, we explained that, in the full data world, globally efficient estimators are not practical but that attractive locally efficient estimators exist. The latter was shown by showing that the orthogonal complement of the nuisance tangent space in the full data model, which identifies all estimating functions, was given by functions $h(X^*)\epsilon(\alpha)$, which thus do not depend on nuisance parameters. In the observed data model $\mathcal{M}(CAR)$, defined by the restrictions (1.3) and (1.18), we claim that it is even impossible to construct any practical estimators at all.

In order to show this, we need to find the orthogonal complement of the nuisance tangent space in the model $\mathcal{M}(CAR)$ and show that each of the elements of this space depends on nuisance parameters that are very hard to estimate with normal sample sizes. Note that in the observed data model $\mathcal{M}(CAR)$, the nuisance parameter consists of the full data nuisance parameter η and G.

Let $\Delta = I(C \geq p)$ be the indicator that the subject does not drop out of the study before p. We have that

$$P(\Delta = 1 \mid X) = \bar{G}(p \mid X) = \prod_{j=0}^{p-1}(1 - \lambda_C(j \mid X)),$$

where $\bar{G}(t \mid X) \equiv P(C \geq t \mid X)$. To begin with, we consider the inverse of probability of censoring weighted estimating functions that are obtained by inverse weighting any full data structure estimating function $D_h(X \mid \alpha) \equiv h(X^*)\epsilon(\alpha)$:

$$\left\{ IC_0(Y \mid G, D) \equiv D_h(X \mid \alpha) \frac{\Delta}{\bar{G}(p \mid X)} : h \right\}. \qquad (1.27)$$

Thus, given an estimator of the nuisance parameter $\bar{G}(p \mid X)$, one could use as estimating equation for α:

$$0 = \frac{1}{n} \sum_{i=1}^{n} h(X_i^*)\epsilon_i(\alpha) \frac{\Delta_i}{\bar{G}_n(p \mid X)}.$$

However, under the sole restriction CAR (1.17), estimation of $\bar{G}$ requires fitting nonparametrically a multinomial regression of very high dimension. As a consequence, these Horvitz–Thompson types of estimating functions do not result in practical estimators that are consistent and asymptotically normal (CAN) over the whole model $\mathcal{M}(CAR)$. We have that (1.27) is a subset of the orthogonal complement of the nuisance tangent space of η in the observed data model with $\bar{G}$ known. However, by CAR, the tangent space $T_{CAR}(P_{F_X,G})$ of G only assuming (1.17) (i.e, CAR) is also contained in the orthogonal complement of the nuisance tangent space of η in the observed data model with G known. In fact, our representation theorem (Theorem 1.3) shows that adding the tangent space $T_{CAR}(P_{F_X,G})$ to (1.27) yields the complete orthogonal complement of the nuisance tangent space of η in the model with G known. The tangent space $T_{CAR}(P_{F_X,G})$ of the conditional distribution G of C, given X, consists of all functions of Y with conditional mean zero, given X, w.r.t. G.

We will now derive a representation of the tangent space $T_{CAR}(P_{F_X,G})$ and determine the projection onto $T_{CAR}(P_{F_X,G})$. Our derivation yields an elegant (and easy-to-understand) proof of a very important fundamental result used throughout this book. We will do this in the general situation where we have observed data $(\tilde{T} = \min(T,C), \Delta = I(C \geq T), \bar{X}(\tilde{T}))$ and the full data structure $\bar{X}(T) = \{X(s) : s \leq T\}$, where T is possibly random: in the current example, we have $T = p$ fixed. We define $C = \infty$ if $C \geq T$ so that C is always observed. In the current example this implies that C can never take value p and $A(p)$ is a deterministic function of $A(p-1)$. Let $A(j) = I(C \leq j)$ so that $dA(j) = I(C = j)$, $j = 0, \ldots, p$. Let $\mathcal{F}(j) = (\bar{A}(j-1), \bar{X}(\min(j,C)))$ be the history observed up and including time j. Let $\alpha(j \mid \mathcal{F}(j)) = E(dA(j) \mid \mathcal{F}(j))$ be the probability that $C = j$, given the history $\mathcal{F}(j)$. Note that

$$\alpha(j \mid \mathcal{F}(j)) = I(\tilde{T} \geq j) P(C = j \mid \mathcal{F}(j), \tilde{T} \geq j) = I(\tilde{T} \geq j) \lambda_C(j \mid \bar{X}(j)),$$

where $\lambda_C(j \mid \bar{X}(j))$ is the hazard of C, given X at time j, which by CAR only depends on X through $\bar{X}(j)$. Under CAR, the G part of the likelihood

1.2. Tour through the General Estimation Problem. 37

of Y is given by

$$g(\bar{A}(p-1) \mid X) = \prod_{j=0}^{p-1} \alpha(j \mid \mathcal{F}(j))^{dA(j)} \{1 - \alpha(j \mid \mathcal{F}(j))\}^{1-dA(j)}. \quad (1.28)$$

Since $\alpha(j \mid \mathcal{F}(j))^{dA(j)} \{1 - \alpha(j \mid \mathcal{F}(j))\}^{1-dA(j)}$ is just a Bernoulli likelihood for the random variable $dA(j)$ with probability $\alpha(j \mid \mathcal{F}(j))$, it follows that the tangent space of $\alpha(j \mid \mathcal{F}(j))$ is the space of all functions of $(dA(j), \mathcal{F}(j))$ with conditional mean zero, given $\mathcal{F}(j)$. Straightforward algebra shows that any such function can be written as

$$\begin{aligned} V(dA(j), \mathcal{F}(j)) - E(V \mid \mathcal{F}(j)) &= \{V(1, \mathcal{F}(j)) - V(0, \mathcal{F}(j))\}(1.29) \\ &\quad \times \{dA(j) - \alpha(j \mid \mathcal{F}(j))\}. \end{aligned}$$

Thus, the tangent space of the parameter $\alpha(j \mid \mathcal{F}(j))$ equals

$$T_{CAR,j} \equiv \{H(\mathcal{F}(j))\{dA(j) - \alpha(j \mid \mathcal{F}(j))\} : H\},$$

where H ranges over all functions of $\mathcal{F}(j)$ for which each element of $T_{CAR,j}$ has finite variance. By factorization of the likelihood (1.28), we have that

$$T_{CAR}(P_{F_X,G}) = T_{CAR,0} \oplus T_{CAR,1} \ldots \oplus T_{CAR,p-1}. \quad (1.30)$$

Equivalently,

$$T_{CAR}(P_{F_X,G}) = \left\{ \sum_{j=0}^{p-1} H(j, \mathcal{F}(j)) dM_G(j) : H \right\},$$

where

$$dM_G(j) = I(C = j) - \lambda_C(j \mid \bar{X}(j)) I(\tilde{T} \geq j).$$

Note that $I(C = j) = I(C = j, \Delta = 0)$ for $j < p$.

Thus, the complete orthogonal complement of the nuisance tangent space of η in the observed data model with G known is given by:

$$\left\{ h(X^*)\epsilon(\alpha) \frac{\Delta}{\bar{G}(p \mid X)} - \sum_{j=0}^{p-1} H(j, \mathcal{F}(j)) dM_G(j) : h, H \right\}. \quad (1.31)$$

This shows that in the observed data model with G known we have access to a rich class (1.31) of estimating functions for α *without* a nuisance parameter, namely any choice of h, H provides an estimating function for α.

The orthogonal complement of the nuisance parameter (η, G) in $\mathcal{M}(CAR)$ is the subspace of (1.31) consisting of the functions in (1.31) which are *also* orthogonal to G. Thus this space is given by:

$$\left\{ h(X^*)\epsilon(\alpha) \frac{\Delta}{\bar{G}(p \mid X)} - \sum_{j=0}^{p-1} H_{opt,h}(j, \mathcal{F}(j)) dM_G(j) : h, H \right\}, \quad (1.32)$$

where $H_{opt,h}$ is chosen so that $\sum_{j=0}^{p} H_{opt,h}(j,\bar{X}(j))dM_G(j)$ equals the projection of $h(X^*)\epsilon(\alpha)\frac{\Delta}{\bar{G}(p|X)}$ onto $T_{CAR}(P_{F_X,G})$ in the Hilbert space $L_0^2(P_{F_X,G})$.

We will now derive this projection. By representation (1.30) of T_{CAR}, we have that

$$\Pi(IC_0(Y \mid G, D) \mid T_{CAR}) = \sum_{j=0}^{p-1} \Pi(IC_0(Y \mid G, D) \mid T_{CAR,j}).$$

The projection onto $T_{CAR,j}$ is obtained by first projecting on all functions of $(dA(j), \mathcal{F}(j))$ and subsequently subtracting its conditional expectation, given $\mathcal{F}(j)$,

$$\Pi(IC_0(D) \mid T_{CAR,j}) = E(IC_0(D) \mid dA(j), \mathcal{F}(j)) \\ - E(E(IC_0(D) \mid dA(j), \mathcal{F}(j)) \mid \mathcal{F}(j)),$$

where we used short hand notation for $IC_0(Y \mid G, D)$. By (1.29), this can be written as

$$\{E(IC_0(D) \mid dA(j) = 1, \mathcal{F}(j)) - E(IC_0(D) \mid dA(j) = 0, \mathcal{F}(j))\} dM_G(j).$$

Finally, we note that $E(IC_0(D) \mid dA(j) = 1, \mathcal{F}(j)) = 0$ since $dA(j) = 1$ implies $\Delta = 0$ for $j \leq p - 1$. This proves that

$$\Pi(IC_0(D) \mid T_{CAR}) = -\sum_{j=0}^{p-1} \{E(IC_0(D) \mid dA(j) = 0, \mathcal{F}(j))\} dM_G(j).$$

This can be represented as $\sum_{j=0}^{p-1} H_{opt,D}(j, \mathcal{F}(j)) dM_G(j)$ with

$$H_{opt,D}(j, \mathcal{F}(j)) = -E(IC_0(Y \mid G, D) \mid C > j, \bar{X}(j)) \\ = -\frac{1}{\bar{G}(j+1 \mid X)} E(D_h(X \mid \alpha) \mid \bar{X}(j), C > j),$$

where, by definition, $\bar{G}(j+1 \mid X) = P(C > j \mid X)$. We also note that by CAR $Q_{X,h} \equiv E(D_h(X \mid \alpha) \mid \bar{X}(j), C > j) = E(D_h(X \mid \alpha) \mid \bar{X}(j))$ which is thus a parameter of the full data distribution F_X.

We conclude that the orthogonal complement of the nuisance parameter (η, G) in the model $\mathcal{M}(CAR)$ is given by

$$\left\{ h(X^*)\epsilon(\alpha)\frac{\Delta}{\bar{G}(p \mid X)} - \sum_{j=0}^{p} Q_{X,h}(j, \bar{X}(j))\frac{dM_G(j)}{\bar{G}(j+1 \mid X)} : h \right\}. \quad (1.33)$$

Each of the elements, indexed by h, in this orthogonal complement of the nuisance tangent space implies an estimating function for α (and a corresponding influence curve) with nuisance parameters being G and the full data parameter $Q_{X,h}$. Without additional assumptions on the full data model and censoring mechanism, neither of these two nuisance parameters can be reasonably well-estimated in practice. This shows that no practical estimators exist in model $\mathcal{M}(CAR)$.

Above, we formally proved the following fundamental results for the general right-censored data structure $(\tilde{T}, \Delta, \bar{X}(\tilde{T}))$ for the case where censoring is discrete:

Theorem 1.1 *Let $R(t) = I(T \leq t)$ for a time variable T. Let $X(t)$ be a time-dependent process including $R(t)$. Let $X = \bar{X}(T)$ be the full data. We have observed data $Y = (\tilde{T} = \min(C, T), \Delta = I(T \leq C), \bar{X}(\tilde{T}))$, where C is a univariate discrete variable with conditional distribution $G(\cdot \mid X)$, given X. Let $A(t) = I(C \leq t)$, where we define $C = \infty$ if $C \geq T$ so that C is always observed. Let $\mathcal{F}(t) = (\bar{A}(t-), \bar{X}(\min(t, C)))$ be the history observed up to time t.*

Assume CAR on G: $E(dA(t) \mid \bar{A}(t-), X) = E(dA(t) \mid \mathcal{F}(t))$ or equivalently, for $t \leq T$,

$$\lambda_{C|X}(t \mid X) \equiv P(C = t \mid C \geq t, X) = m(t, \bar{X}(t))$$

for some measurable function m. Then, the tangent space $T_{CAR}(P_{F_X,G})$ of G is given by

$$T_{CAR}(P_{F_X,G}) = \overline{\left\{\int H(u, \mathcal{F}(u))dM_G(u) : H\right\}} \cap L_0^2(P_{F_X,G}),$$

where $dM_G(u) = I(C \in du, \Delta = 0) - I(\tilde{T} \geq u)\lambda_{C|X}(du \mid X)$. For any function $V(Y)$, we have that $\Pi(V \mid T_{CAR})$ is given by

$$\int \{E(V(Y) \mid dA(u) = 1, \mathcal{F}(u)) - E(V(Y) \mid dA(u) = 0, \mathcal{F}(u))\} dM_G(u).$$

Remark: For the data structure Y of theorem 1.1 any variable $V(Y)$ can be written as $\Delta d_1(X) + (1 - \Delta)V_2(\bar{X}(C), C)$ for some functions d_1 and V_2. It follows that $E[V(Y) \mid dA(u) = 1, F(u)] = V_2(\bar{X}(u), u)$ is actually a deterministic function of $V(Y)$.

If G is actually continuous, then the G part of the likelihood of Y is defined as the partial likelihood of $A(t)$, w.r.t. the left-continuous history $\mathcal{F}(t-)$ as in Andersen, Borgan, Gill and Keiding (1993), if in theorem 1.1 we replace $F(u)$ and $F(t)$ by $F(u-)$ and $F(t-)$.

The formulas for T_{CAR} and the projection onto T_{CAR} in Theorem 1.1 can be applied to the continuous case as well, but the proof of the representation of T_{CAR} involves calculating the scores from this partial likelihood, and the projection formula needs to be formally defined and proved, taking into account possible measurability conditions needed to define the conditional expectations. A formal treatment of the continuous case is given in van der Vaart (2001). Since the latter is beyond the scope and purpose of this book, we will avoid stating these continuous projection results as theorems, but still use them to define the corresponding estimating functions. $\square$

1.2.5 The observed data model

The previous section and the double robustness of estimation functions as established in section 1.6 below, shows that in order to create room for practical estimators, one will often either need to assume a lower-dimensional CAR model $\mathcal{G} \subset \mathcal{G}(CAR)$ for the conditional distribution $G(\cdot \mid X)$ or assume a lower-dimensional full data model $\mathcal{M}^{F,w} \subset \mathcal{M}^F$ for the full data distribution X.

Following Robins, Rotnitzky, and van der Laan (2000), this motivates us to consider the following more general model for the distribution of Y. Given working models $\mathcal{M}^{F,w}$ and $\mathcal{G}$ for the full data structure distribution F_X and censoring mechanism G, respectively, the observed data model is defined as

$$\mathcal{M} = \{P_{F_X,G} : F_X \in \mathcal{M}^F, G \in \mathcal{G}\} \cup \{P_{F_X,G} : F_X \in \mathcal{M}^{F,w}, G \in \mathcal{G}(CAR)\}. \tag{1.34}$$

In other words, either F_X needs to be an element of $\mathcal{M}^{F,w}$ or G needs to be an element of $\mathcal{G}$, but one does not need both working models to contain the true full data structure and censoring distribution. Given this model $\mathcal{M}$ of Y with parameters F_X and G, our goal is to construct a well-behaved estimator of the Euclidean parameter $\mu = \mu(F_X) \in \mathbb{R}^k$ that is locally efficient at the submodel $\{P_{F_X,G} : F_X \in \mathcal{M}^{F,w}, G \in \mathcal{G}\}$.

For many censored data structures, C is low-(e.g., one-) dimensional so that modeling G correctly is much easier than modeling F_X. In particular, in some applications, the censoring mechanism is in control of the experimenter and is thus known. For example, in our missing-covariate example, the missingness mechanism might be known by design. Therefore, the (smaller) model

$$\mathcal{M}(\mathcal{G}) = \{P_{F_X,G} : F_X \in \mathcal{M}^F, G \in \mathcal{G}\} \tag{1.35}$$

is also of interest and will therefore be treated separately.

1.2.6 General method for construction of locally efficient estimators

The class of estimating functions for μ is obtained by mapping full data estimating functions for μ into observed data estimating functions. Let us again review the definition of estimating functions. To be specific, we will do this for the full data model, but it translates immediately into a general definition. Formally, we define a full data (orthogonal) estimating function of the k-dimensional parameter μ as a k-dimensional function $D(X \mid \mu, \rho)$ of X, μ and possibly a nuisance parameter $\rho(F_X)$, where we assume that the estimating function is orthogonal to the nuisance tangent space in the sense that if one evaluates it at $(\mu(F_X), \rho(F_X))$, then it is a vector function of X whose components have both mean zero and covariance zero (w.r.t. F_X) with any nuisance score. In principle, the estimating function only needs to be a well defined function of X for each parameter value in the parameter space $(\mu(F_X), \rho(F_X) : F_X \in \mathcal{M}^F)$, but natural extensions of its domain are typically available (and also needed to define the function for estimators ρ_n of ρ that are not an element of the parameter space). Recall that nuisance scores are scores of one-dimensional submodels $\epsilon \to F_\epsilon$ through F_X at $\epsilon = 0$ for which $d/d\epsilon\, \mu(F_\epsilon)|_{\epsilon=0} = 0$ (i.e one-dimensional submodels which do not perturbate the parameter of interest μ in first order). Consequently, to define such a rich class of estimating functions requires finding a representation of the orthogonal complement of the nuisance tangent space at each F_X. Let $\{D_h(\cdot \mid \mu, \rho) : h \in \mathcal{H}^F\}$ be such a rich set of full data estimating functions indexed by $h \in \mathcal{H}^F$. Here we note that a class of univariate estimating functions $(D_h : h \in \mathcal{H}^F)$ derived from a representation of $T_{nuis}^{F,\perp}$ that satisfies $\{D_h(\cdot \mid \mu(F_X), \rho(F_X)) : h \in \mathcal{H}\} \subset T_{nuis}^{F,\perp}(F_X)$ for all $F_X \in \mathcal{M}^F$ implies a class of k-dimensional estimating functions $(D_h : h \in \mathcal{H}^k)$ by defining $D_{h_1,\ldots,h_k} = (D_{h_1}, \ldots, D_{h_k})$. For well understood full data models, the orthogonal complement of the nuisance tangent space is known, and we derive it for a general class of multivariate generalized linear regression models (i.e., repeated measures) and the class of multiplicative intensity models in Chapter 2.

A practically important feature of estimating functions that are orthogonal to the nuisance tangent space is that the asymptotic limit distribution of the solution of the corresponding estimating equation is not affected by the asymptotic relative efficiency of the consistent estimator of a locally variation-independent nuisance parameter ρ. Under mild conditions, the solution μ_n of any such estimating equation w.r.t. μ, with ρ replaced by an estimate $\hat{\rho}$ (or $\hat{\rho}(\mu)$) that converges to ρ at an appropriate rate, is regular and asymptotically linear with influence curve equal to the standardized estimating function $-[d/d\mu ED(X \mid \mu, \rho)]^{-1} D(X \mid \mu, \rho)$. In fact, in many models, the estimating function does not even depend on nuisance parameters ρ, as in the multivariate generalized linear regression models. Throughout this book we assume that the model M^F is sufficiently small so as not to be affected by curse of dimensionality in the sense that there exists RAL estimators of μ based on the full data structure X whose moderate sample distribution is well approximated by their asymptotic distribution. In particular this implies that we have available estimators ρ_n or $\rho_n(\mu)$ of ρ based on data X that converge at an appropriate rate.

The requirement that the estimating function be orthogonal to the nuisance tangent space does not exclude any regular asymptotically linear estimator in the sense that, given any regular asymptotically linear estimator, there exists an orthogonal estimating function such that an RAL–solution of the corresponding estimating equation (or the corresponding Newton–Raphson one-step estimator if a decent initial estimator is available) is asymptotically equivalent. This follows from the fundamental result that each regular asymptotically linear estimator at F_X has an influence curve $IC(X \mid F_X)$ at F_X whose components are orthogonal to the nuisance tangent space. To summarize, in the full data model, the mapping from the data-generating distribution F_X into the orthogonal complement of the nuisance tangent space at F_X can be used to identify all estimating functions of interest. Similarly, this applies to the observed data model.

Our representation theorem (Theorem 1.3) represents the orthogonal complement of the nuisance tangent space in the model $\mathcal{M}(CAR)$ as the range of a mapping $D(X) \to IC(Y \mid Q(F_X,G), G, D)$ defined on the orthogonal complement of the nuisance tangent space in the full data structure model, where $IC(Y \mid Q(F_X,G), G, D)$ can be any mapping satisfying 1) $E_G(IC(Y \mid Q, G, D) \mid X) = D(X)$ F_X-a.e. for all $D \in T_{nuis}^{F,\perp}(F_X)$ under all possible values of Q and 2) $IC(Y \mid Q(F_X,G), G, D) \perp T_{CAR}(P_{F_X,G})$. This mapping is indexed by a parameter $Q = Q(F_X, G)$ and the censoring mechanism G, and it typically can be chosen to be represented as the projection of an initial (often involving inverse probability of censoring weighting) mapping $IC_0(Y \mid G, D)$, satisfying $E(IC_0(Y \mid G, D) \mid X) = D(X)$ F_X-a.e., onto the orthogonal complement of the tangent space $T_{CAR}(P_{F_X,G})$ of G in model $\mathcal{M}(CAR)$; that is, $IC(Y \mid Q(F_X,G), G, D) = IC_0(Y \mid G, D) - \Pi_{F_X,G}(IC_0(Y \mid G, D) \mid T_{CAR})$. We define $\mathcal{D}(\rho_1(F_X), G)$ as the set of all possible full data functions to be considered for which $E_G(IC(Y \mid Q, G, D) \mid X) = D(X)$ F_X-a.e. for all parameter values Q. This set obviously depends on G, but possibly also on a parameter $\rho_1(F_X)$ of F_X because of the fact that the equality needs to hold F_X-a.e. Thus depending on the model assumptions, condition 1 holds only for a subspace $\mathcal{D}(\rho_1(F_X), G) \cap T_{nuis}^{F,\perp}$ of $T_{nuis}^{F,\perp}(F_X)$. In this case, the set of (influence curve and thereby) regular asymptotically linear estimators of μ at F_X in the full data structure model is larger than the set of regular asymptotically linear estimators of μ at $P_{F_X,G}$ in the observed data structure model $\mathcal{M}(CAR)$, and in each such situation it remains to be verified that the analogue of Theorem 1.3 is true; that is, the range of the mapping defined on this subspace still *equals* $T_{nuis}^{\perp}(\mathcal{M}(CAR))$.

As proved in this chapter in Section 1.6 on double robust estimating functions (and see Chapter 2), these observed data functions satisfy the following crucial identity: given a G_1 with $dG/dG_1 < \infty$ and $D \in \mathcal{D}(\rho_1(F_X), G_1)$ with $E_{F_X} D(X) = 0$, we have

$$E_{F_X,G} IC(Y \mid Q(F_1, G_1), G_1, D) = 0 \text{ if either } F_1 = F_X \text{ or } G_1 = G. \quad (1.36)$$

The protection (of its unbiasedness) against misspecification of G (at a correct F_X) happens to be a consequence of the fact that $IC(Y \mid Q(F_X, G_1), G_1, D)$ is orthogonal to the tangent space of G under a convex model $\mathcal{G}(CAR)$ at P_{F_X,G_1} in the Hilbert space $L_0^2(P_{F_X,G_1})$ (see Lemma 1.8 below). The protection against misspecification of F_X can be seen directly from the fact that $E_G(IC(Y \mid Q(F_1, G), G, D) \mid X) = D(X)$ F_X-a.e. for $D \in \mathcal{D}(\rho_1(F_X), G)$, by assumption, and $E_{F_X} D(X) = 0$.

This mapping (defined at a given F_X, G for all elements in our model) gives rise to a natural mapping $D_h \to IC(Y \mid Q, G, D_h)$ from full data estimating functions $(D_h : h \in \mathcal{H}^F)$ into observed data estimating functions $IC(Y \mid Q, G, D_h(\cdot \mid \mu, \rho))$ for μ with additional nuisance parameters Q and G. To acknowledge that the observed data estimating functions are only unbiased for $D_h(\cdot \mid \mu(F_X), \rho(F_X)) \in \mathcal{D}(\rho_1(F_X), G_1)$ we include this $\mathcal{D}(\rho_1(F_X), G)$ membership requirement for the full data structure estimating functions (assuming that it is not implied by the model) as a nuisance parameter of the full data estimating function. As we will show, this yields a class of unbiased full data estimating functions $(D_h^r(X \mid \mu, \rho, \rho_1, G) : h \in \mathcal{H}^F)$ indexed by a common index set $\mathcal{H}^F$, that are members of $T_{nuis}^{F,\perp}(F_X)$ and $\mathcal{D}(\rho_1(F_X), G)$ when evaluated at the true parameter values. For notational convenience, we denote these estimating functions with $D_h(\cdot \mid \mu, \rho)$ again, but $\rho = \rho(F_X, G)$ now also includes G as a component. This reparametrization procedure will be discussed and illustrated in detail in Chapter 2. As is the case throughout the book, a mapping $D \to IC(Y \mid Q, G, D)$ from univariate full data estimating functions into univariate observed data estimating functions defines a mapping from k-dimensional full data estimating functions into k-dimensional observed data estimating functions by defining $IC(Y \mid Q, G, (D_1, \ldots, D_k)) = (IC(Y \mid Q, G, D_1), \ldots, IC(Y \mid Q(F_X, G), G, D_k))$.

By Theorem 1.3, if $\mathcal{H}^F$ is chosen rich enough, then the optimal estimating function corresponding with $D_{h_{opt}}$ is contained in this class. By CAR, G is orthogonal to F_X so that the semiparametric information bound for μ, and thus the optimal estimating function, is the same for models $\mathcal{M}(\mathcal{G})$ and $\mathcal{M}(CAR)$. This is also the bound for model $\mathcal{M}$ when the model for G is correct. If the dimension of the working models $\mathcal{M}^{F,w}$ and $\mathcal{G}$ for F_X and G, respectively, is such that the nuisance parameters (Q, G) of the estimating functions for μ can be estimated well with a sample of size n, then the asymptotics (in particular, our proposed Wald-type confidence intervals) of our proposed locally efficient estimators in model $\mathcal{M}$ will approximate their finite sample performance. For example, one could choose the working models $\mathcal{M}^{F,w}$ and $\mathcal{G}$ so that the MLE of F_X over $\mathcal{M}^{F,w}$ and G over $\mathcal{G}$ have a good finite sample performance. In particular, if $\mathcal{M}^F$ is already of low enough dimension that estimation of F_X is feasible, then $\mathcal{M}^{F,w} = \mathcal{M}^F$ is appropriate, and similarly, if $\mathcal{G}(CAR)$ is already of low enough dimension that estimation of the censoring mechanism G is feasible, then $\mathcal{G} = \mathcal{G}(CAR)$ is appropriate.

Example 1.15 (Right censored data with covariates; continuation of Example 1.9) If W is continuous, then without smoothness assumptions no globally efficient estimator of μ exists in model $\mathcal{M}(CAR)$. If W is discrete with 20^{25} possible values, then globally efficient estimators of μ exist in $\mathcal{M}(CAR)$, but this efficiency bound does not approximate the finite sample performance. Therefore, in both cases one should try to select working models $\mathcal{M}^{F,w}$ and $\mathcal{G}$ that are small enough that Q and G can be estimated well with a sample of size n. □

Thus, this mapping from full data estimating functions into observed data estimating functions actually yields all estimating functions of interest and each estimating function for μ is orthogonal to its nuisance parameters (Q, G, ρ). Important facts about this mapping are: 1) this mapping is completely determined by the data structure and the assumption CAR on G (i.e., it is not affected by the full data model); and 2) it yields consistent and asymptotically normally distributed (CAN) estimators over the whole model $\mathcal{M}$ due to its double protection property (1.36) given above. Fact 1) means that, given the data structure, the same mapping can be used to generate all estimating functions for any choice of full data model.

Thus, given a choice of full data estimating function indexed by $h_n \in \mathcal{H}^F$, our proposed estimator μ_n of μ is a solution of the estimating equation

$$0 = \frac{1}{n} \sum_{i=1}^{n} IC(Y_i \mid Q_n, G_n, D_{h_n}(\cdot \mid \mu, \rho_n))$$

in μ. Here we estimate the censoring distribution G and F_X (and thereby $Q(F_X, G)$) according to the working models $\mathcal{G}$ and $\mathcal{M}^{F,w}$, respectively. In addition, if the full data estimating function has a nuisance parameter $\rho(F_X, G)$, then the same working models also yield an estimate ρ_n of ρ; we refer to Chapter 2 for additional discussion. In model $\mathcal{M}(\mathcal{G})$, if an initial estimator is available that converges at an appropriate rate, then we propose to use the one-step estimator defined as the first step of the Newton–Raphson procedure for solving this k-dimensional estimating equation, which is already asymptotically equivalent with an iteratively obtained solution of the estimating equation.

The identity (1.36) provides (under regularity conditions) double protection of the consistency of μ_n in the sense that one can misspecify one of the nuisance parameter models for F_X or G, but one cannot misspecify both. Thus, under regularity conditions, μ_n will indeed yield RAL estimators in model $\mathcal{M}$.

We also provide methods for evaluating the optimal index $(F_X, G) \to h_{opt}(F_X, G)$, $F_X \in \mathcal{M}^F$, $G \in \mathcal{G}(CAR)$, where $h_{opt} = h_{opt}(F_X, G)$ is such that $IC(Y \mid Q_X, G, D_{h_{opt}}(\cdot \mid \mu(F_X), \rho(F_X)))$ equals the efficient score for μ and thus the optimal estimating function. The optimal full data estimating function h_{opt} is determined by the data structure, CAR, and $\mathcal{M}^F$. One could, for example, estimate h_{opt} with a substitution estimator $h_{opt}(F_n, G_n)$ where F_n, G_n are estimates of F_X, G according to the working models $\mathcal{M}^{F,w}$ and $\mathcal{G}$. Thus, the working models $\mathcal{M}^{F,w} \subset \mathcal{M}^F$ and $\mathcal{G} \subset \mathcal{G}(CAR)$ have no effect on the mapping IC and no effect on the optimal estimating function, but are only needed to actually be able to effectively estimate the nuisance parameters (Q, G, ρ) of IC and to estimate h_{opt}.

The asymptotic variance of the corresponding estimator μ_n attains the semiparametric variance bound for the model $\{P_{F_X,G} : F_X \in \mathcal{M}^F, G \in \mathcal{G}\}$ when the working model $\mathcal{M}^{F,w}$ for F_X and the working model $\mathcal{G}$ for G are correct and, due to the identity (1.36), the estimator remains consistent and asymptotically normal (CAN) if one of the working models (not both) is misspecified.

1.2.7 Comparison with maximum likelihood estimation

Note that each doubly robust estimator (i.e., indexed by the choice of h) is truly more robust than the maximum likelihood estimator based on model $\mathcal{M}^{F,w}$ and CAR for G; namely, if $\mathcal{M}^{F,w}$ is misspecified, then the maximum likelihood estimator will be inconsistent, while the doubly robust estimator will still be CAN if the working model $\mathcal{G}$ is correct and $D_h(\cdot \mid \mu, \rho) \in \mathcal{D}(\rho_1(F_X), G)$. On the other hand, if $\mathcal{M}^{F,w}$ is correct, then both the maximum likelihood estimator and the doubly robust estimator are CAN (even when $\mathcal{G}$ is a wrong model). To be precise, the consistency of the doubly robust estimator under a correct model $\mathcal{M}^{F,w}$ requires that the limit $D_h(\cdot \mid \mu, \rho(F_X, G_1))$ of $D_h(\cdot \mid \mu, \rho(F_n, G_n))$ is an element of $\mathcal{D}(\rho_1(F_X), G_1)$ so that the doubly robust estimating function is unbiased under (the possibly misspecified) P_{F_X, G_1}. This can typically be arranged by just making sure that the estimated G_n satisfies the needed identifiability condition, where it does not matter that this condition does not hold for the true censoring mechanism.

If one specifies models $\mathcal{M}^{F,w}$ and $\mathcal{G}$ of low enough dimension, then one can estimate F_X and G with a maximum likelihood procedure, assuming an appropriately defined likelihood (see, e.g., Kiefer and Wolfowitz, 1956). By factorization of the observed data likelihood, the maximum likelihood estimators of F_X and G maximize separate likelihoods. In this way, the user can use standard maximum likelihood methodology developed for lower-dimensional full data models $\mathcal{M}^{F,w}$ and $\mathcal{G}$ to obtain our estimator of μ, achieving the information bound for our model $\mathcal{M}$ if both working models are correct. Further, if $\mathcal{G}$ is correct, then the user will be protected against misspecification of $\mathcal{M}^{F,w}$.

In model $\mathcal{M}(\mathcal{G})$, Q_n just represents an index of an estimating function so that it does not need to be compatible with a true full data structure distribution. That is, Q_n need not equal $Q(F_{X,n}, G_n)$ for some full data distribution $F_{X,n}$. In our applications we will display relatively simple-to-compute estimators Q_n, that only require standard software.

Example 1.16 (Repeated measures data with missing covariate; continuation of Example 1.1) Consider an element of (1.26) indexed by a given h. Let us denote it with

$$IC(Y \mid Q_X, G, D_h(\cdot \mid \alpha)) = D_h(X \mid \alpha) \frac{\Delta}{\Pi(W)}$$

46   1. Introduction

$$-(\Delta - \Pi(W))\frac{Q_X(W)}{\Pi(W)},$$

where $Q_X(W) = Q(F_X)(W) \equiv E\{D_h(X \mid \alpha) \mid W\}$. For each choice of h, $IC(Y \mid Q_X, G, D_h(\cdot \mid \alpha))$ identifies an estimating function in α with nuisance parameters (Q_X, Π).

Given working models for $\Pi(W)$ and $Q_X(W)$, consider the corresponding observed data model $\mathcal{M}$ (1.34). For example, we could assume a logistic regression model for $\Pi(W)$ and a linear regression model for $Q_X(W)$. In words, $\mathcal{M}$ assumes the conditional mean model (1.2) for Z, given X^*, and that *either* the logistic regression model for $\Pi(W)$ is correct *or* that the regression model for $Q_X(W)$ is correct. Let Q_n, G_n be estimators of Q_X, G according to these working models. A natural way of estimating $Q_X(W)$ follows by noting that $Q_X(W) = E(D_h(X \mid \alpha) \mid W, \Delta = 1)$, which is due to the fact that Δ is independent of X, given W. As a consequence, one can estimate $Q_X(W)$ by regressing $D_h(X \mid \alpha)$ on W for all subjects with $\Delta = 1$. In spite of the fact that Q_n, G_n are only consistent for the lower-dimensional working models $\mathcal{M}^{F,w}$ and $\mathcal{G}$, the estimating equation

$$0 = \frac{1}{n}\sum_{i=1}^n IC(Y_i \mid Q_n, G_n, D_h(\cdot \mid \alpha))$$

in α with nuisance parameters (Q_X, G) replaced by the estimates (Q_n, G_n) provides CAN estimators for this model $\mathcal{M}$. Thus, if the model for G is correct, then the CAN-property of α_n is protected against misspecification of Q_X and if the model for Q_X is correct, then the CAN property of α_n is protected against misspecification of G.

This nice double protection is the direct consequence of the identity (1.36): if $\Pi_{G_1}(W) > 0$, F_W-a.e., then

$$E_{F_X,G}IC(Y \mid Q(F_{X,1}), G_1, D_h(\cdot \mid \alpha)) = 0 \text{ if either } F_{X,1} = F_X$$

or $G_1 = G$. This can here be explicitly verified. As predicted by our theory, we note that the unbiasedness holds at F_X, G_1 even when the nonparametric identifiability condition $\Pi_G(W) > 0$ F_W-a.e. fails to hold.

If the working models for both Q_X and G are correct, then the estimator α_n will be asymptotically linear with influence curve $IC(Y \mid Q_X, G, D_h(\cdot \mid \alpha))$. By our representation theorem (Theorem 1.3) there exists a choice $h = h_{opt}(F_X, G)$ for which this influence curve equals the efficient influence curve, but as always this optimal choice depends on the truth (F_X, G). This functional $(F_X, G) \to h_{opt}(F_X, G)$ does not exist in closed form but can be implicitly defined in terms of a solution of an integral equation (see Robins, Rotnitzky and Zhao, 1994). In order to yield locally efficient estimators, one needs to choose a data-dependent h_n. For example, if $F_{X,n}, G_n$ are estimates of F_X, G assuming the working models $\mathcal{M}^{F,w}$ and $\mathcal{G}$, then one can set $h_n = h_{opt}(F_{X,n}, G_n)$. Another easier-to-compute, but non optimal

h_n is an estimate of the optimal index (1.8) in the full data world as defined above. □

Example 1.17 (Repeated measures data with right-censoring; continuation of Example 1.2) Consider the element of (1.33) indexed by a given h:

$$D_h(X \mid \alpha) \frac{\Delta}{\bar{G}(p \mid X)} + \sum_{j=0}^{p-1} Q_X(j, \bar{X}(j)) \frac{dM_G(j)}{\bar{G}(j+1 \mid X)}.$$

Here $Q_X(j, \bar{X}(j)) = E(D_h(X \mid \alpha) \mid \bar{X}(j), C \geq j)$ is the full data parameter defined above. Let us denote this element with $IC(Y \mid Q_X, G, D_h(\cdot \mid \alpha))$. For each choice of h, $IC(Y \mid Q_X, G, D_h(\cdot \mid \alpha))$ identifies an estimating function in α with nuisance parameters Q_X, G.

Given a working model for Q_X and G, consider observed data model $\mathcal{M}$ by (1.34). For example, we could assume a logistic regression model for the hazard $P(C = j \mid \bar{X}(j), C \geq j)$ of the discrete $G(\cdot \mid X)$ and a model for $f_\theta(X(t) \mid \bar{X}(t-))$ for the conditional distribution of $X(t)$, given the full-data past $\bar{X}(t-)$, where estimation in this type of working full data structure models is discussed in Chapter 3. Then $\mathcal{M}$ assumes the conditional mean model (1.3) for the conditional distribution of Z, given X^*, and that *either* the logistic regression model for G is correct *or* that the model $\mathcal{M}^{F,w}$ for F_X and thus Q_X is correct. Let $Q_n = Q(F_{\theta_n})$, G_n be estimators of Q_X, G according to these working models. In Subsection 3.5.4 we provide direct ways of estimating Q_X which still yield doubly robust estimators α_n. In spite of the fact that Q_n, G_n are only consistent for the lower-dimensional working models $\mathcal{M}^{F,w}$ and $\mathcal{G}$, under reasonable conditions, the estimating equation

$$0 = \frac{1}{n} \sum_{i=1}^{n} IC(Y_i \mid Q_n, G_n, D_h(\cdot \mid \alpha))$$

in α with nuisance parameters (Q_X, G) replaced by the estimates (Q_n, G_n) provides CAN estimators α_n for this model $\mathcal{M}$. This is a consequence of the general double robustness property: if $\bar{G}_1(p \mid X) > 0$, F_X-a.e., then $E_{F_X, G} IC(Y \mid Q(F_1, G_1), G_1, D_h(\cdot \mid \alpha)) = 0$ if $F_1 = F_X$ or $G_1 = G$. This can also be explicitly verified in this case. Thus, if the model for G is correct, then the CAN property of α_n is protected against misspecification of Q_X, and if the model for Q_X is correct, then the CAN property of α_n is protected against misspecification of G and the nonparametric identifiability condition $\bar{G}(p \mid X) > 0$, F_X-a.e.

If both working models correctly specify Q_X and G, then the estimator α_n will be asymptotically linear with influence curve $IC(Y \mid Q_X, G, D_h(\cdot \mid \alpha))$. Our general representation theorem (Theorem 1.3) shows that there exists a choice $h = h_{opt}(F_X, G)$ for which this influence curve equals the efficient influence curve, but this optimal choice depends on the truth (F_X, G).

Our Theorem 2.11 in Chapter 2 actually provides a closed-form expression of this functional $(F_X, G) \to h_{opt}(F_X, G)$ for the case where the covariates in the regression model are time-independent. Thus, in order to obtain a locally efficient estimator, one needs to choose a data-dependent h_n. For example, if $F_{X,n}, G_n$ are estimates of F_X, G assuming the working models $\mathcal{M}^{F,w}$ and $\mathcal{G}$, then one can set $h_n = h_{opt}(F_{X,n}, G_n)$. □

1.3 Example: Causal Effect of Air Pollution on Short-Term Asthma Response

Consider a longitudinal study involving the follow-up of a population of children with asthma. Suppose that the purpose of the study is to estimate the short-term causal effect of air pollution on asthma symptoms. Let $Z(t)$ denote asthma symptoms on day t, $t = 1, \ldots, p$. Let $A_1(t)$ denote personally monitored air pollution exposure at day t. In addition, let $A_2(t)$ represent rescue medication use, such as steroid inhaler use, measured at day t. More generally, $A_2(t)$ can represent treatment variables that are on the causal pathway from air pollution to asthma or that interact with air pollution (e.g., humidity, temperature) and we wish to estimate a joint treatment effect. Let $A(t) = (A_1(t), A_2(t))$ denote the joint exposure/treatment variable. Thus, for each subject, we observe a realization (i.e., the data) of the vector $\bar{A} = (A(1), \ldots, A(p))$ of exposures and treatments, the vector $\bar{Z} = (Z(1), \ldots, Z(p))$ of outcomes, and a vector $\bar{L} = (L(1), \ldots, L(p))$ of time-dependent covariates. The order in which the variables occur is such that $(Z(j), L(j))$ occurs before $A(j)$ $j = 1, \ldots, p$.

Thus, the observed data structure is given by

$$Y = (\bar{A}, \bar{Z}, \bar{L}).$$

In order to define a causal effect, let $Z_{\bar{a}}(t)$ be the potential asthma symptom response curve that one would have observed if the subject, possibly contrary to the fact, were subject to air pollution-regime $\bar{a}_1 = (a_1(1), \ldots, a_1(p))$ and rescue medication regime $\bar{a}_2 = (a_2(1), \ldots, a_2(p))$, where we assume $Z_{\bar{a}}(t)$ only depends on $\bar{a}$ through $\bar{a}(t-1)$. Since this represents a random variable that one would observe in the world where we would be setting air pollution levels equal to $\bar{a}_1$ and medication-use levels at $\bar{a}_2$, one refers to these treatment-specific variables as potential outcomes or counterfactuals. We consider the general marginal structural repeated measures regression model (analogue to models considered in Robins, 1998b, 1999, Robins, Hernan and Brumback, 2000)

$$E(Z_{\bar{a}}(t) \mid V) = g_t(\bar{a}, V \mid \beta)$$

could be considered, where $g_t(\bar{a}, V \mid \beta)$ is some known regression curve (e.g., linear or logistic regression) indexed by the unknown k-dimensional

1.3. Example: Causal Effect of Air Pollution on Short-Term Asthma Response

vector β and V is the set of baseline covariates. For example, if we do not adjust for V we might choose

$$g_t(\bar{a} \mid \beta) = \beta_0 + \beta_1 a_1(1) + \beta_2(a_1(t-1) - a_1(1)) + \beta_3 a_2(1) + \beta_4(a_2(t-1) - a_2(1)),$$

where one might also include interaction terms if desired. Note that these models model the dependence of the counterfactual treatment-specific population mean of $Z(t)$ adjusted for V on the treatment regime. Thus β represents a causal effect of treatment. The goal is to estimate the causal parameter β based on the observed data $Y_1, \ldots, Y_n$. Note that $(Z(t), L(t))$ is a time-dependent confounder for later treatment in the sense that it predicts future treatment and response. Furthermore, it is affected by past treatment. Adjusting for variables affected by past treatment results in non interpretable regression parameters while adjustment for time-dependent confounders is needed to deal with the confounding. As a consequence, standard adjustment regression methods fail to estimate β consistently. In other words, causal inference methods as presented below are essential.

Let $\mathcal{A}$ be the set of possible sample paths of $\bar{A}$ (i.e., the support of the marginal distribution of $\bar{A}$), where we assume that $\mathcal{A}$ is finite. For each possible treatment regime $\bar{a}$, we define $X_{\bar{a}}(t) = (Z_{\bar{a}}(t), L_{\bar{a}}(t))$ as the data one would observe on the subject, if possibly contrary to the fact, the subject followed treatment regime $\bar{a}$. It is natural to assume $X_{\bar{a}}(t) = X_{\bar{a}(t-1)}(t)$ (i.e., the counterfactual outcome at time t is not affected by treatment given after time t). One refers to $X_{\bar{a}} = \{X_{\bar{a}}(t) : t = 1, \ldots, p\}$ as a counterfactual. The baseline covariates V are included in $L_{\bar{a}}(0) = L(0)$. The observed data can now be represented in terms of counterfactuals as follows:

$$Y = (\bar{A}, \bar{X}_{\bar{A}}) = (\bar{A}, \bar{Z}_{\bar{A}}, \bar{L}_{\bar{A}}).$$

Consequently, the observed data structure Y can be viewed as a missing data structure $Y = \Phi(\bar{A}, X) \equiv (\bar{A}, X_{\bar{A}})$ with full data structure $X = (X_{\bar{a}} : \bar{a} \in \mathcal{A})$. Therefore, as shown by Robins (1999), the general methodology provided in this book can be used to construct locally efficient estimators based on causal inference data structures.

The general methodology requires specifying a class of full data estimating functions for β. Marginal structural models assume a model for the marginal random variable $X_{\bar{a}}$ for *each* $\bar{a}$. Thus $\mathcal{M}^F = \cap_{\bar{a}} \mathcal{M}^F_{\bar{a}}$, where $\mathcal{M}^F_{\bar{a}}$ only assumes the restriction on the distribution of $X_{\bar{a}}$. For example, in the model above, we have $\mathcal{M}^F_{\bar{a}} = \{F_X : E(Z_{\bar{a}}(t) \mid V) = g_t(\bar{a}, V \mid \beta)\}$. Let $T^{F,\perp}_{nuis,\bar{a}}$ be the orthogonal complement of the nuisance tangent space in model $\mathcal{M}^F_{\bar{a}}$. In the previous examples, we found that

$$T^{F,\perp}_{nuis,\bar{a}} = \{h(V)\epsilon_{\bar{a}}(\beta) : h \text{ a } 1 \times p \text{ vector function}\},$$

where $\epsilon_{\bar{a}}(\beta)_{p \times 1} = (\epsilon_{\bar{a},t}(\beta)) : t = 1, \ldots, p)$ is the vector of treatment-specific residuals $Z_{\bar{a}} - g(\bar{a}, V \mid \beta)$. Since $T^F_{nuis} \subset \cap_a T^F_{nuis,a}$, where we typically can prove to also have equality, and the orthogonal complement of an intersection equals the sum of the orthogonal complements, it follows that $T_{nuis}^{F,\perp} \supset \{\sum_{\bar{a}} h(\bar{a},V)\epsilon_{\bar{a}}(\beta) : h\}$. Under appropriate conditions, equality can be proved as well. This yields the following class of full data estimating functions (Robins, 1999):

$$\left\{ D_h(X \mid \beta) = \sum_{\bar{a} \in \mathcal{A}} h(\bar{a},V)\epsilon_{\bar{a}}(\beta) : h \; k \times p \text{ matrix function} \right\}.$$

Let us now consider a model for the censoring/treatment mechanism. We assume that the conditional distribution of $\bar{A}$, given X, satisfies the sequential randomization assumption (SRA):

$$g(\bar{A} \mid X) = \prod_t g(A(t) \mid \bar{A}(t-), X) = \prod_t g(A(t) \mid \bar{A}(t-), \bar{X}_A(t)),$$

where we recall $\bar{X}_A(t) = \bar{X}(t)$. Typically, SRA is locally equivalent with CAR (Robins, 1999). In addition, we pose a model $\mathcal{G} = \{\prod_t g_\eta(A(t) \mid \bar{A}(t-), \bar{X}_A(t)) : \eta\} \subset \mathcal{G}(SRA)$ for $\prod_t g(A(t) \mid \bar{A}(t-), \bar{X}_A(t))$. The observed data likelihood for g is given by $\prod_j g(A(j) \mid \bar{A}(j), \bar{X}_A(j))$, which can be modeled by modeling the conditional distribution of $A(j)$, given the past, for each j separately, or one can use time j as a covariate and assume common parameters for each $g(A(j) \mid \bar{A}(j-), \bar{X}_A(j)), j = 1, \ldots, p$. If $A(j)$ is discrete, then a multinomial logistic regression model extracting covariates from the past is appropriate (Brookhart, and van der Laan, 2002a, provide an implementation and application of this model).

Let us now consider estimation of η in model $\mathcal{M}(\mathcal{G})$, which assumes a correctly specified model for the treatment mechanism. Estimation of the unknown parameter η can be carried out with the maximum likelihood procedure:

$$\eta_n = \max_\eta^{-1} \prod_{i=1}^n \prod_t g_\eta(A_i(t) \mid \bar{A}_i(t-), \bar{X}_{i,A_i}(t)).$$

Since $A(t) = (A_1(t), A_2(t))$ is multivariate, one can further factorize the multivariate probability $g(A(t) \mid \bar{A}(t-), \bar{X}_A(t))$ as $g(A(t) \mid \bar{A}(t-), \bar{X}_A(t)) = g(A_1(t) \mid A_2(t), \bar{A}(t-), \bar{X}_A(t)) g(A_2(t) \mid \bar{A}(t-), \bar{X}_A(t))$. It is now natural to model the different univariate conditional probabilities separately so that the corresponding maximum likelihood estimators also can be obtained separately.

We are now ready to derive a class of observed data estimating functions. To begin with, we define an inverse probability of treatment weighted (IPTW) mapping

$$IC_0(Y \mid G, D_h) = \frac{h(\bar{A}, V)\epsilon(\beta)}{g(\bar{A} \mid X)},$$

1.3. Example: Causal Effect of Air Pollution on Short-Term Asthma Response   51

where $\epsilon(\beta) = \epsilon_{\bar{A}}(\beta)$. By SRA, we have that $g(\bar{A} \mid X)$ is only a function of $Y = (\bar{A}, X_{\bar{A}})$ and thus that $D_h \to IC_0(Y \mid G, D_h)$ indeed maps a full data estimating function into an observed data estimating function. Note also that, if $\max_{\bar{a} \in \mathcal{A}} \frac{h(\bar{a}, V)}{g(\bar{a} \mid X)} < \infty$ F_X-a.e., then

$$E(IC_0(Y \mid G, D_h) \mid X) = \sum_{\bar{a} \in \mathcal{A}} h(\bar{a}, V) \epsilon_{\bar{a}}(\beta) = D_h(X) \; F_X\text{-a.e.}$$

This initial mapping provides a class of unbiased estimating equations for β with nuisance parameter G: Given an estimate of g, one can estimate β by solving

$$0 = \frac{1}{n} \sum_{i=1}^{n} \frac{h(\bar{A}_i, V_i) \epsilon_i(\beta)}{g_n(\bar{A}_i \mid X_i)}.$$

Following Robins (1999), we refer to such an estimator as an inverse probability of treatment weighted (IPTW) estimator.

It is of interest to also provide another type of IPTW estimator. Since h is a $k \times p$ matrix, let $h_1, \ldots, h_p$ be the p k-dimensional vectors spanning column 1 to p of this matrix. Note that

$$h(\bar{A}, V) \epsilon(\beta) = \sum_{j=1}^{p} h_j(\bar{A}, V) \epsilon_j(\beta).$$

Therefore, under the assumption that $h_j(\bar{A}, V)$ is only a function of $\bar{A}(j-1), \bar{V}(j)$, one can also define the IPTW mapping

$$IC_0(Y \mid G, D_h) = \sum_{j=1}^{p} \frac{h_j(\bar{A}(j-1), \bar{V}(j)) \epsilon_j(\beta)}{g(\bar{A}(j-1) \mid X)},$$

where $g(\bar{A}(j) \mid X) = \prod_{l=1}^{j} g(A(l) \mid \bar{A}(l-1), X)$. We believe that, in general, this type of time-dependent weighting yields estimators with better finite sample performance than using a common weight $1/g(\bar{A} \mid X)$ for each time point.

We will now propose a suitable choice for h. Let $g^*(A(j) \mid \bar{A}(j-), \bar{X}_A(j)) = g(A(j) \mid \bar{A}(j-), V)$ be the conditional distribution of $A(j)$, given $(\bar{A}(j-), V)$, and let $g^*(\bar{A} \mid X) = \prod_j g^*(A(j) \mid \bar{A}(j-), \bar{X}_A(j))$. If $g(\bar{A} \mid X) = g^*(\bar{A} \mid X)$, then the causal regression $g_t(\bar{A}, V \mid \beta) = E(Z_{\bar{A}}(t) \mid V, \bar{A}(t-1))$ reduces to a standard repeated regression of $Z(t)$ onto $\bar{A}(t-1), V$. Recall that in the standard repeated regression model the optimal estimating function for β is given by Lemma 2.1:

$$\frac{d}{d\beta} g(\bar{A}, V \mid \beta) E(\epsilon(\beta) \epsilon(\beta)^\top \mid \bar{A}, V)^{-1} \epsilon(\beta). \tag{1.37}$$

If we set

$$h^*_{opt}(\bar{A}, V) = g^*(\bar{A} \mid X) \frac{d}{d\beta} g(\bar{A}, V \mid \beta) E(\epsilon(\beta) \epsilon(\beta)^\top \mid \bar{A}, V)^{-1},$$

then $IC_0(Y \mid G, D_{h^*_{opt}})$ reduces to (1.37) in case the true treatment mechanism happens to be equal to g^*. Let h_n be an estimator of this locally optimal direction h^*_{opt}. With this choice h_n, if the treatment mechanism $g(\bar{A} \mid X)$ is modelled correctly, then the IPTW estimator β_n is (i) consistent and asymptotically normal (CAN), (ii) easy to compute and (iii) it is always more efficient than the usual generalized estimating equation (GEE) when $g(\bar{A} \mid X)$ only depends on X through V. However, it is of interest to note that if $g(\bar{A} \mid X)$ is modelled incorrectly, but, in truth only depends on X through V, then it is possible that the $IPTW$ estimator β_n is inconsistent while the usual GEE estimator is consistent. (Robins, 1999).

In order to obtain the optimal mapping $IC_0(D_h) - \Pi(IC_0(D_h) \mid T_{SRA})$ from full data estimating functions to observed data estimating functions, we need to determine $\Pi(IC_0(D_h) \mid T_{SRA})$, where T_{SRA} is the tangent space of the treatment mechanism under SRA. The following theorem, which generalizes Theorem 1.1, provides us with the desired result.

Theorem 1.2 *Let $A(t) = (A_1(t), A_2(t))$, and assume that the process A is discrete in the sense that it only jumps at time points $j = 1, \ldots, p$. For each possible realization $\bar{a} \in \mathcal{A}$ of $\bar{A}$, define the counterfactual random variable $X_{\bar{a}}$ and let the full data structure be the joint variable $X = (X_{\bar{a}} : \bar{a} \in \mathcal{A})$. We assume that $\bar{X}_{\bar{a}}(t) = \bar{X}_{\bar{a}(t-1)}(t)$. For the observed data, we have $Y = (\bar{A}, X_{\bar{A}})$. Let $X \sim F_X \in \mathcal{M}^F$, and assume the SRA assumption: that is, for all $j \in \{1, \ldots, p\}$,*

$$g(A(j) \mid \bar{A}(j-1), X) = g(A(j) \mid \bar{A}(j-1), \bar{X}_A(j)) \tag{1.38}$$

so that

$$\begin{aligned} g(\bar{A} \mid X) &= \prod_{j=1}^{p} g(A(j) \mid \bar{A}(j-1), X) \\ &= \prod_{j=1}^{p} g(A_1(j) \mid \mathcal{F}_1(j)) \prod_{j=1}^{p} g(A_2(j) \mid \mathcal{F}_2(j)), \end{aligned}$$

where $\mathcal{F}_1(j) = (A_2(j), \bar{A}(j-1), \bar{X}_A(j))$ and $\mathcal{F}_2(j) = (\bar{A}(j-1), \bar{X}_A(j))$. Let $T_{SRA}(P_{F_X,G})$ be the nuisance tangent space of G at $P_{F_X,G}$ under the sole assumption (1.38) on G. We have that

$$T_{SRA} = \sum_{k=1}^{2} \sum_{j=1}^{p} V(A_k(j), \mathcal{F}_k(j)) - E(V(A_k(j), \mathcal{F}_k(j)) \mid \mathcal{F}_k(j)).$$

In addition, we have for any function $V \in L_0^2(P_{F_X,G})$

$$\Pi(V \mid T_{SRA}) = \sum_{k=1}^{2} \sum_{j=1}^{p} \Pi(V \mid T_{SRA,k,j}),$$

1.3. Example: Causal Effect of Air Pollution on Short-Term Asthma Response

where $T_{SRA,k,j} = \{V(A_k(j), \mathcal{F}_k(j)) - E(V \mid \mathcal{F}_k(j)) : V\}$ and

$$\Pi(V \mid T_{SRA,k,j}) = E(V(Y) \mid A_k(j), \mathcal{F}_k(j)) - E(V(Y) \mid \mathcal{F}_k(j)).$$

If $A_k(j)$ is a 1-0 variable, then the latter equals

$$\{E(V(Y) \mid A_k(j) = 1, \mathcal{F}_k(j)) - E(V(Y) \mid A_k(j) = 0, \mathcal{F}_k(j))\} dM_k(j),$$

where $dM_k(j) \equiv A_k(j) - P(A_k(j) = 1 \mid \mathcal{F}_k(j))$.

Proof. By factorization of $g(\bar{A} \mid X)$ in the two products, we have that $T_{SRA} = T_{SRA,1} \oplus T_{SRA,2}$, where $T_{SRA,k}$ is the tangent space for the kth product, $k = 1, 2$. By the same argument, we have that $T_{SRA,k} = T_{SRA,k,1} \oplus \ldots \oplus T_{SRA,k,p}$, where $T_{SRA,k,j}$ is the tangent space for the jth component of the kth product in (1.39). Finally, we have that $T_{SRA,k,j}$ is the space of all functions of $(A_k(j), \mathcal{F}_k(j))$ that have conditional mean zero, given $\mathcal{F}_k(j)$; namely,

$$T_{SRA,k,j} = \{V(A_k(j), \mathcal{F}_k(j)) - E(V \mid \mathcal{F}_k(j)) : V\}.$$

This proves

$$T_{SRA} = \sum_{k=1}^{2} \sum_{j=1}^{p} V(A_k(j), \mathcal{F}_k(j)) - E(V \mid \mathcal{F}_k(j)).$$

and

$$\Pi(V \mid T_{SRA}) = \sum_{k=1}^{2} \sum_{j=1}^{p} \Pi(V \mid T_{SRA,k,j}).$$

It can be directly verified that indeed, for any $V \in L_0^2(P_{F_X,G})$,

$$\Pi(V \mid T_{SRA,k,j}) = E(V(Y) \mid A_k(j), \mathcal{F}_k(j)) - E(V(Y) \mid \mathcal{F}_k(j)). \square$$

We have

$$E(IC_0(Y) \mid \mathcal{F}_k(t)) = E(Q_k(A_k(t), \mathcal{F}_k(t)) \mid \mathcal{F}_k(t)),$$

where

$$Q_k(F_X, G)(A_k(t), \mathcal{F}_k(t)) \equiv E(IC_0(Y) \mid A_k(t), \mathcal{F}_k(t)), \ k = 1, 2.$$

Thus, the projection $\Pi(IC_0 \mid T_{SRA})$ can be represented as

$$IC_{SRA}(Y \mid Q_1, Q_2, G) \equiv \sum_{k=1}^{2} \sum_{t} Q_k(F_X, G)(A_k(t), \mathcal{F}_k(t))$$
$$- \sum_{k=1}^{2} \sum_{t} \sum_{\delta} Q_k(F_X, G)(\delta, \mathcal{F}_k(t)) P(A_k(t) = \delta \mid \mathcal{F}_k(t)).$$

Let $Q = (Q_1, Q_2)$ so that we can denote the proposed estimating function with $IC(Y \mid Q, G, D) = IC_0(Y \mid G, D) - IC_{SRA}(Y \mid Q, G, D)$. This estimating function satisfies the double protection property (1.36): if $D_h(\cdot \mid \mu(F_X), \rho(F_X, G_1)) \in \mathcal{D}(\rho_1(F_X), G_1)$ (i.e., it satisfies $E_{G_1}\{IC(Y \mid Q(F_X, G_1), G_1, D) \mid X\} = D(X)$ F_X-a.e.) and $dG/dG_1 < \infty$, then

$$E_{F_X, G} IC(Y \mid Q(F_1, G_1), G_1, D_h(\cdot \mid \mu(F_X), \rho(F_X, G_1))) = 0$$

if $F_1 = F_X$ or $G_1 = G$.

Given a choice h for the full data estimating function, estimates G_n, Q_n, ρ_n, we would estimate μ by solving

$$0 = \sum_{i=1}^{n} IC(Y_i \mid Q_n, G_n, D_h(\cdot \mid \mu, \rho_n)). \tag{1.39}$$

To fully exploit the protection property against misspecification of G, one would have to estimate $\rho(F_X, G)$ and Q with substitution estimators $\rho(F_n, G_n)$, and $Q_n = Q(F_n, G_n)$, which truly estimate the F_X and G components separately. Such a substitution estimators are provided in Section 1.5 in this chapter and Subsection 6.4.1 in Chapter 6. In the next paragraph, we describe simple methods for estimation of Q that do not separate out the F_X and G components, so that the consistency of μ_n now relies on correct estimation of G.

We can estimate the conditional expectations $E(IC_0(Y) \mid A_k(t) = \delta, \mathcal{F}_k(t))$ (semi) parametrically by regressing an estimate of $IC_0(Y)$ onto t and covariates extracted from the past $(\bar{A}_k(t), \mathcal{F}_k(t))$. For example, we can assume a multivariate generalized linear regression model

$$E(IC_0(Y) \mid A_k(t), \mathcal{F}_k(t)) = m_t(A_k(t), \mathcal{F}_k(t) \mid \alpha)$$

and follow the estimating function methods described in example 1.1. Here, each subject contributes multiple observations $(t, A_k(t), \mathcal{F}_k(t))$, $t = 1, \ldots, p$. Since the first order asymptotics of μ_n is not affected by the efficiency of α_n, one can assume a diagonal covariance matrix and thus simply estimate α by applying a least squares procedure to the pooled sample treating all observations as i.i.d.

Another method would be to regress for each t an estimate of $IC_0(Y)$ onto covariates extracted from $\mathcal{F}_k(t)$ among observations with $A_k(t) = \delta$ as δ varies over the support of $A_k(t)$, and subsequently smooth all of these t-specific regression estimates over t, taking into account the variance of each of these t-specific regression estimates (e.g., by weighting them by 1 over the number of observations used to fit the regression).

In Bryan, Yu and van der Laan (2002) the one-step estimator for solving (1.39) has been implemented for a particular marginal structural logistic regression model defining the causal effect of treatment on time untill death and is used to analyze the causal effect of physical activity on survival in an elderly population. The simulation study in this paper shows that this estimator can be much more efficient (relative efficiencies equal to 4) than the inverse probability of treatment weighted estimator. We discuss this simulation in Chapter 6.

For another application of marginal structural models, we refer the reader to Hernan, Brumback and Robins (2000).

1.4 Estimating Functions

In this section, we will more completely and formally define the orthogonal complement of the nuisance tangent space and review efficiency theory. Subsequently, we link this orthogonal complement of the nuisance tangent space to the construction of estimating functions that are elements of this space when evaluated at the true parameter values and show that the expectation of such estimating functions has a derivative zero w.r.t. to fluctuations of a locally variation-independent nuisance parameter ρ. To avoid additional notation, in our presentation one can consider X as a generic random variable, rather than only as the variable representing the full data. Thus our results can be applied to both full data and observed data models.

1.4.1 Orthogonal complement of a nuisance tangent space

Consider a full data structure model $\mathcal{M}^F$ for the full data distribution F_X. Given F_X, for each g ranging over an index set, let $\epsilon \to F_{\epsilon,g}$ be a one-dimensional submodel of $\mathcal{M}^F$ with parameter $\epsilon \in (-\delta, \delta)$, for some small $\delta > 0$ (δ can depend on g), crossing $F_X = F_{0,g}$ at $\epsilon = 0$, and score $s(X) \in L_0^2(F_X)$, where $L_0^2(F_X)$ is the Hilbert space of functions of X with expectation zero and finite variance endowed with inner product $\langle h_1, h_2 \rangle_{F_X} = \int h_1(x) h_2(x) dF_X(x)$. Here, for simplicity, we define the score s as an $L_0^2(F_X)$ limit :

$$\lim_{\epsilon \to 0} \int \left\{ s(x) - \frac{1}{\epsilon} \frac{dF_{\epsilon,g} - dF_X}{dF_X}(x) \right\}^2 dF_X(x) = 0.$$

One can also define the score pointwise as

$$s(X) = s(g)(X) = \frac{d}{d\epsilon} \log \left(\frac{dF_{\epsilon,g}}{dF_X}(X) \right) \bigg|_{\epsilon=0} \in L_0^2(F_X).$$

For a definition in terms of square roots of densities, we refer to Bickel, Klaassen, Ritov, and Wellner (1993). A typical choice of submodel is of the form $dF_{\epsilon,g}(x) = (1 + \epsilon g(x)) dF_X(x) + o(\epsilon)$ so that $s(g) = g$. Let $\mathcal{S} \subset L_0^2(F_X)$ be the set of scores corresponding with the class $\{F_{\cdot,g} : g\}$ of one-dimensional submodels. Let $T^F(F_X) \subset L_0^2(F_X)$ be the closure of the linear space spanned by $\mathcal{S}$. We refer to this Hilbert space $T^F(F_X)$ as the tangent space of the full data model. It is crucial that one chooses a rich class $\{F_{\cdot,g} : g\}$ of models that locally cover all possible score directions that the model $\mathcal{M}^F$ allows.

Example 1.18 For example, let $\mathcal{M} = \{f_{\mu,\sigma^2} : \mu, \sigma^2\}$ be the family of normal distributions. For each (δ_1, δ_2) we can define a one-dimensional submodel $\{f_{\mu+\epsilon\delta_1, \sigma^2+\epsilon\delta_2} : \epsilon\}$ that has score $\delta_1 S_1(X \mid \mu, \sigma^2) + \delta_2 S_2(X \mid \mu, \sigma^2)$, where S_1, S_2 are the scores for μ (i.e., $d/d\mu \log(f_{\mu,\sigma^2}(X))$) and σ^2, respectively. Thus, the tangent space is the two-dimensional space $\langle S_1, S_2 \rangle$ spanned by these two scores. □

Nuisance tangent space. Let $\mu = \mu(F_X) \in \mathbb{R}^k$ be a Euclidean parameter of interest. We will now define the so-called nuisance tangent space. Since only the score of $F_{\epsilon,g}$ is relevant for the definition of tangent spaces and the efficiency bound, from now on we will index the one-dimensional submodels by their score s, thereby making clear that two different one-dimensional submodels with the same score are only counted as one. In a full data model $\mathcal{M}^F = \{F_{\mu,\eta} : \mu, \eta\}$ with μ and η independently varying parameters over certain parameter spaces, one can directly determine the nuisance tangent space $T^F_{nuis}(F_X)$ as the space generated by all scores of one-dimensional submodels F_{μ,η_ϵ} just varying the nuisance parameter. In general, we define the nuisance tangent space as follows.

Definition 1.1 *Suppose that for each submodel $\{F_{\epsilon,s} : \epsilon\}$ with score s, $s \in \mathcal{S}$, $d/d\epsilon \mu(F_{\epsilon,s})|_{\epsilon=0}$ exists. The nuisance scores are given by the scores of the models $F_{\epsilon,s}$ for which μ does not locally vary:*

$$\left\{ s \in \mathcal{S} : \frac{d}{d\epsilon} \mu(F_{\epsilon,s})|_{\epsilon=0} = 0 \right\}.$$

The nuisance tangent space $T_{nuis}(F_X)$ is now the closure (in $L_0^2(F_X)$) of the linear space generated by these nuisance scores:

$$T^F_{nuis}(F_X) \equiv \overline{\left\{ s \in \mathcal{S} : \frac{d}{d\epsilon} \mu(F_{\epsilon,s})|_{\epsilon=0} = 0 \right\}}.$$

Example 1.19 Suppose that $X \sim F_X$ is a univariate real-valued variable and that the model for F_X is nonparametric. Then, we can choose as the class of one-dimensional submodels $dF_{\epsilon,s}(x) = (1 + \epsilon s(x))dF_X(x)$ with $s \in \mathcal{S} = \{s \in L_0^2(F_X) : s \text{ uniformly bounded}\}$. It follows immediately that the tangent space is saturated: $T^F(F_X) = L_0^2(F_X)$.

Suppose that for a given t_0, $\mu = F(t_0)$ is the parameter of interest. We have

$$\mu(F_{\epsilon,s}) - \mu = \epsilon \int \{I_{(0,t_0]}(x) - \mu\} s(x) dF_X(x).$$

This shows that

$$T^F_{nuis}(F_X) = \{s \in L_0^2(F_X) : \langle s, D_{eff} \rangle_{F_X} = 0\},$$

where $D_{eff}(x) \equiv I_{(0,t_0]}(x) - \mu \in L_0^2(F_X)$. □

Pathwise derivative and gradients. Throughout this book, it is assumed that $\mu \in \mathbb{R}^k$ is pathwise differentiable along each of the one-dimensional submodels in the sense that for each $s \in \mathcal{S}$

$$\lim_{\epsilon \to 0} \frac{1}{\epsilon}(\mu(F_{\epsilon,s}) - \mu(F_X)) = \langle \ell(\cdot \mid F_X), s \rangle_{F_X}$$

for an element $\ell(\cdot \mid F_X) \in L_0^2(F_X)^k$. Note that the right-hand side is a k-dimensional vector. For a k-dimensional function $\ell \in L_0^2(F_X)^k$ and $s \in L_0^2(F_X)$, we define the vector inner product $\langle \ell, s \rangle_{F_X}$ as the vector with jth component $\langle \ell_j, s \rangle_{F_X}$. Similarly, we will define a projection $\Pi(s \mid T^F(F_X))$ of a k-dimensional function $s = (s_1, \ldots, s_k)$ onto a subspace (say) $T^F(F_X)$ of $L_0^2(F_X)$ componentwise as $\Pi(s_j \mid T^F(F_X))_{j=1}^k$. Any such element $\ell(\cdot \mid F_X) \in L_0^2(F_X)^k$ is called a gradient of the pathwise derivative, and the unique gradient $S_{eff}^{*F}(\cdot \mid F_X) \in T^F(F_X)^k$ (i.e., the gradient whose components are elements of the full data tangent space) is called the canonical gradient or efficient influence curve. Notice that $S_{eff,j}^* = \Pi(\ell_j \mid T^F(F_X))$ is the $T^F(F_X)$-component of any gradient component ℓ_j (i.e., the pathwise derivative w.r.t. a class of submodels with tangent space $T^F(F_X)$ only uniquely determines the $T^F(F_X)$-component of the gradient-components of the pathwise derivative). Thus, the set of all gradients is given by

$$\{\ell \in L_0^2(F_X)^k : \langle \ell_j, s \rangle_{F_X} = \langle S_{eff,j}^{F*}(X \mid F_X), s \rangle_{F_X}, s \in T^F(F_X), \forall j\}, \tag{1.40}$$

where $j \in \{1, \ldots, k\}$. Note that if the full data model is nonparametric, then $T^F(F_X) = L_0^2(F_X)$, so $T_{nuis}^{F,\perp}(F_X) = \langle S_{eff}^{*F}(\cdot \mid F_X) \rangle$ is the k-dimensional space spanned by the components of the canonical gradient and the only gradient is the canonical gradient $S_{eff}^{*F}(\cdot \mid F_X)$. Note that for a vector function $a \in L_0^2(F_X)^k$, we define $<a> = \{c^\top a = c_1 a_1(\cdot) + \ldots + c_k a_k(\cdot) : c \in \mathbb{R}^k\} \subset L_0^2(F_X)$ as the k-dimensional space spanned by the components of a. In general, the larger the model, the smaller the set of gradients.

Nuisance tangent space in terms of the canonical gradient. Under the pathwise differentiability condition, the nuisance tangent space is given by

$$T_{nuis}^F(F_X) = \{s \in T^F(F_X) : s \perp S_{eff}^{*F}(\cdot \mid F_X)\}$$

and the tangent space equals

$$T^F(F_X) = < S_{eff}^{*F}(\cdot \mid F_X) > \oplus T_{nuis}^F(F_X). \tag{1.41}$$

Let $T_{nuis}^{F,\perp}(F_X)$ be the orthogonal complement of the nuisance tangent space $T_{nuis}^F(F_X)$ in the Hilbert space $L_0^2(F_X)$. Let $\Pi(\cdot \mid T_{nuis}^F(F_X))$ be the projection operator onto the nuisance tangent space. We have $\Pi(s \mid T_{nuis}^{F,\perp}(F_X)) =$

58   1. Introduction

$s - \Pi(s \mid T^F_{nuis}(F_X))$ and

$$T^{F,\perp}_{nuis} = \{s(X) - \pi(s \mid T^F_{nuis}) : s \in L^2_0(F_X)\}.$$

Alternatively, if $\Pi_{F_X} : L^2_0(F_X) \to T^F(F_X)$ is the projection operator onto $T^F(F_X)$, then it also follows that

$$T^{F,\perp}_{nuis}(F_X) = \{D \in L^2_0(F_X) : \Pi_{F_X}(D \mid T^F(F_X)) \in <S^{*F}_{eff}(\cdot \mid F_X)>\}. \tag{1.42}$$

Example 1.20 Let us continue Example 1.19. Notice that μ is indeed pathwise differentiable with canonical gradient $S^{*F}_{eff}(X) = I_{(0,t_0]}(X) - \mu$. The orthogonal complement of the nuisance tangent space is thus $\langle I_{(0,t_0]}(X) - \mu \rangle$. □

Equivalence between gradients and orthogonal complement of nuisance tangent space. By (1.40), another characterization of a gradient is that each of its components is an element of $T^{F,\perp}_{nuis}$ whose projection onto $T^F(F_X) = T^F_{nuis} \oplus \langle S^{*F}_{eff} \rangle$ equals the corresponding component of S^{*F}_{eff}. Thus, gradients are orthogonal to T^F_{nuis} and need to be appropriately standardized. Since the projection of $D \in L^2_0(F_X)$ onto $\langle S^{*F}_{eff} \rangle$ is given by

$$\Pi(D \mid \langle S^{*F}_{eff} \rangle) = E(DS^{F*\top}_{eff}) E(S^{*F}_{eff} S^{F*\top}_{eff})^{-1} S^{*F}_{eff},$$

it follows that the set of gradients $T^{F,\perp,*}_{nuis}(F_X)$ is given by the following standardized versions of $T^{F,\perp}_{nuis}$:

$$\left\{ E(S^{*F}_{eff}(X) S^{F*\top}_{eff}(X)) \left\{ E(D(X) S^{F*\top}_{eff}(X \mid F_X)) \right\}^{-1} D : D \in T^{F,\perp}_{nuis}(F_X)^k \right\}.$$

This shows that the space spanned by the components of all of the gradients (1.40) equals the orthogonal complement $T^{F,\perp}_{nuis}$ of the nuisance tangent space.

If $D(X)$ plays the role of an estimating function, then the standardization matrix in front of D actually reduces to the much simpler derivative standardization provided in (1.22), as we will now show.

Lemma 1.2 *Suppose that there exists a mapping (i.e., estimating function)* $(h, \mu, \rho) \to D_h(\cdot \mid \mu, \rho)$ *on* $\mathcal{H}^F \times \{(\mu(F_X), \rho(F_X)) : F_X \in \mathcal{M}^F\}$ *into functions of X such that one can represent*

$$T^{F,\perp}_{nuis}(F_X) = \{D_h(\cdot \mid \mu(F_X), \rho(F_X)) : h \in \mathcal{H}^F(F_X)\} \tag{1.43}$$

as the range of an index set $\mathcal{H}^F(F_X) \subset \mathcal{H}^F$ *of* $(h \to D_h(\cdot \mid \mu(F_X), \rho(F_X))$ *for all $F_X \in \mathcal{M}^F$. In addition, assume that for all $h \in \mathcal{H}(F_X)$ and each one-dimensional submodel $F_{\epsilon,s}$, $s \in \mathcal{S}$, we have for $\epsilon \to 0$ $\| D_h(\cdot \mid \mu(F_{\epsilon,s}), \rho(F_{\epsilon,s})) - D_h(\cdot \mid \mu(F_X), \rho(F_X)) \|_{F_X} \to 0$. Assume that μ is a pathwise differentiable parameter at F_X with canonical gradient $S^{*F}_{eff}(\cdot \mid F_X)$ with $\langle S^{*F}_{eff} \rangle \subset \mathcal{S}$.*

1.4. Estimating Functions

Let

$$f_h(s) \equiv \frac{d}{d\epsilon} E_{F_X} D_h(X \mid \mu(F_{\epsilon,s}), \rho(F_{\epsilon,s}))\bigg|_{\epsilon=0}.$$

We have that an element $D = D_h(\cdot \mid \mu(F_X), \rho(F_X)) \in T_{nuis}^{F,\perp}(F_X)^k$ for $h \in \mathcal{H}(F_X)^k$ is a gradient if and only if

$$f_h(s) = \begin{cases} 0 & \text{if } s \text{ is nuisance score} \\ -d/d\epsilon\mu(F_{\epsilon,s})|_{\epsilon=0} & \text{if } s \in \langle S_{eff}^{*F} \rangle \end{cases}.$$

Proof. Firstly, by assumption,

$$\frac{1}{\epsilon} E_{F_X} \{D_h(X \mid \mu(F_{\epsilon,s}), \rho(F_{\epsilon,h})) - D_h(X \mid \mu(F_X), \rho(F_X))\} =$$

$$\int D_h(x \mid \mu(F_{\epsilon,s}), \rho(F_{\epsilon,s})) \frac{1}{\epsilon} \frac{dF_X - dF_{\epsilon,s}}{dF_X}(x) dF_X(x)$$

$$\to -\langle D_h(\cdot \mid \mu(F_X), \rho(F_X)), s \rangle_{F_X} \text{ if } \epsilon \to 0.$$

By definition, D_h is a gradient if and only if for each $s \in T_{nuis}^F(F_X)$ the latter inner product equals zero and for $s \in \langle S_{eff}^{*F} \rangle$ the latter inner product equals $- d/d\epsilon\mu(F_\epsilon)|_{\epsilon=0}$, which proves the lemma. □

Under further smoothness (in μ, ρ) conditions on $(\mu, \rho) \to D_h(\cdot \mid \mu, \rho)$ and under the assumption that μ, ρ are variation-independent parameters, one can now typically show that $D_h(\cdot \mid \mu(F_X), \rho(F_X))$ is a gradient if and only if the Gateaux derivative $ED_g(X \mid \mu(F_X), \rho)$ w.r.t. the nuisance parameter ρ at $\rho = \rho(F_X)$ (in every direction allowed by the model) equals zero and the derivative of $D_h(X \mid \mu, \rho(F_X))$ w.r.t. μ at $\mu(F_X)$ equals minus the identity matrix:

$$\frac{d}{d\mu} E_{F_X} D(X \mid \mu, \rho) = -I, \tag{1.44}$$

$$\frac{d}{d\rho} E_{F_X} D(X \mid \mu, \rho) = 0. \tag{1.45}$$

Formally, we have the following lemma.

Lemma 1.3 *Make the same assumptions as in the previous lemma. Assume that μ and ρ are locally variation independent parameters of F_X. Assume that for all $h \in \mathcal{H}^F(F_X)^k$, $\mu \to E_{F_X} D_h(\cdot \mid \mu, \rho(F_X))$ is differentiable at $\mu(F_X)$ with an invertible derivative matrix. Assume that $E(S_{eff}^{*F}(X) S_{eff}^{*F\top}(X))$ is invertible. If for $h \in \mathcal{H}(F_X)^k$, $D_h(X \mid \mu(F_X, \rho(F_X)) \in T_{nuis}^{F,\perp*}(F_X)$, then*

$$d/d\mu E_{F_X} D_h(X \mid \mu, \rho(F_X)) = -I,$$

where I denotes the $k \times k$ identity matrix. As a consequence, $T_{nuis}^{F,\perp,*}(F_X)$ is given by

$$\left\{-\left\{\frac{d}{d\mu}E_{F_X}D_h(X \mid \mu, \rho(F_X))\right\}\bigg|_{\mu=\mu(F_X)}\right\}^{-1}D_h : h \in \mathcal{H}^F(F_X)\right\}^k. \tag{1.46}$$

Proof. Let $s \in \langle S_{eff}^{*F}\rangle$. Note that $\epsilon \to E_{F_X}D(X \mid \mu(F_{\epsilon,s}), \rho(F_X))$ is a composition $h_1(h_2(\epsilon))$ with $h_2(\epsilon \mid s) = \mu(F_{\epsilon,s})$ and $h_1(\mu) = E_{F_X}D(X \mid \mu, \rho(F_X))$. As in the proof of the previous lemma, we show that

$$d/d\epsilon h_1(h_2(\epsilon))|_{\epsilon=0} = -d/d\epsilon \mu(F_{\epsilon,s})|_{\epsilon=0},$$

where the right-hand side actually equals $-h_2'(0 \mid s)$. By the chain rule, we have that the left-hand side equals $d/d\mu h_1(\mu) * h_2'(0 \mid s)$. Thus, $d/d\mu h_1(\mu) * h_2'(0 \mid s) = h_2'(0 \mid s)$ for all $s \in \langle S_{eff}^{F,*}\rangle$. We now need $h_2'(0 \mid s = S_{eff,j}^{F*})$, $j = 1, \ldots, k$, to be independent vectors. However, the latter vectors are given by $E(S_{eff}^{*F}S_{eff}^{F*j})$, $j = 1, \ldots, k$, so that this independence is a consequence of the assumed invertibility of $E(S_{eff}^{*F}(X)S_{eff}^{F*\top}(X))$. This proves that $d/d\mu h_1(\mu) = -I$. □

Example 1.21 (Parametric model) Consider a parametric model $X \sim f_{\theta,\eta}$, where $\mu = \theta \in \mathbb{R}^k$ is the parameter of interest and $\eta \in \mathbb{R}^m$ is the nuisance parameter. As the class of one-dimensional models, we choose the $k+m$ models just varying one of the parameters: let $a = (\theta, \eta)$. For every $\delta \in \mathbb{R}^{k+m}$, we let $\{f_{a+\epsilon\delta} : \epsilon\}$ be a one-dimensional submodel. The tangent space generated by these one-dimensional models is the $k+m$-dimensional subspace of $L_0^2(F_X)$ spanned by the score components of $h = (h_1, \ldots, h_k)$ of θ and $g = (g_1, \ldots, g_m)$ of η. We can find the orthogonal complement of the nuisance tangent space in two ways. Since the density of X is parametrized naturally with μ and nuisance parameter η, we can calculate the nuisance space directly: $T_{nuis}(F_X) = \langle g_1, \ldots, g_m\rangle$. Since $\Pi(\cdot \mid T_{nuis}(F_X)) : L_0^2(F_X) \to T_{nuis}(F_X)$ is given by

$$\Pi(D \mid T_{nuis}(F_X)) = E(D(X)g(X)^\top)E(g(X)g(X)^\top)^{-1}g(X),$$

we have that the orthogonal complement of the nuisance tangent space is given by

$$T_{nuis}^\perp(F_X) = \{D(X) - E(D(X)g(X)^\top)E(g(X)g(X)^\top)^{-1}g(X) : D \in L_0^2(F_X)\}.$$

Moreover, the efficient score $S_{eff}(X)$ for μ is given by

$$\Pi(h_j \mid T_{nuis}^\perp(F_X))_{j=1}^k = h(X) - E(h(X)g(X)^\top)E(g(X)g(X)^\top)^{-1}g(X), \tag{1.47}$$

and the efficient influence curve/canonical gradient is given by the standardized version of the efficient score:

$$S_{eff}^*(X) = E(S_{eff}S_{eff}^\top(X))^{-1}S_{eff}(X).$$

Let us now find $T_{nuis}^\perp$ and the canonical gradient S_{eff}^* in terms of the pathwise derivative. We have

$$\frac{d}{d\epsilon}\mu(f_{a+\epsilon\delta})\bigg|_{\epsilon=0} = (\delta_1,\ldots,\delta_k)^\top,$$

while the score of $f_{a+\epsilon\delta}$ at $\epsilon = 0$ equals the linear combination $\delta^\top(h,g)^\top$ of the scores and nuisance scores with coefficients given by δ. Thus, the gradients are all functions $\ell \in L_0^2(F_X)^k$ that satisfy

$$(\delta_1,\ldots,\delta_k)^\top = \langle \ell, \delta^\top(h,g)^\top \rangle_{F_X}.$$

To begin with, it follows that $\ell \perp \langle g \rangle$ is orthogonal to the nuisance scores $g_1,\ldots,g_m$. The canonical gradient is the only gradient (and thus orthogonal to $g_1,\ldots,g_m$), which is also an element of the tangent space. It follows that the canonical gradient equals S_{eff}^* defined above. □

1.4.2 Review of efficiency theory

The orthogonal complement of the nuisance tangent space forms the basis of the general estimating function approach presented in this book. It is also a space that is fundamental to efficiency theory. We will now review some of these fundamental results (Bickel, Klaassen, Ritov, and Wellner, 1993). Firstly, we need to recall that an estimator μ_n of μ is called regular relative to the given class of one-dimensional submodels $\{\{F_{\epsilon,s} : \epsilon\} : s \in \mathcal{S}\}$ if for $\epsilon = 1/\sqrt{n}$ the distribution of $\sqrt{n}(\mu_n - \mu(F_{\epsilon,s}))$, under $X_i \sim F_{\epsilon,s}$, $i = 1,\ldots,n$, converges to a limit distribution Z that does not depend on s. Consider now a regular estimator relative to the class of one-dimensional submodels $\{F_{\epsilon,s} : s \in \mathcal{S}\}$ and assume that it is asymptotically linear at F_X with influence curve $IC(X \mid F_X, \mu)$:

$$\mu_n - \mu = \frac{1}{n}\sum_{i=1}^n IC(X_i \mid F_X, \mu) + o_P(1/\sqrt{n}).$$

Then

$$IC(X \mid F_X, \mu) \in T_{nuis}^{F,\perp,*}(F_X);$$

that is, the influence curve of a regular asymptotically linear estimator is a gradient. This shows that the orthogonal complement of the nuisance tangent space identifies asymptotically all regular asymptotically linear estimators of μ in the full data model $\mathcal{M}^F$. More important to us, as heavily exploited in this book, the orthogonal complement of the nuisance tangent space $T_{nuis}^\perp(F_X)$ can be used to define a class of estimating functions defining all estimators of interest.

The canonical gradient $S_{eff}^{*F}(X \mid F_X)$ is of great importance since the asymptotic variance of a regular asymptotically linear estimator of μ at F_X is bounded below by the variance of the canonical gradient, and a

62   1. Introduction

regular estimator is efficient at F_X if and only if it is asymptotically linear with influence curve equal to the canonical gradient (i.e., efficient influence curve) at F_X. The fact that the variance of the efficient influence curve provides a lower bound for the asymptotic variance of any RAL estimator can be understood as follows. For simplicity, consider the situation where μ is univariate. Consider the one-dimensional model $\{F_{\epsilon,s} : \epsilon\}$ with parameter ϵ, and note that the true parameter value is $\epsilon_0 = 0$. Note also that the score for ϵ at ϵ_0 equals $s(X)$. The parameter of interest in this model is the following function of ϵ: $\phi(\epsilon) \equiv \mu(F_{\epsilon,s})$. The Cramer–Rao lower bound for the variance of an unbiased estimator of $\phi(\epsilon) \in \mathbb{R}$ at $\epsilon = \epsilon_0 = 0$ equals

$$\frac{\left(\frac{d}{d\epsilon}\phi(\epsilon)\big|_{\epsilon=0}\right)^2}{E_{F_X} s^2(X)} = \frac{\langle S_{eff}^{*F}, s\rangle_{F_X}}{\langle s, s\rangle_{F_X}}, \qquad (1.48)$$

because $\phi'(0) = d/d\epsilon \mu(F_{\epsilon,s})|_{\epsilon=0}$. Because regularity is the asymptotic version of uniform unbiasedness, any regular asymptotically linear estimator for the model $\mathcal{M}$ should have an influence curve with variance larger than the Cramer–Rao lower bound (1.48) for the one-dimensional submodel $F_{\epsilon,s}$. This is true for every possible one-dimensional submodel. As a consequence, any regular asymptotically linear estimator for the model $\mathcal{M}^F$ should have an influence curve with variance larger than the supremum over all $s \in T^F(F_X)$ of the one-dimensional Cramer–Rao lower bounds (1.48) for the one-dimensional submodel $F_{\epsilon,s}$. By the Cauchy–Schwarz inequality, it follows immediately that this supremum is attained at $s = S_{eff}^{*F}$ with maximum $ES_{eff}^{*F}(X)^2$. This maximum is called the generalized Cramer–Rao lower bound.

Thus, one can view $S_{eff,j}^{F*}$ as the score (index) of the one-dimensional submodel that makes estimation of $\mu_j(F_X)$, $j = 1, \ldots, k$, most difficult, and its variance equals the generalized Cramer–Rao lower bound. An estimator that achieves this bound must be efficient. In addition, the canonical gradients of μ at $F_X \in \mathcal{M}^F$ can be used as the basis for an optimal estimating function.

1.4.3 *Estimating functions.*

Consider a class of k-dimensional estimating functions $\{D_h(X \mid \mu, \rho) : h \in \mathcal{H}^{F^k}\}$ indexed by an index h ranging over a set $\mathcal{H}^{F^k}$. An estimating function $D_h : \mathcal{X} \times \{\mu(F_X), \rho(F_X) : F_X \in \mathcal{M}^F\}$ is a function of X, the parameter of interest μ, and possibly a nuisance parameter $\rho = \rho(F_X)$. An estimating function is (uniformly) unbiased if

$$E_{F_X} D_h(X \mid \mu(F_X), \rho(F_X)) = 0 \text{ for all } F_X \in \mathcal{M}^F.$$

Suppose now that the estimating functions are an element of the orthogonal complement of the nuisance tangent space in the sense that for all $h \in \mathcal{H}^F$

$$D_h(\cdot \mid \mu(F_X), \rho(F_X)) \in T_{nuis}^{F\perp}(F_X) \text{ at all } F_X \in \mathcal{M}^F. \qquad (1.49)$$

1.4. Estimating Functions

We showed in Lemma 1.2 that, if ρ and μ are locally variation-independent parameters, then for any one-dimensional model $F_{\epsilon,s}$, $s \in T^F_{nuis}(F_X)$ (i.e., a one-dimensional model only fluctuating the nuisance parameter so that $\mu(F_{\epsilon,s}) - \mu(F_X) = o(\epsilon)$) we have

$$\frac{d}{d\epsilon} E_{F_X} D_h(X \mid \mu(F_X), \rho(F_{\epsilon,s})) \bigg|_{\epsilon=0} = 0. \qquad (1.50)$$

This is a very nice property of an orthogonal estimating function since it shows that it either does not involve a nuisance parameter ρ or the derivative of the mean of the estimating function w.r.t. ρ (fixing μ) is zero. Consequently, under regularity conditions, for estimator ρ_n that converges to ρ sufficiently quickly, the solution μ_n of the corresponding estimating equation

$$0 = \sum_{i=1}^{n} D_h(X_i \mid \mu, \rho_n)$$

will be asymptotically linear with influence curve

$$IC(X) = -\left\{ \frac{d}{d\mu} E_{F_X} D_h(X \mid \mu, \rho(F_X)) \bigg|_{\mu=\mu(F_X)} \right\}^{-1} D_h(X \mid \mu(F_X), \rho(F_X)). \qquad (1.51)$$

In other words, it will have the same influence curve as in the case where $\rho_n = \rho(F_X)$ is known. This makes statistical inference straightforward, given that we already have the estimating function. Notice that by (1.46) the influence curve $IC(X)$ is indeed a gradient. Finding a class of estimating functions satisfying (1.49) requires computing $T^{F,\perp}_{nuis}(F_X)$ at all $F_X \in \mathcal{M}^F$.

Note that the definition of the orthogonal complement of the nuisance tangent space depends on the class of submodels one specifies. If one chooses the class of one-dimensional submodels allowed by the model too small in the sense that we are excluding certain scores, then the orthogonal complement of the nuisance tangent space will not be truly orthogonal to all directions that the model allows. As a consequence, the corresponding estimating functions will not be orthogonal to all nuisance parameters in the sense that (1.50) is unequal to zero along certain one-dimensional submodels that were excluded from the original class of submodels. There is nothing wrong with using such a class of estimating functions. However, in that case one will not have the influence curve of the corresponding estimators equal the standardized estimating function (1.51).

Example 1.22 Consider the previous example and let us choose too small a class of one-dimensional submodels $F_{\epsilon,h}$ by also requiring that the score h satisfy $\langle h, f - E_{F_X} f(X) \rangle_{F_X} = 0$ for a given function f. The nuisance tangent space equals $\{h \in L^2_0(F_X) : h \perp \langle D^*, f - E_{F_X} f \rangle\}$ so that the orthogonal complement of the nuisance tangent space equals all linear combinations of D^* and $f - E_{F_X} f(X)$. Notice that the estimating function $D(X \mid \mu, \rho) \equiv$

$D^*(X \mid \mu) + f(X) - \rho$ has a nuisance parameter $\rho(F_X) \equiv E_{F_X} f(X)$, and indeed its expected derivative w.r.t. ρ now is not zero: (1.50) now fails. In fact, the solution of the estimating equation $\sum_{i=1}^n D(X_i \mid \mu, \rho_n)$ with $\rho_n = \frac{1}{n} \sum_{i=1}^n f(X_i)$ (the nonparametric estimator of the nuisance parameter) equals the empirical cumulative distribution function at t_0 that solves $0 = \sum_{i=1}^n D^*(X_i \mid \mu)$. □

1.4.4 Orthogonal complement of a nuisance tangent space in an observed data model

Consider the following class of parametric submodels through $G_{Y\mid X}$:

$$\{(1 + \epsilon V(y))dG(y\mid x) : V \in L_0^2(P_{F_X,G}), E(V(Y) \mid X) = 0\}.$$

The tangent space of G in the model $\mathcal{M}(\mathcal{G}_{CAR})$ generated by this class of submodels is given by

$$T_{CAR}(P_{F_X,G}) = \{v \in L_0^2(P_{F_X,G}) : E(v(Y) \mid X) = 0\}.$$

Let $A_{F_X} : L_0^2(F_X) \to L_0^2(P_{F_X,G})$ be the nonparametric score operator for F_X:

$$A_{F_X}(s)(Y) = E(s(X) \mid Y).$$

Let $\{\epsilon \to F_{\epsilon,s} : s \in \mathcal{S}^F\}$ be the class of one-dimensional submodels in the full data model with tangent space $T^F(F_X)$. The one-dimensional submodels $\epsilon \to F_{\epsilon,s}$ imply one-dimensional submodels $P_{F_{\epsilon,s},G}$ with scores

$$A_{F_X}(s)(Y) = E(s(X) \mid Y),$$

as proved in Gill (1989). Therefore, we have that the nuisance tangent space $T_{nuis}(P_{F_X,G})$ in model $\mathcal{M}(CAR)$ is given by

$$T_{nuis}(P_{F_X,G}) = \overline{\{A(s_{nuis}) : s_{nuis} \in T_{nuis}^F(F_X)\}} \oplus T_{CAR}(P_{F_X,G}).$$

The next theorem provides a representation of $T_{nuis}^\perp(P_{F_X,G})$. It will be useful to define the adjoint $A_G^\top : L_0^2(P_{F_X,G}) \to L_0^2(F_X)$ of A_{F_X}, which is given by

$$A_G^\top(V)(X) = E(V(Y) \mid X).$$

Let $\mathbf{I}_{F_X,G} : L_0^2(F_X) \to L_0^2(F_X)$ be defined by $\mathbf{I}_{F_X,G} = A_G^\top A_{F_X}$.

Theorem 1.3 *Since F_X, G is fixed in this theorem, we suppress possible dependence on F_X, G; In particular, U below can depend on both F_X and G.*

Suppose that $U : T_{nuis}^{F,\perp} \to L_0^2(P_{F_X,G})$ satisfies $E(U(D)(Y) \mid X) = D(X)$ for all $D \in T_{nuis}^{F,\perp}$. In the model $\mathcal{M}(CAR)$, we have

$$T_{nuis}^\perp = \{U(D) - \Pi(U(D) \mid T_{CAR}) : D \in T_{nuis}^{F,\perp}\}. \qquad (1.52)$$

1.4. Estimating Functions   65

Specifically, for any $V \in T_{nuis}^{\perp}$, we have that $D_V \equiv A^{\top}(V) \in T_{nuis}^{F,\perp}$ and
$$V = U(D_V) - \Pi(U(D_V) \mid T_{CAR}). \tag{1.53}$$

We also note that in the model $\mathcal{M}(G)$ with G known, we have
$$T_{nuis}^{\perp} = \{U(D) + \Phi : D \in T_{nuis}^{F,\perp}, \Phi \in T_{CAR}\}. \tag{1.54}$$

Finally, we note that for a $D \in R(\mathbf{I})$ (range of linear operator $\mathbf{I}$: $L_0^2(F_X) \to L_0^2(P_{F_X,G})$)
$$U(D) - \Pi(U(D) \mid T_{CAR}) = A\mathbf{I}^{-}(D). \tag{1.55}$$

We also have the following useful representation of the orthogonal complement of the nuisance tangent space at $P_{F_X,G}$ in terms of the orthogonal complement of the nuisance tangent space at P_{F_X,G^*}. This theorem is useful in situations where it is easier to determine the orthogonal complement at censoring mechanisms satisfying certain assumptions.

Theorem 1.4 *Consider the observed data model $\mathcal{M}(G)$ with G known and satisfying CAR for the distribution $P_{F_X,G}$ of Y. Let $G^* \in \mathcal{G}(CAR)$ be given. Assume that $G \equiv G^*$ so that $W \equiv dG^*/dG$ and $1/W$ are uniformly bounded. Then*
$$T_{nuis}^{\perp}(P_{F_X,G}) = W \times T_{nuis}^{\perp}(P_{F_X,G^*}).$$

Proof. By CAR, we have $W = dP_{F_X,G^*}/dP_{F_X,G}$. Thus, by assumption on W, we have that $L^2(P_{F_X,G^*}) = L^2(P_{F_X,G})$. We have that $T_{nuis}(P_{F_X,G}) = \overline{R_{nuis}(A_{F_X})}$ is the closure of the range of the score operator $A_{F_X} : T_{nuis}^F(F_X) \to L_0^2(P_{F_X,G})$. Thus $T_{nuis}(P_{F_X,G}) = T_{nuis}(P_{F_X,G^*})$. Consider now a function $V(Y)$ in $T_{nuis}^{\perp}(P_{F_X,G^*})$. Let $h_{nuis} \in T_{nuis}^{F,\perp}(F_X)$. Then
$$\langle V * W, A_{F_X}(h_{nuis}) \rangle_{P_{F_X,G}} = \langle V, A_{F_X}(h_{nuis}) \rangle_{P_{F_X,G^*}}. \square$$

The constructive statement (1.53) of Theorem 1.3 is a corollary of the following result.

Theorem 1.5 *Let $V \in T_{CAR}^{\perp}$. Let $D_V(X) \equiv E(V(Y) \mid X) \in L_0^2(F_X)$, and let $U(D_V) \in L_0^2(P_{F_X,G})$ satisfy $E_G(U(D_V)(Y) \mid X) = D_V(X)$. Then*
$$V = U(D_V) - \Pi(U(D_V) \mid T_{CAR}).$$

PROOFS OF THEOREMS

Proof of Theorem 1.5. Recall that $A(s) = E(s(X) \mid Y)$ is the nonparametric score operator and $A^{\top}(V) = E(V(Y) \mid X)$ its adjoint. We need to prove that
$$U(A^{\top}(V)) - \Pi(UA^{\top}(V) \mid T_{CAR}) = V \text{ in } L_0^2(P_{F_X,G}). \tag{1.56}$$

By assumption, we have $UA^\top(V) \in L_0^2(P_{F_X,G})$ so that the projection is well-defined. We will prove (1.56) by showing that

$$\langle U(A^\top(V)) - \Pi(UA^\top(V) \mid T_{CAR}) - V, \eta \rangle_{P_{F_X,G}} = 0 \text{ for all } \eta \in L_0^2(P_{F_X,G}).$$

Since T_{CAR} equals the null space of $A^\top : L_0^2(P_{F_X,G}) \to L_0^2(F_X)$, it follows that $T_{CAR}^\perp = \overline{R(A)} \equiv \overline{\{A(s) : s \in L_0^2(F_X)\}}$. Thus $L_0^2(P_{F_X,G}) = \overline{R(A)} \oplus T_{CAR}$ so that we can decompose $\eta = V_1 + \phi$, $V_1 \in \overline{R(A)}$, and $\phi \in T_{CAR}$. Firstly, since $V \in T_{CAR}^\perp$, we have that the left-hand side of (1.56) is orthogonal to T_{CAR}. Thus, the inner product with ϕ is zero. It remains to show that the inner product (1.56) with $V_1 \in \overline{R(A)}$ is zero as well.

We will first prove this for the case where $V_1 \in R(A)$ so that $V_1 = A(s)$, $s \in L_0^2(F_X)$. Since the adjoint of $A : L_0^2(F_X) \to L_0^2(P_{F_X,G})$ is given by $A^\top$, $A^\top U(D) = D$, $A^\top \Pi(\cdot \mid T_{CAR})$ is the zero mapping, and $D_V = A^\top V$, we have

$$\langle U(D_V) - \Pi(U(D_V) \mid T_{CAR}) - V, A(s) \rangle_{P_{F_X,G}} =$$

$$\langle A^\top U(D_V) - A^\top \Pi(U(D_V) \mid T_{CAR}) - D_V, s \rangle_{F_X}$$

$$= \langle D_V - 0 - D_V, s \rangle_{F_X} = 0.$$

Consider now the case where V_1 lies on the boundary of $\overline{R(A)}$ so that there exists a sequence $s_m \in L_0^2(F_X)$ with $V_1 = \lim_{m \to \infty} A(s_m)$. Again, by the same argument, we have

$$\langle U(D_V) - \Pi(U(D_V) \mid T_{CAR}) - V, A(s_m) \rangle_{P_{F_X,G}} = 0.$$

Furthermore, by the Cauchy–Schwarz inequality, $\langle U(D_V) - \Pi(U(D_V) \mid T_{CAR}) - V, A(s_m) - V_1 \rangle$ is bounded by

$$\| U(D_V) - \Pi(U(D_V) \mid T_{CAR}) - V \| \| A(s_m) - V_1 \|_P \to 0,$$

using, by assumption, $\| U(D_V) \|_P < \infty$. This proves Theorem 1.5. $\square$

Proof of Theorem 1.3.
Proof of $\supset$ (1.54). We have that

$$T_{nuis} = \overline{\{A(s_{nuis}) : s_{nuis} \in T_{nuis}^{F,\perp}\}}. \tag{1.57}$$

Now, note that for any $D \in T_{nuis}^{F,\perp}$ and $\Phi \in T_{CAR}$

$$\langle U(D) + \Phi, A(s_{nuis}) \rangle = \langle D, s_{nuis} \rangle = 0,$$

which proves $U(D) + \Phi \in T_{nuis}^\perp$. An alternative proof is the following; If $D \in T_{nuis}^{F,\perp}$, $\Phi \in T_{CAR}$ and Π_{T^F} is the projection operator onto the full data structure tangent space T^F, then $\Pi_{T^F} A^\top (U(D) + \Phi) = \Pi_{T^F} D \in < S_{eff}^{*F} >,$

which proves that $U(D) + \Phi \in T_{nuis}^{\perp}$.
Proof of $\supset$ **(1.52).** We have

$$T_{nuis} = \overline{\{A(s_{nuis}) : s_{nuis} \in T_{nuis}^{F,\perp}\}} \oplus T_{CAR}. \qquad (1.58)$$

Now, note that for any $D \in T_{nuis}^{F,\perp}$ and $\Phi \in T_{CAR}$

$$\langle U(D) - \Pi(U(D) \mid T_{CAR}), A(s_{nuis}) + \Phi \rangle = \langle D, s_{nuis} \rangle = 0,$$

which proves $U(D) - \Pi(U(D) \mid T_{CAR}) \in T_{nuis}^{\perp}$.

Proof of $\subset$ **(1.54).** Let $V \in T_{nuis}^{\perp}$, where we recall that T_{nuis} is given by (1.57). We can write $V = V - \Pi(V \mid T_{CAR}) + \Pi(V \mid T_{CAR})$. Note that $V^{\perp} \equiv V - \Pi(V \mid T_{CAR}) \in T_{CAR}^{\perp}$. Because $V \in T_{nuis}^{\perp}$, we also have $D_{V^{\perp}} = E(V^{\perp}(Y) \mid X) = E(V(Y) \mid X) \in T_{nuis}^{F,\perp}$: for any $s_{nuis} \in T_{nuis}^{F,\perp}$,

$$\langle A^{\top}(V), s_{nuis} \rangle = \langle V, A(s_{nuis}) \rangle = 0.$$

Thus $U(D_{V^{\perp}}) \in L_0^2(P_{F_X,G})$, and it satisfies $E(U(D_{V^{\perp}})(Y) \mid X) = D_{V^{\perp}}(X)$. Thus, we can apply Theorem 1.5, which tells us that $V^{\perp} = U(D_{V^{\perp}}) - \Pi(U(D_{V^{\perp}}) \mid T_{CAR})$. This proves that $V = U(D_{V^{\perp}}) + \Phi_V$ with $\Phi_V = \Pi(V \mid T_{CAR}) - \Pi(U(D_{V^{\perp}}) \mid T_{CAR}) \in T_{CAR}$.

Proof of $\subset$ **(1.52).** Let $V \in T_{nuis}^{\perp}$, where we recall that T_{nuis} is given by (1.58). Thus $V \in T_{CAR}^{\perp}$. Because $V \in T_{nuis}^{\perp}$, we also have $D_V = E(V(Y) \mid X) \in T_{nuis}^{F,\perp}$: for any $s_{nuis} \in T_{nuis}^{F,\perp}$,

$$\langle A^{\top}(V), s_{nuis} \rangle = \langle V, A(s_{nuis}) \rangle = 0.$$

Thus, by the assumption of Theorem 2.6, we have that $U(D_V) \in L_0^2(P_{F_X,G})$ is well-defined and satisfies $E(U(D_V)(Y) \mid X) = D_V(X)$. Thus, we can apply Theorem 1.5, which tells us that $V = U(D_V) - \Pi(U(D_V) \mid T_{CAR})$.

Finally, we will prove (1.55). Let $\overline{R(A_{F_X})}$ denote the closure of the range of A_{F_X}, and let $N(A_G^{\top})$ be the null space of the adjoint $A_G^{\top}$:

$$N(A_G^{\top}) = \{v \in L_0^2(P_{F_X,G}) : E_G(v(Y) \mid X) = 0\} = T_{CAR}(P_{F_X,G}).$$

Then

$$\begin{aligned} IC(\cdot \mid D) &\equiv U(D) - \Pi(U(D) \mid N(A_G^{\top})) \\ &= \Pi(U(D) \mid \overline{R(A_{F_X})}). \end{aligned} \qquad (1.59)$$

The most direct method of computing the projection (1.59) is presented by the Hilbert space analog of the classical least squares formula $Z(Z^{\top}Z)^{-}Z^{\top}W$ of the projection of W onto the space spanned by the columns of a design matrix Z, where now A_{F_X} plays the role of Z and W plays the role of D. Since $A_G^{\top}U(D) = D$, this gives

$$\Pi(U(D) \mid \overline{R(A_{F_X})}) = A_{F_X}\mathbf{I}_{F_X,G}^{-}(D),$$

which proves (1.55). $\square$

1.4.5 Basic useful results to compute projections

The following simple projection results are basic building blocks for finding complicated projection results and, in particular, the orthogonal complement of the nuisance tangent space.

Lemma 1.4 *Suppose that $X \sim F_X$ and $Z = \Phi(X)$ for some given mapping Φ. Let $L^2(F_Z) \subset L_0^2(F_X)$ be the Hilbert space of all functions of Z. Then $\Pi(V \mid L_0^2(F_Z)) = E(V(X) \mid Z)$.*

Lemma 1.5 *Consider a joint random variable $Z = (Z_1, Z_2) \sim F_Z$. Let $H \subset L^2(F_Z)$ be the sub-Hilbert space of all functions of Z with conditional mean zero, given Z_2. Then $\Pi(V \mid H) = V(Z) - E(V(Z) \mid Z_2)$.*

Lemma 1.6 *Consider a model $\{f_{\theta_1, \theta_2} : \theta_1 \in \Theta_1, \theta_2 \in \Theta_2\}$ of densities for a random variable X. Suppose that the likelihood factorizes:*

$$f_{\theta_1, \theta_2}(X) = f_{1,\theta_1}(X) f_{2,\theta_2}(X)$$

for some functions f_{1,θ_1} and f_{2,θ_2}. Consider a class of one-dimensional models that vary either θ_1 or θ_2, but not both. Let $T_j(\theta)$ be the tangent space generated by the scores of the one-dimensional models only varying θ_j, $j = 1, 2$. Let $T(\theta)$ be the tangent space at f_θ and $\Pi(\cdot \mid T(\theta))$ be the projection operator onto $T(\theta)$ in $L_0^2(F_\theta)$. Then $T(\theta) = T_1(\theta) \oplus T_2(\theta)$ is the orthogonal sum of $T_1(\theta)$ and $T_2(\theta)$ so that $\Pi(\cdot \mid T(\theta)) = \sum_{j=1}^{2} \Pi(\cdot \mid T_j(\theta))$.

Lemma 1.7 *Let H_1, H_2 be two sub-Hilbert spaces of $L_0^2(F_X)$ (such as the tangent spaces of two parameters). Let $H_1 + H_2 = \{h_1 + h_2 : h_1 \in H_1, h_2 \in H_2\}$. We have*

$$\overline{(H_1 + H_2)}^\perp = H_1^\perp \cap H_2^\perp. \qquad (1.60)$$

Similarly,

$$\overline{H_1^\perp + H_2^\perp} = (H_1 \cap H_2)^\perp. \qquad (1.61)$$

If H_1 and H_2 are orthogonal, then

$$\overline{H_1 + H_2}^\perp = \overline{\{h - \Pi(h \mid H_2) : h \in H_1^\perp\}}. \qquad (1.62)$$

The second result (1.61) of this lemma is useful to calculate the orthogonal complement of the nuisance tangent space of a model that can be viewed as an intersection of a number of models; Say $\mathcal{M} = \cap \mathcal{M}_j$ is an intersection of K models $\mathcal{M}_j$. It follows immediately that $T_{nuis} \subset \cap_{j=1}^{K} T_{nuis,j}$, and one typically also has that the nuisance tangent space T_{nuis} actually equals the intersection of the nuisance tangent spaces for models $\mathcal{M}_j$ (i.e., $T_{nuis} = \cap_{j=1}^{K} T_{nuis,j}$). Application of (1.61) now teaches us that $T_{nuis}^\perp \supset \sum_{j=1}^{K} T_{nuis,j}^\perp$ always, and typically we have equality:

$$T_{nuis}^\perp = \sum_{j=1}^{K} T_{nuis,j}^\perp.$$

In other words, whenever one is able to view a complicated model as an intersection of simpler models, then, for the purpose of finding the class of estimating functions, it will suffice just to calculate the orthogonal complements of the nuisance tangent space in each of the simpler models.

If the nuisance parameter has various components, then $T_{nuis} = \sum_j T_{nuis,j}$, where $T_{nuis,j}$ is the nuisance tangent space generated by the jth component only (keeping the other components fixed). The first result (1.60) of the lemma teaches us that $T_{nuis}^\perp = \cap_j T_{nuis,j}^\perp$ can be calculated as the intersection of $T_{nuis,j}^\perp$. If $T_{nuis} = T_{nuis,1} \oplus T_{nuis,2}$, then the last result (1.62) of the lemma teaches us that it suffices to compute $T_{nuis,1}^\perp$ and the projection operator onto $T_{nuis,1}^\perp$.

Proof of Lemma 1.7. The first result is standard in Hilbert space theory. Regarding the last result, if H_1, H_2 are orthogonal, then for any $h \in L_0^2(F_X)$

$$\begin{aligned} h - \Pi(h \mid H_1 + H_2) &= h - \Pi(h \mid H_1) - \Pi(h \mid H_2) \\ &= h - \Pi(h \mid H_1) - \Pi(h - \Pi(h \mid H_1) \mid H_2). \end{aligned}$$

Now, note that $H_j^\perp = \{h - \Pi(h \mid H_j) : h \in L_0^2(F_X)\}$, $j = 1, 2$. □

1.5 Robustness of Estimating Functions

1.5.1 Robustness of estimating functions against misspecification of linear convex nuisance parameters.

We showed above that an estimating function that is an element of the orthogonal complement of the nuisance tangent space in the sense defined by (1.49) has a corresponding estimating equation with first derivative (directional) w.r.t. its nuisance parameter equal to zero. In fact, we will now prove that if the data-generating distribution is linear in the nuisance parameter ρ of the estimating function and the nuisance parameter space is convex, then, at the misspecified nuisance parameter, the estimating function remains unbiased *and orthogonal to the tangent space generated by this parameter*. Similar type results have been obtained by Bickel (1982), Bickel, Klaassen, Ritov, and Wellner (1993), Newey (1990), and Robins, Rotnitzky, van der Laan (2000). The following lemma is a slight modification (including now an orthogonality result) of the result in van der Laan, Yu (2001), but uses essentially the same proof.

Lemma 1.8 *Consider an estimating function $D(X \mid \mu, \rho)$ (i.e., a mapping $\mathcal{X} \times \{(\mu(F_X), \rho(F_X)) : F_X \in \mathcal{M}^F\} \to \mathbb{R}$) that satisfies (1.49). Assume that μ is pathwise differentiable at each $F \in \mathcal{M}^F$ along a F-specific class of one-dimensional models including nuisance score lines $F_\epsilon = \epsilon F_1 + (1-\epsilon) F \in \mathcal{M}^F$ indexed by a set of F_1's with 1) $\mu(F_1) = \mu(F)$, 2) $d/d\epsilon \mu(F_\epsilon)|_{\epsilon=0} = 0$, and 3) $dF_1/dF < \infty$ (i.e., being uniformly bounded). In* addition, we assume that these classes of lines satisfy the following "connectivity" property: If we have a line $\epsilon F + (1-\epsilon) F_1$ in the F_1-specific class, and a line $\epsilon F_1^* + (1-\epsilon) F$ in the F-specific class (i.e., $\mu(F) = \mu(F_1) = \mu(F_1^*)$, $dF/dF_1 < \infty$, $dF_1^*/dF < \infty$, and the pathwise derivative of μ at F_1 and F, respectively, equals zero along these lines), then the line $\epsilon F_1^* + (1-\epsilon) F_1$ is an element of the F_1-specific class as well; in other words, beyond the properties 1 and 3 which follow directly it also satisfies property 2. Let $T_1(F_X)$ be the tangent space of this class of one-dimensional submodels at F_X.

Let $F_1 \in \mathcal{M}^F$ be such that $dF/dF_1 < \infty$, $\mu(F_1) = \mu(F)$, and $d/d\epsilon \mu(\epsilon F + (1-\epsilon) F_1)|_{\epsilon=0} = 0$. Then

$$E_{F_X} D(X \mid \mu(F_X), \rho(F_1)) = 0.$$

In fact,

$$D(X \mid \mu(F_X), \rho(F_1)) \in T_1(F_X)^\perp.$$

We note that the connectivity assumption is a natural assumption on the classes of lines. An important corollary of this lemma is that, if the data-generating distribution F_X can be parametrized as $P_{\mu,\eta}$ with $\eta \to P_{\mu,\eta}$ linear, η ranging over a convex parameter space, and ρ a function of η, then $D(X \mid \mu(F_X), \rho_1) \in T_{nuis}^{F,\perp}(F_X)$ for all ρ_1. (Note that the connectivity assumption obviously holds for models with such variation independent parametrizations). This implies that one can treat ρ as the index h of the estimating function.

Note also that, if $\rho = (\rho_1, \rho_2)$ with ρ_1, ρ_2 being variation-independent (w.r.t. to each other and to μ) linear convex parameters (i.e., satisfying the assumptions of Lemma 1.8), then double application of Lemma 1.8 in the model first with ρ_1 known and then with ρ_2 known, respectively, yields the following double robustness property of the estimating function D:

$$E_{F_X} D(X \mid \mu(F_X), \rho_1, \rho_2) = 0 \text{ if either } \rho_1 = \rho_1(F_X) \text{ or } \rho_2 = \rho_2(F_X).$$

However, note that in this case $D(X \mid \mu(F_X), \rho_1, \rho_2(F_X))$ (or $D(X \mid \mu(F_X), \rho_1(F_X), \rho_2)$) is not necessarily still orthogonal to the tangent space corresponding with just varying ρ_2 (or just varying ρ_1).

Lemma 1.8 requires that $F_X \ll F_1$, but it follows straightforwardly that, if $\rho(F_1)$ can be approximated by a $\rho(F_{1m}$ with $F_X \ll F_{1m}$ so that application of this lemma yields $E_{F_X} D(X \mid \mu(F_X), \rho(F_{1m})) = 0$, and $D(X \mid \mu(F_X), \rho(F_{1m}))$ converges to $D(X \mid \mu, \rho(F_1))$ in $L^2(F_X)$, then we will have $E_{F_X} D(X \mid \mu(F_X), \rho(F_1)) = 0$ as well.

Proof of lemma. Let F_1, F be as in the lemma. Thus $\mu(F_1) = \mu(F)$. Then, $F_{1,\epsilon,s} = \epsilon F + (1-\epsilon) F_1$ is a one-dimensional submodel of $\mathcal{M}^F$ with score $s = d(F - F_1)/dF_1$ satisfying

$$0 = \frac{d}{d\epsilon} \mu(F_{1,\epsilon,s}) \bigg|_{\epsilon=0}.$$

By the fact that μ is pathwise differentiable along $F_{1,\epsilon,s}$ at F_1, we have for any gradient $\ell(X \mid \mu(F_1), \rho(F_1))$

$$0 = \int \ell(x \mid \mu(F_1), \rho(F_1)) \frac{d(F - F_1)}{dF_1} dF_1 = \int \ell(x \mid \mu(F_1), \rho(F_1)) dF(x).$$

Since a standardized version of $D(\cdot \mid \mu(F_1), \rho(F_1))$ is a gradient, this implies also that for any such pair F_1, F

$$0 = \int D(x \mid \mu(F_1), \rho(F_1)) dF(x) = \int D(x \mid \mu(F), \rho(F_1)) dF(x),$$

which proves the protection of unbiasedness as stated in the lemma.

This protection will now also provide us with the claimed orthogonality. Any score in $T_1(F_X)$ is of the form $d(F_1^* - F)/dF$ for some F_1^* with $dF_1^*/dF < \infty$, $\mu(F_1^*) = \mu(F)$, and $d/d\epsilon\, \mu(\epsilon F_1^* + (1-\epsilon)F)|_{\epsilon=0} = 0$. We have

$$\int \ell(X \mid \mu, \rho(F_1)) \frac{d(F_1^* - F)}{dF} dF = \int \ell(X \mid \mu, \rho(F_1)) d(F_1^* - F)$$
$$= \int \ell(X \mid \mu, \rho(F_1)) dF_1^* - \int \ell(X \mid \mu, \rho(F_1)) dF.$$

We just proved that the second term equals zero. By the same proof, the first term equals zero if $dF_1^*/dF_1 < \infty$, and $d/d\epsilon\, \mu(\epsilon F_1^* + (1-\epsilon)F_1)|_{\epsilon=0} = 0$. We have $dF_1^*/dF_1 = (dF_1^*/dF) * (dF/dF_1) < \infty$, which proves the first condition. The pathwise derivative conditions holds by our connectivity assumption on the class of lines. This completes the proof. □

Example 1.23 (Mixture models with unspecified mixing distribution) In many applications, the observed data can be thought of as a draw from a distribution indexed by an unobserved label with unknown distribution. Formally, let Y be the observed data and X be the unobserved label. We assume that the density of Y is parametrized as

$$p_{\mu, F_X}(Y) = \int p_\mu(y \mid x) dF_X(x),$$

where F_X is the distribution of X and $p_\mu(y \mid x)$ is the conditional density of Y, given $X = x$, parametrized by a k-dimensional parameter μ. This parametrization could also be employed for conditional mixtures

$$p_{\mu, F}(Y \mid Z) = \int p_\mu(Y \mid x, Z) dF_{X\mid Z}(x \mid Z),$$

where Z is a set of observed covariates. Consider now the semiparametric model:

$$\mathcal{M} = \{p_{\mu, F_X} : \mu \in \mathbb{R}^k, F_X \text{ unspecified}\}.$$

In this example, let μ be the parameter of interest. Note that Lemma 1.8 is applicable to the efficient score for μ in this semiparametric model because p_{μ,F_X} is linear in the nuisance parameter F_X and F_X ranges over the convex space of all possible distributions of X. Let $S^*_{eff}(X \mid \mu, F_X)$ be the efficient score, which is defined as the score for μ minus its projection on the nuisance tangent space $T_{nuis}(P_{\mu,F_X}))$, where the latter space is given by

$$T_{nuis}(P_{\mu,F_X}) = \overline{\left\{ \int p_\mu(y \mid x) s(x) dF_X(x) : s \in L_0^2(F_X) \right\}}.$$

For practical purposes, if X is continuous, then it is convenient to discretize X and consider $T_{nuis}(P_{\mu,F_X})$ as the range of the matrix B corresponding with the discretized linear operator $h \to \int p_\mu(y \mid x) h(x) dF_X(x)$. In this case, the projection operator on the columns of the matrix B is given by the least squares formula $B(B^\top B)^{-1} B^\top$. An alternative way of computing this projection operator is to sample a collection of quite uncorrelated functions of the form $\int p_\mu(y \mid x) h_j(x) dF_X(x)$, $j = 1, \ldots, N$, and approximate the projection with the finite-dimensional projection onto the space spanned by these N functions. The latter method of discretization discretizes the actual space on which we need to project instead of discretizing the underlying space of functions $L_0^2(F_X)$. Since the operator $h \to \int p_\mu(y \mid x) h(x) dF_X(x)$ is typically compact (i.e., maps bounded sets in compact sets), this method might be a sensible strategy.

Application of Lemma 1.8 teaches us that at any F_1 with $F_1 \equiv F_X$, we have

$$E_{P_{\mu,F_X}} S^*_{eff}(Y \mid \mu, F_1) = 0.$$

Depending on the smoothness of S^*_{eff} in F_X, by a standard continuous extension argument, one might be able to extend this result to F_1's that are not equivalent with F_X. Let F_n be an estimator of F_X according to a parametric model, and let μ_n be the solution of the efficient score estimating equation:

$$0 = \sum_{i=1}^n S^*_{eff}(Y_i \mid \mu, F_n).$$

Under regularity conditions, we have that μ_n is asymptotically linear with influence curve $-\left(d/d\mu E S^*_{eff}(Y \mid \mu, F_1)\right)^{-1} S^*_{eff}(Y \mid \mu, F_1)$, where F_1 denotes the limit of F_n. In particular, if F_n is consistent for the true F_X, then μ_n will be asymptotically efficient. In other words, μ_n is a locally efficient estimator of μ.

This general result is not known from the literature and has never been exploited. Because mixtures represent a very large and important class of models, this general result has powerful applications. A well-known and intensively studied example in the literature is a mixture of univariate normal distributions. For example, if one believes that the density of X is a mixture of normals with the same mean but different variance, then F_X is the distribution of the variance σ^2 and μ denotes the mean. Alternatively, if one believes that the density of X is a mixture of normals with different means but equal variance, then μ denotes the variance of the normal distributions and F_X is the distribution of the means.

Other interesting applications occur in change point or signal (such as a binding site in DNA sequence data) detection problems. For example, suppose that one observes a sequence of discrete data that one believes is generated as follows; Firstly, one draws the location of the starting point of the signal, which has length K. Secondly, one draws the signal with a multinomial distribution (independent across locations). Finally, one draws the background of the signal with a multinomial distribution (independent across locations). In other words, the sequence is a mixture of multinomial distributions, where one mixes over the starting point of the signal. Suppose that the vector of all multinomial probabilities is the parameter of interest μ and that the distribution of the starting point is the unspecified nuisance parameter. These models are typically fit with maximum likelihood estimation assuming a known distribution (e.g., uniform) for the starting point. The consistency of this maximum likelihood estimator relies completely on the correct specification of this starting point distribution. Our general result above teaches us that our estimating function approach allows consistent (locally efficient) estimation of the multinomial probabilities in the semiparametric model, which leaves the starting point distribution unspecified. For example, one defines μ_n as a solution of the efficient score equation, where we guess as starting point distribution the uniform distribution. If our guess is wrong, then μ_n will still be consistent and asymptotically linear. $\square$

Example 1.24 (A two-sample semiparametric estimation problem) Suppose that we observe n_0 i.i.d. observations of $X_0 \sim f_0$ and n_1 i.i.d. observations of $X_1 \sim f_1$, where f_0, f_1 are Lebesgue densities. Consider this as a sample of $n = n_0 + n_1$ i.i.d. observations (X_i, ξ_i), $i = 1, \ldots, n$, where $\xi_i \in \{0, 1\}$ indexes the two populations. Let $F_j(x) = P(X \leq x \mid \xi = j)$, $j = 0, 1$, be the corresponding distribution functions. For example, X_0 and X_1 might represent a measurement on a randomly drawn subject from a population of lungcancer patients and a healthy population, respectively. We are concerned with estimation of parameters comparing F_0 and F_1 such as $\mu_1 - \mu_0$, where $\mu_j = EX_j$, $j = 0, 1$. In many applications, n_0 is very small relative to n_1. In these situations, it is beneficial to have a statistical framework that allows one to borrow information from the X_1 sample when estimating F_0. Dominici and Zeger (2001) consider a parametric model for the function $p \to F_1 F_0^{-1}(p)$, $p \in [0, 1]$, and develop a least squares estimation method. In van der Laan, Dominici and Zeger (2002) (see also van der Laan and Yu, 2001) we propose to model the quantile–quantile function (as in the structural nested causal inference models of Robins, 1992) that maps the quantiles of F_0 into the quantiles of F_1,

$$F_1^{-1}F_0(q) = m(q \mid \beta), \qquad (1.63)$$

which yields a simpler parametrization of the likelihood. Here $m(\cdot \mid \beta)$: $[a_0, b_0] \equiv [F_0^{-1}(0), F_0^{-1}(1)] \to [a_1, b_1] \equiv [F_1^{-1}(0), F_1^{-1}(1)]$ is a known increasing absolutely continuous function in q parametrized by a k-dimensional parameter β. Notice that $F_0(x) = P(X_0 \leq x) = P(X_1 \leq F_1^{-1}F_0(x)) = F_1(m(x \mid \beta))$ and that $m(X_0 \mid \beta) \sim F_1$. Assumption (1.63) defines a semiparametric model for the data-generating distribution with infinite-dimensional parameter the cumulative distribution function F_1 and finite-dimensional parameter β.

In order to obtain a monotone parametrisation of $m(q \mid \beta)$ while having no constraints on β one could consider the following model:

$$m(x \mid \beta) = \beta_0 + \int_{a_0}^{x} \exp(\beta^\top W(x))dx, \qquad (1.64)$$

where $\beta = (\beta_1, \ldots, \beta_k)$, $W(x) = (W_1(x), \ldots, W_k(x))$ is a vector of known (basis) functions such as splines or polynomials (i.e. $W_j(x) = x^j$). Notice that $\beta_0 = m(a_0 \mid \beta) = F_1^{-1}(0)$. Therefore one can estimate β_0 with the minimum of the F_1-sample which converges at rate $1/n$ to β_0. Consequently, we can treat β_0 as known so that $\beta = (\beta_1, \ldots, \beta_k)$ is the parameter of interest.

The piecewise-linear-regression model for $m(x \mid \beta)$ is obtained by setting $W_j(x) = I(t_{j-1} < x \leq t_j)$, $j = 1, \ldots, k$, where $t_0 = a_0, \ldots, t_k = b_0$ is a partition of $[a_0, b_0]$. In this case we have

$$\begin{aligned} m(x \mid \beta) &= \beta_0 + \int_{a_0}^{x} \exp(\sum_{j=1}^{k} \beta_j I(t_{j-1} < s \leq t_j))ds \\ &= \beta_0 + \sum_{l=1}^{k} I(x > t_{l-1})(\min(t_1, x) - t_{l-1}) \exp(\beta_l), \end{aligned}$$

which is a piecewise linear function which equals β_0 at $x = 0$ and has slopes $\exp(\beta_j)$ for $x \in (t_{j-1}, t_j]$, $j = 1, \ldots, k$. Let $W_l(x) \equiv I(x > t_{l-1})(\min(t_1, x) - t_{l-1})$, $l = 1, \ldots, k$. Then we have $m(x \mid \beta) = \beta_0 + \sum_{l=1}^{k} W_l(x) \exp(\beta_l)$.

The density of (X, ξ) is given by

$$p_{\beta, f_1}(x, \xi) = \{p_0 f_1(m(x \mid \beta)) m'(x \mid \beta)\}^{\xi=0} \{(1-p_0) f_1(x)\}^{\xi=1},$$

where $m'(x \mid \beta) \equiv d/dx\, m(x \mid \beta)$ denotes the derivative of m w.r.t. x, and $p_0 = P(\xi = 0)$. Thus, the density of the data is linear in the convex nuisance parameter f_1. Application of Lemma 1.8 now teaches us that each estimating function in the orthogonal complement of the nuisance tangent space remains an element of this same space at a misspecified f_1. In particular, the efficient score for β that has as nuisance parameter f_1 remains

1.5. Robustness of Estimating Functions

unbiased at misspecification of f_1. Consequently, using the efficient score as the estimating function for β with a locally consistent estimate (according to some parametric model) of f_1 yields locally efficient estimators of β.

Firstly, we will show that the maximum likelihood estimator of β suffers from the curse of dimensionality. The likelihood of the observed data is given by

$$L(\beta, p_0, f_1) = \prod_{i=1}^{n} \{p_0 f_1(m(X_i \mid \beta)) m'(X_i \mid \beta)\}^{\xi_i=0} \{(1-p_0) * f_1(X_i)\}^{\xi_i=1}.$$

It follows that the maximum likelihood estimator of p_0 is $p_{0n} \equiv \sum_{i=1}^{n} I(\xi_i = 0)/n = n_0/n$ (i.e., the proportion of observations with $\xi = 0$). In addition, given β, we have that the nonparametric maximum likelihood estimator of F_1 is given by

$$F_{1n}(x) = \frac{1}{n} \sum_{i=1}^{n} \{I(X_i \leq x, \xi = 1) + I(m(X_i \mid \beta) \leq x, \xi = 0)\}.$$

These maximum likelihood estimators of p and F_1 are clearly very natural estimates.

It remains to estimate β. Firstly, to define an appropriate maximum likelihood estimator of β, one needs to plug in a density estimator f_{1n} of f_1, which one could obtain by kernel-smoothing F_{1n}. For example, given a density (kernel) k and bandwidth h, we could define

$$f_{1n}(x) = \int k((y-x)/h)/h \, dF_{1n}(y).$$

Now, one can define a regularized maximum likelihood estimator of β as the maximizer of $\beta \to L(\beta, p_n, f_{1n})$. However, below we will show that the efficient score for β depends on f'_1. This suggests that the maximum likelihood estimator of β will involve data adaptively selecting a bandwidth and that, even when selecting a good bandwidth, its finite sample performance will only be reasonable at fairly large sample sizes. This shows the need for locally efficient estimation.

Straightforward calculation of the orthogonal complement of the nuisance tangent space of β yields the following class of estimating functions for β

$$\{D_h(X, \xi \mid \beta) \equiv (\xi = 0) p_0 h(m(X \mid \beta)) - (\xi = 1)(1-p_0) h(X) : h\}, \quad (1.65)$$

where the index $h = (h_1, \ldots, h_k)$ can be any k-dimensional vector of real-valued function. Equation (1.65) represents a class of unbiased estimating functions which generates a subset of $T_{nuis}^{F,\perp}(F_X)$ when evaluated at the true parameter values. This class of estimating functions is indexed by a user-supplied h that does not involve a nuisance parameter f_1. It is straightforward to show that the efficient score for β is given by $D_{h_{opt}}(X, \xi \mid \beta)$

76   1. Introduction

(see also Newey, 1990), where

$$h_{opt}(X \mid f_1, \beta) = \frac{f_1'(x)}{f_1(x)} m^{(1)}(m^{-1}(x)) + \frac{m'^{,(1)}(m^{-1}(x))}{m'(m^{-1}(x))}.$$

Here m' denotes the derivative w.r.t. x, $m^{(1)}(x)$ denotes the k-dimensional vector of first derivatives w.r.t. β_j of $m(x \mid \beta)$, $j = 1, \ldots, k$, and $m'^{,(1)}(x)$ denotes the k-dimensional vector of first derivatives w.r.t. β_j, $j = 1, \ldots, k$, of $m'(x \mid \beta)$. In other words, the class of unbiased estimating functions (1.65) includes, in particular, the efficient score of β, which is the optimal estimating function. One can estimate β with the solution

$$0 = \sum_{i=1}^{n} D_{h_{opt}(f_{1n}, \beta_n^0)}(Y_i \mid \beta),$$

where we assume that (f_{1n}, β_n^0) is the parametric maximum likelihood estimator of (f_1, β) assuming a certain parametric model for f_1. If the parametric model is correct, then the resulting estimator β_n will be efficient, while it remains consistent and asymptotically normally (CAN) distributed if (f_{1n}, β_n^0) converges to a wrong (f^*, β^*). Thus, β_n will be CAN and efficient at the guessed parametric submodel. Note that globally efficient estimation will require estimation of a derivative of the density f_1, which explains why the unregularized maximum likelihood estimator is inconsistent and that a regularized maximum likelihood estimator may perform poorly unless the sample size is large. □

Example 1.25 (Semiparametric bivariate location shift model for failure time data, where one of the failures censors the other) Let T_1 be the log-time until recurrence of cancer and T_2 be the log-time until death. Let Z be a vector of covariates, and consider the bivariate regression model

$$\begin{aligned} T_1 &= \beta_1 Z + e_1 \\ T_2 &= \beta_2 Z + e_2, \end{aligned}$$

where $e = (e_1, e_2)$ is independent of Z. We have as observed data

$$Y = (T \equiv \min(T_1, T_2), \Delta = I(T_1 < T_2), T_2, Z).$$

The parameter of interest is $\beta = (\beta_1, \beta_2)$, and the goal is to construct locally efficient estimators of β based on n i.i.d. observations $Y_1, \ldots, Y_n$.

One can also think of this observed data structure as a censored data structure where the full data structure is (T_1, Z) and the censoring variable is T_2, which right-censors T_1 and is always observed. However, since we make no further assumptions such as CAR, this is not a helpful insight. This model has been introduced and analyzed in Robins (1995a,b) and Lin, Robins and Wei (1996).

The density of the observed data is indexed by the parameter of interest β, the bivariate density g of e, and the density h of Z. Let H be the cumulative probability distribution function of h. The nuisance parameter in this model is (g,h). The density $p_{\beta,g,h}(T,\Delta,T_2,Z)$ of the observed data is given by

$$g(T-\beta_1 Z, T_2 - \beta_2 Z)^\Delta \left\{ \int_{T_2}^\infty g(t_1 - \beta_1 Z, T_2 - \beta_2 Z) dt_1 \right\}^{1-\Delta} h(Z).$$

Thus, the density of the data is linear in the nuisance parameter g, given h, and g varies over the convex parameter space of all bivariate densities. Application of Lemma 1.8 teaches us now that each estimating function that is an element of the orthogonal complement $T_{nuis}^\perp(P_{\beta,g,h})$ of the nuisance tangent space at the true parameter values remains unbiased and orthogonal to the nuisance scores generated by g, at misspecification of g, assuming correct specification of h. In particular, the efficient score $S(Y \mid \beta, g, H)$ for β, which has as nuisance parameter g and the cumulative distribution H of Z, remains unbiased and orthogonal to the nuisance tangent space of g at misspecification of g. Consequently, given the empirical estimate H_n of H and a locally consistent estimate g_n according to some guessed parametric model such as the bivariate normal family of g, we propose to estimate β with the solution β_n of

$$0 = \sum_{i=1}^n S(Y_i \mid \beta, g_n, H_n).$$

By our Lemma 1.8, under regularity conditions, β_n is consistent and asymptotically linear. If g_n is consistent for the true g, then it has influence curve $IC(Y) \equiv -\{d/d\beta ES(Y \mid \beta, g, H)\}^{-1} S(Y \mid \beta, g, H)$ so that it is asymptotically efficient. However, since $S(Y \mid \beta, g_1, H)$ is not necessarily orthogonal to the nuisance tangent space of H at misspecified g_1, the influence curve can have a contribution due to estimating H. Since the tangent space $T_H = \{s(Z) : Es(Z) = 0\}$ generated by the nuisance parameter H is orthogonal to the score of β and the tangent space generated by g, application of Theorem 2.3 in Chapter 2 teaches us that β_n is asymptotically linear with influence curve

$$IC(Y) - \Pi(IC \mid T_H) = IC(Y) - E(IC(Y) \mid Z).$$

This method is introduced, analyzed, and implemented in Scharfstein, Robins and van der Laan (2002).

1.5.2 Double robustness of observed data estimating functions.

Consider now an observed censored data model. We argue as in Section 7 of Robins, Rotnitzky, and van der Laan (2000). Note that the data-generating distribution is linear in the censoring mechanism G. Thus, if we have an estimating function that, when evaluated at its true parameter values, is orthogonal to the tangent space $T_G(P_{F,G})$ of G according to a convex model $\mathcal{G}$, then application of Lemma 1.8 above (with G being the nuisance parameter and F being fixed at the truth) teaches us that if we misspecify G but correctly specify the other nuisance parameters in the estimating function, then the estimating function has expectation zero and is still orthogonal to $T_G(P_{F,G})$. In addition, by factorization of the likelihood (by CAR), this subspace $T_G(P_{F,G})$ of $L_0^2(P_{F,G})$ is a closure of a linear span of a set of scores that is independent of F. Consequently, any function in $T_G(P_{F_1,G})$ that has finite mean w.r.t. $P_{F,G}$ has conditional mean zero, given X, w.r.t. G. The latter observation tells us that, if we misspecify the dependence on F of the projection operator on $T_G(P_{F,G})$, then the misspecified projection will still have conditional mean zero w.r.t. G. This proves the following double robustness property for observed data estimating functions.

Lemma 1.9 (Double robustness of observed data estimating functions) *Consider the observed data model $\mathcal{M}(\mathcal{G}) = \{P_{F,G} : F \in \mathcal{M}^F, G \in \mathcal{G}\}$ for the data-generating distribution of $Y = \Phi(C, X)$ indexed by the full data structure distribution F and the conditional distribution G of C, given X, ranging over parameter spaces $\mathcal{M}^F$ and a convex parameter space $\mathcal{G} \subset \mathcal{G}(CAR)$, respectively. Let $\mu = \mu(F)$ be a parameter of F. Let $T_G(P_{F,G}) \subset T_{CAR}(P_{F_X,G})$ be the tangent space of G generated by the lines $\alpha \to \alpha G_1 + (1-\alpha)G$, $G_1 \in \mathcal{G}$ with $G_1 \ll G$ (and treating F as known).*

Assume that there exists an unbiased estimating function $IC_0(Y \mid G, \mu)$ satisfying $E_{P_{F,G}} IC_0(Y \mid G, \mu(F)) = 0$ for all $F \in \mathcal{M}^F, G \in \mathcal{G}$. Consider now the estimating function $IC(Y \mid F, G, \mu) \equiv IC_0(Y \mid G, \mu) - IC_{nu}(Y \mid F, G)$, where $IC_{nu}(Y \mid F, G)$ is a well-defined function of Y and each possible F, G satisfying $IC_{nu}(Y \mid F, G) = \Pi_{F,G}(IC_0(Y \mid G, \mu(F)) \mid T_G(P_{F,G}))$ in $L_0^2(P_{F_X,G})$. Here $\Pi_{F,G}(\cdot \mid T_G(P_{F,G}))$ is the projection operator onto $T_G(P_{F,G})$ in the Hilbert space $L_0^2(P_{F_X,G})$. Then

$$E_{P_{F,G}} IC(Y \mid F_1, G_1, \mu(F)) = 0$$

if $dG/dG_1 < \infty$ and either $F_1 = F$ or $G_1 = G$.
If $F_1 = F$, then we also have

$$IC(Y \mid F, G_1, \mu(F)) \perp T_G(P_{F,G})$$

at any G_1 satisfying $dG/dG_1 < \infty$.
Suppose now that $IC_0(Y \mid G_1, \mu)$ also satisfies $E_{G_1}(IC_0(Y \mid G_1, \mu(F)) \mid X) \in T_{nuis}^{F,\perp}(F_X)$. If $F_1 = F$, then we have

$$IC(Y \mid F, G_1, \mu(F)) \in T_{nuis}^{\perp}(\mathcal{M}(\mathcal{G}))$$

at any G_1 satisfying $dG/dG_1 < \infty$, where we recall that $T_{nuis}^\perp(\mathcal{M}(\mathcal{G}))$ is the orthogonal complement of the nuisance tangent space (including the nuisance parameter $G \in \mathcal{G}$) of μ in the observed data model $\mathcal{M}(\mathcal{G})$.

Theorem 1.3 below actually teaches us that the orthogonal complement of the nuisance tangent space, $T_{nuis}^\perp(P_{F_X,G})$, of model $\mathcal{M}(CAR)$ consists of all functions of Y that are orthogonal to $T_{CAR}(P_{F_X,G})$ and whose conditional expectation, given X, is an element of $T_{nuis}^{F,\perp}(F_X)$. Thus, Lemma 1.9 yields a desired double robustness property of all estimating functions of interest, including the optimal estimating function. In the next Section 1.6, we will prove that for the last two statements of Lemma 1.9 it is not necessary to have $E_{P_{F,G}}IC_0(Y \mid G, \mu(F)) = 0$, but one only needs $E_{P_{F,G_1}}IC_0(Y \mid G_1, \mu(F)) = 0$; that is, the initial estimating function needs to be unbiased under G_1, but not necessarily under the true G.

1.5.3 Understanding double robustness for a general semiparametric model

Consider a model $\{P_{\theta,\eta} : \theta \in \Theta, \eta \in \Gamma\}$ for the distribution of X, where θ and η are two variation independent parameters. Let $\mu(\theta)$ be a euclidean parameter of interest. We will here provide general conditions under which estimating functions $(X, \mu, \theta, \eta) \to U(X \mid \mu, \theta, \eta)$ satisfying $U(X \mid \mu(\theta), \theta, \eta) \in T_{nuis}^\perp(P_{\theta,\eta})$ for all parameter values of (θ, η) are double robust w.r.t. misspecification of θ and η. The following development is based on Robins and Rotnitzky (2001).

In this model, $T_{nuis}^\perp(P_{\theta,\eta}) \supset T_\eta^\perp(P_{\theta,\eta}) \cap T_\theta^\perp(P_{\theta,\eta})$ (with equality typically), where $T_\eta(P_{\theta,\eta})$ denotes the nuisance tangent space in the model with θ known (i.e., all nuisance scores obtained by varying η only), and $T_\theta(P_{\theta,\eta})$ is the nuisance tangent space in the model with η known (i.e., all nuisance scores obtained by varying θ). Let $(X, \theta) \to U_{1,h_1}(X \mid \theta)$, indexed by h_1 ranging over an index set $\mathcal{H}_1$, be a class of estimating functions satisfying

$$\{U_{1,h_1}(X \mid \theta) : h_1 \in \mathcal{H}_1\} \subset T_\eta^\perp(P_{\theta,\eta})$$

for all parameter values (θ, η). Similarly, let $(X, \mu, \eta) \to U_{2,h_2}(X \mid \mu, \eta)$, indexed by h_2 ranging over an index set $\mathcal{H}_2$, be a class of estimating functions satisfying

$$\{U_{2,h_2}(X \mid \mu, \eta) : h_2 \in \mathcal{H}_2\} \subset T_\theta^\perp(P_{\theta,\eta})$$

for all parameter values (θ, η). Here one aims to choose these classes of estimating functions $\{U_{1,h_1} : h_1\}$ and $\{U_{2,h_2} : h_2 \in \mathcal{H}_2\}$ so that they cover rich subsets of these orthogonal complements. Consider now an estimating function $(X, \mu, \theta, \eta) \to U(X \mid \mu, \theta, \eta)$ satisfying that

$$U(X \mid \mu(\theta), \theta, \eta) \in \{U_{1,h_1}(X \mid \theta) : h_1 \in \mathcal{H}_1\} \cap \{U_{2,h_2}(X \mid \mu(\theta), \eta) : h_2 \in \mathcal{H}_2\}$$

for all parameter values (θ, η). Under this assumption, we have for all possible parameter values of θ, η that $U(X \mid \mu(\theta), \theta, \eta) = U_{1,h_1}(X \mid \theta) = U_{2,h_2}(X \mid \mu(\theta), \eta)$ for some $h_1 = h_1(\theta, \eta) \in \mathcal{H}_1$ and $h_2 = h_2(\theta, \eta) \in \mathcal{H}_2$. Note that here $h_j(\cdot, \cdot)$ maps the parameter space of (θ, η) into $\mathcal{H}_j$, $j = 1, 2$. In addition, we assume that for $(\mu, \theta, \eta) \in \{\mu(\theta) : \theta \in \Theta\} \times \Theta \times \Gamma$, we have

$$U(X \mid \mu, \theta, \eta) = U_{2, h_2(\mu, \theta, \eta)}(X \mid \mu, \eta)$$

for some $(\mu, \theta, \eta) \to h_2(\mu, \theta, \eta) \in \mathcal{H}_2$. It now follows that:

$$U(X \mid \mu(\theta), \theta, \eta_1) = U_{1, h_1(\theta, \eta_1)}(X \mid \theta) \in T_\eta^\perp(P_{\theta, \eta})$$
$$U(X \mid \mu(\theta), \theta_1, \eta) = U_{2, h_2(\mu(\theta), \theta_1, \eta)}(X \mid \mu(\theta), \eta) \in T_\theta^\perp(P_{\theta, \eta}).$$

This proves that for all parameter values (θ, η)

$$U(X \mid \mu(\theta), \theta_1, \eta_1) \in T_\theta^\perp(P_{\theta, \eta}) \cup T_\eta^\perp(P_{\theta, \eta}) \text{ if either } \theta_1 = \theta \text{ or } \eta_1 = \eta.$$

In particular, this yields the desired double robustness property of the estimating function $U(X \mid \mu, \theta, \eta)$:

$$E_{\theta, \eta} U(X \mid \mu(\theta), \theta_1, \eta_1) = 0 \text{ if either } \theta_1 = \theta \text{ or } \eta_1 = \eta.$$

Summary

Let us summarize what we have learned for our censored data model. Firstly, the class of all relevant estimating functions for a parameter μ in the full data model/observed data model can be obtained from the orthogonal complement of the nuisance tangent space in the full data model/observed data model. Theorem 1.3 shows how to map the orthogonal complement of the nuisance tangent space in the full data model into the orthogonal complement of the nuisance tangent space in the observed data model.

Statistical inference for the estimators defined by the corresponding estimating equations is easy if one uses consistent estimators of the nuisance parameters since the influence curve is the standardized version of the estimating function itself. If the nuisance parameters are high-dimensional, then it is important that the estimating function remains unbiased at a misspecified nuisance parameter. Lemma 1.8 shows that this holds, in particular, if the data-generating distribution is linear in the nuisance parameter and the nuisance parameter space is convex. Application of Lemma 1.8 to the corresponding observed data estimating functions yields protection w.r.t. misspecification of convex linear nuisance parameters such as the censoring mechanism G, assuming correct specification of the remaining nuisance parameters. Application of Lemma 1.9 yields a double robust property of our estimating function, allowing either misspecification of G or misspecification of the projection operator into the tangent space of G, but not both.

1.6 Doubly robust estimation in censored data models.

In this section we provide a self-contained proof of the double robustness of T_G-orthogonalized estimating functions in the censored data model with "minimal" conditions, applying the proof of Lemma 1.8, but making precise what is needed at a given misspecified G_1 in our censored data model (Neugebauer, van der Laan, 2002). Subsequently, we provide a generalization of a double robustness result for T_{CAR}-orthogonalized estimating functions in Scharfstein, Rotnitzky, and Robins (1999), which shows that, if the conditional expectation of the T_{CAR}-orthogonalized estimating function, given X, is in the range of the nonparametric information operator, then no further condition is needed. Finally, we present a general method for the implementation of the corresponding doubly robust estimators as proposed and evaluated in Yu, van der Laan (2002).

Consider the censored data structure $Y = \Phi(C, X)$, where X is the full data of interest and C is the censoring or coarsening variable. Here Φ is a known function. Recall that causal inference data structures fall in this category by setting C equal to the observed treatment process A, $X = (X_a : a)$ being the vector of treatment specific counterfactual processes and $Y = \Phi(A, X) \equiv (A, X_A)$. Let $\mathcal{M}^F$ be a model for the distribution F_X of the full-data structure X. In addition, assume that the conditional distribution G of Y given X satisfies coarsening at random (CAR). For notational convenience, we let G denote the conditional distribution of Y given X. Recall that an important consequence of CAR is that it implies factorization $dP_{F_X,G}(Y) = p_{F_X}(Y) dG(Y \mid X)$ in terms of an F_X part and G part of the likelihood so that the consistency of a maximum likelihood estimator under a model for F_X only relies on correct specification of that model.

Let $\mu(F_X)$ be the Euclidean parameter of interest. Let $IC_0(Y \mid G_1, \mu)$ be an initial estimating function which is unbiased under P_{F_X,G_1} (i.e., $E_{P_{F_X,G_1}} IC_0(Y \mid G_1, \mu(F_X)) = 0$ for $F_X \in \mathcal{M}^F$). Consider the orthogonalized estimating function $IC(Y \mid F_X, G_1, \mu)$ for $\mu = \mu(F_X)$, obtained by subtracting from $IC_0(Y \mid G_1, \mu)$ a projection on a tangent space $T_G(P_{F_X,G_1}) \subset T_{CAR}(P_{F_X,G_1})$ of G at P_{F_X,G_1} under a convex model for G. Firstly, these orthogonal estimating functions are unbiased at misspecified F_X as long as G_1 is correct. This follows because the projection operator under P_{F_1,G_1} still maps into functions which have conditional mean zero, given X, w.r.t. G_1. We will now prove a theorem which shows that the estimating functions are also unbiased as long as F_X is correctly specified; that is, $E_{P_{F_X,G}} IC(Y \mid F_X, G_1, \mu(F_X)) = 0$ provided $dG/dG_1 < \infty$. In other words, $P_{F_X,G}$-unbiasedness of $IC(Y \mid F_X, G_1, \mu(F_X))$ holds even at a censoring mechanism G under which the initial estimating function $IC_0(Y \mid G, \mu)$ is biased; that is, $E_{P_{F_X,G}} IC_0(Y \mid G_1, \mu(F_X)) \neq 0$. This

82   1. Introduction

result is very important since it implies that the solution μ_n of the corresponding estimating equation has the same robustness to misspecification of G as the maximum likelihood estimator of $\mu(F_X)$.

Theorem 1.6 *(Neugebauer, van der Laan, 2002) Let $Y = \Phi(X, C)$ for a known function Φ. Let $X \sim F_X \in \mathcal{M}^F$, where $\mathcal{M}^F$ denotes the full data structure model for the distribution of X. Let $Y \mid X \sim G(\cdot \mid X)$, where $G(\cdot \mid X)$ is known to be a member of a convex model $\mathcal{G} \subset \mathcal{G}(CAR)$. Here $\mathcal{G}(CAR)$ denotes the convex model of all conditional distributions satisfying CAR. This implies a model for the observed data structure $Y \sim P_{F_X,G}$. By factorization $dP_{F_X,G}(Y) = p_{F_X}(Y) dG(Y \mid X)$ of the likelihood of Y under CAR, we have that*

$$T_G(P_{F_X,G}) = \overline{\left\{ \frac{d(G_1 - G)(Y \mid X)}{dG(Y \mid X)} : G_1 \in \mathcal{G}, G_1 \ll G \right\}} \subset L_0^2(P_{F_X,G})$$

is the tangent space of G in the observed data model generated by all lines $\alpha \to P_{F_X, \alpha G_1 + (1-\alpha)G} = \alpha P_{F_X,G_1} + (1-\alpha) P_{F_X,G}$ through $P_{F_X,G}$ at $\alpha = 0$.

Let $\mu(F_X) \in \mathbb{R}^k$ be a euclidean parameter of F_X of interest. Consider an estimating function $IC(Y \mid F_X, G, \mu)$ which satisfies at a given $G_1 \in \mathcal{G}$ the following

$$\frac{dG(Y \mid X)}{dG_1(Y \mid X)} < \infty \quad F_X\text{-a.e.} \tag{1.66}$$

$$IC((Y \mid F_X, G_1, \mu(F_X)) \in L_0^2(P_{F_X,G_1}) \tag{1.67}$$

$$IC(Y \mid F_X, G_1, \mu(F_X)) \perp T_G(P_{F_X,G_1}), \tag{1.68}$$

where the tangent space $T_G(P_{F_X,G_1})$ of G at P_{F_X,G_1} is now a subspace of $L_0^2(P_{F_X,G_1})$; that is, the orthogonality relation needs to hold in $L_0^2(P_{F_X,G_1})$. (Note, that (1.67) requires, in particular, $E_{P_{F_X,G_1}} IC(Y \mid F_X, G_1, \mu(F_X)) = 0$) Then

$$E_{P_{F_X,G}} IC(Y \mid F_X, G_1, \mu(F_X)) = 0 \tag{1.69}$$

and

$$IC(Y \mid F_X, G_1, \mu(F_X)) \perp T_G(P_{F_X,G}) \subset L_0^2(P_{F_X,G}). \tag{1.70}$$

Proof. By (1.66) we have that $d(G - G_1)(Y \mid X)/dG_1(Y \mid X) \in T_{G_1}(P_{F_X,G_1})$ is a score of one dimensional submodel $\alpha \to P_{F_X, \alpha G + (1-\alpha) G_1}$ through P_{F_X,G_1} at $\alpha = 0$. Thus by (1.68) we have

$$\begin{aligned} 0 &= E_{P_{F_X,G_1}} IC(Y \mid F_X, G_1, \mu(F_X)) \frac{d(G - G_1)(Y \mid X)}{dG_1(Y \mid X)} \\ &= E_{P_{F_X,G}} IC(Y \mid F_X, G_1, \mu(F_X)) - E_{P_{F_X,G_1}} IC(Y \mid F_X, G_1, \mu(F_X)) \\ &= E_{P_{F_X,G}} IC(Y \mid F_X, G_1, \mu(F_X)) \end{aligned}$$

by (1.67). This proves (1.69).

1.6. Doubly robust estimation in censored data models.

Let $\mu = \mu(F_X)$ and let $G_2 \in \mathcal{G}$ be such that $G_2 \ll G$. We now note that

$$E_{P_{F_X,G}} IC(Y \mid F_X, G_1, \mu) \frac{d(G_2 - G)(Y \mid X)}{dG(Y \mid X)}$$

$$= E_{P_{F_X,G_2}} IC(Y \mid F_X, G_1, \mu) - E_{P_{F_X,G}} IC(Y \mid F_X, G_1, \mu)$$

$$= E_{P_{F_X,G_2}} IC(Y \mid F_X, G_1, \mu) \text{ by (1.69)}.$$

If $dG_2(Y \mid X)/dG_1(Y \mid X) < \infty$, then application of the result (1.69) at $Y \sim P_{F_X,G_2}$ proves that the latter expectation equals zero as well. However, $dG_2/dG_1 = (dG_2/dG) \times (dG/dG_1)$, where dG_2/dG is finite and dG/dG_1 is finite by assumption. Thus, we indeed have dG_1/dG_1 is finite, which proves the theorem. □

Theorem 1.6 teaches us that orthogonalizing an initial function $IC_0(Y \mid G_1, \mu)$ of the observed data Y in $L_0^2(P_{F_X,G_1})$ at a censoring mechanism G_1 under which the initial function has mean zero provides a function $IC_0(Y \mid G_1, \mu) - \Pi(IC_0(\cdot \mid G_1, \mu) \mid T_G(P_{F_X,G_1}))$ which has mean zero under the true data generating distribution $P_{F_X,G}$. Note that Theorem 1.6 assumes that $G \ll G_1$ (i.e., $dG/dG_1 < \infty$). An immediate corollary of Theorem 1.6 is the following.

Corollary 1.1 *Consider the setting of Theorem 1.6. If G_1 can be approximated by a sequence $(G_{1m}, m = 1, \ldots)$ in the sense that $IC(Y \mid F_X, G_{1m}, \mu(F_X)) \to IC(Y \mid F_X, G_1, \mu(F_X))$ for $m \to \infty$ in $L_0^2(P_{F_X,G})$, with G_{1m} satisfying the conditions (1.66), (1.67), and (1.68) (i.e., $G \ll G_{1m}$, $IC(Y \mid F_X, G_{1m}, \mu(F_X)) \in L_0^2(P_{F_X,G_{1m}})$, and $IC(Y \mid F_X, G_{1m}, \mu(F_X)) \perp T_{CAR}(P_{F_X,G_{1m}}))$, then the conclusions (1.69) and (1.70) of Theorem 1.6 hold for $IC(Y \mid F_X, G_1, \mu(F_X))$.*

In other words, the condition $G \ll G_1$ is not a necessary condition, and can , in a particular application, often be deleted by applying this corollary.

The following theorem considers the special case that the estimating function is orthogonalized w.r.t. T_{CAR}, which allows one to exploit additional structure.

Theorem 1.7 *(Generalization of Theorem in Scharfstein, Rotnitzky, and Robins, 1999) Let $Y = \Phi(X, C)$ for a known function Φ. Let $X \sim F_X \in \mathcal{M}^F$, where $\mathcal{M}^F$ denotes the full data structure model for the distribution of X. Let $Y \mid X \sim G(\cdot \mid X)$, where $G(\cdot \mid X)$ is known to be a member of $\mathcal{G}(CAR)$. Here $\mathcal{G}(CAR)$ denotes the convex model of all conditional distributions satisfying CAR. This implies a model for the observed data structure $Y \sim P_{F_X,G}$. By factorization $dP_{F_X,G}(Y) = p_{F_X}(Y) dG(Y \mid X)$ of the likelihood of Y under CAR, we have that*

$$T_{CAR}(P_{F_X,G}) = \overline{\left\{ \frac{d(G_1 - G)(Y \mid X)}{dG(Y \mid X)} : G_1 \in \mathcal{G}(CAR), G_1 \ll G \right\}} \subset L_0^2(P_{F_X,G})$$

84   1. Introduction

is the tangent space of G in the observed data model generated by all lines $\alpha \to P_{F_X,\alpha G_1+(1-\alpha)G} = \alpha P_{F_X,G_1} + (1-\alpha)P_{F_X,G}$ through $P_{F_X,G}$ at $\alpha = 0$ with $dG_1/dG < \infty$, $G_1 \in \mathcal{G}(CAR)$.

Let $\mu(F_X) \in \mathbb{R}^k$ be a euclidean parameter of F_X of interest. Given a $P_{F_X,G}$, let $A_{F_X} : L_0^2(F_X) \to L_0^2(P_{F_X,G})$ be the score operator $A_{F_X}(s)(Y) = E_{F_X}(s(X) \mid Y)$, $A_G : L_0^2(P_{F_X,G}) \to L_0^2(F_X)$ be its adjoint $A_G(v)(X) = E_G(V(Y) \mid X)$, and $I_{F_X,G} : L_0^2(F_X) \to L_0^2(F_X)$ the nonparametric information operator defined by $I_{F_X,G}(s)(X) = E_G(E_{F_X}(s(X) \mid Y) \mid X)$. Let $R(I_{F_X,G})$ denote the range of $I_{F_X,G} : L_0^2(F_X) \to L_0^2(F_X)$.

Consider an estimating function $IC(Y \mid F_X,G,\mu)$ at $G_1 \in \mathcal{G}(CAR)$. Let
$$D(X) \equiv E_{G_1}(IC(Y \mid F_X,G_1,\mu(F_X)) \mid X).$$

Assume

$$IC(Y \mid F_X, G_1, \mu(F_X)) \in L_0^2(P_{F_X,G_1}) \tag{1.71}$$
$$IC(Y \mid F_X, G_1, \mu(F_X)) \perp T_{CAR}(P_{F_X,G_1}) \subset L_0^2(P_{F_X,G_1}) \tag{1.72}$$
$$dG/dG_1 < \infty \text{ or } D \in R(I_{F_X,G_1}). \tag{1.73}$$

(Note, by Theorem 1.3, if $D \in R(I_{F_X,G_1})$, then
$$IC(\cdot \mid F_X, G_1, \mu(F_X)) = A_{F_X} I_{F_X,G_1}^{-}(D), \tag{1.74}$$

where I_{F_X,G_1}^{-} denotes a generalized inverse.)
Then
$$E_{P_{F_X,G}} IC(Y \mid F_X, G_1, \mu(F_X)) = 0 \tag{1.75}$$

and

$$IC(Y \mid F_X, G_1, \mu(F_X)) \perp T_{CAR}(P_{F_X,G}) \subset L_0^2(P_{F_X,G}). \tag{1.76}$$

An element of $L_0^2(P_{F_X,G_1})$ which is orthogonal to $T_{CAR}(P_{F_X,G_1})$ is an element of the closure of the range of the score operator $A_{F_X} : L_0^2(F_X) \to L_0^2(P_{F_X,G_1})$ in $L_0^2(P_{F_X,G_1})$, and, by Theorem 1.3, if it is an element of the range itself, then it equals $A_{F_X} I_{F_X,G_1}^{-1}(D)$ with $D(X) \equiv E_{G_1}(IC(Y \mid F_X, G_1, \mu(F_X)) \mid X)$. Thus conditions (1.71), (1.72) imply that $IC(Y \mid F_X, G_1, \mu(F_X))$ is an element of this closure of the range of the score operator, but do not imply that it is a score and thereby of the form (1.74). Thus one way to interpret Theorem 1.7 is that one does not need the condition $dG/dG_1 < \infty$ if, in fact, $IC(Y \mid F_X, G_1, \mu(F_X))$ is an element of the range of the score operator (i.e., it is a F_X-score itself). Note that $IC(Y \mid F_X, G_1, \mu(F_X))$ being in the range of the score operator $A_{F_X} : L_0^2(F_X) \to L_0^2(P_{F_X,G_1})$ implies that $D \in R(I_{F_X,G_1})$. One immediate application of Theorem 1.7 is that, if I_{F_X,G_1} is 1-1 and onto, then we do not need the condition $dG/dG_1 < \infty$.

Proof. Since $IC(Y \mid F_X, G_1, \mu(F_X)) \perp T_{CAR}(P_{F_X,G_1})$, and $L_0^2(P_{F_X,G_1}) = \overline{R(A_{F_X})} \oplus T_{CAR}(P_{F_X,G_1})$, where $A_{F_X} : L_0^2(F_X) \to L_0^2(P_{F_X,G_1})$ is the score operator defined by $A_{F_X}(s) = E_{F_X}(s(X) \mid Y)$, we have that

$IC(Y \mid F_X, G_1, \mu(F_X)) \in \overline{R(A_{F_X})}$. Thus there exists a sequence $s_m \in L_0^2(F_X)$ such that $IC(Y \mid F_X, G_1, \mu(F_X)) = \lim_{m \to \infty} A_{F_X}(s_m)(Y)$, where the limit is taken in the Hilbert space $L_0^2(P_{F_X,G_1})$. Note that without further conditions, this does not imply convergence in $L^2(P_{F_X,G})$. If $dG/dG_1 < \infty$, then convergence in $L^2(P_{F_X,G_1})$ implies convergence in $L^2(P_{F_X,G})$ and we also have $A_{F_X}(s_m) \in L^2(P_{F_X,G})$. Thus, in this case we have $IC(Y \mid F_X, G_1, \mu(F_X)) = \lim_{m \to \infty} A_{F_X}(s_m)(Y)$ in $L^2(P_{F_X,G})$. If $D(X) = A_{G_1}^\top(IC(\cdot \mid F_X, G_1, \mu(F_X)) \in R(I_{F_X,G_1})$, then $IC(Y \mid F_X, G_1, \mu(F_X)) \in R(A_{F_X})$ and it equals $A_{F_X} I_{F_X,G_1}^-(D)$ (by Theorem 1.3). Thus $s_0 \equiv I_{F_X,G_1}^-(D) \in L_0^2(F_X)$ and $IC(Y \mid F_X, G_1, \mu(F_X)) = A_{F_X}(s_0)$. Since $\| A_{F_X}(s_0) \|_{P_{F_X,G}} \leq \| s_0 \|_{F_X} < \infty$, $A_{F_X}(s_0)$ is an element of $L^2(P_{F_X,G})$. So we can conclude that condition (1.73) implies that either $IC(\cdot \mid F_X, G_1, \mu(F_X)) = A_{F_X}(s_0) \in L^2(P_{F_X,G})$ or $IC(\cdot \mid F_X, G_1, \mu(F_X)) = \lim_{m \to \infty} A_{F_X}(s_m)$ where the convergence is in the Hilbert space $L^2(P_{F_X,G})$. Having established that $A_{F_X}(s_m)$ is integrable w.r.t $P_{F_X,G}$, we can now proceed with noting

$$E_{P_{F_X,G}} A_{F_X}(s_m)(Y)) = E_{P_{F_X,G}} E_{F_X}(s_m(X) \mid Y) = E s_m(X) = 0$$

and, for any score $(dG_2 - dG)/dG$ in $T_{CAR}(P_{F_X,G})$ (with $dG_2/dG < \infty$) we have

$$\begin{aligned}
E_{P_{F_X,G}}\left(A_{F_X}(s_m)(Y) \frac{dG_2 - dG}{dG}(Y \mid X)\right) &= E_{P_{F_X,G_2}} A_{F_X}(s_m)(Y) \\
&\quad - E_{P_{F_X,G}} A_{F_X}(s_m)(Y) \\
&= E_{P_{F_X,G_2}} A_{F_X}(s_m)(Y) \\
&= E_{P_{F_X,G_2}} E_{F_X}(s_m(X) \mid Y) \\
&= E s_m(X) = 0.
\end{aligned}$$

The same equations apply to $A_{F_X}(s_0)$. This completes the proof of the Theorem for the case that $IC(Y \mid F_X, G_1, \mu(F_X)) = A_{F_X}(s_0)$. For the case where we assumed $dG/dG_1 < \infty$, we have shown $A_{F_X}(s_m) \in L_0^2(P_{F_X,G})$, $A_{F_X}(s_m) \perp T_{CAR}(P_{F_X,G})$, and $A_{F_X}(s_m) \to IC(Y \mid F_X, G_1, \mu(F_X))$ with convergence w.r.t. the $L^2(P_{F_X,G})$-norm. Thus

$$E_{P_{F_X,G}} IC(Y \mid F_X, G_1, \mu(F_X)) = \lim_{m \to \infty} E_{P_{F_X,G}} A_{F_X}(s_m)(Y)) = 0. \quad \square$$

If $IC_0(Y \mid G, \mu)$ is not unbiased under $P_{F_X,G}$, then $IC(Y \mid F_X, G, \mu) = IC_0(Y \mid G, \mu) - \Pi(IC_0(Y \mid G, \mu) \mid T_G(P_{F_X,G}))$ will be biased under $P_{F_X,G}$; that is, it equals a non-mean zero function $IC_0(Y \mid G, \mu)$ plus a mean zero function. In the following lemma we show how one can modify this definition of $IC(Y \mid F_X, G, \mu)$ at such a G so that it becomes an unbiased estimating function.

Lemma 1.10 *Let $T_{nuis}^{F,\perp}(F_X)$ be the orthogonal complement of the nuisance tangent space in the full data model $\mathcal{M}^F$. Let $IC_0(Y \mid G, \mu)$ be an initial*

86   1. Introduction

estimating function. At $G_1 \in \mathcal{G}$ s.t.

$$E_{G_1}(IC_0(Y \mid G_1, \mu(F_X)) \mid X) \in T_{nuis}^{F,\perp}(F_X) \qquad (1.77)$$

(and thus has, in particular, mean zero w.r.t. F_X) we define

$$IC(Y \mid F_X, G_1, \mu) = IC_0(Y \mid G_1, \mu) - \Pi(IC_0(\cdot \mid G_1, \mu) \mid T_G(P_{F_X, G_1})),$$

where the projection is defined in $L_0^2(P_{F_X, G_1})$, and $T_G(P_{F_X, G_1})$ is the tangent space of the parameter G at P_{F_X, G_1}. Consider a $G \in \mathcal{G}$ not satisfying (1.77). Assume that there exists a sequence $G_m \in \mathcal{G}$ (converging to G) satisfying (1.77) for each m (i.e., set $G_1 = G_m$ in (1.77)), $dG/dG_m < \infty$, and that $\lim_{m \to \infty} IC(Y \mid F_X, G_m, \mu)$ is a well defined limit in $L_0^2(P_{F_X, G})$

$$IC(Y \mid F_X, G, \mu) \equiv \lim_{m \to \infty} IC(Y \mid F_X, G_m, \mu).$$

Then (since, by theorem 1.6, $E_{P_{F_X, G}} IC(Y \mid F_X, G_m, \mu(F_X)) = 0$) $E_{P_{F_X, G}} IC(Y \mid F_X, G, \mu(F_X)) = 0$.

Maximum likelihood estimation versus estimating functions.

As we have discussed in detail, in most semiparametric models, due to the curse of dimensionality, the full data model $\mathcal{M}^F$ is so large that maximum likelihood estimators of F_X are either not well defined or suffer from poor practical performance. Let $\mathcal{M}^{F,w} \subset \mathcal{M}^F$ be a submodel of the full data model for which maximum likelihood estimators of F_X have good finite sample performance. Let F_n be a maximum likelihood estimator of F_X according to this model $\mathcal{M}^{F,w}$:

$$F_n = \max_{F \in \mathcal{M}^{F,w}}^{-1} \prod_{i=1}^n p_F(Y_i).$$

Let G_n be a maximum likelihood estimator of G according to a convex model $\mathcal{G} \subset \mathcal{G}(CAR)$:

$$G_n = \max_{G \in \mathcal{G}}^{-1} \prod_{i=1}^n dG(Y_i \mid X_i).$$

Let's compare the estimators $\mu(F_n)$ versus the solution $\mu_{n,DR}$ of an estimating equation $0 = \sum_i IC(Y_i \mid F_n, G_n, \mu)$ in μ, whose estimating function is doubly robust in the sense:

$$E_{P_{F_X, G}} IC(Y \mid F_1, G_1, \mu(F_X)) = 0 \text{ if } F_1 = F_X \text{ or}$$

$G_1 = G$ and G satisfies a certain identifiability condition (e.g., the one typically needed for inverse probability censoring weighted estimating functions to be unbiased). If $F_X \in \mathcal{M}^{F,w}$, then $\mu_{n,DR}$ solves asymptotically the always unbiased estimating function $IC(Y \mid F_X, G_1, \mu)$, where G_1 denotes the limit of G_n. Consequently, if $\mathcal{M}^{F,w}$ is correct, then both the maximum likelihood estimator $\mu(F_n)$ and $\mu_{n,DR}$ will be consistent. If $\mathcal{M}^{F,w}$ is misspecified, then the maximum likelihood estimator $\mu(F_n)$ is inconsistent, while $\mu_{n,DR}$ will remain consistent if $G \in \mathcal{G}$ and G satisfies the identifiability condition. This shows that $\mu_{n,DR}$ is more robust than the maximum likelihood estimator $\mu(F_n)$. Of course, $\mu_{n,DR}$ is less efficient than $\mu(F_n)$ if $\mathcal{M}^{F,w}$ is correct.

Application to marginal structural point treatment model.

Let A be a treatment variable with discrete outcome space $\mathcal{A}$. Let $(Z_a : a \in \mathcal{A})$ be the treatment specific outcomes/counterfactuals and let W be a vector of baseline covariates. The full data structure is defined as $X = ((Z_a : a \in \mathcal{A}), W)$ and the observed data structure is $Y = (A, Z = Z_A, W)$. Consider a marginal structural model $E(Z_a \mid V) = m(a, V \mid \beta)$, where V denotes some of the baseline covariates we wish to adjust for in this causal model. We also assume the randomization assumption $g(a \mid X) \equiv P(A = a \mid X) = P(A = a \mid W)$. The inverse probability treatment weighted estimating functions for β are given by:

$$\left\{ IC_0(Y \mid G, h, \beta) = \frac{h(A, V)}{g(A \mid X)} \epsilon(\beta) : h \right\},$$

where $\epsilon(\beta) = Z - m(A, V \mid \beta)$. The conditional expectation of $IC_0(Y \mid G, h, \beta)$, given X, equals $\sum_{a \in \mathcal{A}} h(a, V) \epsilon_a(\beta) \in T_{nuis}^{F,\perp}(F_X)$ if

$$\max_{a \in \mathcal{A}} \frac{h(a, V)}{g(a \mid W)} < \infty \; F_W\text{-a.e.} \quad (1.78)$$

Let's now carry out the general method for constructing doubly robust estimating functions as presented above. Consider a $g_1(a \mid W)$ that satisfies $g_1(a \mid W) > 0$ for all $a \in \mathcal{A}$ F_W-a.e. Orthogonalizing $IC_0(Y \mid G_1, h, \beta)$ w.r.t. $T_{RA}(P_{F_X, G_1}) = \{\Phi(A, W) : E_{G_1}(\Phi(A, W) \mid W) = 0\}$ (i.e., the tangent space of G at G_1 when only assuming the randomization assumption) in the Hilbert space $L_0^2(P_{F_X, G_1})$ yields

$$IC(Y \mid Q, G_1, h, \beta) = IC_0(Y \mid G_1, h, \beta) - \frac{h(A, V)}{g_1(A \mid W)} Q(A, W)$$
$$+ \sum_{a \in \mathcal{A}} h(a, V) Q(a, W),$$

where $Q(A, W) = E(\epsilon(\beta) \mid A, W)$ is a parameter of F_X. Here, we used that a projection of a function IC_0 on $T_{RA}(P_{F_X, G_1})$ is given by the conditional expectation of IC_0, given A, W, minus the conditional expectation of IC_0, given W. Since $g/g_1 < \infty$, application of Theorem 1.6 teaches us that $E_{P_{F_X,G}}(IC(Y \mid Q, G_1, h, \beta)) = 0$, and that it is orthogonal to (i.e. it has covariance zero with) any function $\Phi(A, W)$ which has conditional mean zero, given W (w.r.t. to true G). This can be explicitly verified to be true.

At this point, it is of interest to note that orthogonalizing $IC_0(Y \mid G, h, \beta)$ w.r.t. $T_{RA}(P_{F_X, G})$ in $L_0^2(P_{F_X, G})$ would result in a biased estimating function at any G not satisfying (1.78): one would subtract from a biased estimating function IC_0 a function which has conditional mean zero, given W, which thus results in a biased estimating function. Interestingly enough, orthogonalizing it in the wrong world $L_0^2(P_{F_X,G_1})$, that is, we act as if the true treatment mechanism equals a G_1 satisfying (1.78), results in an unbiased estimating function.

We will now also define the estimating function at a G not satisfying (1.78), as in lemma 1.10. Consider a sequence $(g_{1m}, m = 1, \ldots)$ of conditional probability distributions which satisfies $g_{1m}(a \mid W) > 0$ for all $a \in \mathcal{A}$, F_W-a.e., and $g_{1m}(a \mid W) \to g(a \mid W)$ for $m \to \infty$. For example,

$$g_{1m}(a \mid W) \equiv \frac{g(a \mid W) + \delta_m(a)}{\sum_{a \in \mathcal{A}} g(a \mid W) + \delta_m(a)},$$

where $\delta_m(a) > 0$ for all $a \in \mathcal{A}$ and $\delta_m(a) \to 0$ for $m \to \infty$. Now, note that the limit of $IC(Y \mid Q, G_{1m}, h, \beta)$ in $L_0^2(P_{F_X,G})$ (!), equals

$$IC(Y \mid Q, G, h, \beta) = IC_0(Y \mid G, h, \beta) - \frac{h(A, V)}{g(A \mid W)} Q(A, W)$$
$$+ \sum_{a \in \mathcal{A}} h(a, V) Q(a, W).$$

To show this, one needs to notice that in the world where G is the true treatment mechanism outcomes $A = a$ for which $g(a \mid W) = 0$ simply do not occur and thus do not contribute to the distance in $L_0^2(P_{F_X,G})$. Note also that $IC(Y \mid Q, G, h, \beta)$ does not equal IC_0 minus its projection on $T_{RA}(P_{F_X,G})$ at a G not satisfying (1.78). In fact, the sum of the second and third term does not have mean zero at such a G. We have now defined a doubly robust estimating function $IC(Y \mid Q, G, h, \beta)$ as a function of (Q, G, h, β) and the observed data structure Y.

Doubly robust estimating functions for censored longitudinal data structures.

Let time be discrete $j = 1, \ldots, p+1$. Let $A(j)$ denote treatment and/or censoring actions assigned to the subject at time j, $j = 1, \ldots, p$. For each possible action regime $a = (a(1), \ldots, a(p))$, we define X_a as a time-dependent process one would have observed on the subject if he/she would have followed action regime a. It is assumed that $X_a(j) = X_{\bar{a}(j-1)}(j)$, $j = 1, \ldots, p+1$; that is, only the past of the action process influences the process value at the current time $t = j$. Let $\mathcal{A}$ be the set of possible action regimes and $X = (X_a : a \in \mathcal{A})$ is the vector of action-specific processes, which represents the full data structure. Consider the following observed longitudinal data structure on a randomly sampled subject:

$$Y = (X(1), A(1), X_{A(1)}(2), A(2), \ldots, X_{\bar{A}(p-1)}(p), A(p), X_{\bar{A}(p)}(p+1)).$$

Let F_X be the distribution of X and $G(\cdot \mid X)$ be the distribution of A, given X. We assume that G satisfies the sequential randomization assumption

1.6. Doubly robust estimation in censored data models.

(SRA)
$$g(A(j) \mid \bar{A}(j-1), X) = g(A(j) \mid \bar{A}(j-1), \bar{X}_A(j)), \quad j = 1, \ldots, p.$$

If we define $L(j) \equiv X_{\bar{A}(j-1)}(j)$, then
$$Y = L(1), A(1), \ldots, L(p), A(p), L(p+1)$$

and the likelihood of Y is given by

$$dP_{F_X, G}(Y) = \prod_{j=1}^{p+1} f(L(j) \mid \bar{L}(j-1), \bar{A}(j-1)) \prod_{j=1}^{p} g(A(j) \mid \bar{A}(j-1), \bar{L}(j)).$$

By CAR, and the factorization of the likelihood under CAR, we have that the F_X part of the likelihood is

$$Q(F_X) \equiv \prod_{j=1}^{p} f(L(j) \mid \bar{L}(j-1), \bar{A}(j-1))$$

and the G part of the likelihood is

$$g(\bar{A} \mid X) = \prod_{j=1}^{p} g(A(j) \mid \bar{L}(j), \bar{A}(j-1)).$$

Thus, the data generating distribution $P_{F_X, G}$ can be parametrized as $P_{Q(F_X), G}$, as well.

Consider a particular full data model $\mathcal{M}^F$ for F_X. If A includes treatment variables, then this full-data model could be a causal model such as a marginal structural model. Let $\mu = \mu(F_X) \in \mathbb{R}^q$ be the euclidean parameter of interest.

We are now ready to describe a general methodology for obtaining doubly robust estimating functions for μ and the corresponding doubly robust estimator of μ. Let $IC_0(Y \mid G, \mu)$ be an initial estimating function for μ (e.g., an inverse probability of action weighted estimating function) which satisfies:

$$E_G(IC_0(Y \mid G, \mu) \mid X) \in T_{nuis}^{F, \perp}(F_X) \tag{1.79}$$

under a particular identifiability condition on G. In our examples of inverse probability of action weighted estimating functions (e.g., see Chapter 6), a sufficient condition for (1.79) is that the set

$$\{a(j) : g(a(j) \mid \bar{A}(j-1) = \bar{a}(j-1), \bar{L}(j))) > 0\}, \tag{1.80}$$

does not depend on $\bar{L}(j)$, $j = 1, \ldots, p$. In other words, the set of possible actions at time j, given the observed past, is allowed to be a function of the treatment past $\bar{a}(j-1)$, but should not depend on the confounding covariates of the past. In order to obtain the doubly robust estimating function, we orthogonalize IC_0 w.r.t. to the tangent space T_{SRA} of G under the sole assumption SRA. Consider a $G_1 \in \mathcal{G}(SRA)$ for which (1.79) holds.

By Theorem 1.2, the projection of $IC_0(Y \mid G_1, \mu)$ onto $T_{SRA}(P_{F_X, G_1})$ in the Hilbert space $L_0^2(P_{F_X, G_1})$ is given by

$$IC_{SRA}(Y \mid Q(F_X), G_1) =$$
$$\sum_{j=1}^{p} E_{P_{Q(F_X)}, G_1}(IC_0(Y \mid G_1, \mu(F_X)) \mid \bar{A}(j), \bar{L}(j))$$
$$- \sum_{j=1}^{p} E_{P_{Q(F_X)}, G_1}(IC_0(Y \mid G_1, \mu(F_X)) \mid \bar{A}(j-1), \bar{L}(j)).$$

For j larger than the point at which the subject died or got right-censored the conditional data $\bar{A}(j-1), \bar{L}(j)$ equals Y, so that the conditional expectations reduce to $IC_0(Y \mid G_1, \mu(F_X))$. Thus, the sum over j only runs up till this time point.

Theorem 1.6 teaches us now that

$$IC(Y \mid G_1, Q(F_X), \mu(F_X)) = IC_0(Y \mid G_1, \mu(F_X)) - IC_{SRA}(Y \mid Q(F_X), G_1)$$

has expectation zero under the true data generating distribution $P_{F_X, G} = P_{Q(F_X), G}$ at any G_1 satisfying (1.79) and $dG/dG_1 < \infty$, even when the true G does not satisfy the identifiability condition (1.79) itself. Above, we showed how to define the estimating function $IC(Y \mid Q, G)$ at a G not satisfying (1.80), but we will illustrate this in detail below for a particular example.

Firstly, we will present the general estimating function procedure for μ based on this estimating function. Consider a semiparametric or parametric model for the F_X-part of the likelihood:

$$Q(\theta) = \prod_{j=1}^{p} f_\theta(L(j) \mid \bar{L}(j-1), \bar{A}(j-1)).$$

Let g_η be a semiparametric or parametric model for the G-part of the likelihood:

$$g_\eta(\bar{A} \mid X) = \prod_{j=1}^{p} g_\eta(A(j) \mid \bar{L}(j), \bar{A}(j-1)).$$

Let θ_n and η_n be the maximum likelihood estimators and $Q_n = Q(\theta_n)$, $G_n = G_{\eta_n}$ be the corresponding estimators of $Q(F_X)$ and G, respectively. In order to construct doubly robust estimators we estimate μ with the solution μ_n of

$$0 = \sum_{i=1}^{n} IC(Y_i \mid G_n, Q_n, \mu).$$

Note that the projection term $IC_{SRA}(Y \mid G_n, Q_n)$ of the estimating function does only depend on G_n, Q_n so that it does not need to be reevaluated for each μ (e.g., in a Newton-Raphson algorithm); that is, the μ in $E(IC_0(Y \mid \mu) \mid \bar{A}(j), \bar{L}(j))$ is replaced by the value $\mu(Q_n)$ corresponding with the maximum likelihood estimator. The actual evaluation of $IC_{SRA}(Y \mid G_n, Q_n)$ requires computing, for $j = 1, \ldots, p$ (where for j larger than the point at which the subject died or got right-censored it has a known value, and, in fact, at these j the projection term is zero),

$$E_{P_{Q_n,G_n}}(IC_0(Y \mid G_n, \mu(Q_n)) \mid \bar{A}(j), \bar{L}(j)).$$

We propose to evaluate this conditional expectation under the known law P_{Q_n,G_n} with Monte-Carlo simulation in the following manner.

Algorithm for evaluation of the conditional expectation: Consider a particular observation Y and let j be fixed.
For $b = 1$ till B do Step 1 till Step 5:
Step 1: Set $m = j + 1$.
Step 2: Generate $L(m)$ from $f_{\theta_n}(\cdot \mid \bar{L}(m-1), \bar{A}(m-1))$.
Step 3: Generate $A(m)$ from $g_{\eta_n}(\cdot \mid \bar{A}(m-1), \bar{L}(m))$.
Step 4: Repeat Step 2 and Step 3 till one has observed the complete data structure which we denote with Y_b^*.
Step 5: Evaluate $IC_0(Y_b^* \mid G_n, \mu(Q_n))$ at this observation Y_b^*.
Output: Evaluate

$$\frac{1}{B} \sum_{b=1}^{B} IC_0(Y_b^* \mid G_n, \mu(Q_n)).$$

In Yu, van der Laan (2002) we implemented this Monte-Carlo simulation method to construct doubly robust estimators in a marginal structural model for time-dependent treatment in longitudinal studies. Simulations comparing the maximum likelihood estimator and the doubly robust estimator show that the maximum likelihood estimator is dramatically more sensitive to model misspecification of $Q(F_X)$ than the doubly robust estimator. This even holds up at extreme levels of confounding, under which the IPTW-estimator is inconsistent and the consistency of the doubly robust estimators fully relies on correct specification of $Q(F_X)$.

If the number of time points p is large or $\bar{L}(m)$ and/or $\bar{A}(m)$ is high dimensional, the above algorithm may not be computationally feasible. In that case the methods in Section 6.4 can be used to construct doubly robust estimators.

We will now illustrate with a particular example how to define the projection term $IC_{SRA}(Y \mid G, Q)$ at a G not satisfying the identifiability condition (1.79): recall that it now does not correspond with an actual projection onto T_{SRA} in $L_0^2(P_{F_X,G})$. This involves working out the representation $IC_{SRA}(Y \mid G_1, Q(F_X))$ at a G_1 with $dG/dG_1 < \infty$ satisfying the identifiability condition and subsequently making G_1 approximate G. Consider the inverse probability of treatment weighted mapping for a marginal structural multivariate generalized regression model as covered in section

1.3 of the form:

$$IC_0(Y \mid G_1, \mu) = \sum_{l=1}^{p} \frac{h(\bar{A}(l), V)\epsilon_l(\beta)}{g_1(\bar{A}(l) \mid X)},$$

where $g_1(\bar{A}(l) \mid X) = \prod_{t=1}^{l} g_1(A(t) \mid \bar{A}(t-1), \bar{L}(t))$. Here, the l-th term in the sum is only a function of $\bar{A}(l), \bar{L}(l)$. Under condition (1.80) on G_1, we have $E_{G_1}(IC_0(Y \mid G_1, \mu) \mid X) \in T_{nuis}^{F,\perp}(F_X)$ and, thus, in particular, that $IC_0(Y \mid G, \mu)$ is an unbiased estimating function for μ. Under this condition on G_1, we have:

$$E_{Q(F_X), G_1}(IC_0(Y) \mid \bar{A}(j), \bar{L}(j)) = \sum_{l=1}^{j} \frac{h(\bar{A}(l), V)\epsilon_l(\beta)}{g_1(\bar{A}(l) \mid X)} + \frac{1}{g_1(\bar{A}(j)\mid X)} \sum_{l=j+1}^{p} \int h(\bar{A}(l), V)\epsilon_l(\beta) dP(\underline{A}(j+1), \underline{L}(j+1)),$$

where $dP(\underline{A}(j+1), \underline{L}(j+1))$ is defined as

$$\prod_{t>j} f(L(t) \mid \bar{L}(t-1), \bar{A}(t-1)) \prod_{t>l} g_1(A(t) \mid \bar{A}(t-1), \bar{L}(t)).$$

Here we used the notation $\underline{L}(j+1) = (L(j+1), \ldots, L(p))$ to denote the future sample path of L. The integral over $A(t)$, given $\bar{L}(t), \bar{A}(t-1)$, sums up over all possible outcomes of $A(t)$, given $\bar{A}(t-1)$ (which is thus a set independent of $\bar{L}(t)$), $t = j+1, \ldots, p$. If we would have worked out this conditional expectation under a G not satisfying (1.80), then we would only have summed over the $A(t)$ which occur with positive probability under $g(A(t) \mid \bar{L}(t), \bar{A}(t-1))$. Consequently, at a g_1 not satisfying (1.80), the last integral is not equal to the actual conditional expectation, and the corresponding IC_{SRA} expression does not equal the projection onto T_{SRA}. We can evaluate this integral with the Monte-Carlo simulation method described above, but where we choose a uniform distribution for the $A(t)$, $t = j+1, \ldots, l$.

Let $IC_{SRA}(Y \mid G, Q)$ be defined by this latter integral. We claim that this definition of IC_{SRA} indeed satisfies that $IC_{SRA}(Y \mid G, Q) = \lim_{m \to \infty} IC_{SRA}(Y \mid G_{1m}, Q)$ for a sequence G_{1m} satisfying (1.80), where the limit holds in $L_0^2(P_{F_X,G})$, as required. In other words, $IC_{SRA}(Y \mid G, Q)$ actually equals the projection of $IC_0(Y \mid G, \mu)$ onto $T_{SRA}(P_{F_X,G})$ at a G satisfying (1.79), but it is something else at a G not satisfying (1.79).

Remark

Suppose that the nonparametric identifiability condition (1.80) is practically (but not theoretically) violated; that is, the conditional probability $g(\bar{a} \mid X)$ on certain possible treatment regimes $\bar{a}$ is extremely small relative to the sample size so that the data cannot be distinguished from the data from an action mechanism g^* which theoretically violates the identifiability condition. In this case, the solution of the IPTW estimating equation $0 = \sum_i IC_0(Y_i \mid G, \mu)$ will suffer from large finite sample bias, comparable with the bias of the estimator solving the biased estimating equation $0 = \sum_i IC_0(Y_i \mid G^*, \mu)$ at G^*. However, if the number B of replicates in the Monte-Carlo simulation method for evaluating the conditional expectations is very large, then, one will still have that the doubly robust estimating function gives approximately unbiased estimators for finite samples. In other words, the practical violation affects the finite sample bias of the IPTW-estimator, but not the finite sample bias of the doubly robust estimator, while the theoretical violation would make the doubly robust estimator biased as well. This explains a finding in our simulations (Yu, van der Laan, 2002) which showed that the T_{SRA}-orthogonalized estimating functions, using the Monte-Carlo simulation method with B large relative to sample size, would still be unbiased at a treatment mechanism suffering from extreme confounding which caused the IPTW-estimator to be very biased. On the other hand, the practical violation of the identifiability condition can have a dramatic impact on the variance of the doubly robust estimator. Therefore, we believe it is still beneficial to artificially truncate the weights used in the IPTW-estimating function. In either case, in spite of the practical violation of the nonparametric identifiability condition, there is no need to do the algebraic evaluation of IC_{SRA} as carried out above to modify the definition of IC_{SRA}.

1.7 Using Cross-Validation to Select Nuisance Parameter Models

Consider the censored data structure $Y = \Phi(C, X) \sim P_{F_X, G}$, and let us consider the model $\mathcal{M}(\mathcal{G})$. Let $\mu = \mu(F_X) \in \mathbb{R}^k$ be the Euclidean parameter of interest. The estimating equation methodology presented in the previous examples and in the book in general defines estimators μ_n as a solution of an estimating equation $0 = \sum_{i=1}^n IC(Y_i \mid Q_n, G_n, D_h(\cdot \mid \mu))$. Beyond the index h of the full data structure estimating function, this estimating equation is indexed by an estimator G_n of the censoring mechanism G according to the model $\mathcal{G}$ and an estimator Q_n of another large nuisance parameter $Q = Q(F_X, G)$ according to a model $\mathcal{Q}^w$.

The efficiency and/or the consistency of μ_n is affected by the choice of these models $\mathcal{G}, \mathcal{Q}^w$. For example, consider the missing covariate data structure of Example 1.1. In this case, $\mathcal{G}$ might represent a logistic regression for the missingness indicator conditional on the observed covariates, and $Q = E(D(X) \mid W, \Delta = 1)$ is a regression among the complete observations for which we can assume a linear regression model $\mathcal{Q}^w$. The selection of the covariates for each of the two models and the flexibility in which they enter these models are choices to be made by the user.

An important point that we need to make is that asymptotics does not guide us in selecting these working models for the nuisance parameters of the estimating function for μ. For example, by the asymptotics presented in Chapter 2, for any model $\mathcal{G}$ containing the true G, μ_n is consistent and asymptotically linear, but the larger the working model $\mathcal{G}$, the more asymptotically efficient μ_n will be. Thus, asymptotics would suggest setting $\mathcal{G} = \mathcal{G}(CAR)$, which results, by the curse of dimensionality, in miserable finite sample performance of μ_n. On the other hand, given a correct model $\mathcal{G}$, our asymptotics teaches us that any working model $\mathcal{Q}^w$ results in a consistent and asymptotically linear estimator μ_n, and a correctly specified working model $\mathcal{Q}^w$ achieves maximal asymptotic efficiency of μ_n. Thus, asymptotics suggests making sure that $\mathcal{Q}^w$ contains the true parameter $Q(F_X, G)$. Similarly, the choice of full data index h can have a substantial effect on the efficiency, and the asymptotically optimal index is $h_{opt}(F_X, G)$, but, by the curse of dimensionality, nonparametric estimation of this optimal index h_{opt} results in poor estimators μ_n. Since asymptotics fails to assist the user in selecting nuisance parameter models, we need a criterion that aims to guide us in choosing working models that maximize the *finite sample* efficiency of μ_n.

In the next subsection, we propose a distance-based cross-validation method minimizing a particular criterion over the potential working models for G and Q. We will refer to this criterian as a semiparametric model selection criterion. This method was originally introduced, in general, in Pavlic and van der Laan (2002). Pavlic, van der Laan (2002) study this method for the purpose of selecting the number of components in mixture models. Brookhart and van der Laan (2002b) applied this method for selecting regression models for the treatment mechanism G and Q in a marginal structural causal model. The expected value of our proposed cross-validation criterion is minimized by the nuisance parameter model $\mathcal{G}, \mathcal{Q}^w$ that minimizes the finite sample mean squared error of the estimator μ_n based on a sample of size $n*p$ for the parameter of interest μ, where, p is the proportion used for trainings sample (and $1 - p$ is the proportion used for the validation sample) . Brookhart and van der Laan (2002b) carry out a simulation study examining the performance of this criterion for selecting a treatment mechanism model in a marginal structural model of point treatment data. They also propose a forward/backward selection algorithm for selecting covariates in the treatment model and Q based on this cross-validation criterion. They apply this forward/backward selection method to select a treatment mechanism model and regression model for Q in a marginal structural model analysis of the causal relationship between boiled water use and diarrhea in HIV-positive men. We propose to use this model selection method in practice for any of the proposed estimators in this book.

1.7.1 A semiparametric model selection criterian

Let $P = P_{F_X, G}$ be the true data-generating distribution. The methods discussed in this section assume we have available an initial estimator $u_{n,0}$

with no or minimal finite sample bias for estimating μ. In observational studies in which data are missing by happenstance and subjects self-select treatment, even if we are willing to assume the data are CAR (i.e impose model $M(CAR)$), we have seen that, because of the curse of dimensionality, no such estimator exists unless we further assume we have available a correct lower dimensional model for either g or F_X (but we do not have to know which of two candidate models is correct) i.e. unless we further assume model M holds. In other word the estimation of μ from model $M(CAR)$ without addiitonal assumptions is an ill-posed problem. In settings in which we cannot guarantee near unbiasedness of our initial estinmator $u_{n,0}$, our methods are still useful for finding estimators of the mean of $u_{n,0}$ that haven smaller MSE than $u_{n,0}$ itself . Of course, even when $u_{n,0}$ is known to be unbiased it is only sometimes desirable to try to find, as we do here, an estimator with smaller mean squared error ; for example if, in the future, many studies will be combined in a meta-analysis, it may preferable to report an unbiased estimator with its associated variance for each study rather than a biased estimator with smaller MSE. In additon to $u_{n,0}$ we suppose we have candidiate estimators $\mu_{n,l}$ of $\mu \in \mathbb{R}^k$, $l = 1, \ldots, L$, where l indexes a particular choice of working models for these nuisance parameters Q and G.

Regarding the choice $\mu_{n,0}$, for example, $\mu_{n,0}$ could be an inverse probability of censoring weighted estimator including in the censoring model $\mathcal{G}$ all variables explaining informative censoring. In Brookhart and van der Laan (2002b), it is noticed in simulations that it is beneficial to use a quite efficient estimator $\mu_{n,0}$ since the variance of $\mu_{n,0}$ affects the variability of the proposed criteria. From that point of view, one might choose $\mu_{n,0}$ to be a doubly robust estimator itself, obtained by solving a T_{CAR}-orthogonalized inverse probability of censoring weighted estimating function using ad hoc choices for the working models $\mathcal{M}^{F,w}$ and $\mathcal{G}$.

The method for selecting l requires a choice of distance $d(\mu_1, \mu_2)$ between two vectors $\mu_1, \mu_2 \in \mathbb{R}^k$. We will choose $d(\mu_1, \mu_2) = \sum_{j=1}^{k}(\mu_{1j} - \mu_{2j})^2$. Let $p \in (0, 1)$ be given. Clearly, one wants to choose p close to 1 to make the expectation of the proposed criterion $c_n(l)$ below approximate the MSE of the estimator based on the full data set, but choosing p too close to one, results in a more variable criterion. This is a problem common to model cross-validation and further research is needed to understand the trade off. Let $S_j \subset \{Y_1, \ldots, Y_n\}$ be a random subset of average size np, and let $T_j = \{Y_1, \ldots, Y_n\}/S_j$ be the remaining set of observations, $j = 1, \ldots, J$. We refer to S_j as a training sample and T_j as a test sample corresponding with the jth split of the sample. Let $\mu_{n,l}(S_j)$ and $\mu_{n,0}(T_j)$ be the estimator $\mu_{n,l}$ and μ_n^0 applied to the sample S_j and T_j, respectively, with $l = 1, \ldots, L$.

We propose to estimate μ with μ_{n,l^*}, where l^* is the minimizer of

$$l \to c_n(l) \equiv \sum_{j=1}^{J} d(\mu_{n,l}(S_j), \mu_{n,0}(T_j)).$$

It is straightforward to show that

$$Ec_n(l)/J = d(E\mu_{n,l}, E\mu_{n,0}) + \text{VAR}(\mu_{n,l}(S_j)) + \text{Constant},$$

where $\text{VAR}(\mu_{n,l}(S_j))$ is the variance of $\mu_{n,l}$ based on np observations. Thus, if $E\mu_{n,0} = \mu$, then minimizing $Ec_n(l)$ corresponds exactly with minimizing the finite sample mean squared error of $\mu_{n,l}$ over l, but based on np rather than the actual n observations. So there is some prejudice against biased estimators.

Establishing a "confidence measure" of l^*

We can also report an l_j^* for each sample split, $j = 1, \ldots, J$, where l_j^* is the minimizer of

$$l \to d(\mu_{n,l}(S_j), \mu_{n,0}(T_j)).$$

The variability of l_j^* gives us a sense of the variability of l^* due to sample splits. At minimum, it can be used to compare results across different analyses (e.g., using different sequences of models). In addition, the voting majority rule $\ell^* = \max_l^{-1} \#\{j : \ell_j^* = l\}$ provides an alternative method of selecting l.

Remark

An interesting suggestion is to estimate G and Q, as needed in the estimators $\mu_{n,l}(S_j)$ and $\mu_{n,0}(T_j)$, with estimators $G_{n,l}, G_{n,0}, Q_{n,l}, Q_{n,0}$ based on the whole sample. If $\mu_{n,l}$ is based on solving an estimating function that is asymptotically an element of $T_{nuis}^{\perp}(\mathcal{M}(CAR))$, then one can argue that this will not cause a significant bias in the criterion $c_n(l)$, while it certainly results in a significant reduction of its variance (and computing time). In addition, even when the estimating function is not completely orthogonal, we have seen in some preliminary simulations that the finite sample bias in the criterion has no significant effect on the bias of its minimizer.

Remark

A model selection criterian $l \to c_n(l)$ is a random function in $l \in \{1, \ldots, L\}$, where L is the number of models considered. So even when the minimum of $l \to Ec_n(l)$ identifies an optimal model indexed by l^*, the probability of selecting this best model l^* by minimizing the random function $c_n(\cdot)$, and the probability of selecting a truly bad model, are affected by the number of models L considered, and the multivariate distribution of $(c_n(1), \ldots, c_n(L))$. In principle, by identifying the influence curves of $\mu_{n,0}$ and the l-specific estimates based on the training sample, we could obtain an estimate $\hat{\Sigma}$ of a covariance matrix of $(c_n(1), \ldots, c_n(L))$. Assuming that $c_n(\cdot)$ follows a multivariate normal distribution $N(Ec_n, \hat{\Sigma})$, the problem becomes to estimate the minimizer of Ec_n based on a single observation from this multivariate normal distribution. We do not consider the optimal solution to this estimation problem in this book. In addition, it seems sensible to redefine the estimation problem as a subset selection problem in which one wants to determine a subset of $\{1, \ldots, L\}$ which contains with large probability the minimizer of Ec_n based on a single observation from the L-variate normal distribution $N(Ec_n, \hat{\Sigma})$. We raise these issues as topics for future research.

1.7.2 Forward/backward selection of a nuisance parameter model based on cross-validation with respect to the parameter of interest.

To be specific, let G be the nuisance parameter, and suppose that the models for G that we consider are regression models defined by the set of covariates that we enter in the model. For example, if $Y = (\min(C, T), \Delta = I(T < C), \bar{X}(\min(C, T)))$ is right-censored data on a full data process X that includes the failure time process $I(T \leq \cdot)$, then we might consider fitting the hazard $\lambda_{c|X}(t \mid X)$ of C, given X, with a Cox proportional hazards model $\lambda_{c|X}(t \mid X) = \lambda_0(t) \exp(\beta W(t))$ including time-independent and time-dependent covariates $W(t)$ extracted from the observed past $\bar{X}(t)$. In this subsection, we propose a forward/backward selection algorithm selecting this set of covariates $W(t)$ based on the cross-validation criteria described above (Brookhart and van der Laan, 2002b).

Let us index the set of p covariates that we consider with $\{1, \ldots, p\}$. For a subset $A \subset \{1, \ldots, p\}$, let β_A be the p-dimensional regression parameter with jth component set equal to zero for all $j \notin A$. Each subset A defines a lower-dimensional multivariate regression model. Let $\mu_{n,A}$ be the corresponding estimator of the parameter of interest μ. Let $\mu_{n,0}$ be an approximately unbiased estimator of μ. For example, $\mu_{n,0}$ might be based on fitting G with a standard forward selection algorithm adding the next best covariate if its regression coefficient is marginally significant. Thus, we are not concerned with slightly overfitting since our goal is to obtain an approximately unbiased estimator.

Let $S_j \cup T_j = \{1, \ldots, n\}$ be a split of the sample in a training sample S_j and test sample T_j, $j = 1, \ldots, J$. Define as criteria

$$c_n(A) \equiv \sum_{j=1}^{J} (\mu_{n,A}(S_j) - \mu_{n,0}(T_j))^2.$$

As remarked above, in a particular version of this method, $\mu_{n,A}(S_j)$, $\mu_{n,0}(T_j)$ would use an estimate $G_{n,A}$ of the nuisance parameter G based on the whole sample. The distance-based cross-validation method above suggests minimizing $c_n(A)$ over all subsets A. Since this is a computationally infeasible problem, we propose to use the following forward/backward selection algorithm with cross-validation for obtaining a good data adaptively selected set of covariates identified by $\hat{A}$.

Initialization of forward selection. Let $k = 0$, $A(0)$ be empty, and $A^+(j,k) = A(k) \cup \{j\}$ is defined as the set $A(k)$ augmented with the singleton $\{j\}$.

Forward selection. We have that $A(k)$ is given. Let
$$j^* = \min_j{}^{-1} c_n(A^+(j,k))$$
be the best singleton $\{j\}$ to add to $A(k)$ w.r.t. the criteria $c_n(\cdot)$. If $c_n(A^+(j^*,k)) < c_n(A(k))$, then $k = k+1$, $A(k) = A^+(j^*,k)$, and repeat the previous step. Otherwise, we stop with this forward selection and proceed to backward selection with this set $A(k)$ as start.

Backward selection. From the forward selection algorithm, we obtain a set $A(k)$. Let $A^-(j,k) = A(k)/\{j\}$ be the set $A(k)$ excluding the singleton $\{j\}$. Let $j^* = \min^{-1}_{j \in A(k)} c_n(A^-(j,k))$ be the best singleton $\{j\}$ to delete from $A(k)$. If $c_n(A^-(j^*,k)) < c_n(A(k))$, then $k = k - 1$, $A(k) = A^-(j^*,k)$, and repeat the previous step. Otherwise, we stop with this backward selection and stop or proceed with forward selection with this set $A(k)$.

Iterate forward/backward selection until convergence. Let $\hat{A} = A(k)$ be the final subset resulting from this algorithm.

Note that the algorithm converges since it strictly decreases the semiparametric model selection criterian $c_n(\cdot)$ at each carried out step. Alternatively, at each k, we can calculate both the best forward and best backward step and carry out the best of these two moves. We will now generalize this forward/backward selection method to the case where we want to maximize the criteria jointly over two regression models for both Q and G. Let us index the set of all p covariates with $\{1,\ldots,p\}$. For a subset $A = A_1 \times A_2 \subset \{1,\ldots,p\}^2$, A_1 defines a lower-dimensional multivariate regression model for G, and A_2 defines a lower-dimensional multivariate regression model for Q. Let $\mu_{n,A}$ be the corresponding estimator of the parameter of interest μ. Let μ_{n,A_0} be an approximately unbiased estimator of μ, where $A_0 = A_{01} \times A_{02}$. We use the same criteria:

$$c_n(A) \equiv \sum_{j=1}^{J}(\mu_{n,A}(S_j) - \mu_{n,0}(T_j))^2.$$

The algorithm is now described as follows.

1.7. Using Cross-Validation to Select Nuisance Parameter Models

Initialization of forward selection. Let $k = 0$, and let $A_1(0)$ and $A_2(0)$ be empty. Given a $j \in \{1, \ldots, p\}$ and $\delta \in \{1, 2\}$ indicating G and Q, respectively, we define

$$A^+(j, \delta, k) = \begin{cases} (A_1(k) \cup \{j\}) \times A_2(k) & \text{if } \delta = 1 \\ A_1(k) \times (A_2(k) \cup \{j\}) & \text{if } \delta = 2. \end{cases}$$

Thus, $A^+(j, \delta, k)$ is the set $A(k)$ either with covariate j added to the censoring model defined by $A_1(k)$ ($\delta = 1$) or covariate j added to the Q-model defined by $A_2(k)$ ($\delta = 2$).

Forward selection. We have that $A(k)$ is given. Let

$$(j^*, \delta^*) = \min_{j, \delta}^{-1} c_n(A^+(j, \delta, k)).$$

Thus (j^*, δ^*) represents the best covariate addition to $A(k)$, where additions to the censoring model defined by $A_1(k)$ and additions to the Q-model defined by $A_2(k)$ are competing with each other. If $c_n(A^+(j^*, k)) < c_n(A(k))$, then $k = k + 1$, $A(k) = A^+(j^*, \delta^*, k)$, and repeat the previous step. Otherwise, we stop with this forward selection and proceed to backward selection starting with this set $A(k)$.

Backward selection. From the forward selection algorithm, we obtain a set $A(k)$. Given $j \in \{1, \ldots, p\}$ and $\delta \in \{1, 2\}$, we define

$$A^-(j, \delta, k) = \begin{cases} (A_1(k)/\{j\}) \times A_2(k) & \text{if } \delta = 1 \\ A_1(k) \times (A_2(k)/\{j\}) & \text{if } \delta = 2. \end{cases}$$

Thus $A^-(j, \delta, k)$ is the set $A(k)$ either with covariate j deleted from the censoring model defined by $A_1(k)$ ($\delta = 1$) or covariate j deleted from the Q-model defined by $A_2(k)$ ($\delta = 2$). Let $(j^*, \delta^*) = \min_{j \in A(k)}^{-1} c_n(A^-(j, \delta, k))$. Thus (j^*, δ^*) represents the best covariate deletion from $A(k)$, where deletions to the censoring model defined by $A_1(k)$ and deletions to the Q-model defined by $A_2(k)$ are competing with each other. If $c_n(A^-(j^*, \delta^*, k)) < c_n(A(k))$, then $k = k - 1$, $A(k) = A^-(j^*, \delta^*, k)$ and repeat the previous step. Otherwise, we stop with this backward selection and stop or proceed with forward selection with this set $A(k)$.

Iterate forward/backward selection until convergence. Let $\widehat{A} = A(k)$ be the final subset resulting from this algorithm.

1.7.3 Data analysis example: Estimating the causal relationship between boiled water use and diarrhea in HIV-positive men

In this subsection, we illustrate the use of the cross-validation criterion in combination with the forward model selection algorithm to select covariates for a treatment mechanism model used in the definition of the IPTW estimator in a marginal structural logistic regression model of point treatment data. The data that we consider were gathered to estimate the causal effect of boiled water use on the incidence of diarrhea among 499 HIV-positive men in San Francisco. The data and sample are described in detail in Eisenberg et al. (2002). The data consist of a treatment indicator A (boiled water use), an outcome Y (diarrhea during the past seven days), and 26 additional covariates that are potential confounders. These include variables such as ethnicity, presence of pets in the home, consumption of high-risk foods, anal sexual contact, medication and homelessness. As potential confounders, these variables may both predict the use of boiled water and be independently related to diarrhea incidence.

We employ a marginal structural model $P(Y_a = 1) = 1/\exp(-\{\psi_0 + \psi a\})$, where $\exp(\psi)$ represents the causal odds ratio due to the treatment "boiled water use". We assume that the 26 covariates contain all possible confounders, and as the model for the treatment mechanism, we assume a linear logistic regression model in these covariates. We define $\widehat{\psi}_0$ (the approximate unbiased estimator) to be the IPTW estimator of ψ associated with the treatment mechanism model using all of these 26 covariates.

We used bootstrap resampling (based on 250 resamples) to compare the estimate $\widehat{\psi}$ from the treatment mechanism model selected by the forward selection method with cross-validation described above to $\widehat{\psi}_0$. Smoothed kernel density estimates of the bootstrap distribution of $\widehat{\psi}_p^*$ and $\widehat{\psi}_0$ are depicted in Figure 1.7.3. The estimated variance of $\widehat{\psi}_p^*$ is 0.034, while the estimated variance of $\widehat{\psi}_0$ was nearly twice that at 0.064. We also note that the bias of $\widehat{\psi}_p^*$ relative to the bootstrap mean of $\widehat{\psi}_0$ only equals 0.05.

1.7. Using Cross-Validation to Select Nuisance Parameter Models   101

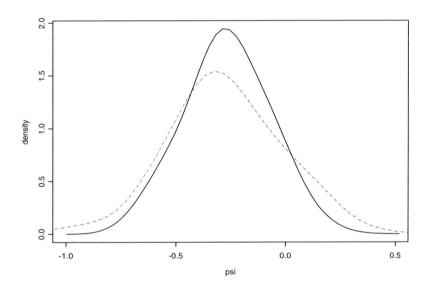

Figure 1.1. Smoothed kernel density estimates of the bootstrap distribution of $\widehat{\psi}_0$ (dotted line) and $\widehat{\psi}_p^*$ (solid line) based on 250 bootstrap samples.

2
General Methodology

2.1 The General Model and Overview

Let X be the full data structure for one subject, and it is assumed that the full data distribution F_X is an element of a model $\mathcal{M}^F$. Let $Y = \Phi(X, C)$ be the observed data for one subject, where Φ is a known many to one mapping and C is a censoring variable. Typically, in most of our applications we parametrize the data structure such that C is always observed, but this is not required; obviously, this is always possible, since one can define $C = Y$, in particular. Let $G(\cdot \mid X)$ be the conditional distribution of C, given X, which is assumed to satisfy coarsening at random. The set of all conditional distributions satisfying coarsening at random will be denoted with $\mathcal{G}(CAR)$. Because of the curse of dimensionality, it typically will not suffice to assume only that $F_X \in \mathcal{M}^F$ and $G \in \mathcal{G}(CAR)$. In this chapter, we develop estimating functions and corresponding locally efficient estimators for two models. Firstly, given working models $\mathcal{M}^{F,w} \subset \mathcal{M}^F$ for F_X and $\mathcal{G} \subset \mathcal{G}(CAR)$ for G, we consider the following model for the distribution of Y:

$$\mathcal{M} = \{P_{F_X,G} : F_X \in \mathcal{M}^F, G \in \mathcal{G}\} \cup \{P_{F_X,G} : F_X \in \mathcal{M}^{F,w}, G \in \mathcal{G}(CAR)\}.$$

In other words, either F_X needs to be an element of $\mathcal{M}^{F,w}$ or G needs to be an element of $\mathcal{G}$. We will also consider the less nonparametric model

$$\mathcal{M}(\mathcal{G}) = \{P_{F_X,G} : F_X \in \mathcal{M}^F, G \in \mathcal{G}\},$$

which assumes a correctly specified model for the censoring mechanism. The data consist of n i.i.d. copies $Y_1, \ldots, Y_n$ of Y. Let $\mu = \Phi(F_X) \in \mathbb{R}^k$ be a k-dimensional Euclidean parameter of interest.

In this chapter, we propose general mappings from full data estimating functions into observed data estimating functions. In the next section, we study full data estimating functions for two general classes of full data models: multivariate generalized linear regression models and multiplicative intensity models. In Section 2.3 we propose methods for constructing mappings from full data estimating functions into observed data estimating functions for model $\mathcal{M}(\mathcal{G})$ and a doubly robust mapping for model $\mathcal{M}$. These doubly robust mappings are $\mathcal{G}$-orthogonalized initial mappings in the sense that they are defined as an initial mapping minus its projection onto a nuisance tangent space of G corresponding to a convex model $\mathcal{G}$. In Section 2.4 we define the optimal mapping (based on (1.52) in Theorem 1.3) from full data estimating functions into observed data estimating functions, which can be used for both models $\mathcal{M}$ and $\mathcal{M}(\mathcal{G})$. The optimal mapping is optimal in the sense that it is an $\mathcal{G}(CAR)$-orthogonalized initial mapping, and by Theorem 1.3 it covers all estimating functions, including the optimal one.

Since this optimal mapping does not always exist in closed form, the methods of Section 2.3 can be preferable and are therefore still very important as well. Section 2.5 defines the corresponding estimating equations and, in model $\mathcal{M}(\mathcal{G})$, we show how to adjust the estimating equation to obtain an estimator that is guaranteed more efficient than an initial estimator. Section 2.6 proposes confidence intervals, and Section 2.7 presents two asymptotic theorems for the one-step estimator based on the estimating equation of Section 2.5 in model $\mathcal{M}(\mathcal{G})$ and in model $\mathcal{M}$, respectively, which provide templates for proving local efficiency of the one-step estimator. Section 2.8 presents representations of the optimal index $h_{opt}(F_X, G)$ of the full data estimating functions. In particular, we prove a theorem for general censored data that provides a closed-form expression of the optimal index if the full data model is a multivariate generalized linear regression model with uncensored covariates. In Section 2.9 we derive a general reparametrization of h_{opt} and propose a corresponding substitution estimator h_n. Finally, in Section 2.10 we present a general locally efficient estimator based on the representation of the efficient influence curve in terms of score and information operators as presented in Bickel, Klaassen, Ritov and Wellner (1993).

2.2 Full Data Estimating Functions.

Given a full data model $\mathcal{M}^F$ and parameter $\mu = \Phi(F_X) \in \mathbb{R}^k$ of interest, finding the class of estimating functions requires finding the orthogonal complement of the nuisance tangent space at F_X for each $F_X \in \mathcal{M}^F$. We refer the reader to Chapter 1 for an overview of the relevant efficiency and estimating functions theory. Here we will provide a short summary. Subsequently, we will derive the orthogonal complement of the nuisance tangent space in multivariate generalized linear regression models and multiplicative intensity models. These two general models form two of the most important full data models in the literature and will act as possible full data models in this book. Finally, we show how one links the orthogonal complement of the nuisance tangent space to a class of estimating functions.

It is assumed that the parameter $\mu = \Phi(F_X) \in \mathbb{R}^k$ of interest is pathwise differentiable in the full data model $\mathcal{M}^F$ with canonical gradient $S_{eff}^{*F}(\cdot \mid F_X) \in L_0^2(F_X)$ relative to a class of parametric submodels with tangent space $T^F(F_X)$. The canonical gradient is also called the efficient influence curve. The canonical gradient $S_{eff}^{*F}(X \mid F_X)$ is of great importance since the asymptotic variance of a regular asymptotically linear estimator of β at $P_{F_X,G}$ is bounded below by the variance of the canonical gradient and a regular estimator is efficient at $P_{F_X,G}$ if and only if it is asymptotically linear with influence curve equal to the canonical gradient (i.e., efficient influence curve) at $P_{F_X,G}$. Let $T_{nuis}^F(F_X) \subset L_0^2(F_X)$ be the nuisance tangent space in the full data model $\mathcal{M}^F$ (i.e., the closure of the linear span of all scores of 1-dimensional submodels F_ϵ through F at $\epsilon = 0$ for which $d/d\epsilon \mu(F_\epsilon)|_{\epsilon=0} = 0$). Let $T_{nuis}^{F,\perp}(F_X)$ be the orthogonal complement of $T_{nuis}^F(F_X) \subset L_0^2(F_X)$.

We will index each element of $T_{nuis}^\perp(F_X)$ with an index h running over an index set $\mathcal{H}^F(F_X)$. Specifically, assume we can represent

$$T_{nuis}^{F,\perp}(F_X) = \{D_h(X \mid \mu(F_X), \rho(F_X)) : h \in \mathcal{H}^F(F_X)\}, \qquad (2.1)$$

where $\rho(F_X)$ is a parameter defined on $\mathcal{M}^F$. Note that these index sets $\mathcal{H}^F(F_X)$ will typically depend on F_X. For example, in the multivariate generalized linear regression model $E(Z \mid X^*) = g(X^* \mid \beta)$ of Lemma 2.1 below, we have $T_{nuis}^{F,\perp}(F_X) = \{D_h(X \mid \beta) = h(X^*)\epsilon(\beta) : h \in \mathcal{H}^F(F_X)\}$ with $\mathcal{H}^F(F_X) = \{h(X^*) : E_{F_X}\{h(X^*)\epsilon(\beta)\}^2 < \infty\}$. In words, in this case the index h is allowed to be any function of X^* so that $h(X^*)\epsilon(\beta)$ has finite variance w.r.t. F_X. Let $h_{ind,F_X} : L_0^2(F_X) \to \mathcal{H}^F(F_X)$ be the index mapping defined by

$$\Pi(V \mid T_{nuis}^{F,\perp}(F_X)) = D_{h_{ind,F_X}(V)}(\cdot \mid \mu(F_X), \rho(F_X)). \qquad (2.2)$$

Let $h_{eff}(F_X) = h_{ind,F_X}(S_{eff}^{*F}(\cdot \mid F_X))$ be the index of the full data canonical gradient. In general, the mapping h_{ind,F_X} is determined by the mapping $\Pi(\cdot \mid T_{nuis}^\perp(F_X))$ and the representation (2.1) in the same manner as above.

As an illustration we consider the generalized linear regression example. Lemma 2.1 teaches us that for $D \in L_0^2(F_X)$

$$\Pi(D \mid T_{nuis}^{F,\perp}) = E(D(X)\epsilon^\top \mid X^*)E(\epsilon\epsilon^\top \mid X^*)^{-1}\epsilon.$$

Thus, we have that the index mapping is given by
$$h_{ind,F_X}(D) = E(D(X)\epsilon^\top \mid X^*)E(\epsilon\epsilon^\top \mid X^*)^{-1}.$$
In particular, $h_{eff}(F_X) = h_{ind,F_X}(S_{eff}^F)$, which can be simplified as in Lemma 2.1 below.

2.2.1 Orthogonal complement of the nuisance tangent space in the multivariate generalized linear regression model (MGLM)

The following lemma provides the orthogonal complement of the nuisance tangent space in multivariate generalized linear regression models $Z = g(X^* \mid \alpha) + \epsilon$, the projection onto this space, and the efficient score. We allow these models to model a user-supplied location parameter of the conditional error distribution by requiring that $E(K(\epsilon) \mid X^*) = 0$ for a user-supplied monotone function $K(\epsilon)$. For example, if $K(\epsilon) = \epsilon$, then the regression curve $g(X^* \mid \alpha)$ models the mean, if $K(\epsilon) = I(\epsilon > 0) - 1/2$, then it models the median, and, in general, if $K(\epsilon) = I(\epsilon > 0) - (1 - p)$, then it models the pth quantile of the conditional error distribution of ϵ, given X^*. Allowing this flexibility is particularly crucial for the censored data models since estimation of a mean based on censored data might not be possible due to lack of data in the tails of the distribution, while the median might not be a smooth enough functional of the observed data (e.g., see Chapter 4). By truncating $K(\epsilon) = \epsilon$ for $\mid \epsilon \mid > M$ (i.e., set it equal to M), one obtains a truncated mean, and by setting $K(\epsilon)$ equal to a smooth approximation of $I(\epsilon > 0) - 1/2$, one obtains a smooth median.

Lemma 2.1 *Let Z be a p-dimensional vector of outcomes. Suppose that we observe n i.i.d. observations of $X = (Z, X^*)$ for some vector of covariates X^*. Consider the multivariate regression model of Z on X^*,*
$$Z = g(X^* \mid \alpha) + \epsilon, \quad E(K(\epsilon) \mid X^*) = 0, \tag{2.3}$$
where $g = (g_1, \ldots, g_p)^\top$ is a p-dimensional vector of functions $g_j(X^* \mid \alpha)$, ϵ is a p-dimensional vector of residuals, K is a given real-valued monotone increasing function with $K(-\infty) < 0$ and $K(\infty) > 0$, and $\alpha = (\alpha_1, \ldots, \alpha_q)$ is a q-dimensional regression parameter. Here $K(\epsilon) = (K(\epsilon_1), \ldots, K(\epsilon_p))^\top$ is a p-dimensional vector.

The orthogonal complement of the nuisance tangent space at F_X is given by
$$T_{nuis}^{F,\perp}(F_X) = \{h(X^*)K(\epsilon) : h \; 1 \times p \; vector\}.$$
The projection $\Pi(V \mid T_{nuis}^{F,\perp})$ onto this subspace of the Hilbert space $L_0^2(F_X)$, endowed with inner product $\langle f, g \rangle_{F_X} = E_{F_X} f(X)g(X)$, is given by
$$E(\{V(X) - E(V \mid X^*)\}K(\epsilon)^\top \mid X^*)E(K(\epsilon)K(\epsilon)^\top \mid X^*)^{-1}K(\epsilon). \tag{2.4}$$

Assume that the conditional distribution of ϵ, given X^*, has a Lebesgue p-variate density $f(\epsilon \mid X^*)$. The score for α_j is given by

$$S_j(X) = -\frac{d}{d\alpha_j}g(X^* \mid \alpha)^\top \frac{f'(\epsilon \mid X^*)}{f(\epsilon \mid X^*)},$$

where $f'(\epsilon \mid X^*)$ is a p-dimensional vector containing the p partial derivatives w.r.t. $\epsilon_1,\ldots,\epsilon_p$. We can represent the q-dimensional score vector $S(X) = (S_1(X),\ldots,S_q(X))^\top$ as

$$S(X) = -\frac{d}{d\alpha}g(X^* \mid \alpha)^\top_{q\times p} \frac{f'(\epsilon \mid X^*)}{f(\epsilon \mid X^*)}.$$

The efficient score is given by

$$\begin{aligned} S^* &\equiv \Pi(S_j \mid T^{F,\perp}_{nuis}(F_X))^q_{j=1} \\ &= -\frac{d}{d\alpha}g(X^* \mid \alpha)^\top_{q\times p} A(X^*)_{p\times p} E(K(\epsilon)K(\epsilon)^\top \mid X^*)^{-1}_{p\times p} K(\epsilon), \end{aligned}$$

where $A(X^*) \equiv E\left(\frac{f'(\epsilon|X^*)}{f(\epsilon|X^*)} K(\epsilon)^\top \mid X^*\right)_{p\times p}$. If we assume that $f(\epsilon \mid X^*)$ equals zero at the end of its support and K is absolutely continuous w.r.t. the Lebesgue measure, then by integration by parts it follows that

$$A(X^*) = -\mathrm{diag}\left(E(K'(\epsilon) \mid X^*)\right)_{p\times p},$$

where $\mathrm{diag} E(K'(\epsilon) \mid X^*)$ denotes the $p\times p$ diagonal matrix with jth diagonal element $E(K'(\epsilon_j) \mid X^*)$. As a consequence, under this assumption, we have that the efficient score vector is given by

$$S^* = \frac{d}{d\alpha}g(X^* \mid \alpha)^\top_{q\times p}\mathrm{diag}\left(E(K'(\epsilon) \mid X^*)\right)_{p\times p} E(K(\epsilon)K(\epsilon)^\top \mid X^*)^{-1}_{p\times p} K(\epsilon).$$

For example, if $p=1$ and $K(\epsilon) = (I(\epsilon > 0) - 1/2)$, which corresponds with median regression, then

$$S^*_j(X) = f_{\epsilon|X^*}(0 \mid X^*)\frac{d}{d\alpha_j}g(X^* \mid \alpha)^\top E(K^2(\epsilon) \mid X^*)^{-1} K(\epsilon).$$

Proof. The density of X can be written as

$$f_X(X) = f(Z \mid X^*)f_{X^*}(X^*) = f_{\epsilon|X^*}(\epsilon(\alpha) \mid X^*)f_{X^*}(X^*).$$

This density is indexed by the parameter of interest α, f_{X^*} and the conditional distribution of $\epsilon = \epsilon(\alpha)$, given X^*, where the latter ranges over all conditional distributions with conditional expectation of $K(\epsilon)$, given X^*, equal to zero. Here f_{X^*} and $f_{\epsilon|X^*}$ are the nuisance parameters.

Let α be fixed. For any uniformly bounded function $s(X^*)$ with $E(s(X^*)) = 0$ and uniformly bounded function $s(\epsilon \mid X^*)$ with $E(s(\epsilon \mid X^*) \mid X^*) = E(s(\epsilon \mid X^*)K(\epsilon) \mid X^*) = 0$, we have that

$$f_\delta(X) = (1 + \delta s(X^*))f_{X^*}(X^*)(1 + \delta s(\epsilon \mid X^*))f_{\epsilon|X^*}(\epsilon \mid X^*)$$

is a one-dimensional submodel of the full data model with parameter δ going through the truth f_X at $\delta = 0$. Notice that these one-dimensional models provide a rich class of fluctuations for our nuisance parameter. The nuisance tangent space is defined by the closure of the linear span of the scores of this class of one-dimensional submodels in the Hilbert space $L_0^2(F_X) = \{s(X) : Es(X) = 0, Es^2(X) < \infty\}$ endowed with the inner product $\langle f, g \rangle_{F_X} = E_{F_X} f(X) g(X)$. It is given by the orthogonal sum of the two spaces generated by the $s(X^*)$'s and $s(\epsilon \mid X^*)$'s,

$$T_{nuis}(F_X) = L_0^2(F_{X^*}) \oplus H,$$

where $H \subset L_0^2(F_X)$ is the Hilbert space of functions s satisfying $E(s(\epsilon \mid X^*) \mid X^*) = E(s(\epsilon \mid X^*) K(\epsilon) \mid X^*) = 0$.

We have that $\Pi(V \mid L_0^2(F_{X^*})) = E(V \mid X^*)$. Let $H^+ \supset H$ be the Hilbert space of functions s only satisfying $E(s(\epsilon \mid X^*) \mid X^*) = 0$. We have $\Pi(V \mid H^+) = V - E(V \mid X^*)$. Now note that H consists of the orthogonal complement of the p-dimensional space $\langle K(\epsilon_1), \ldots, K(\epsilon_p) \rangle$ in the world where X^* is fixed. Thus, the projection operator onto this space is the identity operator minus the projection onto $\langle K(\epsilon_1), \ldots, K(\epsilon_p) \rangle$. The projection onto a p-dimensional space of functions $(K(\epsilon_j) : j = 1, \ldots, p)$ is given by the formula

$$E(V(X) K(\epsilon)^\top) E(K(\epsilon) K(\epsilon)^\top)^{-1} K(\epsilon).$$

Now, we simply need to apply this formula in the world with X^* fixed, so we have for any function $\eta \in H^+$

$$\Pi(\eta \mid H) = \eta(X) - E(\eta(X) K(\epsilon) \mid X^*)^\top \left\{ E(K(\epsilon) K(\epsilon)^\top \mid X^*) \right\}^{-1} K(\epsilon).$$

The rest of the proof is straightforward. □

2.2.2 Orthogonal complement of the nuisance tangent space in the multiplicative intensity model

Suppose that the full data $X = \bar{X}(T) = (X(t) : 0 \leq t \leq T)$ is a stochastic time-dependent process up to a possibly random time T. In addition, suppose that $X(t) = (N(t), V_1(t), V_2(t))$, where $N(t)$ is a counting process of interest and $V(t) = (V_1(t), V_2(t))$ is a time-dependent covariate process. Let $R(t) = I(T \leq t)$ be a component of $N(t)$ so that observing the process $X(t)$ up to T includes observing T itself. Let $Z(t) = (N(t), V_1(t))$. In these settings, there is often interest in modeling the intensity of $N(t)$ w.r.t. history $\bar{Z}(t-) = (Z(s) : s < t)$. The following lemmas provide us with the orthogonal complement of the nuisance tangent space for this multiplicative intensity model, the projection operator onto this space, and the efficient score.

Lemma 2.2 *Consider the setting above. Consider the model for the distribution of $X = \bar{X}(T)$ defined by the multiplicative intensity model (for a* continuous counting process $N(t)$) assumption:

$$\lambda(t)dt \equiv E(dN(t) \mid \bar{Z}(t-)) = Y(t)\lambda_0(t)\exp(\beta W(t))dt,$$

where $Y(t)$ and the k-dimensional vector $W(t)$ are uniformly bounded functions of $\bar{Z}(t-)$. Here $Y(t)$ is the indicator that $N(t)$ is still at risk of jumping right before time t. Here $\beta \in \mathbb{R}^k$ and λ_0 are unspecified. Let β be the parameter of interest and let (λ_0, η) represent the nuisance parameter (so β, λ_0, η identify f_X). Let $dM(t) = dN(t) - E(dN(t) \mid \bar{Z}(t-))$. The orthogonal complement of the nuisance tangent space in the model in which λ_0 is known is given by

$$T_\eta^\perp \equiv \overline{\left\{\int H(t, \bar{Z}(t-))dM(t) : H\right\}} \cap L_0^2(F_X).$$

The nuisance tangent space of $\Lambda_0 = \int_0^{\cdot} \lambda_0$ is given by

$$T_{\Lambda_0} \equiv \overline{\left\{\int g(t)dM(t) : g\right\}} \cap L_0^2(F_X).$$

We have

$$\Pi\left(\int H(t, \bar{Z}(t-))dM(t) \mid T_{\Lambda_0}\right) = \int g(H)(t)dM(t),$$

where

$$g(H)(t) = \frac{E\left\{H(t, \bar{Z}(t-))Y(t)\exp(\beta W(t))\right\}}{E\{Y(t)\exp(\beta W(t))\}}. \tag{2.5}$$

Thus, the orthogonal complement of the nuisance tangent space of β $T_{nuis}^{F,\perp} = T_\eta^\perp \cap T_{\Lambda_0}^\perp$ is given by

$$T_{nuis}^{F,\perp} = \overline{\left\{\int \{H(t, \bar{Z}(t-)) - g(H)(t)\}dM(t) : H\right\}} \cap L_0^2(F_X).$$

We have

$$\Pi\left(\int H(t, \bar{Z}(t-))dM(t) \mid T_{nuis}^{F,\perp}\right) = \int \{H(t, \bar{Z}(t-)) - g(H)\}dM(t).$$

The score for β is given by $S_\beta = \int W(t)dM(t)$. Thus the efficient score for β is given by

$$S_{eff}^F = \int \left\{W(t) - \frac{E\left\{W(t)Y(t)\exp(\beta W(t))\right\}}{E\{Y(t)\exp(\beta W(t))\}}\right\}dM(t).$$

This efficient score formula is due to Ritov, and Wellner (1988). We want to have an expression for the projection onto $T_{nuis}^{F,\perp}$ of any function $D(X)$. The previous lemma provides the projection of full data functions of the form $\int H(t, \bar{Z}(t-))dM(t)$. In the next lemma, we establish the projection in the case where $N(t)$ can only jump at a given set of points, thereby avoiding technical measurability conditions. Since continuous processes can be arbitrarily well-approximated by discrete processes, it will also provide us with a formula for the general projection operator onto $T_{nuis}^{F,\perp}$ for the continuous multiplicative intensity model. Note that the multiplicative intensity model makes only sense for discrete data on a relatively fine grid of points so that the modeled probabilities are bounded by 1.

Lemma 2.3 *Assume that the counting process $N(t)$ can only jump at given points t_j, $j = 1,\ldots,p$, and consider the multiplicative discrete intensity model $\lambda(t_j) = P(dN(t_j) = 1 \mid \bar{Z}(t_j-)) = Y(t_j)\lambda_0(t_j)\exp(\beta W(t_j))$, where $W(t_j)$ are uniformly bounded functions of $\bar{Z}(t_j)$, $j = 1,\ldots,p$. Let $dM(t) = dN(t) - \lambda(t)$ for $t \in \{t_1,\ldots,t_p\}$. Then, the statements in Lemma 2.2 hold and, in addition, we have that for any $D \in L^2(F_X)$*

$$\Pi(D \mid T_\eta^\perp) = \int H_D(t, \bar{Z}(t-))dM(t), \qquad (2.6)$$

where

$$H_D(t, \bar{Z}(t-)) = E(D(X) \mid dN(t) = 1, \bar{Z}(t-)) - E(D(X) \mid dN(t) = 0, \bar{Z}(t-)).$$

Thus

$$\Pi(D \mid T_{nuis}^{F,\perp}) = \int \{H_D(t, \bar{Z}(t-)) - g(H_D)\}dM(t), \qquad (2.7)$$

where the mapping $g(h)$ is defined in (2.5).

We conjecture that, given appropriate measurability conditions so that the conditional expectations are properly defined, this projection formula (2.6) and thereby (2.7) holds in the continuous setting of Lemma 2.2 as well.

A direct proof of the representation $T_{nuis}^{F,\perp}$ given in Lemma 2.2 is obtained by directly computing the nuisance tangent space from the likelihood $f(X) = f(X \mid Z)\prod_t f(Z(t) \mid \bar{Z}(t-))$ which can be further factorized by $f(Z(t) \mid \bar{Z}(t-)) = f(dN(t) \mid \bar{Z}(t-))f(Z(t) \mid N(t), \bar{Z}(t-))$. Here $\prod_t f(dN(t) \mid \bar{Z}(t-)) = \prod_t \lambda(t)^{dN(t)}(1-\lambda(t))^{1-dN(t)}$ is the partial likelihood, where this product integral representation of the likelihood is formally defined in Andersen, Borgan, Gill and Keiding (1993). The proof Lemma 2.3 below provides an intuitive non-formal way of understanding Lemma 2.2 and provides a formal proof of Lemma 2.3 in which $N(t)$ is a discrete counting process.

Proof of Lemma 2.3. Let $\mathcal{M} = \{F_X : E(dN(t) \mid \bar{Z}(t-)) = Y(t)\lambda_0(t)\exp(\beta W(t))$ all $t\}$ be this model. Let (η, λ_0) represent the nuisance parameter of β. We have that the nuisance tangent space T_{η,λ_0} equals the sum of the nuisance tangent space T_η in the model with λ_0 known and the nuisance tangent space T_{λ_0} in the model with η known: $T_{\eta,\lambda_0} = T_\eta + T_{\lambda_0}$. Thus $T_{\eta,\lambda_0}^\perp = T_\eta^\perp \cap T_{\lambda_0}^\perp$. It follows directly from differentiating the log-partial-likelihood

$\log \prod_t \lambda(t)^{dN(t)}(1 - \lambda(t))^{1-dN(t)}$ along one-dimensional fluctuations $\lambda_0(\cdot) + \epsilon h(\cdot)$ of λ_0 that $T_{\lambda_0} = \overline{\{\int g(t)dM(t) : g\}}$.

We will now prove that $T_\eta^\perp = \overline{\{\int H(t, \bar{Z}(t-))dM(t) : H\}}$. Notice that $\mathcal{M} = \cap_{t=1}^p \mathcal{M}_t$, where $\mathcal{M}_t = \{F_X : \lambda(t) = Y(t)\lambda_0(t)\exp(\beta W(t))\}$. In other words, $\mathcal{M}$ can be viewed as an intersection of t-specific models only restricting the intensity $\lambda(t) = E(dN(t) \mid \bar{Z}(t-))$ at a fixed point t. The orthogonal complement of the nuisance tangent space of β in model $\mathcal{M}_t$ equals $\overline{\{H(\bar{Z}(t-))dM(t) : H\}}$. This is proved directly from the likelihood representation in the same manner as we proved that in the regression model $E(Z \mid X^*) = m(X^* \mid \beta)$ the orthogonal complement of the nuisance tangent space equals $\{H(X^*)(Z - m(X^* \mid \beta)) : H\}$. In fact, since N can only jump at predetermined grid points $\mathcal{M}_t$ can be viewed as a regression model of $Z = dN(t)$ on $X^* = \bar{Z}(t-)$ with $m(X^* \mid \beta) = Y(t)\lambda_0(t)\exp(\beta W(t))$. The orthogonal complement of the nuisance tangent space of the intersection of models $\mathcal{M}_t$ equals the sum (integral) of the orthogonal complements of the nuisance tangent spaces for the models $\mathcal{M}_t$, where the nuisance tangent space for $\mathcal{M}$ equals the intersection of the nuisance tangent spaces for model $\mathcal{M}_t$. Thus, the orthogonal complement of the nuisance tangent space in the model with λ_0 known equals

$$T_\eta^\perp = \overline{\left\{\int H(t, \bar{Z}(t-))dM(t) : H\right\}} \cap L_0^2(F_X).$$

Therefore, we can conclude that

$$T_\eta^\perp \cap T_{\lambda_0}^\perp = \overline{\left\{\int (H(t, \bar{Z}(t-)) - g(H)(t))dM(t) : H\right\}},$$

where $\int g(H)(t)dM(t) = \Pi(\int HdM \mid T_{\lambda_0})$. It can be directly verified that $g(H)(t) = E\{H(t, \bar{Z}(t-))Y(t)\exp(\beta W(t))\}/E\{Y(t)\exp(\beta W(t))\}$.

We will now prove the projection formula (2.6). Firstly, we note that $T_\eta^\perp = \{\int H(t, \bar{Z}(t-))dM(t) : H\} = H_1 \oplus \ldots \oplus H_k$ is an orthogonal sum of subspaces $H_j \equiv \{H(\bar{Z}(t_j-))dM(t_j) : H\}$. Therefore, we have that $\Pi(D \mid T_\eta^\perp) = \sum_{j=1}^k \Pi(D \mid H_j)$. As explained above, we can apply Lemma 2.4 with $\epsilon = dM(t_j)$, $X^* = \bar{Z}(t_j-)$, and $K(\epsilon) = \epsilon$ to obtain that $\Pi(D \mid H_j)$ is given by

$$E(\{D(X) - E(D(X) \mid \bar{Z}(t_j-))\}dM(t_j) \mid \bar{Z}(t_j-)) \times$$
$$\frac{1}{E(dM(t_j)^2 \mid \bar{Z}(t_j-))}dM(t_j).$$

We have

$E(D(X) \mid dN(t_j), \bar{Z}(t_j-)) - E(D(X) \mid \bar{Z}(t_j-)) =$
$\{E(D(X) \mid dN(t_j) = 1, \bar{Z}(t_j-)) - E(D(X) \mid dN(t_j) = 0, \bar{Z}(t_j-))\}dM(t_j)$

This proves that $\Pi(D \mid H_j)$ is given by

$\{E(D(X) \mid dN(t_j) = 1, \bar{Z}(t_j-)) - E(D(X) \mid dN(t_j) = 0, \bar{Z}(t_j-))\} dM(t_j),$

which proves Lemma 2.3. □

Suppose now that the counting process is discrete on a sparse set of points so that one might want to assume the logistic regression intensity model. The proof of the previous lemma proves, in particular, a simple representation of $T_{nuis}^{F,\perp}$ and the projection operator onto $T_{nuis}^{F,\perp}$ for parametric discrete intensity models such as the logistic regression intensity model. The results are stated in the following lemma.

Lemma 2.4 *Assume that the counting process $N(t)$ can only jump at given points t_j, $j = 1, \ldots, p$, and consider a discrete intensity model $\lambda(t_j) = P(dN(t_j) = 1 \mid \bar{Z}(t_j-)) = Y(t_j)m(W(t_j), t_j \mid \beta)$, where $m(W(t_j), t_j \mid \beta)$ is parametrized by a k-dimensional regression parameter β and is uniformly bounded: For example, $m(W(t), t \mid \beta) = 1/(1 + \exp(-(\beta_0 + \beta_1 * t + \beta_2 W(t))$. Let $dM(t) = dN(t) - \lambda(t)$ for $t \in \{t_1, \ldots, t_p\}$. Then, the orthogonal complement of the nuisance tangent space at F_X is given by*

$$T_{nuis}^{F,\perp}(F_X) = \overline{\left\{ \int H(t, \bar{Z}(t-))dM(t) : H \right\}} \cap L_0^2(F_X).$$

In addition, we have that for any $D \in L^2(F_X)$

$$\Pi(D \mid T_{nuis}^{F,\perp}) = \int H_D(t, \bar{Z}(t-))dM(t), \qquad (2.8)$$

where

$$H_D(t, \bar{Z}(t-)) = E(D(X) \mid dN(t) = 1, \bar{Z}(t-)) - E(D(X) \mid dN(t) = 0, \bar{Z}(t-)).$$

2.2.3 Linking the orthogonal complement of the nuisance tangent space to estimating functions

Consider the full data structure model $\mathcal{M}^F$ with parameter of interest $\mu = \mu(F_X)$. Given representations of $T_{nuis}^{F,\perp}(F_X) = \{D_h(\cdot \mid \mu(F_X), \rho(F_X)) : h \in \mathcal{H}^F(F_X)\}$ at all $F_X \in \mathcal{M}^F$, the goal is to define a class of full data estimating functions $\{(X, \mu, \rho) \to D_h(X \mid \mu, \rho) : h \in \mathcal{H}^F\}$ for μ with a (possibly different) nuisance parameter $\rho = \rho(F_X)$ and an index set $\mathcal{H}^F$ independent of F_X so that

$$\{D_h(\cdot \mid \mu(F_X), \rho(F_X)) : h \in \mathcal{H}^F\} \subset T_{nuis}^{F,\perp}(F_X) \text{ for all } F_X \in \mathcal{M}^F. \quad (2.9)$$

Recall that it yields estimating functions indexed by $\mathcal{H}^{Fk}$ for $\mu \in \mathbb{R}^k$ by defining $D_h = (D_{h_1}, \ldots, D_{h_k})$ for any $h = (h_1, \ldots, h_k) \in \mathcal{H}^{Fk}$.

In this subsection, we provide a template for deriving such a class of estimating functions from these representations of $T_{nuis}^{F,\perp}(F_X)$. Firstly, let $\mathcal{H}^F$ be an index set containing each $\mathcal{H}^F(F_X)$, $F_X \in \mathcal{M}^F$, and $(D_h^1 : h \in \mathcal{H}^F)$ be a class of estimating functions $D_h^1 : \mathcal{X} \times \{(\mu(F_X), \rho(F_X)) : F_X \in \mathcal{M}^F\} \to \mathbb{R}$ so that

$$\{D_h^1(\cdot \mid \mu(F_X), \rho(F_X)) : h \in \mathcal{H}^F(F_X)\} = T_{nuis}^{F,\perp}(F_X) \text{ for all } F_X \in \mathcal{M}^F.$$

For example, $\mathcal{H}^F = \cup_{F_X \in \mathcal{M}^F} \mathcal{H}^F(F_X)$. Since $T_{nuis}^{F,\perp}(F_X)$ is defined in $L_0^2(F_X)$, we mean that for each element in $T_{nuis}^{F,\perp}(F_X)$ there exists a function $D_h^1(X \mid \mu(F_X), \rho(F_X))$ that is equal to this element in $L_0^2(F_X)$. Now, $D_h^1(\cdot \mid \mu, \rho)$, $h \in \mathcal{H}^F$, is a class of (biased and unbiased) full data estimating functions.

Since $\mathcal{H}^F(F_X)$ possibly depends on unknown parameters of F_X, the membership indicator $I(h \in \mathcal{H}^F(F_X))$, which guarantees the unbiasedness, represents a nuisance parameter of the estimating function $D_h^1(\cdot \mid \mu, \rho)$. In order to acknowledge this fact, we reparametrize $D_h^1(\cdot \mid \mu, \rho)$ as follows. Let $\Pi(\cdot \mid \mathcal{H}^F(F_X))$ be a user-supplied mapping from $\mathcal{H}^F$ into $\mathcal{H}^F(F_X)$ satisfying $\Pi(h \mid \mathcal{H}^F(F_X)) = h$ if $h \in \mathcal{H}^F(F_X)$. We now redefine the class of full data estimating functions $\{D_h^1(\cdot \mid \mu, \rho) : h \in \mathcal{H}^F\}$

$$\{D_h^2(\cdot \mid \mu, \rho') \equiv D_{\Pi(h \mid \mathcal{H}^F(F_X))}(\cdot \mid \mu, \rho) : h \in \mathcal{H}\}, \qquad (2.10)$$

where ρ' denotes ρ augmented with the parameters indexing $\Pi(h \mid \mathcal{H}^F(F_X))$. For the sake of notational simplicity, we redefine $D_h^2(\cdot \mid \mu, \rho')$ as $D_h(\cdot \mid \mu, \rho)$ again. Note that we can now state

$$\{D_h(\cdot \mid \mu(F_X), \rho(F_X)) : h \in \mathcal{H}^F\} = T_{nuis}^{F,\perp}(F_X).$$

If $\Pi(\cdot \mid \mathcal{H}^F(F_X))$ were not required to be the identity on $\mathcal{H}^F(F_X)$, it might have a range that is a strict subset of $\mathcal{H}^F(F_X)$. Even so, we still would have

$$\{D_h(\cdot \mid \mu(F_X), \rho(F_X)) : h \in \mathcal{H}^F\} \subset T_{nuis}^{F,\perp}(F_X).$$

One might choose such a mapping $\Pi(\cdot \mid \mathcal{H}^F(F_X))$ to simplify the parametrization of the estimating function, where one now takes the risk of excluding (e.g.) the optimal estimating function.

As a side remark here, we mention that ρ plays the role of a nuisance parameter that will be estimated with external (relative to the estimating function) procedures. For example, in the full data world, we would be solving $0 = \sum_{i=1}^n D_h(X_i \mid \mu, \rho_n)$ for a given estimator ρ_n of ρ. Thus, one wants to choose ρ as variation-independent of μ as possible in order to maximize efficiency of the estimator of μ that solves the estimating equation. If $\rho = \rho(\mu, \eta)$ for two variation independent parameters μ, η, then one redefines the full data estimating functions as $D_h(\cdot \mid \mu, \eta) = D_h(\cdot \mid \mu, \rho(\mu, \eta))$. We conjecture that it essentially will always be possible to parametrize the estimating function so that μ and ρ are locally variation independent.

Such a collection $\{D_h : h \in \mathcal{H}^F\}$ represents a set of full data structure estimating functions. We want to choose the index set as large as possible in the sense that if $\rho = (\rho_1, \rho_2)$ with

$$E_{F_X} D_h(X \mid \mu(F_X), \rho_1, \rho_2(F_X)) \in T_{nuis}^{F,\perp}(F_X) \text{ for all possible } \rho_1$$

and $F_X \in \mathcal{M}^F$, then one should make ρ_1 a component of the index h.

2.2. Full Data Estimating Functions. 113

In most full data models, the estimating functions D_h and index set $\mathcal{H}^F$ are naturally implied by the representation of $F_X \to T_{nuis}^{F,\perp}(F_X) = \{D_h(\cdot \mid \mu(F_X), \rho(F_X)) : h \in \mathcal{H}^F(F_X)\}$ and does not require much thinking.

Because it is of interest to be able to map a full data estimating function into its corresponding index, we also want to extend the index mapping h_{ind,F_X} (2.2) to be well-defined on pointwise well-defined functions of X. Let $\mathcal{D} = \{D_h(\cdot \mid \mu, \rho) : \mu, \rho, h \in \mathcal{H}^F\}$ be the set of full data functions. Let $\mathcal{L}(\mathcal{X})$ be the space of functions of X with finite supremum norm over a set K for which we know that $P(X \in K) = 1$ w.r.t. the true F_X. It will be assumed that $\mathcal{D} \subset \mathcal{L}(\mathcal{X})$. Let $h_{ind,F_X} : \mathcal{L}(\mathcal{X}) \to \mathcal{H}$ be an index mapping satisfying for any $D \in \mathcal{L}(\mathcal{X})$

$$D_{h_{ind,F_X}(D)}(\cdot \mid \mu(F_X), \rho(F_X)) = \Pi(D \mid T_{nuis}^{F,\perp}(F_X)),$$

where we formally mean that the equality holds in $L_0^2(F_X)$ (since the right-hand side is defined in $L_0^2(F_X)$).

Example 2.1 (Multivariate generalized linear regression; continuation of Example 2.1) In our multivariate generalized linear regression example, a natural candidate for the index set $\mathcal{H}^F$ is simply all functions of X^*:

$$\mathcal{H}^F \equiv \{h(X^*) : \text{ any h}\}.$$

A possible mapping into $\mathcal{H}^F(F_X) = \{h \in \mathcal{H}^F : E_{F_X}\{h(X^*)K(\epsilon(\alpha))\}^2 < \infty\}$ (here α is the true parameter value corresponding with F_X) is given by

$$\Pi(h \mid \mathcal{H}^F(F_X))(X^*) = \min(h(X^*), M),$$

where the truncation constant M is user-supplied. Notice that indeed the finite supremum norm of this index (say) h^* guarantees that $h^*(X^*)\epsilon(\alpha)$ has finite variance for any $F_X \in \mathcal{M}^F$. Note also that the range of this mapping does not necessarily cover $\mathcal{H}^F(F_X)$. This mapping has no unknown nuisance parameters. Thus, the corresponding set of full data estimating functions (2.10) is given by

$$\{(X, \alpha) \to \min(h(X^*), M)K(\epsilon(\alpha)) : h \in \mathcal{H}^F\}.$$

If the full data structure model $\mathcal{M}^F$ assumes that, for a specified k, $X^{*k}\epsilon(\beta)$ has finite variance, then one can define

$$\Pi(h \mid \mathcal{H}^F(F_X)) = \min(h(X^*), X^{*k}).$$

For any $D \in \mathcal{D} = \{\min(h(X^*), M)K(\epsilon(\alpha)) : h \in \mathcal{H}^F, \alpha\}$, we define

$$h_{ind,F_X}(D)(X^*) = E_{F_X}(D(X)K(\epsilon)^\top \mid X^*)E_{F_X}(K(\epsilon)K(\epsilon)^\top \mid X^*)^{-1},$$

where $\epsilon = \epsilon(\alpha(F_X))$. □

2.3 Mapping into Observed Data Estimating Functions

In this section, we provide a variety of methods to construct mappings from full data estimating functions to observed data estimating functions. The first five sections are focused on mappings that one can use to construct estimators in model $\mathcal{M}(\mathcal{G})$, and they can form the basis of an orthogonalized mapping such as the optimal mapping in the next section. In Subsection 2.3.6, we will show that making a given mapping orthogonal to the tangent space of G for a convex model containing $\mathcal{G}$ yields the double robustness property so that it can be used to obtain RAL estimators in model $\mathcal{M}$ as well.

2.3.1 Initial mappings and reparametrizing the full data estimating functions

Let $D_h \to IC_0(Y \mid Q_0, G, D_h)$ be a mapping from full data estimating functions $\{D_h : h \in \mathcal{H}^F\}$ into observed data estimating functions indexed by nuisance parameters $Q_0(F_X, G)$ and G. Let $\mathcal{Q}_0 \equiv \{Q_0(F_X, G) : F_X \in \mathcal{M}^{F,w}, G \in \mathcal{G}\}$ be the parameter space of this nuisance parameter Q_0, where F_X ranges over a submodel $\mathcal{M}^{F,w}$ of $\mathcal{M}^F$. For each possible parameter value $(\mu, \rho) \in \{(\mu(F_X), \rho(F_X)) : F_X \in \mathcal{M}^F\}$ and $G \in \mathcal{G}$, let $\mathcal{H}^F(\mu, \rho, \rho_1, G) \subset \mathcal{H}^F$ be a collection of h for which

$$E_G(IC_0(Y \mid Q, G, D_h(\cdot \mid \mu, \rho)) \mid X) = D_h(X \mid \mu, \rho) \ F_X\text{-a.e. for all } Q \in \mathcal{Q}^0 \tag{2.11}$$

and

$$\text{VAR}_{P_{F_X},G} IC_0(Y \mid Q, G, D_h(\cdot \mid \mu(F_X), \rho(F_X))) < \infty \text{ for all } Q \in \mathcal{Q}^0. \tag{2.12}$$

Note that the statement F_X-a.e. in (2.11) also creates dependence on F_X. Since the latter restriction only affects the variance of the estimating function (it is unbiased by (2.11)) it can often be arranged by a simple truncation of h (see e.g., Example 2.1). Therefore, we suppressed the possible dependence of $\mathcal{H}^F(\mu, \rho, \rho_1, G)$ on another nuisance parameter needed to guarantee (2.12). This dependence is expressed by the parameter ρ_1 of F_X.

It is also natural to make (2.12) a model assumption or, equivalently, a regularity condition in an asymptotics theorem. Note that, if we ignore the (2.12) constraint, then the maximal set $\mathcal{H}^F(\mu, \rho, \rho_1, G)$ is given by

$$\left\{ h \in \mathcal{H}^F : \sup_{Q_0 \in \mathcal{Q}_0} \mid E_G(IC_0(Y \mid Q_0, G, D_h(\cdot \mid \mu, \rho)) \mid X) - D_h(X \mid \mu, \rho) \mid = 0 \right\},$$

where the equality needs to hold F_X-a.e.

It will be convenient to also define the set of allowed full data estimating functions directly (instead of in terms of the index sets).

Definition 2.1 *Let $\mathcal{D} = \{D_h(\cdot \mid \mu, \rho) : h \in \mathcal{H}^F, (\mu, \rho)\}$ with (μ, ρ) ranging over the parameter space $\{\mu(F_X), \rho(F_X) : F_X \in \mathcal{M}^F\}$. Let $\mathcal{Q}_0 = \{Q_0(F_X, G) : F_X \in \mathcal{M}^F, G \in \mathcal{G}\}$. For each $G \in \mathcal{G}$ and $F_X \in \mathcal{M}^F$, we define the set $\mathcal{D}(\rho_1(F_X), G)$ as*

$$\{D \in \mathcal{D} : E_G(IC_0(Y \mid Q, G, D) \mid X) = D(X) \; F_X\text{-a.e. for all } Q \in \mathcal{Q}_0. \tag{2.13}$$

Given an initial mapping IC_0, the dependence of $\mathcal{D}(\rho_1, G)$ on F_X, G typically has to do with the support of $D(X)$; that is the possible values of X at which $D(X)$ is non zero relative to the support of G. As a consequence, under strong conditions on G, one will typically have $\mathcal{D}(\rho_1, G) = \mathcal{D}$.

Example 2.2 (Right censored data structure with time-dependent covariates) Consider the right-censored data structure $Y = (\tilde{T} = \min(T, C), \Delta = I(\tilde{T} = T), \bar{L}(\tilde{T}))$. For $D(X)$ we define $\Delta(D) = I(D(X) \text{ observed})$. There exists a real-valued random variable $V(D) \leq T$ so that $I(D(X) \text{ is observed}) = I(C \geq V(D))$. We define

$$IC_0(Y \mid G, D) = \frac{D(X)\Delta(D)}{P_G(\Delta(D) = 1 \mid X)} = \frac{D(X)\Delta(D)}{\bar{G}(V(D) \mid X)},$$

where $\bar{G}(t \mid X) \equiv P(C \geq t \mid X)$. Note that if $\bar{G}(T \mid X) > \delta > 0$ F_X-a.e. for some $\delta > 0$, then one has $\mathcal{D}(\rho_1, G) = \mathcal{D}$, but this condition might not be necessary for identification of a particular parameter μ. □

Having identified an appropriate mapping IC_0, in many models it is indeed the case that $E_G(IC_0(Y \mid Q, G, D_h(\cdot \mid \mu(F_X), \rho(F_X))) \mid X) = D_h(X \mid \mu(F_X), \rho(F_X))$ only holds for $D_h(\cdot \mid \mu(F_X), \rho(F_X))$ ranging over a true (not even dense) subset of $T_{nuis}^{F,\perp}(F_X)$ (i.e., $\mathcal{H}^F(\mu(F_X), \rho(F_X), \rho_1(F_X), G) \subset \mathcal{H}^F$). In this case, there exist many full data structure estimating functions (i.e., full data structure model gradients) that cannot be mapped into an observed data estimating function (i.e., observed data model $\mathcal{M}(G)$ gradients).

Typical candidates of the mapping $D_h \to IC_0(Y \mid Q_0, G, D_h)$ are so-called inverse probability of censoring weighted mappings, as we provided in Chapter 1 and will provide below for various censored data structures. These mappings involve a censoring probability or density in the denominator. By assuming that this censoring probability is uniformly bounded away from zero, one will typically have $\mathcal{H}^F(\mu, \rho, \rho_1, G) = \mathcal{H}^F$ (i.e., all full data structure estimating functions satisfy (2.11)). On the other hand, a given censoring distribution not satisfying this property can still allow estimation of the particular parameter of interest or, equivalently, there is still a real subset $\mathcal{H}^F(\mu, \rho, \rho_1, G)$ of $\mathcal{H}^F$ for which (2.11) holds. For example, in the current status data location (mean, smooth median, truncated mean)

116   2. General Methodology

regression model covered in Chapter 4, the class of allowed full data structure estimating functions is a function of the support of the monitoring mechanism and the support of the location parameter. The next example illustrates this for linear regression with a right-censored outcome.

Example 2.3 (Linear regression with right-censored outcome)
Suppose that one is interested in estimating a linear regression parameter $\mu = \beta$ of log-survival on a treatment dose Z. We denote the log survival and log censoring time by T and C. Our model is $T = \beta_0 + \beta_1 Z + \epsilon$, $E(\epsilon \mid Z) = 0$. Let $X = (T, Z)$ be the full data structure. We assume that the right-censoring time C is conditionally independent of survival, given treatment dose Z. We observe n i.i.d. copies of $Y = (\tilde{T} = \min(T,C), \Delta = I(T \leq C), Z)$. A rich class of full data structure estimating functions is $\{D_h(T, Z \mid \beta) = \min(h(Z), M)\epsilon(\beta) : h\}$ for a bound $M < \infty$ to guarantee that all of these estimating functions have finite variance. Let $IC_0(Y \mid G, D_h) = \min(h(Z), M)\epsilon(\beta)\Delta/\bar{G}(T \mid Z)$ which equals zero if $\Delta = 0$, regardless of the denominator, where $\bar{G}(t \mid Z) = P(C \geq t \mid Z)$.

Suppose that T, given Z, has compact support $[\alpha_Z, \alpha^Z]$. For example, if ϵ has known support $[-\tau, \tau]$, then we have $\alpha^Z = \beta_0 + \beta_1 Z + \tau$. Note that

$$E\left(h(Z)\epsilon(\beta)I(T \leq C)/\bar{G}(T \mid Z) \mid T, Z\right) = h(Z)\epsilon(\beta)I(\bar{G}(T \mid Z) > 0).$$

Define for some fixed small $\delta > 0$

$$\mathcal{Z}(\beta, G) = \{z : \bar{G}(\alpha^Z \mid Z) > \delta > 0\}$$

as the set of treatment values z for which the conditional probability (given treatment) $\bar{G}(T \mid Z = z)$ that a subject's survival time is observed is bounded away from zero. It follows that for all functions $h(Z)$ that are zero for $Z \notin \mathcal{Z}(\beta, G)$

$$E_G(IC_0(Y \mid G, D_h(\cdot \mid \beta)) \mid X) = D_h(X \mid \beta) \text{ for all } G \text{ and } \beta.$$

Thus, we can set

$$\begin{aligned}\mathcal{H}^F(\mu, \rho, \rho_1, G) &= \mathcal{H}(\beta, G) = \{h(Z) : h(Z) = h(Z)I(Z \in \mathcal{Z}(\beta, G))\},\\ \mathcal{D}(\beta, G) &= \{h(Z)\epsilon(\beta) : h(Z) = 0 \text{ if } \bar{G}(\alpha^Z \mid Z) = 0\}.\end{aligned}$$

In other words, one can estimate β by simply throwing away all subjects with a treatment dose outside $\mathcal{Z}(\beta, G)$. This example can be directly generalized to the general location regression model: $T = \beta_0 + \beta_1 Z + \epsilon$, $E(K(\epsilon) \mid Z) = 0$ for a monotone function K that has derivative zero outside an interval, say $(-\tau, \tau)$. □

Reparametrizing the full data structure estimating functions

Since $\mathcal{H}^F(\mu, \rho, \rho_1, G)$ possibly depends on the unknown parameters (μ, ρ, ρ_1, G), this makes the index h essentially a nuisance parameter of the estimating function $IC_0(Y \mid Q, G, D_h(\cdot \mid \mu, \rho))$. In other words, to estimate μ, we need to estimate the set $\mathcal{H}^F(\mu, \rho, \rho_1, G)$ and try to make sure that our choice h_n converges to an element in $\mathcal{H}(\mu, \rho, \rho_1, G)$. In order to acknowledge this fact, we reparametrize $D_h(\cdot \mid \mu, \rho)$ in the following manner, which is completely analogous to (2.10).

Let $\Pi(\cdot \mid \mathcal{H}^F(\mu, \rho, \rho_1, G))$ be a user-supplied mapping from $\mathcal{H}^F$ into $\mathcal{H}^F(\mu, \rho, \rho_1, G)$ that only depends on the unknown (μ, ρ, ρ_1, G), which equals the identity on a rich subset (preferably all) of $\mathcal{H}^F(\mu, \rho, \rho_1, G)$. We now redefine the class of full data estimating functions $\{D_h(\cdot \mid \mu, \rho) : h \in \mathcal{H}^F\}$ so that it is guaranteed to satisfy (2.11) for all $h \in \mathcal{H}^F$:

$$\{D_h^r(\cdot \mid \mu, \rho' = (\rho, \rho_1, G)) \equiv D_{\Pi(h \mid \mathcal{H}^F(\mu, \rho, \rho_1, G))}(\cdot \mid \mu, \rho) : h \in \mathcal{H}^F\}. \quad (2.14)$$

For the sake of notational simplicity, we will denote the parameter ρ' with ρ, again, and we denote $D_h^r(\cdot \mid \mu, \rho')$ with $D_h(\cdot \mid \mu, \rho)$ again, but we now need to remind ourselves that ρ possibly also includes G as a component and that $h \to D_h$ can be a many-to-one mapping in the sense that many $h \in \mathcal{H}^F$ are mapped into the same full data structure estimating function. The reparametrized class of estimating functions are now elements of $T_{nuis}^{F,\perp}(F_X)$ and $\mathcal{D}(\rho_1(F_X), G)$ when evaluated at the true parameter values. Consequently, we now have for *all $h \in \mathcal{H}^F$*

$$E_G(IC_0(Y \mid Q, G, D_h(\cdot \mid \mu, \rho)) \mid X) = D_h(X \mid \mu, \rho) \text{ for all } Q \in \mathcal{Q}^0. \quad (2.15)$$

This and (2.12) imply that

$$\{IC_0(Y \mid Q, G, D_h(\cdot \mid \mu(F_X), \rho(F_X, G))) : h \in \mathcal{H}^F, Q \in \mathcal{Q}^0\} \subset T_{nuis}^\perp(\mathcal{M}(G));$$

that is, IC_0 maps full data structure estimating functions into observed data estimating functions that are orthogonal to the nuisance tangent space in the model with G known. Consequently, the estimating function still has the property that the first-order asymptotics of the locally (variation-independent of μ) F_X components of ρ_n will not affect the influence curve of the estimator μ_n solving $0 = \sum_i IC_0(Y_i \mid Q_n, G_n, D_h(\cdot \mid \mu, \rho_n))$.

Example 2.4 (Linear regression with right-censored outcome; continuation of Example 2.3) The class of full data structure estimating functions is $\{D_h(X \mid \beta) = \min(h(Z), M)\epsilon(\beta) : h \in \mathcal{H}^F\}$, where $\mathcal{H}^F$ denotes all functions of Z. We derived in the previous example a subclass $\mathcal{H}^F(\mu, \rho, \rho_1, G) = \mathcal{H}^F(\beta, G) = \{\min(h(Z), M) : h(Z) = h(Z)I(Z \in \mathcal{Z}(\beta, G))\}$ so that for all $h \in \mathcal{H}^F(\beta, G)$ $E_G(IC_0(Y \mid G, D_h(\cdot \mid \beta)) \mid X) = D_h(X \mid \beta)$. To reparametrize the estimating functions $\{IC_0(Y \mid G, D_h(\cdot \mid \beta)) : h \in \mathcal{H}^F(\beta, G)\}$ in terms of a class of unbiased estimating functions with an index h running over an index set independent of any unknown parameters, we define the mapping $\Pi(h \mid \mathcal{H}^F(\beta, G)) = h(Z)I(Z \in \mathcal{Z}(\beta, G))$. This yields the reparametrized full data structure estimating functions

$$D_h^r(X \mid \mu = \beta, G) = \min(h(Z), M)I(Z \in \mathcal{Z}(\beta, G))\epsilon(\beta).$$

For notational convenience, we denote this latter full data structure estimating function with $D_h(X \mid \beta, G)$. □

This mapping can be viewed as a mapping from full data estimating functions D_h for μ into observed data estimating functions $IC_0(\cdot \mid Q_0, G, D_h(\cdot \mid \mu, \rho))$ for μ indexed by an unknown nuisance parameter G and unknown (but) protected nuisance parameter Q_0. Therefore, it can be used to construct an initial estimator in the model $\mathcal{M}(\mathcal{G})$ in which we assume that $G \in \mathcal{G}$. For a given $h \in \mathcal{H}^{F^k}$, an estimator ρ_n of ρ, G_n of G and Q_{0n} of Q_0, let μ_n^0 be the solution of the estimating equation

$$0 = \sum_{i=1}^{n} IC_0(Y_i \mid Q_n^0, G_n, D_h(\cdot \mid \mu, \rho_n)). \tag{2.16}$$

Here, the G component of ρ is estimated with the same G_n. One can solve the estimating equation with the Newton–Raphson algorithm. Let μ_n^0 be an initial guess or estimator. Set $l = 0$. The first step of the Newton–Raphson procedure involves estimation of a derivative (matrix) w.r.t. μ at μ_n^l of the estimating equation. This derivative at $\mu = \mu_1$ is defined by

$$c(\mu_1) = c(h, \mu_1, \rho, Q_0, G, P) = \left.\frac{d}{d\mu} PIC_0(Y \mid Q_0, G, D_h(\cdot \mid \mu, \rho))\right|_{\mu=\mu_1},$$

where we used the notation $Pf \equiv \int f(y)dP(y)$. Note that $c(\mu)$ is a $k \times k$ matrix with $c_{ij}(\mu) = \frac{d}{d\mu_j} PIC_{0,i}(Y \mid Q_0, G, D_{h_n}(\mu, \rho))$. Its estimate at $\mu = \mu_1$ is given by

$$\begin{aligned} c_n(\mu_1) &\equiv c(h_n, \mu_1, \rho_n, Q_{0n}, G_n, P_n) \\ &= \left.\frac{1}{n}\sum_{i=1}^{n} \frac{d}{d\mu} IC_0(Y_i \mid Q_{0n}, G_n, D_{h_n}(\mu, \rho_n))\right|_{\mu=\mu_1}. \end{aligned}$$

If $IC_0(Y \mid Q_{0n}, G_n, D_{h_n}(\cdot \mid \mu, \rho_n))$ is not differentiable in μ, but the integral of $IC_0(Y)$ w.r.t. $P_{F_X,G}$ is differentiable w.r.t. μ, then we replace the analytical derivative $d/d\mu$ by a numerical derivative: for a given function $f : \mathbb{R} \to \mathbb{R}$, the numerical derivative w.r.t. x at $x = x_1$ is defined as

$$\frac{f(x_1 + \Delta_n) - f(x_1)}{\Delta_n} \quad \text{for a sequence } \Delta_n = O(n^{-1/2}).$$

The $(l+1)$th step of the Newton–Raphson procedure is given by

$$\mu_n^{l+1} = \mu_n^l - c_n(\mu_n^l)^{-1} \frac{1}{n} \sum_{i=1}^{n} IC(Y_i \mid Q_{0n}, G_n, D_{h_n}(\cdot \mid \mu_n^l, \rho_n)). \tag{2.17}$$

If μ_n^0 is a decent consistent estimator of μ (if a second-order Taylor expansion in μ exists, one needs $\| \mu_n^0 - \mu \| = o_P(n^{-1/4})$ and otherwise $\| \mu_n^0 - \mu \| = O_P(n^{-1/2})$ suffices), then further iteration beyond the one-step estimator μ_n^1 will not result in first-order improvements (i.e., μ_n^0 does now only affects the second-order asymptotics of μ_n^1). Therefore, in this case one can just use μ_n^1. If no consistent initial estimator is available, then one can repeat these updating steps until convergence is established. To guarantee

2.3. Mapping into Observed Data Estimating Functions

convergence, the following modification of the algorithm is often needed. For a given vector norm $\|\cdot\|$, we can define

$$l(\mu) \equiv \| \sum_{i=1}^{n} IC_0(Y_i \mid G_n, D_h(\cdot \mid \mu, \rho_n)) \|.$$

For example, we could use the Euclidean norm or average of absolute value norm. Now, if $l(\mu_n^{l+1}) < l(\mu_n^l)$, then we accept the update μ_n^{l+1}, but otherwise we take as update $\epsilon\mu_n^l + (1-\epsilon)\mu_n^{l+1}$ with ϵ chosen to be the minimizer of $\epsilon \to l(\epsilon\mu_n^l + (1-\epsilon)\mu_n^{l+1})$. It actually is not necessary to determine the exact minimizer, but one needs to find an ϵ that improves the update w.r.t. the criterion l. This minimization problem can be carried out with the S-plus function nlminb().

In this book, we will not be concerned with the existence of solutions and or multiple solutions o estimating equations, but we would like to make the following suggestions. The existence of solutions has been a non issue in our experience, but we have experienced cases where estimating equations had multiple solutions. In this case, it is very helpful if either a consistent initial estimator μ_n^0 is available so that the one-step estimator suffices or that an initial ad hoc guess is available so that certain solutions can be ruled out right away. A useful idea to deal with multiple solutions comes from noting that it is unlikely that the same wrong solution will consistently come up in different estimating equations. Therefore, solving a number of estimating equations can be a sensible approach to rule out certain solutions. More formally, a promising method is to solve a number of estimating equations simultaneously. In other words, let $U(\beta)$ be a stack (i.e., vector) of estimating equations, and we estimate β by minimizing $U(\beta)^\top E(U(\beta)U(\beta)^\top)^{-1}U(\beta)$ over β. By incorporating enough estimating equations, this method will often uniquely identify the true β. By Hansen (1982), the efficiency of the resulting estimator corresponds with the estimator solving the optimal k-dimensional linear combination of the components of $U(\beta)$, provided the number of components in $U(\beta)$ does not increase too quickly with sample size.

Example 2.5 (Linear regression with right-censored outcome; continuation of Example 2.3) Let β_n be the solution of

$$0 = \sum_{i=1}^{n} \min(h(Z_i), M) I(Z_i \in \mathcal{Z}(\beta, G_n)) \epsilon_i(\beta) \frac{\Delta_i}{\bar{G}_n(T_i \mid Z_i)},$$

where G_n is an estimator of the conditional distribution $G(t \mid Z) = P(C \geq t \mid Z)$. For example, we could assume the Cox proportional hazards model for $\lambda_C(t \mid Z)$ and estimate G accordingly. We have

$$\mathcal{Z}(\beta, G_n) = \{z : \bar{G}_n(\beta_0 + \beta_1 z + \tau \mid z) > \delta > 0\}.$$

Instead of enforcing $\bar{G}_n$ to be larger than $\delta > 0$, we could also just require positivity. In this case,

$$I(Z \in \mathcal{Z}(\beta, G)) = I(\beta_0 + \beta_1 Z + \tau < \alpha^Z).$$

We will now verify that, under some smoothness conditions, the changes of the order σ in β and α^Z only have an effect of order σ^2 on $E\left\{\min(h(Z), M)I(Z \in \mathcal{Z}(\beta, G))\epsilon(\beta)\frac{\Delta}{\bar{G}(T|Z)}\right\}$. Let us denote the set $\mathcal{Z}(\beta, G)$ with $\mathcal{Z}(\beta, \alpha^Z)$. Define the set $A(\sigma)$ as all elements $z \in \mathcal{Z}(\beta + \sigma, \alpha^Z + \sigma)$ that are not an element of $\mathcal{Z}(\beta, \alpha^Z)$, where $\vec{x} + \sigma$ denotes adding the constant σ to each component of $\vec{x}$. By noting that the conditional expectation, given $Z = z \in \mathcal{Z}(\beta, G)$, of the estimating function equals zero, it follows that

$$E\left(h(Z)\{I(Z \in \mathcal{Z}(\beta + \sigma, \alpha^Z + \sigma)) - I(Z \in \mathcal{Z}(\beta, \alpha^Z))\}\epsilon(\beta)\frac{I(T \leq C)}{\bar{G}(T \mid Z)}\right)$$

$$\leq \int_{Z \in A(\sigma)} \left\{\int_T h(Z)(T - \beta Z)I(\bar{G}(T|Z) > 0)dF(T|Z)\right\} dF_Z(Z)$$

$$\equiv \int_{Z \in A(\sigma)} g(Z)dF_Z(Z).$$

Now, note that $g(Z) = 0$ for $Z \in \mathcal{Z}(\beta, \alpha^Z)$. Thus, if g is a smooth function in Z, then $g(Z) = O(\sigma)$ for $Z \in \mathcal{Z}(\beta + \sigma, \alpha^Z + \sigma)$ and, in particular, for $Z \in A(\sigma)$. This shows that the last term equals $\int_{A(\sigma)} O(\sigma)dF_Z(z) = F_Z(A(\sigma))O(\sigma) = O(\sigma^2)$.

As a consequence of this result, the asymptotics of β_n is not affected by the first-order behavior of $\mathcal{Z}(\beta_n, G_n)$. Thus, under weak conditions, β_n will be asymptotically equivalent with the estimator using $\mathcal{Z}(\beta, G)$ as given and known. This is a helpful insight for derivation of the influence curve of β_n. □

A general initial mapping only indexed by the censoring distribution.

Firstly, consider a censored data model for which

$$P(X \text{ is observed} \mid X = x) > 0 \text{ for almost all } x. \tag{2.18}$$

Given a $D(X)$, define a random variable that is 1 if $D(X)$ is observed and zero otherwise:

$$\Delta(D) = \begin{cases} 1 & \text{if } D(X) \text{ is observed.} \\ 0 & \text{if } D(X) \text{ is censored.} \end{cases}$$

Define $\Pi_{G,D}(x) = P(\Delta(D) = 1 \mid X = x)$. Now, define for $D \in L_0^2(F_X)$ the following inverse probability of censoring weighted mapping

$$IC_0(Y \mid G, D) = \frac{D(X)\Delta(D)}{\Pi_{G,D}(X)}.$$

Notice that indeed $E(IC_0(Y \mid G, D) \mid X) = D(X)$ for all $D(X)$. If (2.18) only holds on a subset of the support of X, then, as in our linear regression Example 2.3, $E_G(IC_0(Y \mid G, D) \mid X) = D(X)$ can still hold for a subset of D's covering full data structure estimating functions for a parameter of interest.

In censored data models in which X is never completely observed, such as in the current status data example below, it might not be so easy to find an initial mapping $IC_0(\cdot \mid G, D)$. In this case, the following theorem provides a general representation of an initial mapping IC_0.

Theorem 2.1 *Let $A_{F_X} : L_0^2(F_X) \to L_0^2(P_{F_X,G})$ be the nonparametric score operator for F_X:*

$$A_{F_X}(s)(Y) = E(s(X) \mid Y).$$

The adjoint $A_G^\top : L_0^2(P_{F_X,G}) \to L_0^2(F_X)$ of A_{F_X} is given by

$$A_G^\top(V)(X) = E(V(Y) \mid X).$$

Let $\mathbf{I}_{F_X,G} = A_G^\top A_{F_X} : L_0^2(F_X) \to L_0^2(F_X)$ which will be referred to as the nonparametric information operator.

Let F_1 be given. Let $(\mathcal{L}(\mathcal{X}), \|\cdot\|_\infty)$ be the space of all functions of X defined on set K with $P(X \in K) = 1$ with finite supremum norm over this set K. We have that $\mathbf{I}_{F_1,G} : (\mathcal{L}(\mathcal{X}), \|\cdot\|_\infty) \to (\mathcal{L}(\mathcal{X}), \|\cdot\|_\infty)$. Assume that $D \in \mathcal{L}(\mathcal{X})$; that is, D has finite supremum norm in X, and either (i) D lies in the range of $\mathbf{I}_{F_1,G} : (\mathcal{L}(\mathcal{X}), \|\cdot\|_\infty) \to (\mathcal{L}(\mathcal{X}), \|\cdot\|_\infty)$ or (ii) in the range of $\mathbf{I}_{F_1,G} : L_0^2(F_X) \to L_0^2(F_X)$. Then

$$IC_0(Y \mid G, D) \equiv A_{F_1} \mathbf{I}_{F_1,G}^-(D)(Y) \in L_0^2(P_{F_X,G})$$

satisfies $E(IC_0(Y \mid G, D) \mid X) = D(X)$ for all values of $X \in K$ (if (i) holds) or with probability one (if (ii) holds).

By Theorem 1.3 we also have

$$A_{F_1} \mathbf{I}_{F_1,G}^{-1}(D) = U_{F_1,G}(D) - \Pi_{F_1,G}(U_{F_1,G}(D) \mid T_{CAR}(P_{F_1,G}))$$

for any $U_{F_1,G}(D)$ satisfying $E(U_{F_1,G}(D)(Y) \mid X) = D(X)$.

Proof. Given assumption (i), for each $x \in K$ we have

$$E(A_{F_1} \mathbf{I}_{F_1,G}^-(D)(Y) \mid X = x) = \mathbf{I}_{F_1,G} \mathbf{I}_{F_1,G}^-(D)(x) = D(x).$$

Similarly, given assumption (ii), we prove this statement with probability one. □

Condition (i) is stronger than condition (ii), but the supremum norm invertibility condition (i) is needed to prove most asymptotic theorems for the estimator solving the corresponding estimating equation.

Example 2.6 (Current status data structure) Consider a carcinogenicity experiment in which the time T until onset of a tumor in a

122   2. General Methodology

mouse is the random variable of interest. Suppose that one collects time-independent covariates $L(0)$ and possibly time-dependent covariates (such as the weight of the mouse) $L(t)$ up to the sacrificing time C. Then, the full data structure is $X = (T, L(\cdot))$ and the observed data structure is $Y = (C, \Delta = I(T \leq C), \bar{L}(C))$.

To begin with, we will consider the current status data structure (C, Δ, L) with time-independent covariates L. In this case, $X = (T, L)$ and CAR is equivalent with assuming $G(\cdot \mid X) = G(\cdot \mid L)$. Below we will derive an explicit form of $IC_0(Y \mid G, D) = A_{F_1}\mathbf{I}^-_{F_1,G}(D)$ that will provide an $IC_0(Y \mid G, D)$ for the general data structure $(C, \Delta, \bar{L}(C))$ by simply replacing $G(\cdot \mid L)$ by the true G only satisfying CAR w.r.t. the general data structure. We actuall suggest this as a general method for finding such mappings IC_0; that is, first obtain a mapping for a marginal data structure (e.g., not involving covariates or not involving time-dependent covariates) and subsequently simply replace the censoring mechanism for the marginal data structure by the true censoring mechanism. The latter type of method will be discussed in more detail in the next subsection.

We have

$$A_{F_1}(h) = \frac{\int_0^C h(t,L)dF_1(t \mid L)}{F_1(C \mid L)}\Delta + \frac{\int_C^\infty h(t,L)dF_1(t \mid L)}{1 - F_1(C \mid L)}(1-\Delta),$$

and its adjoint is given by

$$A_G^\top(V) = \int_0^T V(c, 0, L)dG(c \mid L) + \int_T^\infty V(c, 1, L)dG(c \mid L).$$

Thus

$$\begin{aligned}\mathbf{I}_{F_1,G}(h)(T,L) &= \int_0^T \frac{\int_0^c h(t,L)dF_1(t \mid L)}{F_1(c \mid L)} dG(c \mid L) \\ &+ \int_T^\infty \frac{\int_c^\infty h(t,L)dF_1(t \mid L)}{1 - F_1(c \mid L)} dG(c \mid L).\end{aligned}$$

Consider the equation $\mathbf{I}_{F_1,G}(h)(t,L) = D(t,L)$ for a D that is differentiable in the first coordinate. We assume that $dG(t \mid L) = g(t \mid L)dt$. Differentiation w.r.t. t yields

$$\frac{\int_0^t h(s,L)dF_1(s \mid L)}{F_1(t \mid L)} - \frac{\int_t^\infty h(s,L)dF_1(s \mid L)}{1 - F_1(t \mid L)} = \frac{D_1(t,L)}{g(t \mid L)},$$

where $D_1(t,L) = d/dt D(t,L)$. Now, we write $\int_0^t h(s,L)dF_1(s \mid L) = \int_0^\infty h(s,L)dF_1(s \mid L) - \int_t^\infty h(s,L)dF_1(s \mid L)$. Solving for $\int_t^\infty h(s,L)dF_1(s \mid L)$ in terms of D_1 and $\Phi_h(L) \equiv \int_0^\infty h(s,L)dF_1(s \mid L)$ now yields

$$\int_t^\infty h(s,L)dF_1(s \mid L) = \frac{D_1(t,L)}{g(t \mid L)} F_1(1-F_1)(t \mid L) + \{1 - F_1(t \mid L)\}\Phi_h(L).$$

2.3. Mapping into Observed Data Estimating Functions

The last equality gives us also

$$-\int_0^t h(s,L)dF_1(s\mid L) = \frac{D_1(t,L)}{g(t\mid L)}F_1(1-F_1)(t\mid L) - F_1(t\mid L)\Phi_h(L).$$

Thus

$$A_{F_1}\mathbf{I}_{F_1,G}^-(D) = \frac{D_1(C,L)}{g(C\mid L)}\{F_1(C\mid L) - \Delta\} + \Phi_h(L).$$

Consider now the equation $\mathbf{I}_{F_1,G}(h)(\alpha_L, L) = D(\alpha_L, L)$, where α_L is the most leftmost point of the support of $g(\cdot \mid L)$. This equation reduces to

$$\Phi_h(L) = D(\alpha_L, L) - \int_0^\infty D_1(c,L)\{1 - F_1(c,L)\}dc.$$

We conclude that (here $\bar{F}_1 = 1 - F_1$):

$$\begin{aligned}IC_0(Y\mid G,D) &= \frac{D_1(C,L)}{g(C\mid L)}\{\bar{F}_1(C\mid L) - (1-\Delta)\} \\ &\quad - \int D_1(c,L)\bar{F}_1(c\mid L)dc + D(\alpha_L, L).\end{aligned} \quad (2.19)$$

Consider now the general data structure $(C, \Delta, \bar{L}(C))$. We still assume the full data estimating functions D to depend only on data $(T, W = L(0))$. For this data structure, $g(C\mid X)$ satisfies CAR if $g(C\mid X) = h(C, \bar{L}(C))$ for some measurable function h. In (2.19), replace $g(C\mid L)$ by $g(C\mid X)$, and we can replace $\bar{F}_1(C\mid L)$ by any function $\phi(C, \bar{L}(C))$. Assume that $D_1(c,L)I(T > c)/g(c\mid L) < \infty$ for all c, F_X-a.e. We will now verify that $IC_0(Y\mid G, D)$ indeed satisfies the desired property: for any $D(T, W = L(0))$, we have

$$\begin{aligned}E(IC_0(Y\mid G,D)\mid X) &= \int D_1(c,W)\phi(c,\bar{L}(c))dc + \int_{\alpha_L}^T D_1(c,W)dc \\ &\quad - \int D_1(c,W)\phi(c,\bar{L}(c))dc + D(\alpha_L, W) \\ &= D(T,W).\end{aligned}$$

By setting $\phi = 1$, we obtain the mapping

$$IC_0(Y\mid G, D) = \frac{D_1(C,L)(1-\Delta)}{g(C\mid L)} + D(\alpha_L, L).$$

One can also treat the conditional distribution $F_1(\cdot \mid L(0))$ as a nuisance parameter of the mapping IC_0 and thus define

$$\begin{aligned}IC_0(Y\mid F, G, D) &= \frac{D_1(C,L)}{g(C\mid X)}\{\bar{F}(C\mid L(0)) - (1-\Delta)\} \\ &\quad - \int D_1(c,L)\bar{F}(c\mid L(0))dc + D(\alpha_L, L).\end{aligned}$$

Since $E(IC_0(Y \mid F_1, G, D) \mid X) = D(X)$ for all F_1, the resulting estimator will remain CAN under misspecification of $F(\cdot \mid L(0))$. Therefore, the latter is an example of an initial mapping indexed by the censoring mechanism and a protected nuisance parameter Q_0. By Theorem 1.3, if there are no time-dependent covariates (i.e., $L = L(0)$), and $D = D_{opt}$ is the optimal full data estimating function choice, then $IC_0(Y \mid F, G, D)$ is the efficient influence curve. □

2.3.2 Initial mapping indexed by censoring and protected nuisance parameter

By Theorem 2.1, we have $I_{F,G} : (\mathcal{L}(\mathcal{X}), \|\cdot\|_\infty) \to (\mathcal{L}(\mathcal{X}), \|\cdot\|_\infty)$ for all F, G. Let $R^\infty(I_{F,G})$ denote its range. Consider as mapping

$$IC_0(Y \mid F_X, G, D) \equiv A_{F_X} \mathbf{I}^-_{F_X, G}(D)(Y), \quad (2.20)$$

which can also be represented as $IC_0(Y \mid G, D) - \Pi(IC_0 \mid T_{CAR})$ for any $IC_0(Y \mid G, D)$ satisfying $E(IC_0(Y \mid G, D) \mid X) = D(X)$ (Theorem 1.3 Chapter 1). Given a working model $\mathcal{M}^{F,w}$, suppose that

$$\mathcal{D}(\rho_1, G) = \{ D \in \mathcal{D} : D \in R^\infty(I_{F_1,G}) \text{ for all } F_1 \in \mathcal{M}^{F,w} \}.$$

is non empty. By Theorem 2.1, for any $D \in \mathcal{D}(\rho_1, G)$ it satisfies $E(IC_0(Y \mid F, G, D) \mid X) = D(X)$ F_X-a.e. for all $F \in \mathcal{M}^{F,w}$. Thus, this mapping indeed satisfies (2.11) with $Q_0(F_X) = F_X$ for appropriately chosen $\mathcal{H}^F(\mu, \rho, \rho_1, G)$ (e.g., defined by the conditions of Theorem 2.1 at a fixed F_X, G).

Again, when applied to full data estimating functions for a particular parameter of interest, IC_0 yields a mapping from full data estimating functions $D_h(\cdot \mid \mu, \rho)$ for μ into observed data estimating functions $IC_0(\cdot \mid Q_0, G, D_h(\cdot \mid \mu, \rho))$ for μ indexed by unknown nuisance parameter $G \in \mathcal{G}$ and Q_0. As in the previous subsection, one needs 1) to identify a subset $\mathcal{H}^F(\mu, \rho, \rho_1, G) \subset \mathcal{H}^F$ so that for all $h \in \mathcal{H}^F(\mu, \rho, \rho_1, G)$ $E_G(IC_0(Y \mid F, G, D_h(\cdot \mid \mu, \rho)) \mid X) = D_h(X \mid \mu, \rho)$ F_X-a.e. (for all possible μ, ρ, G) and 2) to reparametrize this restricted class of full data structure estimating functions $\{D_h : h \in \mathcal{H}^F(\mu, \rho, \rho_1, G)\}$ as $\{D_h^r : h \in \mathcal{H}^F\}$ by incorporating the extra nuisance parameters ρ_1, G (needed to map any $h \in \mathcal{H}^F$ into $\mathcal{H}^F(\mu, \rho, \rho_1, G)$) in the nuisance parameter of D_h^r. Subsequently, we denote this reparametrized class of estimating functions with $\{D_h(\cdot \mid \mu, \rho) : h \in \mathcal{H}^F\}$ again, where ρ includes the old ρ, ρ_1, and G.

This mapping is actually the optimal mapping of the next section, which can be used to construct locally efficient estimators of μ in model $\mathcal{M}$. We highlight this in this section as a special choice that one can use to construct estimators in $\mathcal{M}(\mathcal{G})$, where one might even consider extremely small parametric models $\mathcal{M}^{F,w}$ since one already assumed correct specification of G.

2.3.3 Extending a mapping for a restricted censoring model to a complete censoring model

The basic goal in this section is to find a mapping $IC_0(Y \mid Q_0, G, D)$ such that for a reasonable set of full data structure functions D (i.e., $\mathcal{D}(\rho_1, G)$ is rich enough) and all $G \in \mathcal{G}$

$$E_G(IC_0(Y \mid Q_0, G, D) \mid X) = D(X) \ F_X\text{-a.e. for all possible } Q_0. \quad (2.21)$$

For each particular full data structure model and parameter of interest, one still needs to specify the actual class $\mathcal{D}(\rho_1, G)$ of full data structure estimating functions for which (2.21) holds (see (2.11)) and specify the corresponding index sets $\mathcal{H}^F(\mu, \rho, \rho_1, G)$. Thus, (2.21) is not a formal property, but we want to separate the construction of sensible (i.e., in principle satisfying (2.21)) initial mappings from the verification of (2.21) for a particular set of full data estimating functions.

The mapping (2.20) is the optimal mapping defined in the next section, which might not always be easy to calculate. Therefore, we proceed with discussing various useful approaches for obtaining ad hoc mappings $IC_0(Y \mid Q_0, G, D)$ satisfying (2.21). Suppose that one has obtained a particular mapping satisfying (2.21) for G in a restricted censoring model $\mathcal{G}^* \subset \mathcal{G}$ of the true model $\mathcal{G}$: for a desired set of full data structure functions D

$$E_G(IC_0(Y \mid Q_0, G, D) \mid X) = D(X) \ F_X\text{-a.e. for all } Q_0, \ G \in \mathcal{G}^*.$$

For example, one might develop such a mapping under the assumption that censoring C is completely independent of X: in particular, one can set $IC_0(Y \mid Q_0, G, D)$ equal to the influence curve of an ad hoc RAL estimator under such an independent censoring model. In this case, the mapping $IC_0(Y \mid Q_0, G, D_h)$ straightforwardly extended to all $G \in \mathcal{G}$ typically satisfies (2.21) at all G. When formulating the extension, one might want to note that $IC_0(Y \mid Q_0, G, D_h)$ depends on (F_X, G) only through the law $P_{F_X, G} \in \mathcal{M}(\mathcal{G}^*)$ of the observed data when the conditional distribution of C, given X, is given by an element of $\mathcal{G}^*$. Thus, one needs to extend this mapping defined on $\mathcal{M}(\mathcal{G}^*)$ to $\mathcal{M}(\mathcal{G})$, but a straightforward ad hoc substitution typically works. This method provides a powerful way of obtaining initial mappings from full data estimating functions into observed data estimating functions since it only requires understanding a strongly simplified version (e.g., independent censoring) of the true data-generating experiment.

Example 2.7 (Right censored data structure: continuation of Example 2.2) Consider the right-censored data structure $(\tilde{T} = \min(T, C), \Delta, \bar{X}(\tilde{T}))$ and suppose that μ is a parameter of the marginal distribution F of T. Firstly, assume the independent censoring model $\mathcal{G}^* = \{G(\cdot \mid X) = G(\cdot)\}$, where C is independent of X under G^*. In this model, one can use the optimal mapping $A_F I_{F,G}^{-1}(D)$ for the *marginal* right-censored data structure $(\tilde{T}, \Delta)$, which is given by

$$IC_0(Y \mid F, G, D) = D(T)\Delta/\bar{G}(T) + \int E(D(T) \mid T > u) dM_G(u)/\bar{G}(u),$$

where $dM_G(u) = I(\tilde{T} \in du, \Delta = 0) - I(\tilde{T} \geq u) dG(u)/\bar{G}(u)$ and $\bar{G}(u) \equiv P(C \geq u)$. Simply replacing the independent censoring $G \in \mathcal{G}^*$ by a $G \in \mathcal{G}(CAR)$ now yields an extension $IC_0(Y \mid F, G, D)$ with protected nuisance parameter F satisfying the desired property (2.21) for all $G \in \mathcal{G}(CAR)$ provided $D(T)/\bar{G}(T \mid X) < \infty$ F_X-a.e. □

Example 2.8 (Multivariate right censored data structure) Let (T_1, T_2) be a bivariate survival time of interest, and let μ be a parameter of the bivariate cumulative distribution function F of (T_1, T_2). Let $C = (C_1, C_2)$ be a bivariate censoring variable. Suppose that we observe $(\tilde{T}_j = \min(T_j, C_j), \Delta_j = I(T_j \leq C_j), \bar{L}_j(\tilde{T}_j))$, $j = 1, 2$, where $L_j(\cdot)$ are covariate processes. We have for full data $X = (T_1, \bar{L}_1(T_1), T_2, \bar{L}(T_2))$. The observed data distribution is indexed by the full data distribution F_X and the conditional bivariate distribution G of (C_1, C_2), given X. CAR is a complicated concept for this data structure, but nice rich submodels of CAR are provided in Chapter 6, where we study this data structure in detail.

Firstly, assume the independent censoring model $\mathcal{G}^* = \{G : G(\cdot \mid X) = G(\cdot)\}$. In this model, one can use the optimal mapping $A_F I_{F,G}^{-1}(D)$ for the *marginal* bivariate right-censored data structure $(\tilde{T}_j, \Delta_j)$, $j = 1, 2$. The inverse $I_{F,G}^{-1}(D) = \sum_{k=0}^{\infty} (I - I_{F,G})^k(D)$ can be represented by a Neumann series mapping, which has been implemented in (Quale, van der Laan and Robins, 2001, see also Chapter 5). Replacing the marginal G by $G \in \mathcal{G}(CAR)$ now yields a mapping $IC_0(Y \mid F, G, D) = A_F I_{F,G}^{-1}(D)$ from full data estimating functions into observed data estimating functions with protected nuisance parameter F (bivariate cumulative distribution function) satisfying the desired property (2.21) for all $G \in \mathcal{G}(CAR)$. □

2.3.4 Inverse weighting a mapping developed for a restricted censoring model

We will now provide an alternative to the previous method. Again, consider a particular mapping $IC_0(Y \mid Q_1, G, D_h)$ developed under a restricted censoring model $\mathcal{G}^* \subset \mathcal{G}$ of the true model $\mathcal{G}$. Thus, it satisfies (2.21) at $G \in \mathcal{G}^* \subset \mathcal{G}$. For each $G \in \mathcal{G}$, let $G^* = G^*(G) \in \mathcal{G}^*$ be an approximation of G defined by a mapping $\Pi : \mathcal{G} \to \mathcal{G}^*$. For example, if G is an element of a multiplicative intensity model, then Π might correspond with setting some or all of the regression coefficients equal to zero. Alternatively, Π can be an unknown mapping defined by the Kullback–Leibner projection of G onto $\mathcal{G}^*$: the latter would be estimated by maximizing the likelihood over the restricted model $\mathcal{G}^*$. In addition, suppose that for each $G \in \mathcal{G}$ it is known that the Radon–Nykodim derivative dG^*/dG exists and is uniformly

bounded:
$$G^*(\cdot \mid X) \ll G(\cdot \mid X) \ F_X\text{-a.e.}$$

In this case, the mapping

$$IC_0(Y \mid Q_0, G, D_h) \equiv IC_0(Y \mid Q_0, G^*, D_h) \frac{dG^*(Y \mid X)}{dG(Y \mid X)} \quad (2.22)$$

satisfies (2.21) at all $G \in \mathcal{G}$.

Example 2.9 (Marginal structural models, continued) Consider the previously covered example in Section 1.3 of Chapter 1. Thus, for each subject, we observe a realization (i.e., the data) of vector $\bar{A} = (A(1), \ldots, A(p))$ of exposures and treatments, a vector of outcomes $\bar{Z} = (Z(1), \ldots, Z(p))$, and the covariates $L(\cdot)$ (including many time-dependent covariates) of interest. For observed data we have

$$Y = (\bar{A}, \bar{Z}, \bar{L}),$$

which in terms of counterfactuals is represented as the missing data structure:

$$Y = (\bar{A}, \bar{X}_{\bar{A}}) = (\bar{A}, \bar{Z}_{\bar{A}}, \bar{L}_{\bar{A}}).$$

It is assumed that the missingness mechanism (i.e., the conditional distribution of $\bar{A}$, given X) satisfies the SRA,

$$g(\bar{A} \mid X) = \prod_t g(A(t) \mid \bar{A}(t-), X) = \prod_t g(A(t) \mid \bar{A}(t-), \bar{X}_{\bar{A}}(t)), \quad (2.23)$$

and we consider a marginal structural repeated measures regression model as the full data model,

$$E(Z_{\bar{a}}(t) \mid V) = g_t(\bar{a}, V \mid \beta),$$

where $g_t(\bar{a}, V \mid \beta_j)$ is some specified regression curve (e.g., linear or logistic regression) indexed by the unknown regression coefficient vector, β, and V is the set of adjustment covariates (i.e., variables not affected by $\bar{a}$ by which one wants to stratify). The goal is to estimate the causal parameter β based on the observed data Y.

Let $\mathcal{A}$ be the set of possible sample paths of $\bar{A}$, where we assume that $\mathcal{A}$ is finite. In Example 1.3, we showed that the set of full data estimating functions is given by

$$\left\{ D_h(X \mid \beta) = \sum_{\bar{a}} h(\bar{a}, V) \epsilon_{\bar{a}}(\beta) : h \right\}.$$

Let $\mathcal{G}^* = \{g : g(A(j) \mid \bar{A}(j-1), \bar{X}_A(j)) = g(A(j) \mid \bar{A}(j-1), V)\}$ assume SRA w.r.t. treatment past and V. Thus, for each $g \in \mathcal{G}^*$, we have $g(\bar{A} \mid X) = g(\bar{A} \mid V)$. We define $IC_0(Y \mid G, D_h) = \frac{h(\bar{A}, V)}{g(\bar{A} \mid V)} \epsilon_A(\beta)$. Note that, indeed, at any $G \in \mathcal{G}^*$ we have

$$E_G(IC_0(Y \mid G, D_h) \mid X) = \sum_{\bar{a}} h(\bar{a}, V)\epsilon_{\bar{a}}(\beta) = D_h(X).$$

Given $g \in \mathcal{G}(SRA)$, let $g^* = g^*(g) \in \mathcal{G}^*$ be its projection (in some sense) of g onto $\mathcal{G}^*$ satisfying $\max_{\bar{a} \in \mathcal{A}}\{h(\bar{a}, V)g^*(\bar{a} \mid V)\}/g(\bar{a} \mid X) < \infty$ F_X-a.e. Then

$$IC_0(Y \mid G, D_h) \equiv IC_0(Y \mid G^*, D_h)\frac{g^*(\bar{A} \mid X)}{g(\bar{A} \mid X)} = \frac{h(\bar{A}, V)\epsilon(\beta)}{g(\bar{A} \mid X)}$$

is the IPTW mapping presented in Example 1.3, which satisfies the desired property $E_G(IC_0(Y \mid G, D_h) \mid X) = D_h(X)$ F_X-a.e. and at each $G \in \mathcal{G}(SRA)$. Note that this condition on h defines the set of allowed indexes $\mathcal{H}(\mu, \rho, \rho_1, G)$ and the allowed set of full data functions $\mathcal{D}(\rho_1, G)$. Notice that we would have obtained the same IPTW mapping by simply extending $IC_0(Y \mid G, D_h) = \frac{h(\bar{A}, V)}{g(\bar{A}|V)}\epsilon_A(\beta)$ to $\mathcal{G}(SRA)$. Thus, the methods of the previous subsection and this subsection yield identical results for this example.

In Chapter 6, we also apply this method to obtain the class of all estimating functions in marginal structural nested models, another class of causal inference models that allows one to estimate dynamic treatment-regime-specific outcome distributions. Other important applications of this method in causal inference are covered in Murphy, van der Laan and Robins (2001) and van der Laan, Murphy and Robins (2002). □

2.3.5 Beating a given RAL estimator

We will now show, given an RAL estimator of μ, how one can obtain a mapping $D_h \to IC_0(Y \mid F, G, D_h)$ from full data estimating functions into observed data estimating functions so that for a specified full data estimating function D_h it provides an estimating function that when evaluated at the true parameter values equals the influence curve of the given RAL estimator (and thus results in an estimator that is asymptotically equivalent with the given RAL estimator). Let μ_n be a given RAL estimator, and let $IC(Y \mid F_X, G)$ be its influence curve. Since $IC(Y \mid F_X, G)$ is a gradient of the pathwise derivative of μ, we have that $E_G(IC(Y \mid F, G) \mid X) \in T_{nuis}^{F, \perp, *}(F)$ for all $F \in \mathcal{M}^F$. Thus, by taking a conditional expectation, given X, $IC(Y \mid F, G)$ maps into a particular full data estimating function for μ. Let $h^* \equiv h_{ind, F_X}(E(IC(Y \mid F_X, G) \mid X))$ be the corresponding index of this estimating function:

$$D_{h^*}(X \mid \mu(F_X), \rho(F_X)) = E(IC(Y \mid F_X, G) \mid X).$$

For a multivariate full data function $D = (D_1, \ldots, D_k)$, one defines $h_{ind, F_X}(D) = (h_{ind, F_X}(D_1), \ldots, h_{ind, F_X}(D_k))$. Note that $h^* = h^*(F_X, G)$. Let $D_h \to IC_0(Y \mid G, D_h)$ be an initial mapping from full data estimating functions into observed data estimating functions satisfying $E_G(IC_0(Y \mid G, D_{h^*(F_X,G)}(\cdot \mid \mu(F_X), \rho(F_X, G))) \mid X) = D_{h^*(F_X,G)}(\cdot \mid \mu(F_X), \rho(F_X, G))$ for all $F_X \in \mathcal{M}^F$ and $G \in \mathcal{G}$. We now define $IC_{CAR}(Y \mid F_X, G)$ as

$$IC(Y \mid F_X, G) - IC_0(Y \mid G, D_{h^*(F_X,G)}(\cdot \mid \mu(F_X), \rho(F_X))).$$

Note that $E(IC_{CAR}(Y \mid F, G) \mid X) = 0$ for all $F \in \mathcal{M}^F$.

We now define as mapping from full data estimating functions into observed data estimating functions

$$IC(Y \mid F_X, G, D_h) = IC_0(Y \mid G, D_h) + IC_{CAR}(F_X, G).$$

Note that it satisfies (2.21) and, in addition, $IC(Y \mid F_X, G, D_{h^*}) = IC(Y \mid F_X, G)$. Consequently, under the regularity conditions of our asymptotic Theorem 2.4, the estimating equation with index h^* (or a consistent estimator thereof) yields an estimator that is asymptotically equivalent with μ_n. Other choices of h might result in more efficient estimators than μ_n.

In the following example, we combine this method described above with the extension method of Subsection 2.3.3 into a powerful application for the bivariate right-censored data structure.

Example 2.10 (Multivariate right-censored data structure; continuation of Example 2.8) We refer to Example 2.8. Thus, we observe $(\tilde{T}_j = \min(T_j, C_j), \Delta_j = I(T_j \leq C_j), \bar{L}_j(\tilde{T}_j))$, $j = 1, 2$, where $L_j(\cdot)$ are covariate processes. The parameter of interest is $\mu = S(t_1, t_2) = P(T_1 > t_1, T_2 > t_2)$. Let F be the bivariate cumulative distribution of (T_1, T_2). For full data, we have $X = (T_1, \bar{L}_1(T_1), T_2, \bar{L}(T_2))$. The observed data distribution is indexed by the full data distribution F_X and the conditional bivariate distribution G of (C_1, C_2), given X, which is assumed to be modeled with some submodel $\mathcal{G}$ of CAR, as provided in Chapter 6. Let the full data model be nonparametric so that the only full data estimating function is $D(X \mid \mu) = I_{(t_1,\infty) \times (t_2,\infty)}(T_1, T_2) - \mu$. Firstly, assume the independent censoring model $\mathcal{G}^* = \{G(\cdot \mid X) = G(\cdot)\}$.

A well-known estimator of $\mu = S(t_1, t_2)$ based on marginal bivariate right-censored data in the independent censoring model is the Dabrowska estimator (Dabrowska, 1988,1989). We want to apply the method above to find an estimating function for μ that yields an estimator that is asymptotically equivalent with Dabrowska's estimator. Subsequently, extending this mapping to $G \in \mathcal{G}$ yields an estimating function for our extended bivariate data structure only assuming our posed model $\mathcal{G}$ for G. The influence curve $IC_{Dab}(Y \mid F, G, (t_1, t_2))$ of Dabrowska's estimator is derived in Gill, van der Laan and Wellner (1995) and van der Laan (1990) and is given by

$$IC(Y) = \bar{F}(t_1, t_2) \left\{ -\int_0^{t_1} \frac{I(\tilde{T}_1 \in du, \Delta_1 = 1) - I(\tilde{T}_1 \geq u)\Lambda_1(du)}{P_{F,G}(\tilde{T}_1 \geq u)} \right.$$

$$\left. -\int_0^{t_2} \frac{I(\tilde{T}_2 \in du, \Delta_2 = 1) - I(\tilde{T}_2 \geq u)\Lambda_2(du)}{P_{F,G}(\tilde{T}_2 \geq u)} \right.$$

$$+ \int_0^{t_1} \int_0^{t_2} \frac{I(\tilde{T}_1 \in du, \tilde{T}_2 \in dv, \Delta_1 = 1, \Delta_2 = 1)}{P_{F,G}(\tilde{T}_1 \geq u, \tilde{T}_2 \geq v)}$$

$$- \int_0^{t_1} \int_0^{t_2} \frac{I(\tilde{T}_1 \geq u, \tilde{T}_2 \geq v)\Lambda_{11}(du, dv)}{P_{F,G}(\tilde{T}_1 \geq u, \tilde{T}_2 \geq v)}$$

$$- \int_0^{t_1} \int_0^{t_2} \frac{I(\tilde{T}_1 \in du, \tilde{T}_2 \geq v, \Delta_1 = 1)\Lambda_{01}(dv, u)}{P_{F,G}(\tilde{T}_1 \geq u, \tilde{T}_2 \geq v)}$$

$$+ \int_0^{t_1} \int_0^{t_2} \frac{I(\tilde{T}_1 \geq u, \tilde{T}_2 \geq v)\Lambda_{10}(du, v)\Lambda_{01}(dv, u)}{P_{F,G}(\tilde{T}_1 \geq u, \tilde{T}_2 \geq v)}$$

$$- \int_0^{t_1} \int_0^{t_2} \frac{I(\tilde{T}_1 \geq u, \tilde{T}_2 \in dv, \Delta_2 = 1)\Lambda_{10}(du, v)}{P_{F,G}(\tilde{T}_1 \geq u, \tilde{T}_2 \geq v)}$$

$$+ \int_0^{t_1} \int_0^{t_2} \frac{I(\tilde{T}_1 \geq u, \tilde{T}_2 \geq v)\Lambda_{10}(du, v)\Lambda_{01}(dv, u)}{P_{F,G}(\tilde{T}_1 \geq u, \tilde{T}_2 \geq v)} \Bigg\},$$

where $\Lambda_j(du) = P(T_j \in du \mid T_j \geq u)$, $j = 1, 2$, $\Lambda_{10}(du \mid v) = P(T_1 \in du \mid T_1 \geq u, T_2 \geq v)$, $\Lambda_{01}(dv, u) = P(T_2 \in dv \mid T_1 \geq u, T_2 \geq v)$, and $\Lambda_{11}(du, dv) = P(T_1 \in du, T_2 \in dv \mid T_1 \geq u, T_2 \geq v)$. Here $P_{F,G}(\tilde{T}_1 > s, \tilde{T}_2 > t) = S(s,t)\bar{G}(s,t)$. Firstly, we note that it is straightforward to verify that, if $\bar{G}(t_1, t_2) > 0$, then $E_G(IC_{Dab}(Y \mid F, G, (t_1, t_2)) \mid X) = D(X \mid \mu)$ for all $G \in \mathcal{G}^*$ satisfying independent censoring. In addition, if we replace G by any $G \in \mathcal{G}(CAR)$ satisfying CAR, then we still have

$$E_G(IC_{Dab}(Y \mid F, G, (t_1, t_2)) \mid X) = I_{(t_1, \infty) \times (t_2, \infty)}(T_1, T_2) - \mu$$

for all bivariate distributions F, as predicted in Subsection 2.3.3.

Let $IC_0(Y \mid G, D) = D(X)\Delta_1\Delta_2/\bar{G}(T_1, T_2 \mid X)$. We now define

$$IC_{CAR}(Y \mid F, G) \equiv IC_{Dab}(Y \mid F, G) - IC_0(Y \mid G, D(\cdot \mid \mu(F))).$$

Note that $E_G(IC_{CAR}(Y \mid F, G) \mid X) = 0$ for all bivariate distributions F and all $G \in \mathcal{G}(CAR)$.

We now define an observed data estimating function for μ indexed by the true censoring mechanism G and a bivariate distribution F:

$$IC(Y \mid F, G, D(\cdot \mid \mu)) = IC_0(Y \mid G, D(\cdot \mid \mu)) + IC_{CAR}(F, G). \quad (2.24)$$

It follows that this estimating function for μ satisfies $E_G(IC(Y \mid F, G, D(\cdot \mid \mu)) \mid X) = D(X \mid \mu)$ for all $G \in \mathcal{G}(CAR)$ and, at the true μ and F, it reduces to Dabrowska's influence curve. Given consistent estimators F_n of F and G_n of G according to model $\mathcal{G}$, let μ_n be the solution of

$$0 = \frac{1}{n} \sum_{i=1}^n IC(Y_i \mid F_n, G_n, D(\cdot \mid \mu)).$$

Under the regularity conditions of Theorem 2.4, μ_n is asymptotically linear with influence curve $IC(Y) \equiv \Pi(IC(\cdot \mid F, G, D(\cdot \mid \mu)) \mid T_2(P_{F_X, G}))$, where $T_2(P_{F_X, G}) \subset T_{CAR}$ is the observed data tangent space of G under the posed model $\mathcal{G}$. Firstly, assume that $\mathcal{G}^*$ is the independent censoring model. Since $IC(Y \mid F, G, D(\cdot \mid \mu))$ is already orthogonal to the tangent space $T(\mathcal{G}^*)$ of G for the independent censoring model $\mathcal{G}^*$, we have that $IC(Y) = IC_{Dab}(Y)$. Secondly, if the tangent space $T_2(P_{F_X,G})$ contains scores that are not in $T(\mathcal{G}^*)$, then it will result in an estimator more efficient than Dabrowska's estimator, even when (C_1, C_2) is independent of X. In Chapter 5, we provide a simulation study comparing this estimator with Dabrowska's estimator and further improve on this estimating function by orthogonalizing w.r.t. a tangent space of a rich submodel $\mathcal{G}$ of $\mathcal{G}(CAR)$ for G.

Note that the method used in this example can be used, in general, to generalize an estimator for a marginal data structure into an estimator for an extended data structure. □

2.3.6 Orthogonalizing an initial mapping w.r.t. G: Double robustness

Consider the following class of parametric submodels through the censoring mechanism $G_{Y|X}$:

$$\{(1 + \epsilon V(y))dG(y|x) : V \in L_0^2(P_{F_X,G}), E(V(Y) \mid X) = 0\}.$$

It is straightforward to show that the tangent space of G in the model $\mathcal{M}(\mathcal{G}_{CAR})$ generated by this class of parametric submodels is given by

$$T_{CAR}(P_{F_X,G}) = N(A_G^\top) = \{v \in L_0^2(P_{F_X,G}) : E(v(Y) \mid X) = 0\}.$$

An initial mapping can be orthogonalized w.r.t. $T_{CAR}(P_{F_X,G})$ itself, resulting in the optimal mapping in the next section, or w.r.t. subspaces of $T_{CAR}(P_{F_X,G})$ as in this subsection.

We will now present a general way of obtaining a mapping of estimating functions $IC_0(Y \mid Q_0, G, D)$ indexed by nuisance parameters Q_0, G with a double robustness property. Let $H(P_{F_X,G})$ be a tangent space of G according to some submodel of $\mathcal{G}(CAR)$. Thus $H(P_{F_X,G}) \subset T_{CAR}(P_{F_X,G})$ is a subspace of $T_{CAR}(P_{F_X,G})$ for all $P_{F_X,G} \in \mathcal{M}$. For example, one can set $H(P_{F_X,G})$ equal to the observed data tangent space $T_2(P_{F_X,G})$ of G in model $\mathcal{M}(\mathcal{G})$.

Since $T_{CAR}(P_{F_X,G}) = \{V(Y) \in L_0^2(P_{F_X,G}) : E_G(V(Y) \mid X) = 0\}$ only depends on F_X to make sure that the elements have finite variance w.r.t. $P_{F_X,G}$, it is always possible to find a rich common subset of $T_{CAR}(P_{F_X,G})$ only depending on G. By the same argument, one will also always be able to choose a rich common subset $H(G)$ of $H(P_{F_X,G})$. Let $\mathcal{Q}_0$ be an index set (independent of (F_X, G)) for $H(G)$ so that

$$H(G) \equiv \{IC_{nu}(\cdot \mid Q_0, G) : Q_0 \in \mathcal{Q}_0\} \subset H(P_{F_X,G}) \text{ for all } G \in \mathcal{G},$$

where $IC_{nu}(\cdot \mid Q_0, G)$ denotes the Q_0 indexed element of $H(G)$. It will be possible to define $(Q_0, G) \to (Y \to IC_{nu}(Y \mid Q_0, G))$ as a mapping from

$\mathcal{Q}_0 \times \mathcal{G}$ into pointwise well-defined functions of Y, which we will need in order to define the estimating function $IC_0(Y \mid Q_0, G, D)$ below.

We can now make a mapping $IC_0(Y \mid G, D)$ satisfying (2.21) orthogonal (at the truth) to $H(P_{F_X,G})$ by introducing another nuisance parameter $Q_0 = Q_0(F_X, G)$ as follows:

$$IC_0(Y \mid Q_0, G, D) = IC_0(Y \mid G, D) - IC_{nu}(Y \mid Q_0, G),$$

where the unknown parameter $Q_0(F_X, G)$ is defined by

$$IC_{nu}(\cdot \mid Q_0(F_X, G), G) = \Pi_{F_X, G}(IC_0(\cdot \mid G, D) \mid H(P_{F_X,G}))$$

and the equality holds in $L_0^2(P_{F_X,G})$.

This mapping $D \to IC_0(Y \mid Q_0, G, D)$ maps full data estimating functions $D_h(\cdot \mid \mu, \rho)$ for μ into observed data estimating functions $IC_0(\cdot \mid Q_0, G, D_h(\cdot \mid \mu, \rho))$ for μ with unknown nuisance parameters $Q_0 = Q_0(F_X, G)$ and G. It has the property $E_G(IC_0(Y \mid Q_0, G, D) \mid X) = D(X)$ for all possible Q_0, and thus it remains unbiased when Q_0 is misspecified. Therefore, it can be used to construct an initial estimator in the model $\mathcal{M}(\mathcal{G})$ in which we assume that $G \in \mathcal{G}$: for a given $h \in \mathcal{H}$, an estimator ρ_n of ρ, Q_{0n} of Q_0, G_n of G, let μ_n^0 be the solution of the estimating equation

$$0 = \sum_{i=1}^{n} IC_0(Y_i \mid Q_{0n}, G_n, D_h(\cdot \mid \mu, \rho_n)). \quad (2.25)$$

If Q_{0n} converges to some Q_0 not necessarily equal to $Q_0(F_X, G)$, then application of Theorem 2.4 yields, under regularity conditions, that the estimator is asymptotically linear with influence curve $-\Pi(c^{-1} IC_0(\cdot \mid Q_0, G, D_h(\cdot \mid \mu, \rho)) \mid T_2(P_{F_X,G})^{\perp})$, where c is the derivative matrix w.r.t. μ of the expectation of IC_0. In particular, if $Q_0 = Q_0(F_X, G)$ and $H(P_{F_X,G}) = T_2(P_{F_X,G})$, then this influence curve equals $-c^{-1} IC_0(\cdot \mid Q_0(F_X, G), G, D, D_h(\cdot \mid \mu, \rho))$.

Finally, we note that the mapping $IC_0(Y \mid F, G, D) = A_F I_{F,G}^-(D)$ considered in the previous subsection is also of this type since

$$A_{F_X} I_{F_X,G}^-(D) = IC_0(Y \mid G, D) - \Pi_{F_X,G}(IC_0(Y \mid G, D) \mid T_{CAR})$$

for any initial $IC_0(Y \mid G, D)$ satisfying $E(IC_0(Y \mid G, D) \mid X) = D(X)$. In other words, if we set $H(P_{F_X,G}) = T_{CAR}(P_{F_X,G})$, then $IC_0(Y \mid Q_1, G, D)$ reduces to $IC_0(Y \mid F, G, D) = A_F I_{F,G}^-(D)$.

Example 2.11 (Right-censored data structure; continuation of Example 2.2) Consider the right-censored data structure $Y = (\tilde{T} = \min(T, C), \Delta = I(\tilde{T} = T), \bar{L}(\tilde{T}))$. Suppose that $H(P_{F_X,G})$ is the tangent space of G in the independent censoring model. We have that $H(P_{F_X,G}) = \overline{\{\int H(u) dM_G(u) : H\}} \cap L_0^2(P_{F_X,G})$, where $dM_G(u) = I(\tilde{T} \in du, \Delta = 0) - I(\tilde{T} \geq u) \Lambda_C(du)$. If $\int \mid dM_G(u) \mid < \infty$, then one can choose $H(G) = \{\int H(u) dM_G(u) : \parallel H \parallel_\infty < \infty\}$. Let $IC_0(Y \mid G, D) = \frac{D(X)\Delta(D)}{G(V(D)\mid X)}$,

2.3. Mapping into Observed Data Estimating Functions

where $\Delta(D)$ is the indicator that $D(X)$ is observed, $V(D)$ is the minimum time at which D is fully observed, and $\bar{G}(V(D) \mid X)$ is the probability that $\Delta(D) = 1$, given X.

Application of Lemma 3.2, formula (3.17) from the next chapter, yields

$$\Pi_{F_X,G}(IC_0 \mid H(P_{F_X,G})) = -\int \frac{E_{F_X,G}\left(\frac{D(X)\Delta(D)}{\bar{G}(V(D)\mid X)}I(T \geq u)\right)}{P(\tilde{T} \geq u)} dM_G(u)$$

so that, for any function $Q_0(u)$, we can define

$$IC_0(Y \mid Q_0, G, D) = \frac{D(X)\Delta(D)}{\bar{G}(V(D) \mid X)} + \int Q_0(u) dM_G(u),$$

where $Q_0(F_X, G)(u) = E_{F_X,G}(D(X)\Delta(D)I(T \geq u)/\bar{G}(V(D) \mid X))/P(\tilde{T} \geq u) = E_{F_X}(D(X) \mid T > u)/\bar{G}(u)$.

Let us now consider the special case in which $\mu = F(t) = P(T \leq t)$, $D(X) = I(T \leq t) - F(t)$, and we assume the independent censoring model $G(\cdot \mid X) = G(\cdot)$ for G. Then $IC_0(Y \mid Q_0(F_X, G), G, D)$ equals the influence curve IC_{KM} of the Kaplan–Meier estimator. The corresponding estimating equation results in an estimator μ_n that is asymptotically equivalent with the Kaplan–Meier estimator. If one assumes the Cox proportional hazards model for G with covariates extracted from the observed past, then μ_n is asymptotically linear with influence curve $IC_{KM} - \Pi(IC_{KM} \mid T_2(P_{F_X,G}))$, where $T_2(P_{F_X,G})$ denotes the tangent space of the Cox proportional hazards model. Thus, in the last case, μ_n will be more efficient than the Kaplan–Meier estimator. □

Double protection (robustness) when orthogonalizing w.r.t. convex censoring models

If $H(P_{F_X,G})$ is the tangent space of G for a *convex* model $\mathcal{G}(conv) \subset \mathcal{G}(CAR)$ containing $\mathcal{G}$, then the mapping $D \to IC_0(\cdot \mid Q_0, G, D)$ from full data estimating functions to observed data estimating functions satisfies a double protection property against misspecification of G and F_X defined by (2.27) below. This follows from Theorem 1.6 and Lemma 1.9. As a consequence, in this case it actually yields estimating functions in model $\mathcal{M}$. A special case is $H(P_{F_X,G}) = T_{CAR}(P_{F_X,G})$, where $T_{CAR}(P_{F_X,G})$ is the tangent space of G for the model $\mathcal{G}(CAR)$, which makes IC_0 corresponded with the optimal mapping $A_F I_{F,G}^-(D)$ as introduced above. The latter mapping will actually be the mapping proposed in the next section and applied in all subsequent chapters, which will allow locally efficient estimation. For some data structures, the projection on $T_{CAR}(P_{F_X,G})$ does not exist in closed form. In that case, the estimating function $IC_0(\cdot \mid Q_0, G, D_h(\cdot \mid \mu, \rho))$ with $H(P_{F_X,G}) \subset T_{CAR}(P_{F_X,G})$ chosen so that the projection operator on $H(P_{F_X,G})$ exists in closed form provides an interesting alternative. Such a mapping is used in Chapter 5 to provide estimators for the extended bivariate right-censored data structure and in Chapter 6 to identify causal and non causal parameters in complex longitudinal data structures involving censoring and time-dependent informative treatment assignments.

Let us prove the double protection property (2.27) to make this section self-contained. By definition, $IC_0(\cdot \mid Q_0(F_X, G), G, D)$ is actually orthogonal to the tangent space $H(P_{F_X,G})$. By the convexity of $\mathcal{G}(conv)$, we know that for all $G_1 \in \mathcal{G}(conv)$ with $dG_1/dG < \infty$, $\alpha G_1 + (1-\alpha)G$ is a submodel of $\mathcal{G}(conv)$. Consequently, the line $dP_{F_X, \alpha G_1 + (1-\alpha)G}$ is a submodel of $\mathcal{M}(\mathcal{G}(conv))$ that has score (by linearity of $G \to P_{F_X,G}$) $(dP_{F_X,G_1} - dP_{F_X,G})/dP_{F_X,G}$. Thus, the latter score is an element of $H(P_{F_X,G})$. Thus, the orthogonality of $IC_0(Y \mid Q_0(F_X,G), G, D)$ to $(dP_{F_X,G_1} - dP_{F_X,G})/dP_{F_X,G}$ now yields

$$\begin{aligned} 0 &= E_{P_{F_X,G}} IC_0(Y \mid Q_0(F_X,G), G, D) \frac{dP_{F_X,G_1} - dP_{F_X,G}}{dP_{F_X,G}}(Y) \\ &= E_{P_{F_X,G_1} - P_{F_X,G}} IC_0(Y \mid Q_0(F_X,G), G, D) \\ &= E_{P_{F_X,G_1}} IC_0(Y \mid Q_0(F_X,G), G, D) \text{ if } D \in \mathcal{D}(\rho_1(F_X), G) \end{aligned}$$

and $E_{F_X} D(X) = 0$. Here we used that $D \in \mathcal{D}(\rho_1(F_X), G)$ guarantees that $E_{P_{F_X,G}} IC_0(Y \mid Q(F_X,G), G, D) = E_{F_X} D(X) = 0$. Exchanging the role of G and G_1 proves the following result: for all pairs $G, G_1 \in \mathcal{G}(conv)$ with $dG/dG_1 < \infty$, we have for all $D \in \mathcal{D}(\rho_1(F_X), G_1)$ with $E_{F_X} D(X) = 0$

$$0 = E_{P_{F_X,G}} IC_0(Y \mid Q_0(F_X, G_1), G_1, D).$$

We note that this provides a sufficient, but not necessary condition. For example, if the identity holds at $G_1 = G_{1m}$ for a sequence at G_{1m}, $m = 1, \ldots$, which approximates a G^* in the sense that $E_{P_{F_X,G}} IC_0(Y \mid Q_0(F_X, G_{1m}), G_{1m}, D) \to E_{P_{F_X,G}} IC_0(Y \mid Q_0(F_X, G^*), G^*, D)$, then it follows that the identity also holds at $G_1 = G^*$. Therefore, it is not surprising that in many applications the identity also holds for pairs G_1, G not satisfying $dG/dG_1 < \infty$. This identity gives us protection against misspecification of G when the Q_0 component of IC is correctly estimated in the sense that if G_n converges to some $G_1 \in \mathcal{G}(conv)$ with $dG/dG_1 < \infty$, then μ_n^0 (2.25) will still be consistent.

Given $D \in \mathcal{D}(\rho_1(F_X), G)$, the conditional expectation of $IC_0(Y \mid Q_0, G, D)$, given X, equals $D(X)$, which proves that for any $Q_0 \in \mathcal{Q}_0$ $E_{F_X,G} IC(Y \mid Q_0, G, D) = 0$. This gives us protection against misspecification of $Q_0(F_X, G)$ when G is correctly estimated. To summarize, our definition of the mapping $IC_0(\cdot \mid Q_0, G, D)$ of full data estimating functions to observed data estimating function depends on the unknown $Q_0(F_X, G)$ and G, but it is protected by misspecification of either F_X or G in the following sense.

Theorem 2.2 *We have*

$$\begin{aligned} E_{F_X,G} IC_0(Y \mid Q_0(F_X, G_1), G_1, D) &= E_{F_X} D(X) \text{ for } D \in \mathcal{D}(\rho_1(F_X), G_1) \\ &\text{and all } G_1 \in \mathcal{G}(conv) \text{ with } G \ll G_1. \end{aligned} \quad (2.26)$$

$$E_{F_X,G} IC_0(Y \mid Q_0, G, D) = E_{F_X} D(X)$$
$$\text{for all } Q_0 \in \mathcal{Q}_0 \text{ and } D \in \mathcal{D}(\rho_1(F_X), G). \tag{2.27}$$

Note that the protection against misspecification of G can be exploited by estimating Q_0 and the nuisance parameter $\rho(F_X, G)$ in $D_h(\cdot \mid \mu, \rho)$ with substitution estimators $Q_0(F_n, G_n)$ and $\rho(F_n, G_n)$.

2.3.7 Ignoring information on the censoring mechanism improves efficiency

Let $T_2(P_{F_X,G})$ be the tangent space of G in model $\mathcal{M}(\mathcal{G})$. Application of Theorem 2.4 below shows that, under regularity conditions, μ_n^0 (2.25) is asymptotically linear with influence curve

$$\Pi(c^{-1} IC_0(\cdot \mid Q_0, G, D_h(\cdot \mid \mu, \rho)) \mid T_2^{\perp}(P_{F_X,G})), \tag{2.28}$$

where $c = d/d\mu E IC_0(Y \mid Q_0, G, D_h(\cdot \mid \mu, \rho))$ and Q_0 is the limit of Q_{0n}. In particular, this teaches us that μ_n^0 will become more efficient if one estimates G more nonparametrically. Thus, if G is known and one sets $G_n = G$ in the estimating equation (2.25), then μ_n^0 is asymptotically linear with influence curve $c^{-1} IC_0(\cdot \mid G, c(\mu), D_h(\cdot \mid \mu, \rho))$, which can have much larger variance than the influence curve (2.28) for a reasonable size model $\mathcal{G}$.

To understand this feature of the estimator, we prove the following general result. The proof of this theorem actually shows, in general, that optimal estimation of an orthogonal nuisance parameter leads to an asymptotic improvement of the estimator. Application of this theorem with $\mu_n(G_n) = \mu_n^0$ and $\mu_n(G)$ being the solution of the estimating equation (2.25) with $G_n = G$ known explains the result (2.28).

Theorem 2.3 *Let $\mathcal{M}(G) = \{P_{F_X,G} : F_X \in \mathcal{M}^F\}$ be the model $\mathcal{M}$ with G known. Let $\mu_n(G)$ be a regular asymptotically linear estimator of μ in the model $\mathcal{M}(G)$ with G known with influence curve $IC_0(Y \mid F_X, G)$. Assume now that for an estimator G_n*

$$\mu_n(G_n) - \mu = \mu_n(G) - \mu + \Phi(G_n) - \Phi(G) + o_P(1/\sqrt{n})$$

for some functional Φ of G_n. Assume that $\Phi(G_n)$ is an asymptotically efficient estimator of $\Phi(G)$ for the model $\mathcal{M}(\mathcal{G})$ with tangent space generated by G given by $T_2(P_{F_X,G})$. Then $\mu_n(G_n)$ is regular asymptotically linear with influence curve

$$IC_1(F_X, G) = \Pi(IC_0(F_X, G) \mid T_2(P_{F_X,G})^{\perp}).$$

Proof. We decompose $L_0^2(P_{F_X,G})$ orthogonally in $T_1(P_{F_X,G}) + T_2(P_{F_X,G}) + T^{\perp}(P_{F_X,G})$, where $T^{\perp}(P_{F_X,G})$ is the orthogonal complement of $T_1 + T_2$, and $T_1 = T_1(P_{F_X,G})$ and $T_2(P_{F_X,G})$ are the tangent spaces corresponding to F_X and G, respectively. The assumptions in the lemma imply that $\mu_n(G_n)$ is asymptotically linear with influence curve $IC = IC_0 + IC_{nu}$, where IC_{nu} is an influence curve corresponding with an estimator of the nuisance parameter $\Phi(G)$ estimated under the model with nuisance tangent space T_2. Let $IC_0 = a_0 + b_0 + c_0$ and $IC_{nu} = a_{nu} + b_{nu} + c_{nu}$ according to the orthogonal decomposition of $L_0^2(P_{F_X,G})$ above. From now on, the proof uses the following two general facts about influence curves of regular asymptotically linear estimators (see Bickel, Klaassen, Ritov and Wellner, 1993): an influence curve is orthogonal to the nuisance tangent space, and the efficient influence curve lies in the tangent space. Since IC_{nu} is an influence curve of $\Phi(G)$ in the model where nothing is assumed on F_X it is orthogonal to T_1; that is, $a_{nu} = 0$. Since $\Phi(G_n)$ is efficient, IC_{nu} lies in the tangent space T_2 and hence $c_{nu} = 0$ as well. We also have that $IC_0 + IC_{nu}$ is an influence curve for an estimator of μ and hence is orthogonal to T_2, so $b_0 + b_{nu} = 0$. Consequently, we have that

$$IC_1 = IC_0 + IC_{nu} = a_0 + c_0 = \Pi(IC_0 \mid T_2^\perp).$$

This completes the proof. □

Example 2.12 (Marginal right-censored data) Suppose that we observe n i.i.d. observations of $Y = (\tilde{T} = T \wedge C, \Delta = I(\tilde{T} = T) = I(C \geq T))$. Let F be the cumulative distribution function of the full data T, and let G be the conditional distribution of C, given T, satisfying CAR. In this case, CAR is equivalent with assuming that the censoring hazard $\lambda_{C\mid T}(t \mid T)$ only depends on $\bar{X}(t)$, where $X(t) = I(T \leq t)$.

Let us first consider the observed data model with G known. In that model, we could estimate $\mu = F(t)$ with the inverse probability of censoring weighted estimator

$$\mu_n(G) = \frac{1}{n} \sum_{i=1}^{n} I(T_i \leq t) \frac{\Delta_i}{\bar{G}(T_i)},$$

where $\bar{G}(t) = P(C \geq t)$. We have that $\mu_n(G)$ is regular and asymptotically linear with influence curve $IC_0(Y \mid G, \mu) = I(T \leq t)\Delta/\bar{G}(T) - \mu$. Consider now the model where we only assume CAR on G. Let G_n be the Kaplan–Meier estimator of G based on the n censored observations $(\tilde{T}, 1 - \Delta)$. It is well-known that G_n is an efficient estimator of G in the model $\mathcal{M}(CAR)$. Application of Lemma 2.3 yields that $\mu_n(G_n)$ is a regular and asymptotically linear estimator with influence curve $IC_0(Y \mid G, \mu)$ minus its projection on the tangent space $T_{CAR}(P_{F_X,G})$ for G when only assuming CAR.

Let $A_F : L_0^2(F) \to L_0^2(P_{F,G})$ $A_F(h)(Y) = E_F(h(T) \mid Y)$ be the nonparametric score operator, and let $A_G(V)(X) = E_G(V(Y) \mid X)$ be its adjoint. Since the full data model is nonparametric, we actually have that the closure of the range of A_F is the tangent space of F in the model $\mathcal{M}(CAR)$. We have that $T_{CAR}^\perp = N(A_G^\top)^\perp = \overline{R(A_F)}$. This proves that the influence curve of $\mu_n(G_n)$ is an element of the tangent space $\overline{R(A_F)}$ and thus must equal the efficient influence curve; Here, we use the fact that the efficient influence curve (which equals the canonical gradient of the pathwise derivative) is the only influence curve which is an element of the tangent space. This proves that $\mu_n(G_n)$ is an efficient estimator of μ, while $\mu_n(G)$ is far from efficient. In this particular example, we have the remarkable coincidence that $\mu_n(G_n)$ equals the Kaplan–Meier estimator algebraically, assuming that we define the Kaplan-Meier estimator to be zero after the last uncensored observation. □

2.4 Optimal Mapping into Observed Data Estimating Functions

Let $D_h \rightarrow IC_0(Y \mid Q_0, G, D_h)$ be an initial mapping from full data estimating functions into observed data estimating functions satisfying (2.21). Let $IC_{CAR}(\cdot \mid Q, G)$ with Q ranging over a parameter space $\mathcal{Q}$ be pointwise well defined functions of Y satisfying

$$\{IC_{CAR}(\cdot \mid Q, G) : Q \in \mathcal{Q}\} \subset T_{CAR}(P_{F_X, G}) \text{ for all } P_{F_X, G} \in \mathcal{M}. \quad (2.29)$$

Let $IC_{CAR}(\cdot \mid Q(F_X, G), G, D)$ be a pointwise well-defined function of Y that equals the projection

$$\Pi_{F_X, G}(IC_0(\cdot \mid Q_0, G, D) \mid T_{CAR}(P_{F_X, G}))$$

of $IC_0(\cdot \mid Q_0, G, D)$ onto $T_{CAR}(P_{F_X, G})$ in the Hilbert space $L^2(P_{F_X, G})$. Then, for any $D \in \mathcal{D}, Q_0 \in \mathcal{Q}_0, Q \in \mathcal{Q}, F_X \in \mathcal{M}^F, G \in \mathcal{G}$,

$$IC(Y \mid Q_0, Q, G, D) \equiv IC_0(Y \mid Q_0, G, D) - IC_{CAR}(Y \mid Q, G, D)$$

is a pointwise well-defined function of Y. Note that if $IC_0(Y \mid Q_0, G, D) = IC_0(Y \mid G, D) + IC_{nu}(Y \mid Q_0, D)$ with $IC_{nu}(Y \mid Q_0, G, D) \in T_{CAR}$, such as the orthogonalized mapping of the previous subsection, then $IC(Y \mid Q_0, Q, G, D)$ does not depend on Q_0. For simplicity, let Q include Q_0 if needed so that we can denote $IC(Y \mid Q_0, Q, G, D)$ with $IC(Y \mid Q, G, D)$.

Again, this mapping can be viewed as a mapping from full data estimating functions $D_h(\cdot \mid \mu, \rho)$ for μ into observed data estimating functions $IC(\cdot \mid Q, G, D_h(\cdot \mid \mu, \rho))$ for μ, indexed by unknown nuisance parameters $Q(F_X, G)$ and G. Theorem 1.3 proves that, if the set $\{D_h(\cdot \mid \mu(F_X), \rho(F_X)) : h \in \mathcal{H}^F(\mu(F_X), \rho(F_X), \rho_1(F_X), G)\}$ of full data functions satisfying $E_G(IC(Y \mid Q(F_X, G), G, D_h(\cdot \mid \mu(F_X), \rho(F_X))) \mid X) = D_h(X \mid \mu(F_X), \rho(F_X))$ equals $T_{nuis}^{F, \perp}(F_X)$, then $\{IC(Y \mid Q(F_X, G), G, D) : D \in T_{nuis}^{F, \perp}(F_X)\}$ equals the orthogonal complement of the nuisance tangent space $T_{nuis}^{\perp}(P_{F_X, G})$ in model $\mathcal{M}(CAR)$, which includes the efficient influence curve $IC(Y \mid Q(F_X, G), G, D_{h_{opt}(F_X, G)}(\cdot \mid \mu(F_X), \rho(F_X, G)))$. This mapping generates a class of estimating functions for the model $\mathcal{M}$ because

138   2. General Methodology

of the double protection property proved above:
$$E_{F_X,G}IC(Y \mid Q(F_X,G_1), G_1, D) = E_{F_X}D(X)$$
for all $D \in \mathcal{D}(\rho_1(F_X), G_1)$ and $G_1 \in \mathcal{G}$ with $dG/dG_1 < \infty$. (2.30)
$$E_{F_X,G}IC(Y \mid Q, G, D) = E_{F_X}D(X)$$
for all $Q \in \mathcal{Q}$, $D \in \mathcal{D}(\rho_1(F_X), G)$. (2.31)

Implications of protection property (2.30) for estimation of Q and ρ.

In model $\mathcal{M}(\mathcal{G})$, one only needs to rely on (2.31), which allows one to estimate $Q(F_X, G)$ with any estimator Q_n, and one needs to estimate $\rho = \rho(F_X, G)$ with a consistent estimator. However, in model $\mathcal{M}$, one needs to exploit (2.30). Let F_n be an estimator of F_X according to a working model $\mathcal{M}^w$, and assume that we use a substitution estimator $Q_n = Q(F_n, G_n)$, and $\rho_n = \rho(F_n, G_n)$ of $\rho(F_X, G)$. Consider the situation that $F_n \to F_X$ but $G_n \to G_1$ for a possibly wrong G_1. Then (2.30) teaches us that we need $Q_n \to Q(F_X, G_1)$, which naturally will hold, and $D \in \mathcal{D}(\rho_1(F_X), G_1)$. We will now explain why the latter condition can also be expected to hold. Recall that the nuisance parameter ρ in the full data structure estimating function $D_h(X \mid \mu, \rho)$ includes G as a component, which we needed to make sure that the estimating function at the true parameter values is an element of $\mathcal{D}(\rho_1(F_X), G)$. Since we estimate G with G_n, $G_n \to G_1$, and $F_n \to F_X$, we would precisely obtain that
$$D_h(\cdot \mid \mu_n, \rho_n) \to D_h(\cdot \mid \mu(F_X), \rho(F_X, G_1)) \in \mathcal{D}(\rho_1(F_X), G_1),$$
in the limit, as required.

Note also, as stressed in the discussion after Theorem 1.6, one does not need that $D_h(\cdot \mid \mu(F_X), \rho(F_X, G)) \in \mathcal{D}(\rho_1(F_X), G))$ necessarily; that is, $IC_0(Y \mid G, D(\cdot \mid \mu(F_X), \rho(F_X, G)))$ is allowed to be biased under the true data generating distribution $P_{F_X,G}$, but we do need that $IC_0(Y \mid G_1, D(\cdot \mid \mu(F_X), \rho(F_X, G_1)))$ needs to be unbiased under the possibly misspecified P_{F_X,G_1}, which holds if $D_h(\cdot \mid \mu(F_X), \rho(F_X, G_1)) \in \mathcal{D}(\rho_1(F_X), G_1)$.

A score operator representation

Let $A_{F_X} : L_0^2(F_X) \to L_0^2(P_{F_X,G})$ be the nonparametric score operator for F_X:
$$A_{F_X}(s)(Y) = E(s(X) \mid Y).$$
The adjoint $A_G^\top : L_0^2(P_{F_X,G}) \to L_0^2(F_X)$ of A_{F_X} is given by
$$A_G^\top(V)(X) = E(V(Y) \mid X).$$
Let $\mathbf{I}_{F_X,G} = A_{F_X} A_G^\top : L_0^2(F_X) \to L_0^2(F_X)$ which will be referred to as the nonparametric information operator. As shown in Theorem 1.3 (Chapter 1), for $D \in R(\mathbf{I}_{F_X,G})$ we have
$$IC(Y \mid Q(F_X, G), G, D) = A_{F_X} \mathbf{I}_{F_X,G}^{-1}(D). \quad (2.32)$$

2.4. Optimal Mapping into Observed Data Estimating Functions

Double protection property

The least squares representation $D \to IC(\cdot \mid Q(F_X, G), G, D) = IC(\cdot \mid F_X, G, D) \equiv A_{F_X}\mathbf{I}^-_{F_X, G}(D)$ from full data estimating functions to observed data estimating equations indexed by nuisance parameters F_X, G satisfies the double protection property (see Theorem 1.7 for the fact that we do not need the condition $dG/dG_1 < \infty$):

$$E_{F_X, G} IC(Y \mid F_X, G_1, D) = E_{F_X} D(X) \text{ for } D \in \mathcal{D}(F_X, G_1)$$
$$\text{for all } G_1 \in \mathcal{G}(CAR),$$
$$E_{F_X, G} IC(Y \mid F_{X1}, G, D) = E_{F_X} D(X)$$
$$\text{for } F_{X1} \in \mathcal{M}^F, D \in \mathcal{D}(F_X, G),$$

where

$$\mathcal{D}(F_X, G) = \{D \in \mathcal{D} : D \in R(\mathbf{I}_{F_1, G}) \text{ for all } F_1 \in \mathcal{M}^F\}$$

plays the role of $\mathcal{D}(\rho_1(F_X), G)$. Here $D \in R(\mathbf{I}_{F_1, G})$ denotes that D is an element of the range of the information operator $\mathbf{I}_{F_1, G} : L^2_0(F_X) \to L^2_0(F_X)$. Alternatively, we could require $D \in R_\infty(\mathbf{I}_{F_1, G})$ for all $F_1 \in \mathcal{M}^F$, as defined in Theorem 2.1.

2.4.1 The corresponding estimating equation

Consider the optimal mapping $IC(Y \mid Q, G, D)$ from full data structure estimating functions $\{D_h : h \in \mathcal{H}^F\}$ into observed data estimating functions. As described in detail in the previous section, given such a mapping, one first needs to identify the index set $\mathcal{H}^F(\mu, \rho, \rho_1, G) \subset \mathcal{H}^F$ so that

$$\{D_h(\cdot \mid \mu(F_X), \rho(F_X)) : h \in \mathcal{H}^F((\mu, \rho, \rho_1)(F_X), G)\} \subset \mathcal{D}(\rho_1(F_X), G).$$

Subsequently, one reparametrizes the allowed full data structure estimating functions $\{D_h : h \in \mathcal{H}^F(\mu, \rho, \rho_1, G)\}$ as $\{D^r_h : h \in \mathcal{H}^F\}$ by including the membership $I(D_h(\cdot \mid \mu(F_X), \rho(F_X)) \in \mathcal{D}(\rho_1(F_X), G))$ as an additional nuisance parameter as in (2.14). In this manner, one obtains a set of full data estimating functions that satisfy $E_G(IC(Y \mid Q(F_X, G), G, D^r_h) \mid X) = D^r_h(X)$ F_X-a.e. when D^r_h is evaluated at the true parameter values. As we mentioned, for notational convenience, this reparametrized set of allowed full data structure estimating functions is denoted with $D_h(\cdot \mid \mu, \rho)$, where ρ now also includes G as a component.

Consider estimators G_n and Q_n. In model $\mathcal{M}$, we assume that $Q_n = Q(F_n, G_n)$ is a substitution estimator, where F_n is an estimator of F_X that is consistent at $F_X \in \mathcal{M}^{F,w}$ so that either G_n or F_n will be consistent. Assume also that we have available an estimator ρ_n that is consistent for $\rho(F_X, G_1)$, where G_1 is the limit of G_n; that is, ρ_n is consistent for $\rho(F_X, G)$ in model $\mathcal{M}(\mathcal{G})$, and consistent for $\rho(F_X, G_1)$ in model $\mathcal{M}$. Thus, in model $\mathcal{M}$ one should use a substitution estimator $\rho_n = \rho(F_n, G_n)$. In the next

140   2. General Methodology

paragraph we provide a general strategy for providing such a estimator ρ_n in model $\mathcal{M}$. Note that in essence we require the existence of a doubly robust estimator of the F_X-parameter $\rho(F_X, G_1)$, which might itself require the doubly robust estimation methodology we present for estimation of μ.

Remark: Doubly robust estimation of nuisance parameter ρ in model $\mathcal{M}$.

For simplicity, consider the case where the nuisance parameter $\rho = \rho(F_X)$ does not have a G-component. As pointed out above, if ρ includes a G-component and G_n converges to a G_1, then we need that ρ_n converges to $\rho = \rho(F_X, G_1)$. As a consequence, in this case one just applies the following to the F_X-parameter $\rho_1(F_X) = \rho(F_X, G_1)$, where G_1 is estimated with G_n. We can obtain consistent estimator (i.e. doubly robust estimator) ρ_n of ρ under Model M, even when ρ is a non-regular parameter (i.e., a parameter for which the semiparametric information bound is 0) in model M^F. To do so, we express the non-regular parameter ρ as the limit of a regular parameter ρ_σ as $\sigma \to 0$, where σ is a bandwidth or other regularization parameter. See van der Laan and Robins (1998) for an example, and van der Laan, van der Vaart (2002). Because ρ_σ is a regular parameter of F_X we can often construct consistent estimators of $\rho(\sigma)$ in Model M (i.e., doubly robust estimators of ρ_σ). Let σ_n be an appropriate bandwidth or regularization parameter corresponding to sample size n and let $\hat{\rho}_{\sigma_n}$ be the corresponding doubly robust estimator of ρ_{σ_n}. Then, as in Robins and Rotnitzky (2001), we obtain a doubly robust estimator of μ using the approach discussed above by using $\hat{\rho}_{\sigma_n}$ as an estimator of ρ

To achieve higher efficiency, it makes sense to use a data-dependent index h_n. We use as the estimating equation for μ

$$0 = \frac{1}{n} \sum_{i=1}^{n} IC(Y_i \mid Q_n, G_n, D_{h_n}(\cdot \mid \mu, \rho_n)). \qquad (2.33)$$

Note that h indexes a whole class of estimating functions. In Section 2.8, we identify the optimal index $h_{opt}(F_X, G)$, which yields the optimal estimating function, given that we know the true (F_X, G). In model $\mathcal{M}$, one estimates $h_{opt}(F_X, G)$ with a plug-in estimator $h_n = h_{opt}(F_{X,n}, G_n)$, assuming our working models $\mathcal{M}^{F,w}$ and $\mathcal{G}$. This estimator h_n will be consistent for $h_{opt}(F_X, G)$ if both working models $\mathcal{M}^{F,w}$ and $\mathcal{G}$ are correctly specified.

One can solve the estimating equation (2.33) with the Newton–Raphson procedure described in Section 2.3. Let μ_n^0 be an initial estimator or guess. The first step of the Newton–Raphson procedure involves estimation of a derivative (matrix) w.r.t. μ_n^0. This derivative is defined by

$$c(\mu) = c(h, \mu, \rho, Q, G, P) = \frac{d}{d\mu} PIC(Y \mid Q, G, D_{h_n}(\cdot \mu, \rho)),$$

2.4. Optimal Mapping into Observed Data Estimating Functions

where we used the notation $Pf \equiv \int f(y)dP(y)$. Let

$$IC(Y \mid Q, G, c, D_h(\cdot \mu, \rho)) = c^{-1}IC(Y \mid Q, G, D_h(\cdot \mu, \rho)) \qquad (2.34)$$

be the standardized estimating function in the sense that it has the derivative minus the identity.

Note that $c(\mu)$ is a $k \times k$ matrix with $c_{ij}(\mu) = P\frac{d}{d\mu_j}IC_i(Y \mid Q, G, D_{h_n}(\mu, \rho))$. Its estimate $c_n(\mu_n^0)$ is given by

$$c(h_n, \mu_n^0, \rho_n, Q_n, G_n, P_n) = \frac{1}{n}\sum_{i=1}^{n} \frac{d}{d\mu}IC(Y_i \mid Q_n, G_n, D_{h_n}(\mu, \rho_n))\bigg|_{\mu=\mu_n^0}.$$

If $IC(Y \mid Q_n, G_n, D_{h_n}(\cdot \mid \mu, \rho_n))$ is not differentiable in μ, but the integral of $IC(Y)$ w.r.t. $P_{F_X,G}$ is differentiable w.r.t. μ, then the derivative $d/d\mu$ is defined as a numerical derivative. The first step of the Newton–Raphson procedure is now defined by

$$\mu_n^1 = \mu_n^0 - c_n(\mu_n^0)^{-1} \frac{1}{n} \sum_{i=1}^{n} IC(Y_i \mid Q_n, G_n, D_{h_n}(\cdot \mid \mu_n^0, \rho_n)). \qquad (2.35)$$

If one has a decent initial estimator μ_n^0 available, then one can use this one-step estimator μ_n^1. Otherwise, one iterates until convergence is established and we possibly need to use the line-search modification as provided in Section 2.3.

2.4.2 Discussion of ingredients of a one-step estimator

At this stage, it is appropriate to discuss the ingredients of our proposed estimator (2.35). To begin with, let us discuss estimation of $Q = Q(F_X, G)$ and the censoring mechanism G. Under coarsening at random, the likelihood of Y actually factorizes in a likelihood parametrized by F_X and a likelihood parametrized by G. In model $\mathcal{M}$, one assumes that the user has supplied a lower-dimensional model $\mathcal{M}^{F,w}$ for F_X and a lower-dimensional model $\mathcal{G}$ for G. If these models are of low enough dimension, then one can estimate F_X and G by maximizing their corresponding likelihoods. In all applications covered in this book, we can estimate G with maximum likelihood methods. For example, in the right-censored data structures, we estimate G with the maximum partial likelihood estimator for the multiplicative intensity (i.e., Cox proportional hazards) model. However, since one does not need to estimate the whole full data distribution F_X but just the component $Q(F_X, G_n)$, other direct methods for estimation of $Q(F_X, G_n)$ are often available. We provide such methods in Chapters 3 and 6.

In model $\mathcal{M}(\mathcal{G})$, one does not need to estimate Q by substituting estimators F_n of F_X and G_n of G. Instead, one can often estimate Q directly with standard software, which will be illustrated in our examples.

142   2. General Methodology

Another issue is the choice h of the full data estimating function. The efficiency of the proposed estimator depends on this choice. In particular, in Section 2.8 we provide a choice $h_{opt} = h_{opt}(F_X, G)$, which makes the estimating function optimal. In model $\mathcal{M}$, one estimates h_{opt} with $h_n = h_{opt}(F_n, G_n)$, while in model $\mathcal{M}(\mathcal{G})$, other direct methods are often available. In particular, Theorem 2.8 establishes such a direct easy-to-estimate representation of h_{opt} for the multivariate generalized linear regression full data model. If the full data model is locally saturated then the optimal choice of full data structure estimating function is actually the optimal estimating function one would use in the full data model. In that case, $D_{h_{opt}}(X \mid \mu(F_X), \rho(F_X))$ equals the efficient score or efficient influence function $S_{eff}^{*F}(X \mid F_X)$ of μ in the full data structure model.

In general, evaluating $D_{h_{opt}}$ requires inverting a linear Hilbert space operator (i.e., a possibly infinite-dimensional system of linear equations). In Section 2.8, we provide a Neumann series algorithm for evaluating $D_{h_{opt}}$ for a given (F_X, G) and useful characterizations of the inversion problem that have resulted in closed-form solutions in many of our examples.

2.5 Guaranteed Improvement Relative to an Initial Estimating Function

If one assumes model $\mathcal{M}(\mathcal{G})$, then it will be possible to construct an estimating function that yields estimators at least as efficient as a given initial estimator.

Define

$$IC(\cdot \mid Q_0, Q, G, c_{nu}, D) = IC_0(\cdot \mid Q_0, G, D) - c_{nu} IC_{nu}(\cdot \mid Q, G, D), \quad (2.36)$$

where $IC_{nu}(Y \mid Q(F_X, G), G, D)$ parametrizes the projection of $IC_0(Y \mid Q_0, G, D)$ onto a subspace $H(P_{F_X,G})$ of T_{CAR}, as in Section 2.3. Given functions $IC_0(Y)$ and $IC_{nu}(Y)$, we define $c_{nu} = c_{nu}(IC_0, IC_{nu}, P_{F_X,G})$ as the projection matrix

$$E_{P_{F_X,G}}(IC_0(Y) IC_{nu}^\top(Y)) E_{P_{F_X,G}} \{IC_{nu}(Y) IC_{nu}^\top(Y)\}^{-1}$$

so that $c_{nu} IC_{nu} = \Pi(IC_0 \mid \langle IC_{nu} \rangle)$. Note that the j-th component of $c_{nu} IC_{nu}$ equals the projection of IC_{0j} on the space $\langle IC_{nu,l}, l = 1, \ldots, k \rangle_{j=1}^k$ spanned by $IC_{nu,l}$, $l = 1, \ldots, k$. Note also that if IC_{nu} equals the projection of IC_0 onto a subspace of $L_0^2(P_{F_X,G})$, then $c_{nu} = I$, where I denotes the identity matrix. Estimation of c_{nu} only involves taking empirical expectations of the already estimated IC_0, IC_{nu}, and it will guarantee that the estimating function is more efficient than the estimating function $IC_0(\cdot \mid Q_0, G, D_h(\cdot \mid \mu, \rho))$, even when Q_n is an inconsistent estimator of

2.5. Guaranteed Improvement Relative to an Initial Estimating Function

$Q(F_X, G)$. We estimate c_{nu} with

$$c_{nu,n} = \left[1/n \sum_{i=1}^{n} \widehat{IC_0}(Y_i)\widehat{IC}_{nu}^\top(Y_i)\right]\left[1/n \sum_{i=1}^{n} \widehat{IC}_{nu}(Y_i)\widehat{IC}_{nu}(Y_i)^\top\right]^{-1},$$

where $\widehat{IC_0}(Y) = IC_0(Y \mid Q_{0n}, G_n, D_h(\mu, \rho_n))$ and similarly we define $\widehat{IC}_{nu}$. With this c_{nu} extension, the estimating equation (2.33) for μ becomes

$$0 = \frac{1}{n} \sum_{i=1}^{n} IC(Y_i \mid Q_{0n}, Q_n, G_n, c_{nu,n}, D_{h_n}(\cdot \mid \mu, \rho_n)). \tag{2.37}$$

If the parameter $Q_0(F_X, G)$ of the initial estimating function $IC_0(\cdot \mid Q_0, G, D(\cdot \mid \mu, \rho))$ is already easy to estimate in the model $\mathcal{M}^F$, then we recommend estimating $Q_0(F_X, G)$ consistently. In that case, the proposed one-step estimator μ_n^1 corresponding with our estimating function (2.37) is asymptotically linear with an influence curve with smaller variance than $c^{-1}IC_0(\cdot \mid Q_0(F_X, G), G, D_h(\cdot \mid \mu, \rho))$, even when Q_n is inconsistent. Note that $IC_0(\cdot \mid Q_0(F_X, G), G, D_h(\cdot \mid \mu, \rho))$ can be chosen to represent the influence curve of a good initial estimator μ_n^0 (e.g., inverse probability of censoring weighted estimator estimating G according to a model $\mathcal{G}$) so that μ_n^1 is guaranteed to be more efficient than μ_n^0. It is also of interest to note that inspecting $c_{nu,n}$ for a number of fits $\widehat{IC}_{nu}$ can provide insight into which fit Q_n results in the best approximation of $\Pi(\widehat{IC}_0 \mid H(P_{F_X,G}))$; that is, one selects the fit which makes $c_{nu,n}$ closest to the identity matrix.

If one assumes the more nonparametric model $\mathcal{M}$, then the c_{nu} extension is not a good idea since it will destroy the protection w.r.t. misspecification of G at correctly specified guessed full data structure model $\mathcal{M}^{F,w}$.

Example 2.13 (Multivariate right censored data structure; continuation of Example 2.8) Let (T_1, T_2) be a bivariate survival time of interest, and let $\mu = S(t_1, t_2) = P(T_1 > t_1, T_2 > t_2)$. Let F be the bivariate cumulative distribution function of (T_1, T_2). Let $C = (C_1, C_2)$ be a bivariate censoring variable. Suppose that we observe $(\tilde{T}_j = \min(T_j, C_j), \Delta_j = I(T_j \leq C_j), \bar{L}_j(\tilde{T}_j))$, $j = 1, 2$, where $L_j(\cdot)$ are covariate processes. We have for full data $X = (T_1, \bar{L}_1(T_1), T_2, \bar{L}(T_2))$. The observed data distribution is indexed by the full data distribution F_X and the conditional bivariate distribution G of (C_1, C_2), given X, which is assumed to be modeled with some submodel of CAR (e.g., see Chapter 6). Let the full data model be nonparametric so that the only full data estimating function is $D(X \mid \mu) = I_{(t_1, \infty) \times (t_2, \infty)}(T_1, T_2) - \mu$.

In the previous coverage of this example, we derived an estimating function $IC(Y \mid F, G, D(\cdot \mid \mu))$ (2.24) for μ indexed by a marginal bivariate distribution F and the censoring mechanism G, which yields an influence curve equal to or better than the influence curve of Dabrowska's estimator. We propose now to use this as the initial influence curve IC_0 in the estimating function $IC_0 - c_{nu}IC_{nu}$, where IC_{nu} denotes the projection of IC_0 onto a subspace of T_{CAR}.

In this multivariate right-censored data model (no common censoring time), the CAR model $\mathcal{G}(CAR)$ for the censoring mechanism is hard to understand and, in particular, projections on its tangent space $T_{CAR}(P_{F_X,G})$ do not exist in closed form. However, in Chapter 6, we consider an interesting submodel of CAR, only assuming that censoring actions at time t are sequentially randomized w.r.t. the observed past. This submodel of $\mathcal{G}(CAR)$ has a closed-form observed data tangent space $T_{SRA}(P_{F_X,G}) \subset T_{CAR}$. In Chapter 6, we also propose a semiparametric multiplicative intensity model $\mathcal{G}$ of this SRA model that yields an estimator of G with standard software. A closed-form representation of its tangent space T_{SRA} and the projection operator on this tangent space are provided in Chapter 6. Thus $IC_{nu} = \Pi(IC_0 \mid T_{SRA})$ exists in closed form. The estimating function $IC_0 - c_{nu}IC_{nu}$ now yields an RAL estimator of μ based on the extended bivariate right-censored data structure in model $\mathcal{M}(\mathcal{G})$, which is guaranteed to be more efficient than the Dabrowska estimator under independent censoring, even for the marginal data structure in which data on the covariate processes $L_j(\cdot)$ are not available. □

2.6 Construction of Confidence Intervals

Firstly, consider model $\mathcal{M}(\mathcal{G})$; that is, we are willing to assume that the censoring mechanism is correctly specified so that $\mathcal{G}$ contains the true G. Let $T_2(P_{F_X,G})$ denote the corresponding tangent space generated by G. Given an initial estimator μ_n^0 that converges to μ at an appropriate rate, we consider the one-step estimator (2.35) that is given by $\mu_n^0 + 1/n \sum_{i=1}^n \widehat{IC}(Y_i)$, where $\widehat{IC}(Y) \equiv IC(Y \mid Q_n, G_n, c_{nu,n}, c_n, D_{h_n}(\cdot \mid \mu_n^0, \rho_n))$ defined by (2.34). Under the conditions of Theorem 2.4, μ_n^1 is asymptotically linear with influence curve $IC_1(Y) - \Pi(IC_1 \mid T_2)$, where $IC_1(Y) = IC(Y \mid Q^1, G, c, D_h(\cdot \mid \mu, \rho))$ represents the limit for $n \to \infty$ of $\widehat{IC}(Y)$. Thus, estimation of the influence curve requires computing an expression for the projection formula of IC_1 onto the tangent space generated by the censoring mechanism in the observed data model $\mathcal{M}(\mathcal{G})$. We provide this projection formula in Lemma 3.2 for the case where C is identified with a counting process and one uses a multiplicative intensity model to model the intensity of this counting process w.r.t. the observed past. Alternatively, one can note that this influence curve has variance smaller than or equal to the variance of $IC_1(Y) \equiv IC(Y \mid Q^1, G, c_{nu}, c, D_h(\cdot \mid \mu, \rho))$ and use a conservative estimate of the asymptotic covariance matrix of μ_n^1:

$$\widehat{\Sigma} = \frac{1}{n} \sum_{i=1}^n \widehat{IC}(Y_i)\widehat{IC}(Y_i)^\top.$$

This can be used to construct a conservative 95% confidence interval for μ,

$$\mu_{nj}^1 \pm 1.96 \frac{\widehat{\Sigma}_{jj}}{\sqrt{n}}. \tag{2.38}$$

This confidence interval is asymptotically correct if one consistently estimates $Q(F_X, G)$, and it is asymptotically conservative otherwise. However, if one uses the $c_{nu,n}$ adjustment and guarantees that Q_{0n} is consistent, then it is always less conservative than using as the influence curve $c^{-1}IC_0(Y \mid Q_0(F_X, G), G, D_h(\mu, \rho))$; see Section 2.5. This confidence interval (2.38) is practical since one gets it for free after having computed the estimator μ_n^1.

Consider now the more nonparametric model $\mathcal{M}$ only assuming that either the censoring mechanism model $\mathcal{G}$ or the $\mathcal{M}^{F,w}$ is correctly specified. Under the conditions of Theorem 2.5, μ_n^1 is asymptotically linear with an influence curve equal to a sum of two components of which one is consistently estimated by $\widehat{IC}$. The other component of this influence curve will depend on the linear expansion of the estimators of a smooth functional of the unknown parameters in model $\mathcal{M}^{F,w}$. If one wants to avoid the $\mathcal{M}^{F,w}$-specific technical exercise and wants a confidence interval that is also correct when G is misspecified (and $\mathcal{M}^{F,w}$ is correctly specified), then we recommend using the semiparametric or nonparametric bootstrap (e.g., Gill, 1989; Efron, 1990; Gine and Zinn, 1990; Efron and Tibshirani, 1993; van der Vaart and Wellner; 1996).

2.7 Asymptotics of the One-Step Estimator

An estimator μ_n of μ is asymptotically linear at $P_{F_X,G}$ with influence curve $IC(Y \mid F_X, G)$ if $\mu_n - \mu = n^{-1} \sum_{i=1}^n IC(Y_i \mid F_X, G) + o_P(n^{-1/2})$. From Bickel, Klaassen, Ritov and Wellner (1993), we have that an estimator is asymptotically efficient if it is asymptotically linear with the influence curve the so-called efficient influence curve, $IC^*(Y \mid F_X, G)$. The efficient influence curve is also called the canonical gradient and $IC^*(Y \mid F_X, G) = IC(Y \mid Q(F_X, G), G, D_{h_{opt}(F_X,G)}(\cdot \mid \mu(F_X), \rho(F_X)))$ for a specified (next section) index $h_{opt}(F_X, G)$.

We prove two asymptotics theorems for the one-step estimator μ_n^1 corresponding with the estimating equation (2.37), one for model $\mathcal{M}(\mathcal{G})$ and one for model $\mathcal{M}$. We note that the estimating function $IC(Y \mid Q_0, G, c_{nu}, D_h) = IC_0(Q_0, G, D_h) - c_{nu}IC_{nu}(Q, G, D_h)$ captures all proposed estimating functions in the previous sections, where one can set $c_{nu} = I$ and/or $IC_{nu} = 0$ and/or IC_0 equal to the optimal mapping to obtain the various proposed estimating functions. In particular, in model $\mathcal{M}$ we set $c_{nu} = I$. Theorem 2.4 for $\mathcal{M}(\mathcal{G})$ below assumes consistent estimation of the censoring mechanism. Theorem 2.5 for $\mathcal{M}$ assumes *either* consistent estimation of the censoring mechanism *or* consistent estimation of F_X. This does not require choosing which of the two quantaties are consistently estimated. Obviously, the last theorem provides the most nonparametric consistency and asymptotic normality result, but the price one has to pay is that one cannot use the conservative confidence interval (2.38). Because of this and the fact that for many censored data structures it is easier to estimate the censoring mechanism than it is to estimate the full data distribution, we feel that the theorem for $\mathcal{M}(\mathcal{G})$ deserves a separate treatment.

We note that Theorem 2.4 can be applied to any one-step estimator corresponding with the non optimal estimating equations $0 = \sum_i IC_0(Y_i \mid Q_{1n}, G_n, D_{h_n}(\cdot \mid \mu, \rho_n))$ provided in Section 2.3. Similarly, Theorem 2.5 can be applied to any IC_0 that is orthogonalized w.r.t. the tangent space $T_2(P_{F_X,G})$ of G so that it satisfies (2.30).

2.7.1 Asymptotics assuming consistent estimation of the censoring mechanism

The following theorem provides a template for proving asymptotic linearity with specified influence curve of this one-step estimator μ_n^1 (2.35) (i.e., set $c_{nu,n} = c_{nu} = 1$) or, if one uses the adjustment constant $c_{nu,n}$, then it is the one-step estimator corresponding with (2.37). Recall the following Hilbert space terminology: $L_0^2(P_{F_X,G})$ is the Hilbert space of functions of Y with finite variance and mean zero endowed with the covariance inner product $<v_1, v_2>_{P_{F_X,G}} \equiv \sqrt{\int v_1 v_2 dP_{F_X,G}}$. The tangent space $T_2 = T_2(P_{F_X,G})$ for the parameter G is the closure of the linear extension in $L_0^2(P_{F_X,G})$ of the scores at $P_{F_X,G}$ from all correctly specified parametric submodels (i.e., submodels of the assumed semiparametric model $\mathcal{G}$) for the distribution G.

Theorem 2.4 *Consider the observed data model $\mathcal{M}(\mathcal{G})$. Let $Y_1, \ldots, Y_n$ be n i.i.d. observations of $Y \sim P_{F_X,G} \in \mathcal{M}(\mathcal{G})$. Consider a one-step estimator of the parameter $\mu \in \mathbb{R}^k$ of the form $\mu_n^1 = \mu_n^0 - P_n IC(\cdot \mid Q_n, G_n, c_{nu,n}, c_n, D_{h_n}(\mu_n^0, \rho_n))$ corresponding with (2.37). Assume that the limit of $IC(Q_n, G_n, c_{nu,n}, D_{h_n}(\mu_n^0, \rho_n))$ specified in (ii) below satisfies*

$$E_G(IC(Y \mid Q^1, G, c_{nu}, D_h(\cdot \mid \mu, \rho)) \mid X) = D_h(X \mid \mu, \rho) \quad F_X\text{-}a.e \quad (2.39)$$

$$D_h(\cdot \mid \mu, \rho) \in T_{nuis}^{F,\perp}(F_X). \quad (2.40)$$

Let $f_n(\mu) \equiv P_n IC(\cdot \mid Q_n, G_n, c_{nu,n}, D_{h_n}(\mu, \rho_n))$. Assume (we write $f \approx g$ for $f = g + o_P(1/\sqrt{n})$)

$$c_n^{-1}\{f_n(\mu_n^0) - f_n(\mu)\} \approx \mu_n^0 - \mu. \quad (2.41)$$

and

$$E_{P_{F_X,G}} IC(Y \mid Q_n, G, c_{nu,n}, D_{h_n}(\mu, \rho_n)) = o_P(1/\sqrt{n}). \quad (2.42)$$

2.7. Asymptotics of the One-Step Estimator

where the G component of ρ_n is set equal to G as well.

In addition, assume

(i) $IC(\cdot \mid Q_n, G_n, c_{nu,n}, c_n, D_{h_n}(\cdot \mid \mu_n^0, \rho_n))$ falls in a $P_{F_X,G}$-Donsker class with probability tending to 1.

(ii) Let $IC_n(\cdot) = IC(\cdot \mid Q_n, G_n, c_{nu,n}, c_n, D_{h_n}(\cdot \mid \mu_n^0, \rho_n))$. For some (h, Q^1), we have

$$\| IC_n(\cdot) - IC(\cdot \mid Q^1, G, c_{nu}, c, D_h(\cdot \mid \mu, \rho)) \|_{P_{F_X,G}} \to 0,$$

where the convergence is in probability. Here (suppressing the dependence of the estimating functions on parameters) $c_{nu} = \langle IC_0, IC_{nu}^\top \rangle \langle IC_{nu}, IC_{nu}^\top \rangle^{-1}$ is such that $c_{nu} IC_{nu}$ equals the projection of IC_0 onto the k-dimensional space $< IC_{nu,j}, j = 1, \ldots, k >$ in $L_0^2(P_{F_X,G})$.

(iii) Define for a G_1

$$\Phi(G_1) = P_{F_X,G} IC(\cdot \mid Q^1, G_1, c_{nu}, c, D_h(\mu, \rho)).$$

For notational convenience, let

$$IC_n(G) \equiv IC(\cdot \mid Q_n, G, c_{nu,n}, c_n, D_{h_n}(\mu, \rho_n)),$$
$$IC(G) \equiv IC(\cdot \mid Q^1, G, c_{nu}, c, D_h(\mu, \rho)).$$

Assume

$$P_{F_X,G}\{IC_n(G_n) - IC_n(G)\} \approx \Phi(G_n) - \Phi(G).$$

(iv) $\Phi(G_n)$ is an asymptotically efficient estimator of $\Phi(G)$ for the CAR model $\mathcal{G}$ containing the true G with tangent space $T_2(P_{F_X,G}) \subset T_{CAR}(P_{F_X,G})$.

Then μ_n^1 is asymptotically linear with influence curve given by

$$IC \equiv \Pi(IC(\cdot \mid Q^1, G, c_{nu}, c, D_h(\cdot \mid \mu, \rho)) \mid T_2^\perp(P_{F_X,G})).$$

If $Q^1 = Q(F_X, G)$ and $IC(Y \mid Q(F_X, G), G, c_{nu}, D_h(\cdot \mid \mu, \rho)) \perp T_2(P_{F_X,G})$, then this influence curve equals $IC(\cdot \mid Q(F_X, G), G, c_{nu} = 1, c, D_h(\mu, \rho))$. In particular, if $h = h_{opt}$ so that $IC(Y \mid Q(F_X, G), G, D_{h_{opt}}(\cdot \mid \mu(F_X), \rho(F_X, G)))$ equals the efficient influence curve $S_{eff}^{*F}(Y \mid F_X, G)$, then μ_n^1 is asymptotically efficient.

Discussion of asymptotic linearity Theorem 2.4

We will discuss the assumptions of Theorem 2.4 and illustrate that the assumptions are natural. Firstly, note that the structural conditions (2.39) and (2.40) hold for our estimating functions by (2.31) and the fact that we choose the full data estimating functions to be elements of $T_{nuis}^{F,\perp}(F_X)$ at the true parameter values. Note also that these conditions imply that the estimating function is orthogonal to all F_X nuisance parameters in the sense that it is an element of $T_{nuis}^\perp(\mathcal{M}(G))$ in the model with G known at any Q_1. This explains why condition (2.42) is a natural condition; see Subsection 1.4.3.

Condition (2.41) is a natural condition as well, which is illustrated as follows. Define $f_n(\mu) \equiv P_n IC(\cdot \mid Q_n, G_n, D_{h_n}(\cdot \mid \mu, \rho_n))$. By definition, we have

$$c_n = f_n'(\mu_n^0) \equiv d/d\mu f_n(\mu)|_{\mu=\mu_n^0}.$$

In this notational setting, condition (2.41) translates to

$$\{f_n'(\mu_n^0)\}^{-1}\{f_n(\mu_n^0) - f_n(\mu)\} = \mu - \mu_n^0 + o_P(1/\sqrt{n}). \tag{2.43}$$

Under regularity conditions (e.g., a Taylor expansion of $f_n(\mu)$ at μ_n^0), one expects to have a first-order expansion

$$f_n(\mu) - f_n(\mu_n^0) = f_n'(\mu_n^0)(\mu_n^0 - \mu) + o(|\mu_n^0 - \mu|). \tag{2.44}$$

If the second-order term is $o_P(n^{-1/2})$ and the determinant $f_n'(\mu_n^0)$ is bounded away from zero uniformly in n, then this expansion proves (2.43) and thus (2.41). If $f_n(\mu)$ is continuously differentiable in μ with bounded derivative, then the second order term is $o_P(|\mu_n^0 - \mu|)$, while if it is twice continuously differentiable, then the second-order term is $O(|\mu_n^0 - \mu|^2)$. Consider now the case where $f(\mu) = P_{F_X,G} IC(\cdot \mid Q, G, D_h(\cdot \mid \mu, \rho))$ is continuously differentiable but $f_n(\mu)$ is not differentiable. In that case, one still expects this expansion (2.44) to hold with $f_n'(\mu_n^0)$ now being a numerical derivative. In many of our censored data models with a nonparametric full data model, we actually have that $f_n(\mu)$ is linear in μ so that (2.41) holds with remainder zero. However, in general, we can conclude that condition (2.41) typically requires a convergence rate of the initial estimator μ_n^0.

Condition (i) can often be arranged by choosing truly lower-dimensional working models $\mathcal{G}$ and $\mathcal{M}^{F,w}$ when estimating G and F_X. This condition formally represents the "asymptotic curse of dimensionality" since if one uses as working models $\mathcal{M}^{F,w} = \mathcal{M}^F$ and $\mathcal{G} = \mathcal{G}(CAR)$, then the class of functions of $IC(\cdot \mid Q_n, G_n, D_{h_n}(\cdot \mid \mu_n^0, \rho_n))$ of Y generated by varying Q_n, G_n over all possible parameter values will typically be very large (meaning that for finite samples the first-order asymptotics is irrelevant) or not even be a Donsker class. Condition (ii) is a weak consistency condition requiring that G_n be consistent and Q_n converge to something. This condition will hold if our model $\mathcal{M}(\mathcal{G})$ contains the true $P_{F_X,G}$. Regarding condition (iii), we have

$$P_{F_X,G} IC_n(G_n) - IC_n(G) \approx P_{F_X,G} IC_n(G_n) \text{ by (2.42)}$$
$$\approx P_{F_X,G-G_n} IC_n(G_n),$$

where the latter approximation is expected to hold because of the protection (2.31) against misspecification of Q with the data-generating distribution being P_{F_X,G_n}. Thus, condition (iii) requires that second-order terms involving integrals of differences $(G_n-G)(Q_n-Q^1)$, $(G_n-G)(\rho_n-\rho)$ be $o_P(1/\sqrt{n})$. Thus, if G_n converges to G at a rate $n^{-1/2}$, then this condition typically only requires consistency of the other nuisance parameter

2.7. Asymptotics of the One-Step Estimator

estimates Q_n, ρ_n, μ_n^0, but if G_n converges at a very low rate to G, then the other nuisance parameter estimates will have to compensate for this by converging at an appropriate rate.

Condition (iv) just requires that one estimates G with an efficient procedure such as maximum likelihood estimation. Condition (iv) is not needed to establish that μ_n^1 is RAL, but it is needed to obtain the elegant formula of its influence curve.

This finishes our discussion of the assumptions. Let us now consider the conclusions of Theorem 2.4. It is interesting to consider what the limit distribution of μ_n^1 would be when $G(\cdot \mid x)$ is known and is used in the one-step estimator. In that case, the nuisance tangent space T_2 is empty. Thus, by Theorem 2.4, the influence curve of μ_n^1 is then given by $IC(\cdot \mid Q^1, G, c_{nu}, c, D_h(\cdot \mid \mu, \rho))$, which has variance greater than or equal to that of the influence curve IC based on an efficient estimator of $G(\cdot \mid X)$ according to a (any) model for G. Lemma 2.3 provides the general understanding of the fact that efficient estimation of a known orthogonal nuisance parameter (such as G) improves efficiency of estimation of a parameter μ of the distribution of the full data structure X.

We also note that, due to the c_{nu}-adjustment, $IC(\cdot \mid Q^1, G, c_{nu}, c, D_h(\cdot \mid \mu, \rho))$ has variance smaller than or equal to the variance of $IC_0(\cdot \mid Q_0, G, c, D_h(\cdot \mid \mu, \rho))$. Thus, by choosing $IC_0(\cdot \mid Q_0(F_X, G), G, c, D_h(\cdot \mid \mu, \rho))$ equal to an influence curve of a given estimator, the one-step estimator will always be asymptotically more efficient than this estimator. Therefore, the inclusion of c_{nu} in the definition of the one-step estimator is only really useful if one sets $IC_0(\cdot \mid Q_0, G, c, D_h(\mu, \rho))$ equal to a challenging influence curve. Note that one can always make the choice IC_0 more challenging by redefining a new IC_0 as the old IC_0 minus the projection of the old IC_0 onto any given subset of scores in T_{CAR}.

Finally, we make some comments about the efficiency condition. We have that $h_{opt} = h_{opt}(F_X, G)$ is a functional of the true (F_X, G). In some examples, one has available a closed-form representation of h_{opt} that will imply natural methods of estimation. In general, we provide a Neumann series algorithm for calculating $h_{opt}(F_X, G)$ for a given (F_X, G). Let $F_{X,n}$ and G_n be the estimates of F_X and G assuming the lower dimensional working models $\mathcal{M}^{F,w} \subset \mathcal{M}^F$ and $\mathcal{G} \subset \mathcal{G}(CAR)$. Then, one can estimate h_{opt} with the plug-in method:

$$h_n = h_{opt}(F_{X,n}, G_n).$$

If the working model contains the truth, then (h_n, Q_n) consistently estimates $(h_{opt}, Q(F_X, G))$ so that under the "regularity" conditions (i)–(iv) μ_n^1 is asymptotically efficient. Otherwise, (h_n, Q_n) will still converge to some (h, Q^1) so that μ_n^1 will still be consistent and asymptotically linear.

2.7.2 Proof of Theorem 2.4

For notational convenience, we give the proof for $c_{nu,n} = 1$ and use obvious short-hand notation. We have

$$\mu_n^1 = \mu_n^0 + c_n^{-1} P_n \left\{ IC(Q_n, G_n, D_{h_n}(\mu_n^0, \rho_n)) - IC(Q_n, G_n, D_{h_n}(\mu, \rho_n)) \right\}$$
$$+ c_n^{-1} P_n IC(Q_n, G_n, D_{h_n}(\mu, \rho_n)).$$

By condition (2.41), the difference on the right-hand side equals $\mu - \mu_n^0 + o_P(1/\sqrt{n})$. Thus, we have

$$\mu_n^1 - \mu = (P_n - P) c_n^{-1} IC(Q_n, G_n, D_{h_n}(\mu, \rho_n))$$
$$+ c_n^{-1} P IC(Q_n, G_n, D_{h_n}(\mu, \rho_n)).$$

For empirical process theory, we refer to van der Vaart and Wellner (1996). Conditions (i) and (ii) in the theorem imply that the empirical process term on the right-hand side is asymptotically equivalent with $(P_n - P_{F_X,G}) c^{-1} IC(\cdot \mid Q^1, G^1, D_h(\mu, \rho))$, so it remains to analyze the term

$$c_n^{-1} P IC(Q_n, G_n, D_{h_n}(\mu, \rho_n)).$$

Now, we write this term as a sum of two terms $A + B$, where

$$A = c_n^{-1} P \left\{ IC(Q_n, G_n, D_{h_n}(\mu, \rho_n)) - IC(Q^1, G, D_h(\mu, \rho)) \right\},$$
$$B = c_n^{-1} P IC(Q^1, G, D_h(\mu, \rho)).$$

By (2.39) and (2.40), we have $B = 0$. As in the theorem, let

$$IC_n(G) \equiv IC(\cdot \mid Q_n, G, D_{h_n}(\mu, \rho_n(G))),$$
$$IC(G) \equiv IC(\cdot \mid Q^1, G, D_h(\mu, \rho)).$$

We decompose $A = A_1 + A_2$ as follows:

$$A = P_{F_X, G}\{IC_n(G_n) - IC(G)\}$$
$$= P_{F_X, G}\{IC_n(G) - IC(G)\} + P_{F_X, G}\{IC_n(G_n) - IC_n(G)\}.$$

By assumption (2.42), we have $A_1 = o_P(1/\sqrt{n})$. By assumption (iii),

$$A_2 = \Phi_2(G_n) - \Phi_2(G) + o_P(1/\sqrt{n}).$$

By assumption (iv), we can conclude that μ_n^1 is asymptotically linear with influence curve $IC(\cdot \mid Q^1, G, c, c_{nu}, D_h(\mu, \rho)) + IC_{nuis}$, where IC_{nuis} is the influence curve of $\Phi_2(G_n)$. Now, the same argument as given in the proof of Theorem 2.3 proves that this influence curve of μ_n^1 is given by

$$\Pi(IC(\cdot \mid Q^1, G, c, c_{nu}, D_h(\mu, \rho)) \mid T_2^\perp).$$

This completes the proof. □

2.7.3 Asymptotics assuming that either the censoring mechanism or the full data distribution is estimated consistently

If one is only willing to assume that either the censoring mechanism or the full data distribution is modeled correctly (but not necessarily both), then one can apply the following asymptotic theorems.

Theorem 2.5 *Consider the observed data model $\mathcal{M}$. Let $Y_1, \ldots, Y_n$ be n i.i.d. observations of $Y \sim P_{F_X,G} \in \mathcal{M}$. Consider a one-step estimator $\mu_n^1 = \mu_n^0 + P_n IC(Y_i \mid Q_n, G_n, c_n, D_{h_n}(\mu_n^0, \rho_n))$ (e.g., (2.35) or the one-step estimator corresponding with estimating equation (2.37) with $c_{nu} = I$) of the parameter $\mu \in \mathbb{R}^k$. Assume that the limit of $IC(\cdot \mid Q^1, G^1, c, D_h(\mu, \rho(F_X, G^1)))$ in (ii) satisfies*

$$P_{F_X,G} IC(Y \mid Q^1, G^1, c_n, D_{h_n}(\mu(F_X), \rho(F_X, G^1))) = 0. \tag{2.45}$$

Let $f_n(\mu) = P_n \{IC(\cdot \mid Q_n, G_n, D_{h_n}(\mu, \rho_n))\}$. Assume that

$$c_n^{-1}\{f_n(\mu_n^0) - f_n(\mu)\} = \mu_n^0 - \mu + o_P(1/\sqrt{n}). \tag{2.46}$$

In addition, assume that
(i) $IC(\cdot \mid Q_n, G_n, c_n, D_{h_n}(\mu_n^0, \rho_n))$ falls in a $P_{F_X,G}$-Donsker class with probability tending to 1.
(ii) Let $IC_n(\cdot) = IC(\cdot \mid Q_n, G_n, c_n, D_{h_n}(\cdot \mid \mu_n^0, \rho_n))$. For some (h, Q^1, G^1) with either $Q^1 = Q(F_X, G^1)$ or $G^1 = G$, we have

$$\| IC_n(\cdot) - IC(\cdot \mid Q^1, G^1, c, D_h(\cdot \mid \mu, \rho(F_X, G^1))) \|_{P_{F_X,G}} \to 0,$$

where the convergence is in probability.
(iii) Let $\rho = \rho(F_X, G) = (\rho^*, G)$ for a F_X-parameter $\rho^*(F_X)$. Define

$$\begin{aligned}
\Phi_1(Q) &= P_{F_X,G} IC(\cdot \mid Q, G^1, c, D_h(\cdot \mid \mu, (\rho^*, G^1))), \\
\Phi_2(G') &= P_{F_X,G} IC(\cdot \mid Q^1, G', c, D_h(\cdot \mid \mu, (\rho^*, G'))), \\
\Phi_3(\rho^*) &= P_{F_X,G} IC(\cdot \mid Q^1, G^1, c, D_h(\cdot \mid \mu, (\rho^*, G^1))).
\end{aligned}$$

Assume that

$$P_{F_X,G} \{IC(\cdot \mid Q_n, G_n, c_n, D_{h_n}(\mu, \rho_n)) - IC(Q^1, G^1, c_n, D_{h_n}(\mu, \rho^*, G^1))\}$$

$$= \Phi_1(Q_n) - \Phi_1(Q^1) + \Phi_2(G_n) - \Phi_2(G^1) + \Phi_3(\rho_n^*) - \Phi_3(\rho^*) + o_P(1/\sqrt{n}).$$

(iv) Assume that $\Phi_1(Q_n)$ is a regular asymptotically linear estimator at $P_{F_X,G}$ of $\Phi_1(Q^1)$ with influence curve $IC_1(Y \mid F_X, G)$, $\Phi_2(G_n)$ is a regular asymptotically linear estimator at $P_{F_X,G}$ of $\Phi_2(G^1)$ with influence curve $IC_2(Y \mid F_X, G)$, and $\Phi_3(\rho_n^*)$ is a regular asymptotically linear estimator at $P_{F_X,G}$ of $\Phi_3(\rho^*(F_X))$ with influence curve $IC_3(Y \mid F_X, G)$.

Then μ_n^1 is a regular asymptotically linear estimator with influence curve

$$IC \equiv IC(\cdot \mid Q^1, G^1, c, D_h(\cdot \mid \mu, \rho)) + (IC_1 + IC_2 + IC_3)(Y \mid F_X, G).$$

Now, also assume

$$\Phi_1(Q_n) = o_P(1/\sqrt{n}) \text{ at } G^1 = G, \tag{2.47}$$
$$\Phi_2(G_n) = o_P(1/\sqrt{n}) \text{ at } Q^1 = Q(F_X, G^1), \tag{2.48}$$
$$\Phi_3(\rho_n^*) = o_P(1/\sqrt{n}) \text{ at } G^1 = G. \tag{2.49}$$

If $G^1 = G$, then $IC_1 = IC_3 = 0$. If $Q^1 = Q(F_X, G)$, then $IC_2 = 0$. If $G^1 = G$ and $Q^1 = Q(F_X, G)$, then $IC = IC(\cdot \mid Q(F_X, G), G, c, D_h(\cdot \mid \mu, \rho))$. In particular, if also $h = h_{opt}$ so that $IC(Y \mid Q(F_X, G), G, D_{h_{opt}}(\cdot \mid \mu(F_X), \rho(F_X, G))) = S^*_{eff}(Y \mid F_X, G)$, then μ_n^1 is asymptotically efficient.

Note that condition (2.45) relies on the double robustness of the estimating function. One expects (2.47) and (2.48) to hold by the protection (2.31) against misspecification of Q and protection (2.30) against misspecification of G, respectively. In addition, one often expects (2.49) to hold since the estimating function at G is orthogonal to all F_X nuisance parameters in the sense that it is an element of $T^\perp_{nuis}(\mathcal{M}(G))$ in the model with G known at any Q_1. Specifically we would expect (2.49) to hold when regular estimators of μ can be constructed based on full data structure X, and consistent estimators of $\rho(F_X, G^1)$ can be constructed in model $\mathcal{M}$ using the approach described in the remark in Section 2.4.1. This shows that all structural conditions in this theorem are natural.

2.7.4 Proof of Theorem 2.5

We have

$$\mu_n^1 = \mu_n^0 + c_n^{-1} P_n IC(Q_n, G_n, D_{h_n}(\mu_n^0, \rho_n)) - IC(Q_n, G_n, D_{h_n}(\mu, \rho_n)) \\ + c_n^{-1} P_n IC(Q_n, G_n, D_{h_n}(\mu, \rho_n)).$$

By condition (2.41), the difference on the right-hand side equals $\mu - \mu_n^0 + o_P(1/\sqrt{n})$. Thus, we have

$$\mu_n^1 - \mu = (P_n - P)c_n^{-1} IC(Q_n, G_n, D_{h_n}(\mu, \rho_n)) \\ + c_n^{-1} P IC(Q_n, G_n, D_{h_n}(\mu, \rho_n)).$$

For empirical process theory, we refer to van der Vaart and Wellner (1996). Conditions (ii) and (iii) in the theorem imply that the empirical process term on the right-hand side is asymptotically equivalent with $(P_n - P_{F_X,G})IC(\cdot \mid Q^1, G^1, D_h(\mu, \rho))$, so it remains to analyze the term

$$c_n^{-1} P IC(Q_n, G_n, D_{h_n}(\mu, \rho_n)).$$

Now, we write this term as a sum of two terms $A + B$, where

$$A = c_n^{-1} P IC(Q_n, G_n, D_{h_n}(\mu, \rho_n)) - IC(Q^1, G^1, D_{h_n}(\mu, (\rho^*, G^1))),$$
$$B = c_n^{-1} P IC(Q^1, G^1, D_{h_n}(\mu, (\rho^*, G^1))).$$

We have $B = 0$ by (2.45). By conditions (iii) and (iv), we have that A equals in first order $(P_n - P)\{IC(Q^1, G^1, D_h(\mu, \rho(G^1))) + IC_1 + IC_2 + IC_3\}$. The other statements are true by assumption. □

2.8 The Optimal Index

Consider representations $T_{nuis}^{F,\perp}(F_X) = \{D_h(X \mid \mu(F_X), \rho(F_X)) : h \in \mathcal{H}^F(F_X)\}$ of the orthogonal complement of the full data nuisance tangent space for all $F_X \in \mathcal{M}^F$. Let $h_{ind, F_X} : L_0^2(F_X) \to \mathcal{H}^F(F_X)$ be the index mapping (2.2) from $L_0^2(F_X)$ to the index set $\mathcal{H}^F(F_X)$. Let $h_{eff}(F_X) = h_{ind, F_X}(S_{eff}^F(\cdot \mid F_X))$ be the index of the full data canonical gradient.

Consider the optimal mapping $D_h \to IC(Y \mid Q(F_X, G), G, D_h)$ characterized by the conditions $E_G(IC(Y \mid Q, G, D_h) \mid X) = D_h(X)$ F_X-a.e. and $IC(Y \mid Q(F_X, G), G, D_h) \perp T_{CAR}(P_{F_X, G})$. For simplicity, we will here assume that this mapping satisfies these conditions for all $D \in T_{nuis}^{F,\perp}(F_X)$. Due to its double robustness property, Theorem 2.5 for model $\mathcal{M}$ shows, under regularity conditions, that if both working models are correctly specified, then our proposed estimator μ_n^1 is regular and asymptotically linear at $P_{F_X, G} \in \mathcal{M}$ with influence curve $IC(Y \mid Q(F_X, G), G, D_h(\cdot \mid \mu(F_X), \rho(F_X)))$. The following corollary of Theorem 1.3 in Chapter 1 shows that, given any influence curve $IC(Y \mid F_X, G)$ of a regular asymptotically linear estimator of μ at $P_{F_X, G}$, we can choose $D_{h(F_X, G)}(\cdot \mid \mu, \rho) \in T_{nuis}^{F,\perp}(F_X)$ in such a way that $IC(Y \mid Q(F_X, G), G, D_{h(F_X, G)}(\cdot \mid \mu, \rho)) = IC(Y \mid F_X, G)$. In particular, it shows that for an appropriate choice $D_{h_{opt}(F_X, G)}(\cdot \mid \mu, \rho) \in T_{nuis}^{F,\perp}(F_X)$ we have that $IC(Y \mid Q(F_X, G), G, D_{h_{opt}}(F_X, G)(\cdot \mid \mu, \rho))$ equals the efficient influence curve $S_{eff}^*(Y \mid F_X, G)$ of μ at $P_{F_X, G}$.

Theorem 2.6 *Consider the model $\mathcal{M}(CAR)$. Let $IC(Y \mid Q(F_X, G), G, D) \perp T_{CAR}$ and $E(IC(Y \mid Q(F_X, G), G, D) \mid X) = D(X)$ F_X-a.e. for all $D \in T_{nuis}^{F,\perp}$. Let $IC(Y \mid F_X, G)$ be a gradient of μ in the model $\mathcal{M}(CAR)$. We have that*

$$D(X) \equiv E(IC(Y \mid F_X, G) \mid X) \in T_{nuis}^{F,\perp}(F_X)$$

and

$$IC(Y \mid Q(F_X, G), G, D) = IC(Y \mid F_X, G).$$

In particular, if $S_{eff}^*(Y \mid F_X, G)$ is the canonical gradient (i.e., the efficient influence curve) of μ at $P_{F_X, G}$, then

$$D_{opt}(X) = E(S_{eff}^*(Y \mid F_X, G) \mid X) \in T_{nuis}^{F,\perp}(F_X)$$

154   2. General Methodology

and

$$IC(Y \mid Q(F_X,G), G, D_{opt}) = S^*_{eff}(Y \mid F_X, G).$$

Equivalently, but in terms of indexes, if $h(F_X, G) \equiv h_{ind, F_X}(E(IC(Y \mid F_X, G) \mid X))$, then

$$IC(Y \mid Q(F_X,G), G, D_{h(F_X,G)}(\cdot \mid \mu(F_X), \rho(F_X))) = IC(Y \mid F_X, G),$$

and if $h_{opt}(F_X, G) = h_{ind, F_X}(E(S^*_{eff}(Y \mid F_X, G) \mid X))$, then

$$IC(Y \mid Q(F_X,G), G, D_{h_{opt}(F_X,G)}(\cdot \mid \mu(F_X), \rho(F_X))) = S^*_{eff}(Y \mid F_X, G).$$

Thus, the optimal index $h_{opt}(F_X, G)$ is uniquely identified as the index $h \in \mathcal{H}^F(F_X)$, for which

$$D_h(X \mid \mu(F_X), \rho(F_X)) = E(S^*_{eff}(Y \mid F_X, G) \mid X). \tag{2.50}$$

If the full data model is locally saturated, then $T^{F, \perp *}_{nuis}(F_X) = \{S^{*F}_{eff}(X \mid F_X)\}$ so that the right-hand side of (2.50) equals $S^{*F}_{eff}(X \mid F_X)$ and $h_{opt} = h_{eff}(F_X)$ is the index of the full data canonical gradient.

Since S^*_{eff} is not always trivially computed, we will now provide algorithms for determining the optimal index $h_{opt}(F_X, G)$.

Theorem 2.7 *In this theorem, we will suppress in the notation the dependence on F_X, G of Hilbert space operators, Hilbert spaces, index sets, and indexes (such as h_{eff} and h_{opt}). Let $A(s) = E(s(X) \mid Y)$ and $A^\top(V) = E(V(Y) \mid X)$. Let $\mathbf{I} = A^\top A : L_0^2(F_X) \to L_0^2(F_X)$. Let $\mathbf{I}^* \equiv \Pi_{T^F} \mathbf{I} : T^F \to T^F$, where Π_{T^F} is the projection operator onto the full data tangent space T^F in the Hilbert space $L_0^2(F_X)$. It is assumed that both operators $\mathbf{I}^*$ and $\mathbf{I}$ are 1-1. Assume that the efficient score $S^F_{eff} = D_{h_{eff}} \in R(\mathbf{I}^*)$. Let $h_{ind} : L_0^2(F_X) \to \mathcal{H}^F(F_X)$ be the index mapping. Then, we have the following representations of h_{opt}.*

- *(Robins and Rotnitzky, 1992) Consider the mapping $B : T^{F, \perp}_{nuis} \cap R(\mathbf{I}) \to T^{F, \perp}_{nuis}$ defined by*

$$B(D) = \Pi(\mathbf{I}^{-1}(D) \mid T^{F, \perp}_{nuis}).$$

Then

$$h_{opt} = h_{ind} B^{-1} D_{h_{eff}}.$$

An alternative way to define h_{opt} is the following. Define $B' : \mathcal{H}^F(F_X) \to \mathcal{H}^F(F_X)$ by

$$B'(h) = h_{ind} \mathbf{I}^{-1} D_h.$$

Then

$$h_{opt} = B'^{-1} h_{eff}.$$

- *(van der Vaart, 1991)* We have

$$h_{opt} = h_{ind}\mathbf{II}^{*-1}D_{h_{eff}}.$$

In full notation, this theorem provides us with the following representations of h_{opt}:

$$h_{opt}(F_X,G) = h_{ind,F_X}\left\{B_{F_X,G}^{-1}D_{h_{eff}(F_X)}(\cdot \mid \mu(F_X),\rho(F_X))\right\}, \quad (2.51)$$

$$h_{opt}(F_X,G) = B_{F_X,G}^{\prime-1}(h_{eff}(F_X)), \quad (2.52)$$

$$h_{opt}(F_X,G) = h_{ind,F_X}\mathbf{I}_{F_X,G}\mathbf{I}_{F_X,G}^{*-}D_{h_{eff}(F_X)}(\cdot \mid \mu(F_X),\rho(F_X)). \quad (2.53)$$

Thus, we have two mappings, $B_{F_X,G}^{-1}$ and $\mathbf{I}_{F_X,G}\mathbf{I}_{F_X,G}^{*-1}$, mapping $D_{h_{eff}(F_X)}$ into the optimal full data function $D_{h_{opt}(F_X,G)}$. Although, by definition $B_{F_X,G}^{-1}$ maps $T_{nuis}^{F,\perp}(F_X)$ into itself, it might be less obvious to see that $\mathbf{I}_{F_X,G}\mathbf{I}_{F_X,G}^{*-1}$ maps $D_{h_{eff}}$ into an element of $T_{nuis}^{F,\perp}$. We will now give a proof of this fact. We parametrize the projection operator on the full data tangent space as

$$\Pi(D \mid T^F) = \Pi(D \mid \langle D_{h_{eff}}\rangle) + D - \Pi(D \mid T_{nuis}^{F,\perp}).$$

Note that, for any $D \in T_{nuis}^{F,\perp}$, we have

$$D - \Pi(D \mid T^F) \in T_{nuis}^{F,\perp}.$$

Define $D = \mathbf{I}_{F_X,G}\mathbf{I}_{F_X,G}^{*-}(D_{h_{eff}})$. Now write

$$D = \{D - \Pi(D \mid T^F)\} + \Pi(D \mid T^F),$$

and note that the second term equals $D_{h_{eff}} \in T_{nuis}^{F,\perp}$. This proves that $\mathbf{I}_{F_X,G}\mathbf{I}_{F_X,G}^{*-1}D_{h_{eff}(F_X)}(\cdot \mid \mu(F_X),\rho(F_X)) \in T_{nuis}^{F,\perp}(F_X)$. Since $T_{nuis}^{F,\perp}(F_X) = \{D_h(\cdot \mid \mu(F_X),\rho(F_X)) : h \in \mathcal{H}^F(F_X)\}$, we have that $\mathbf{I}_{F_X,G}\mathbf{I}_{F_X,G}^{*-1}D_{h_{eff}(F_X)}(\cdot \mid \mu(F_X),\rho(F_X)) = D_{h_{opt}(F_X,G)}(\cdot \mid \mu(F_X),\rho(F_X))$ for some $h_{opt}(F_X,G) \in \mathcal{H}^F(F_X)$.

The proof in the preceding paragraph actually shows which arguments in

$$\mathbf{I}_{F_X,G}\mathbf{I}_{F_X,G}^{*-1}D_{h_{eff}(F_X)}(\cdot \mid \mu(F_X),\rho(F_X)) = D_{h_{opt}(F_X,G)}(\cdot \mid \mu(F_X),\rho(F_X)) \quad (2.54)$$

determine that the left-hand side of (2.54) is an element of $T_{nuis}^{F,\perp}(F_X)$, and which arguments determine h_{opt}. The $\mu(F_X),\rho(F_X)$ in $D_{h_{eff}(F_X)}(\cdot \mid \mu(F_X),\rho(F_X))$ and in $T_{nuis}^{F,\perp}(F_X) = \{D_h(\cdot \mid \mu(F_X),\rho(F_X)) : h \in \mathcal{H}^F(F_X)\}$ determine that the left-hand side of (2.54) is an element of $T_{nuis}^{F,\perp}(F_X)$ while 1) (F_X,G) in $\mathbf{I}_{F_X,G}$, 2) F_X in $h_{eff}(F_X)$ and 3) F_X in h_{ind,F_X} determine the index of $\Pi_{F_X}(\cdot \mid T_{nuis}^\perp(F_X))$ and the index $h_{opt}(F_X,G)$.

Proof of Theorem 2.7. If $S_{eff}^{*F} \in R(\mathbf{I}^*)$, then by van der Vaart (1991) $S_{eff}^* = A\mathbf{I}^{*-1}(S_{eff}^{*F})$. This can be written as

$$S_{eff}^* = A\mathbf{I}^{-1}(\mathbf{II}^{*-1})(S_{eff}^{*F}),$$

156   2. General Methodology

which proves by Theorem 1.3 that $D_{opt} = \mathbf{II}^{*-}(S^{*F}_{eff})$ and proves the second expression for $h_{opt}(F_X, G)$.

We will now prove the first statement. Since $\mathbf{I}^{*-1}(S^{*F}_{eff}) \in \langle S^{*F}_{eff} \oplus T^F_{nuis}(F_X)$, it follows that $\Pi(\mathbf{I}^{*-1}(S^{*F}_{eff}) \mid T^{F,\perp}_{nuis}(F_X)) = S^{*F}_{eff}$, and thus that $D_{opt} = \mathbf{II}^{*-}(S^{*F}_{eff})$ solves

$$\Pi(\mathbf{I}^{-1}(D) \mid T^{\perp}_{nuis}) = S^{*F}_{eff}. \tag{2.55}$$

In addition, by definition, it is an element of $R(\mathbf{I})$ and $\Pi_{T^F} D_{opt} = S^{*F}_{eff}$ so that it is indeed an element of $R(\mathbf{I}) \cap T^{F,\perp}_{nuis}$. We will now show that if $D \in T^{F,\perp}_{nuis} \cap R(\mathbf{I})$ and solves (2.55), then $A\mathbf{I}^{-1}(D) = S^*_{eff}$ and thus $D = D_{opt}$.

Firstly, if $D \in T^{F,\perp*}_{nuis}$, then it follows that $A\mathbf{I}^{-1}(D) \in T^{\perp*}_{nuis}$. Consider the following representation:

$$\mathbf{I}^{-1}(D) = \Pi(\mathbf{I}^{-1}(D) \mid T^F) - \Pi(\mathbf{I}^{-1}(D) \mid S^F_{eff}) + \Pi(\mathbf{I}^{-1}(D) \mid T^{F,\perp}_{nuis}).$$

Thus, (2.55) teaches us that $\mathbf{I}^{-1}(D) \in T^F$. Therefore $A\mathbf{I}^{-1}(D)$ is an element of the tangent space T in $\mathcal{M}(G)$. It is well known that if a gradient is an element of the tangent space, then it equals the canonical gradient. This proves that if $D \in T^{F,\perp*}_{nuis}$ and solves (2.55), then $A\mathbf{I}^{-1}(D) = S^*_{eff}$, which proves the first statement. □

We will provide two examples in which we solve for $h_{opt}(F_X, G)$ using representation (2.51).

Example 2.14 (Current status data structure; continuation of Example 2.6) Consider the current status data structure $Y = (C, \Delta = I(T \leq C), \bar{L}(C))$, where we have for the full data $X = (T, \bar{L})$. Assume as the full data model the univariate linear regression model $T = \beta Z + \epsilon$, where it is assumed that, for a given monotone function K, $E(K(\epsilon(\beta)) \mid Z) = 0$. Lemma 2.1 tells us $T^{F,\perp}_{nuis}(F_X) = \{h(Z)K(\epsilon(\beta)) : h\}$ and

$$\Pi(\mathbf{I}^-_{F_X,G}(D) \mid T^{F,\perp}_{nuis}(F_X)) = \frac{E(\mathbf{I}^{-1}_{F_X,G}(D)(X)K(\epsilon) \mid Z)}{E(K(\epsilon)^2 \mid Z)} K(\epsilon).$$

By (2.51), we have that $h_{opt}(Z)$ is the solution $h(Z)$ of

$$\frac{E(\mathbf{I}^{-1}_{F_X,G}(hK)(X)K(\epsilon) \mid Z)}{E(K(\epsilon)^2 \mid Z)} K(\epsilon) = h_{eff}(Z)K(\epsilon),$$

where $h_{eff}(Z) = Z/E(K(\epsilon)^2 \mid Z)$ is the index of the efficient score S^F_{eff} of β. Since Z is always observed, we have that $\mathbf{I}^-_{F_X,G}(hK)(X) = h(Z)\mathbf{I}^-_{F_X,G}(K)(X)$. Thus, this proves the following representation of h_{opt}:

$$h_{opt}(Z) = \frac{h_{eff}(Z)}{E(\mathbf{I}^{-1}_{F_X,G}(K)(X)K(\epsilon) \mid Z)} E(K(\epsilon)^2 \mid Z).$$

2.8. The Optimal Index

If L is time-independent, then $\mathbf{I}_{F_X,G}^-$ has a simple closed-form expression derived in Example 2.6. However, if L is time-dependent, then this inverse is very involved. Therefore, the following derivation is very useful. Let $\langle f, g \rangle_Z = E(f(X)g(X) \mid Z)$. Using that $A_G^\top$ is also the adjoint of A_{F_X} in the world where one conditions on Z, it follows that

$$\begin{aligned}
\langle \mathbf{I}_{F_X,G}^-(K), K \rangle_Z &= \langle \mathbf{I}_{F_X,G}^-(K), \mathbf{I}_{F_X,G} \mathbf{I}_{F_X,G}^-(K) \rangle_Z \\
&= \langle A_{F_X} \mathbf{I}_{F_X,G}^-(K), A_{F_X} \mathbf{I}_{F_X,G}^-(K) \rangle_Z \\
&= \langle IC(\cdot \mid Q(F_X, G), G, K), IC(\cdot \mid Q(F_X, G), G, K) \rangle_Z \\
&= E\left\{ IC(Y \mid Q(F_X, G), G, K)^2 \mid Z \right\}.
\end{aligned}$$

This proves the representation of h_{opt}

$$h_{opt}(Z) = \frac{Z E(K(\epsilon)^2 \mid Z)}{E\left\{ IC(Y \mid Q(F_X, G), G, K)^2 \mid Z \right\}},$$

where the denominator is actually straightforward to estimate by regressing $IC(Y_i \mid Q_n, G_n, K)$ onto Z_i, $i = 1, \ldots, n$. □

Example 2.15 (Generalized linear regression with missing covariate; continuation of Example 1.1) We refer to Example 1.1 in Chapter 1 for a description of this example and the optimal mapping (1.24) $IC(\cdot \mid Q(F_X), G, D) = \frac{D(X)\Delta}{\Pi(W)} - (\Delta - \Pi(W))\frac{E(D(X)|W)}{\Pi(W)}$. Thus, we have for the observed data $Y = (\Delta, \Delta X + (1 - \Delta W))$, $W \subset X$, and we consider a univariate generalized linear regression model $Z = g(X^* \mid \beta) + \epsilon$, where $E(K(\epsilon) \mid X^*) = 0$. Here $Z \subset W$ is always observed, while $X^* \subset X$ has missing components. We have $T_{nuis}^{F,\perp}(F_X) = \{h(X^*)K(\epsilon) : h\}$ and $\Pi(D \mid T_{nuis}^{F,\perp}(F_X)) = \frac{E(D(X)K(\epsilon)|X^*)}{E(K^2(\epsilon)|X^*)} K(\epsilon)$. Our first goal is to determine a closed-form expression for $\mathbf{I}_{F_X,G}^{-1} : L_0^2(F_X) \to L_0^2(F_X)$. By Theorem 1.3, we have

$$\begin{aligned}
A_{F_X} \mathbf{I}_{F_X,G}^{-1}(D) &= IC(\cdot \mid Q(F_X), G, D) \\
&= \frac{D(X)\Delta}{\Pi(W)} - (\Delta - \Pi(W)) \frac{E(D(X) \mid W)}{\Pi(W)}.
\end{aligned}$$

By definition of A_{F_X}, we have

$$A_{F_X} \mathbf{I}_{F_X,G}^{-1}(D) = \mathbf{I}_{F_X,G}^-(D)\Delta + E(\mathbf{I}_{F_X,G}^-(D)(X) \mid W)(1 - \Delta).$$

Combining these two identities yields

$$\mathbf{I}_{F_X,G}^-(D) = \frac{D(X)}{\Pi(W)} + \left(1 - \frac{1}{\Pi(W)}\right) E(D(X) \mid W).$$

158   2. General Methodology

Thus $\Pi(\mathbf{I}_{F_X,G}^-(D_{h_{opt}}) \mid T_{nuis}^{F,\perp}(F_X)) = D_{h_{eff}}$ translates into

$$\frac{E(\{D_{h_{opt}}(X)/\Pi(W) + E(D_{h_{opt}}(X) \mid W) - 1\}K(\epsilon) \mid X^*)}{E(K^2(\epsilon) \mid X^*)}K(\epsilon)$$

$$= h_{eff}(X^*)K(\epsilon).$$

Since $D_{h_{opt}}(X) = h_{opt}(X^*)K(\epsilon)$, this reduces to

$$h_{opt}(X^*)E(K^2(\epsilon)/\Pi(W) \mid X^*) + E\left(E(h_{opt}(X^*)K(\epsilon) \mid W)K(\epsilon) \mid X^*\right)$$

$$= h_{eff}(X^*)E(K^2(\epsilon) \mid X^*) + E(K(\epsilon) \mid X^*).$$

Thus, the function $x^* \to h_{opt}(x^*)$ is the solution of an integral equation, first derived in Robins, Rotnitzky, Zhao (1994). □

In the current status data example above, we made use of the following general lemma for any censored data model.

Lemma 2.5 Let $Y = \Phi(X, C)$, $X \sim F_X$, $C \mid X \sim G(\cdot \mid X)$ and assume that the conditional distribution G satisfies CAR. Consider the nonparametric information operator $I_{F_X,G} : L_0^2(F_X) \to L_0^2(F_X)$ defined by $I_{F_X,G}(s) = A_G^\top A_{F_X}(s) = E_G E_{F_X}(s(X) \mid Y) \mid X)$. Let $X^* \subset X$ and $X^* \subset Y$ (i.e., X^* is part of the full data structure and is always observed). Then, for any pair of functions $D_1, D_2 \in L_0^2(F_X)$ in the range of $I_{F_X,G}$, we have

$$E(I_{F_X,G}^{-1}(D_1)D_2 \mid X^*) = E(A_{F_X} I_{F_X,G}^{-1}(D_1) A_{F_X} I_{F_X,G}^{-1}(D_2) \mid X^*).$$

Proof. In the Hilbert space with X^* fixed, we need to prove

$$\langle I^{-1}(D_1), D_2 \rangle = \langle AI^{-1}(D_1), AI^{-1}(D_2) \rangle.$$

Since $A^\top$ is still the adjoint of A conditional on X^*, moving the first A to the other side and noting that $A^\top A I^{-1}$ is the identity operator gives the desired result. □

The closed-form representation of the optimal full data index h_{opt} in the current status example above can be generalized to general censored data structures with the full data model being the multivariate generalized linear regression model with covariates always observed.

Theorem 2.8 Let $Y = \Phi(X, C)$, $X \sim F_X$, $C \mid X \sim G(\cdot \mid X)$ and assume that the conditional distribution G satisfies CAR. Let the full data model be the p-variate generalized regression model $Z = g(X^* \mid \beta) + \epsilon$, $\beta \in \mathbb{R}^k$, $E(K(\epsilon) \mid X^*) = 0$, and $K(\epsilon) = (K(\epsilon_1), \ldots, K(\epsilon_p))$. We refer to Lemma 2.1 for 1) the orthogonal complement of the nuisance tangent space in the full data model given by $\{D_h(X) = h(X^*)K(\epsilon) : h\ 1 \times p\ vector\}$, 2) the index h_{eff} ($k \times p$ matrix) so that $h_{eff}(X^*)K(\epsilon)$ is the efficient score of β, and

3) the index mapping given, for a function $D \in L_0^2(F_X)^k$, by

$$h_{ind,F_X}(D) \equiv E(\{D(X) - E(D(X) \mid X^*)\}K(\epsilon)^\top \mid X^*)E(K(\epsilon)K(\epsilon)^\top \mid X^*)^{-1}.$$

Note that $h_{ind,F_X}(D)$ is an $k \times p$ matrix function of X^*.

Assume that X^* is always observed (i.e., X^* is a component of the full data X, which is also a function of Y). Consider the nonparametric information operator $I_{F_X,G} : L_0^2(F_X) \to L_0^2(F_X)$ defined by $I_{F_X,G}(s) = A_G^\top A(s) = E_G E_{F_X}(s(X) \mid Y) \mid X)$. Define $IC(Y \mid F_X, G, D) = A_{F_X} I_{F_X,G}^{-1}(D)$. We have that the $p \times p$ matrix $\left\{h_{ind,F_X} I_{F_X,G}^{-1} K\right\}$ is given by

$$E(IC(Y \mid F_X, G, K) IC(Y \mid F_X, G, K)^\top \mid X^*) E(K(\epsilon) K(\epsilon)^\top \mid X^*)^{-1}.$$

If

$$h_{opt}(X^*) \equiv h_{eff}(X^*) \left\{h_{ind,F_X} I_{F_X,G}^{-1} K\right\}_{p \times p}^{-1}, \qquad (2.56)$$

where we assume that the inverse exists a.e., then $IC(Y \mid F_X, G, D_{h_{opt}})$ equals the efficient influence curve for β.

This is clearly an important result since it allows us to compute closed form locally efficient estimators of regression parameters in univariate and multivariate generalized linear regression models under any type of censoring of the full data structure as long as the covariates X^* in the regression model are always observed.

2.8.1 Finding the optimal estimating function among a given class of estimating functions

Consider a class of estimating functions $IC(Y \mid Q, G, D_h(\cdot \mid \mu, \rho))$, $h \in \mathcal{H}^F$. If for all $F_X \in \mathcal{M}^F$ and $G \in \mathcal{G}$ $\{IC(Y \mid Q(F_X, G), G, D_h(\cdot \mid \mu(F_X), \rho(F_X, G))) : h \in \mathcal{H}^F\} \subset T_{nuis}^\perp(P_{F_X,G})$ in model $\mathcal{M}(\mathcal{G})$, then $c^{-1} IC(Y \mid Q(F_X,G), G, D_h(\cdot \mid \mu, \rho))$ denotes the influence curve corresponding with the estimating function $IC(Y \mid Q, G, D_h(\cdot \mid \mu, \rho))$, assuming correct specification of the nuisance parameters Q, G. Theorem 2.9 below, based on Newey and McFadden (1994), provides us with a formula identifying the estimating function whose corresponding influence curve has minimal variance among the class of estimating functions.

Theorem 2.9 *Consider the censored data structure $Y = \Phi(C, X)$, $X \sim F_X \in \mathcal{M}^F$, and $C \mid X \sim G(\cdot \mid X) \in \mathcal{G} \subset \mathcal{G}(CAR)$. Let μ be a k-dimensional real-valued parameter of F_X. Consider a class of k-dimensional full data structure estimating functions $D_h(\cdot \mid \mu, \rho)$ for μ indexed by h ranging over a set $\mathcal{H}^k$ that satisfies for all $F_X \in \mathcal{M}^F$ and all $G \in \mathcal{G}$ $T_{nuis}^{F,\perp}(F_X) \supset \{D_h(\cdot \mid \mu(F_X), \rho(F_X, G)) : h \in \mathcal{H}\}$. Let $(H, \langle \cdot, \cdot \rangle_H)$ be a Hilbert space defined by* the closure of the linear span of $\mathcal{H}$, which is assumed to be embedded in a Hilbert space with inner product $\langle \cdot, \cdot \rangle_H$.

Consider a class of k-dimensional observed data estimating functions $IC(Y \mid Q, G, D_h)$ indexed by $h \in \mathcal{H}^k$, where $IC(Y \mid Q, G, D_h) = (IC(Y \mid Q, G, D_{h_1}), \ldots, IC(Y \mid Q, G, D_{h_k}))$. Here $Q = Q(F_X, G)$ and G denote the true parameter values for Q and G. Define for $h \in \mathcal{H}^k$

$$\kappa(h) = -\frac{d}{d\mu} E_{P_{F_X,G}} IC(Y \mid Q(F_X, G), G, D_h(\cdot \mid \mu, \rho(F_X, G)))\Big|_{\mu=\mu(F_X)},$$

where we assume that this $k \times k$ derivative matrix is well-defined. Assume that $\kappa(\cdot)$ is bounded and linear, so that (by the Riesz Representation theorem) there exists $h^* \in H^k$ so that for all $h \in \mathcal{H}^k$

$$\kappa(h)_{ij} = \langle h_i^*, h_j \rangle_H, (i,j) \in \{1,\ldots,k\}^2.$$

For notational convenience, define $\tilde{A} : (H, \langle \cdot, \cdot \rangle_H) \to L_0^2(P_{F_X,G})$ by $\tilde{A}(h) \equiv IC(\cdot \mid Q(F_X, G), G, D_h)$. Let $\tilde{A}^\top : L_0^2(P_{F_X,G}) \to (H, \langle \cdot, \cdot \rangle_H)$ be the adjoint of $\tilde{A}$. By applying these operators to each component of a multivariate function, we can also define these operators on multivariate functions so that $\tilde{A} : H^k \to L_0^2(P_{F_X,G})^k$ and $\tilde{A}^\top : L_0^2(P_{F_X,G})^k \to H^k$. Define

$$\Sigma(h) \equiv E(\kappa(h)^{-1} \tilde{A}(h)(Y)(\kappa(h)^{-1} \tilde{A}(h)(Y))^\top).$$

Assume that h^* is an element of the range of $\tilde{A}^\top \tilde{A} : H^k \to H^k$ and that $(\tilde{A}^\top \tilde{A}) : H \to H$ is 1-1. Then

$$h_{opt} \equiv \min{}^{-1}_{h \in H^k} c^\top \Sigma(h) c \text{ for all } c \in \mathbb{R}^k$$

exists, and is given by

$$h_{opt} = (\tilde{A}^\top \tilde{A})^-(h^*).$$

Thus

$$\tilde{A}(h_{opt}) = \tilde{A}(\tilde{A}^\top \tilde{A})^{-1} h^*.$$

Proof. Firstly, note that

$$\kappa(h) = \langle h^*, h \rangle_H = \langle \tilde{A}(\tilde{A}^\top \tilde{A})^{-1}(h^*), \tilde{A}(h) \rangle_{P_{F_X,G}},$$

where the inner product $\langle h_1, h_2 \rangle_H$ is defined as the matrix with (i,j)th element $\langle h_{1i}, h_{2j} \rangle_H$. Using this notation for inner products of vectors, it follows that

$$c^\top E(\kappa(h)^{-1} \tilde{A}(h)(Y)(\kappa(h)^{-1} \tilde{A}(h)(Y))^\top) c$$
$$= c^\top \kappa(h)^{-1} \langle \tilde{A}(h), \tilde{A}(h) \rangle_{P_{F_X,G}} \kappa(h)^{-1\top} c$$
$$= c^\top D(\tilde{A}(h)) \langle \tilde{A}(h), \tilde{A}(h) \rangle_{P_{F_X,G}} D(\tilde{A}(h))^\top c,$$

where $D(\tilde{A}(h)) = \langle \tilde{A}(\tilde{A}^\top \tilde{A})^{-1}(h^*), \tilde{A}(h) \rangle_{P_{F_X,G}}^{-1}$. By the Cauchy–Schwarz inequality, this expression in $\tilde{A}(h)$ is minimized by $\tilde{A}(h_{opt}) = \tilde{A}(\tilde{A}^\top \tilde{A})^{-1} h^*$. □

A special case of Theorem 2.9 is obtained by letting the index set $\mathcal{H}$ be the class of full data estimating functions itself. Application of this theorem to our T_{CAR}-orthogonalized mapping from full data structure estimating functions to observed data estimating functions results in the formula for the efficient influence curve (and efficient score) as presented in Theorem 1.3 and originally derived in Robins, and Rotnitzky (1992). However, note the next theorem is more general since it can be applied to any mapping from full-data structure estimating functions to observed data estimating functions.

Theorem 2.10 *Consider the censored data structure $Y = \Phi(C, X)$, $X \sim F_X \in \mathcal{M}^F$, and $C \mid X \sim G(\cdot \mid X) \in \mathcal{G} \subset \mathcal{G}(CAR)$. Let μ be a k-dimensional real-valued parameter of F_X. Consider a class of k-dimensional full data structure estimating functions $D_h(\cdot \mid \mu, \rho)$ for μ indexed by h ranging over a set $\mathcal{H}^k$ that satisfies for all $F_X \in \mathcal{M}^F$ and $G \in \mathcal{G}$ $T_{nuis}^{F,\perp}(F_X) \supset \{D_h(\cdot \mid \mu(F_X), \rho(F_X, G)) : h \in \mathcal{H}\}$. Let $(H, \langle \cdot, \cdot \rangle_{F_X}) \subset L_0^2(F_X)$ be the sub-Hilbert space of $L_0^2(F_X)$ defined by the closure of the linear span of $\{D_h(\cdot \mid \mu(F_X), \rho(F_X)) : h \in \mathcal{H}\}$. Consider a class (not necessarily T_{CAR}-orthogonalized) of k-dimensional observed data estimating functions $IC(Y \mid Q, G, D_h(\cdot \mid \mu, \rho))$ indexed by $h \in \mathcal{H}^k$ with nuisance parameters $Q(F_X, G)$, G and $\rho(F_X, G)$.*

Define for $h \in \mathcal{H}^k$

$$\kappa(D_h) = -\frac{d}{d\mu} E_{P_{F_X,G}} IC(Y \mid Q(F_X, G), G, D_h(\cdot \mid \mu, \rho(F_X, G)))\bigg|_{\mu=\mu(F_X)},$$

where we assume that this $k \times k$ derivative matrix is well-defined. Assume that $\kappa : (H, \langle \cdot, \cdot \rangle_{F_X}) \to \mathbb{R}$ is bounded and linear, so that (by the Riesz Representation theorem) there exists $D^* \in H^k$ so that for all $h \in \mathcal{H}^k$

$$\kappa(D_h) = \langle D_h, D^* \rangle_{F_X} \equiv E(D_h(X) D^{*\top}(X)).$$

For notational convenience, define $\tilde{A} : (H, \langle \cdot, \cdot \rangle_H) \to L_0^2(P_{F_X,G})$ by $\tilde{A}(D) \equiv IC(\cdot \mid Q(F_X, G), G, D)$. Let $\tilde{A}^\top : L_0^2(P_{F_X,G}) \to (H, \langle \cdot, \cdot \rangle_H)$ be the adjoint of A. By applying these operators to each component of a multivariate function, we can also define these operators on multivariate functions so that $\tilde{A} : H^k \to L_0^2(P_{F_X,G})^k$ and $\tilde{A}^\top : L_0^2(P_{F_X,G})^k \to H^k$. Define the covariance matrix

$$\Sigma(D) \equiv E(\kappa(D)^{-1} A(D)(Y)(\kappa(D)^{-1} A(D)(Y))^\top).$$

Assume that D^* is an element of the range of $\tilde{A}^\top \tilde{A} : H^k \to H^k$ and that $\tilde{A}^\top \tilde{A} : H \to H$ is 1-1. Then

$$D_{opt} \equiv \min_{D \in H^k}{}^{-1} c^\top \Sigma(D) c \text{ for all } c \in \mathbb{R}^k$$

162   2. General Methodology

exists, and is given by

$$D_{opt} = (\tilde{A}^\top \tilde{A})^{-1}(D^*).$$

Thus

$$\tilde{A}(D_{opt}) = \tilde{A}(\tilde{A}^\top \tilde{A})^{-1} D^*.$$

Remark:

Suppose that we apply this theorem to the T_{CAR}-optimal mapping into observed data estimating functions satisfying $IC(Y \mid Q(F_X,G), G, D_h(\cdot \mid \mu(F_X), \rho(F_X,G))$ satisfies for all D_h $E_G(IC(Y \mid Q(F_X,G), G, D_h) \mid X) = D_h(X)$, $IC(Y \mid Q(F_X,G), G, D_h(\cdot \mid \mu(F_X), \rho(F_X,G))) \perp T_{CAR}(P_{F_X,G})$, and $\{D_h(\cdot \mid \mu(F_X), \rho(F_X,G)) : h \in \mathcal{H}\} = T_{nuis}^{F,\perp}(F_X)$. Then $\tilde{A}(\tilde{A}^\top \tilde{A})^{-1}(D^*)$ has to equal the efficient influence curve $S_{eff}^*(\cdot \mid P_{F_X,G}) = A_{F_X} I_{F_X,G}^{*-1}(S_{eff}^{F*})$ for μ at $P_{F_X,G}$, Off course, this identity is a consequence of (by Theorem 1.3) the fact that in this case $\tilde{A}(D_h) = AI^{-1}D_h$. It follows that $D^* = S_{eff}^{*F}$ and $D_{opt} = (\tilde{A}^\top \tilde{A})^{-1}(D^*)$ corresponds with the optimal full data function defined by $D_{opt} = I_{F_X,G} I_{F_X,G}^{*-1}(S_{eff}^{*F})$ or the solution in $T_{nuis}^{F,\perp}$ satisfying $\Pi(I_{F_X,G}^{-1}(D) \mid T_{nuis}^{F,\perp}) = S_{eff}^{*F}$.

Closed-form optimal estimating functions for MGLM

We will now apply Theorem 2.9 to obtain a closed-form representation of the optimal estimating function among a general class (not necessarily the class of all estimating functions including the efficient influence curve as in Theorem 2.8) of estimating functions in a multivariate generalized linear regression model with covariates always observed. In such models, classes of estimating functions obtained by mapping full data estimating functions $h(X^*)K(\epsilon(\beta))$ into observed data estimating functions $IC(Y \mid Q, G, D_h)$ will have the property that $IC(Y \mid Q, G, D_h) = h(X^*)IC(Y \mid Q, G, K_\beta)$, where $K_\beta(X) = K(\epsilon(\beta))$. This special property combined with Theorem 2.9 results in a closed-form representation of the optimal estimating function. The result is a generalization of Theorem 2.8 since it specifies the optimal estimating function among any given class of estimating functions, not necessarily the class including the efficient influence curve and/or a T_{CAR}-orthogonalized class of estimating functions. For example, if one uses non optimal mappings only orthogonalizing w.r.t. a subspace of T_{CAR}, as provided in this chapter, then Theorem 2.11 below can be used to find the optimal choice.

Theorem 2.11 *Let $Y = \Phi(X,C)$, $X \sim F_X$, $C \mid X \sim G(\cdot \mid X)$, and assume that the conditional distribution G satisfies CAR. Let the full data model be the p-variate generalized regression model $Z = g(X^* \mid \beta) + \epsilon$, $\beta \in \mathbb{R}^k$, $E(K(\epsilon) \mid X^*) = 0$, and $K(\epsilon) = (K(\epsilon_1), \ldots, K(\epsilon_p))$. Assume that $g(X^* \mid \beta)$ is differentiable in β for each possible X^* and that K is differentiable. Consider the full data estimating functions $\{D_h(X \mid \beta) =$

2.8. The Optimal Index

$h(X^*)^\top K(\epsilon(\beta)) : h \in \mathcal{H}\}$, where $\mathcal{H}$ is an index set of $1 \times p$ vector-valued functions of X^*. Consider a class of k-dimensional observed data estimating functions $IC(Y \mid Q, G, D_h(\cdot \mid \mu, \rho))$ with unknown nuisance parameters $Q(F_X, G), G, \rho(F_X, G)$ indexed by $h \in \mathcal{H}^k$, where h denotes a $k \times p$ matrix valued function of X^*. Suppose that for each $k \times p$ matrix-valued function $h \in \mathcal{H}^k$ of X^*,

$$IC(Y \mid Q, G, D_h(\cdot \mid \beta)) = h(X^*)IC(Y \mid Q, G, K_\beta).$$

Here $K_\beta(X) = K(\epsilon(\beta))$. For each $h \in \mathcal{H}^k$, we define the $k \times k$ derivative matrix $\kappa(h)$:

$$\kappa(h) = -E(d/d\beta IC(Y \mid Q, G, D_h)) = -E(h(X^*)d/d\beta IC(Y \mid Q, G, K_\beta)).$$

For each $h \in \mathcal{H}^k$, let $\Sigma(h) = E(\kappa(h)^{-1}IC(Y \mid Q, G, D_h)(\kappa(h)^{-1}IC(Y \mid Q, G, D_h)^\top)$ be the covariance matrix of $\kappa(h)_{k \times k}^{-1}IC(Y \mid Q, G, D_h)$. Let H be the sub-Hilbert space defined by the closure of the linear span of $\mathcal{H}$ w.r.t. the norm in $L_0^2(F_X^*)$. Consider

$$h^* = -E(d/d\beta IC(Y \mid K_\beta) \mid X^*)_{k \times p} E(IC(Y \mid K_\beta)IC(Y \mid K_\beta)^\top \mid X^*)^{-1},$$

where we used shorthand notation $IC(Y \mid K_\beta) = IC(Y \mid Q, G, K_\beta)$. Assume h^* is well defined (i.e., derivative and inverse exist) and $h^* \in H^k$. Then

$$h_{opt} \equiv \min_{h \in H^k}{}^{-1} c^\top \Sigma(h) c \text{ for all } c \in \mathbb{R}^k$$

exists, and is given by $h_{opt} = h^*$.

This theorem is a straightforward consequence of Theorem 2.9. In a typical application of this theorem one would have that $H = L_0^2(F_X^*)$ so that the last condition holds.

Example 2.16 (Optimal IPTW estimating function) Let $A(t)$ represent a time-dependent treatment process that potentially changes value at a finite prespecified set of points. Let $\mathcal{A}$ be the set of possible sample paths of A, where we assume that $\mathcal{A}$ is finite. For each possible treatment regime $\bar{a}$, we define $X_{\bar{a}}(t)$ as the data that one would observe on the subject if, possibly contrary to the fact, the subject had followed treatment regime $\bar{a}$. It is natural to assume that $X_{\bar{a}}(t) = X_{\bar{a}(t-)}$ (i.e., the counterfactual outcome at time t is not affected by treatment given after time t). One refers to $X_{\bar{a}} = (X_{\bar{a}}(t) : t)$ as counterfactual. Suppose that $X_{\bar{a}} = (Z_{\bar{a}}, L_{\bar{a}})$ consists of an outcome process $Z_{\bar{a}}$ and covariate process $L_{\bar{a}}$. The baseline covariates are included in $L_{\bar{a}}(0) = L(0)$. Let $X = (X_{\bar{a}}, \bar{a} \in \mathcal{A})$ be the full data structure, and the observed data structure is given by

$$Y = (\bar{A}, X_{\bar{A}}) = (\bar{A}, Z_{\bar{A}}, L_{\bar{A}}).$$

Let $Y_{\bar{a}}^*$ be a counterfactual outcome of interest such as $Z_{\bar{a}}(\tau)$ at an endpoint τ. Consider a marginal structural generalized linear regression model:

$$Y_{\bar{a}}^* = m(\bar{a}, V \mid \beta) + \epsilon_{\bar{a}}, \text{ where } E(\epsilon_{\bar{a}} \mid V) = 0,$$

where V is a subset of the baseline covariates and $m(\bar{a}, V \mid \beta)$ denotes a parametrization of the conditional mean of $Y_{\bar{a}}^*$, given V, parametrized by the parameter of interest β. Assume that $g(\bar{a} \mid X)$ satisfies the SRA (i.e., $P(A(t) = a(t) \mid \bar{A}(t-), X) = P(A(t) = a(t) \mid \bar{A}(t-), \bar{X}_{\bar{a}}(t)))$. Consider the class of IPTW estimating functions

$$\left\{ IC(Y \mid G, D_h) = \frac{h(\bar{A}, V)\epsilon(\beta)}{g(\bar{A} \mid X)} : h \right\}$$

indexed by real-valued functions h of $\bar{A}, V$, where $\epsilon(\beta) = Y^* - m(\bar{A}, V \mid \beta)$ is the observed residual. An interesting choice of h is the h that gives an optimal covariance matrix $E(IC(Y \mid G, D_h) IC(Y \mid G, D_h)^\top)$ when g is known. In the same way as one proves Theorem 2.11, application of Theorem 2.9 teaches us that this optimal index is given by

$$h^*(\bar{A}, V) = \frac{d}{d\beta} m(\bar{A}, V \mid \beta) \frac{E(1/g(\bar{A} \mid X) \mid \bar{A}, V)}{E(\epsilon^2(\beta)/g^2(\bar{A} \mid X) \mid \bar{A}, V)}.$$

It is interesting to compare this choice with the computationally simple choice recommended in Robins (1999), given by

$$h(\bar{A}, V) = \frac{g^*(\bar{A} \mid V) d/d\beta m(\bar{A}, V \mid \beta)}{E(\epsilon^2(\beta) \mid \bar{A}, V)},$$

where $g^*(\bar{A} \mid V)$ is the conditional density of $\bar{A}$, given V. Note that both choices reduce to the optimal weighted least squares estimating function that is optimal among all estimating functions whose weights only depend on $\bar{A}, V$ in the situation where $g(\bar{A} \mid X) = g(\bar{A} \mid V)$ is only a function of V. Robins (1999, Section 4.1) provides the efficient choice $h_{opt}(\bar{A}, V)$ for this model in the special case where A is time independent. However, $h_{opt}(\bar{A}, V)$ is the solution to a Fredholm integral equation of the second kind which does not admit a closed form solution. Thus an easily computed alternative, although less efficient, is useful. □

An algorithm for evaluating the representations of the optimal full data structure function

Consider the representations $\mathbf{I}_{F_X, G} \mathbf{I}_{F_X, G}^{*-}(D_{h_{eff}})$ and $B_{F_X, G}^{-1}(D_{h_{eff}})$ for $D_{h_{opt}}$. The following two lemmas prove that under reasonable conditions these inverses exist and provide general simple algorithms for determining them.

Lemma 2.6 *For notational convenience, in this lemma we suppress the dependence on (F_X, G) of the Hilbert space operators. Let $\mathbf{I}^* = \Pi_{T^F} \mathbf{I} : T^F \to T^F$ be the information operator. Assume that for all $h \in T^F$ with $\| h \|_{F_X} > 0$ we have $\| A(h) \|_{P_{F_X}, G} > 0$. Then $\mathbf{I}^*$ is 1-1.*

Suppose that for some $\delta > 0$

$$\inf_{\|h\|_{F_X}=1, h \in T^F} \| A(h) \|^2_{P_{F_X},G} \geq \delta. \quad (2.57)$$

Then $\inf_{\|h\|_F=1} \| \mathbf{I}^*(h) \|_{F_X} \geq \delta$, $(I - \mathbf{I}^*)$ has operator norm bounded by $1 - \delta$, $\mathbf{I}^*$ is onto and has bounded inverse with operator norm smaller than or equal to $1/\delta$, and its inverse is given by

$$\mathbf{I}^{*-1} = \sum_{i=0}^{\infty} (I - \mathbf{I}^*)^i.$$

In addition, the following algorithm converges to $\mathbf{I}^{*-1}(f)$: Set $k = 0$

$$\begin{aligned} h^0 &= 0, \\ h^{k+1} &= f - \mathbf{I}^*(h^k) + h^k, \end{aligned}$$

and iterate until convergence. The convergence rate is bounded by

$$\| h^k - \mathbf{I}^{*-}(f) \|_{F_X} \leq \frac{(1-\delta)^k}{\delta} \| f \|_{F_X}.$$

If $\Delta = I(X \text{ observed})$ and $\inf_x P(\Delta = 1 \mid X = x) > 0$, then the condition for bounded invertibility above holds with $\delta \geq \inf_x P(\Delta = 1 \mid X = x)$. Finally, we note that

$$\begin{aligned} \mathbf{I}^*(h) &= \Pi(\mathbf{I}(h) \mid < S^F_{eff} > \oplus T^F_{nuis}) \\ &= \Pi(\mathbf{I}(h) \mid < S^F_{eff} >) + \{\mathbf{I}(h) - \Pi(\mathbf{I}(h) \mid T^{F,\perp}_{nuis})\}. \end{aligned}$$

The condition $\inf_x P(\Delta = 1 \mid X = x) > 0$ is not a necessary condition for the bounded invertibility of $\mathbf{I}^*$. This lemma does not prove that the Neumann series converges if $\| A(h) \| > 0$ for all $h \neq 0$ (thus I^* is 1-1), but $\inf_{\|h\|=1} \| A(h) \|^2 = 0$. We conjecture that if $D_{h_{eff}} \in R(\mathbf{I}^*)$ and I^* is 1-1, then the Neumann series applied to $D_{h_{eff}}$ will converge to $\mathbf{I}^{*-}(S^{*F}_{eff})$. We feel (based on our empirical findings) comfortable recommending this algorithm in practice.

Proof. This lemma can be found in van der Laan (1998) except the actual convergence rate. The convergence rate is proved as follows. Firstly, we have that if $\| \mathbf{I}^*(h) \|_F \geq \delta \| h \|_F$, then

$$\| \mathbf{I}^*(h^k - \mathbf{I}^{*-}(f)) \| \geq \delta \| h^k - \mathbf{I}^{*-}(f) \|.$$

This proves that

$$\| h^k - \mathbf{I}^{*-}(f) \| \leq 1/\delta \| f - \mathbf{I}^*(h^k) \|.$$

Now, note that $f - \mathbf{I}^*(h^k) = h^{k+1} - h^k$. We have

$$h^{k+1} - h^k = (I - \mathbf{I}^*)(h^k - h^{k-1}) = (I - \mathbf{I}^*)^k (h^1 - h^0) = (I - \mathbf{I}^*)^k (f).$$

Since $I - \mathbf{I}^*$ is a contraction with operator norm $1-\delta$, this shows that

$$\|h^k - \mathbf{I}^{*-}(f)\| \le \frac{1}{\delta}(1-\delta)^k \|f\|. \quad \square$$

Similarly, one proves the following algorithm for inverting $B_{F_X,G}$.

Lemma 2.7 *Consider the operator $B_{F_X,G} : T_{nuis}^\perp(F_X) \to T_{nuis}^\perp(F_X)$ defined by $B(D) = \Pi(\mathbf{I}_{F_X,G}^-(D) \mid T_{nuis}^\perp(F_X))$. We have that with $D \in T_{nuis}^{F,\perp}(F_X)$ and $D_1 \equiv \mathbf{I}_{F_X,G}^-(D)$,*

$$\begin{aligned} B_{F_X,G}(D) &= \Pi(\mathbf{I}^-(D) \mid T_{nuis}^{F,\perp}(F_X)) \\ &= D_1 - \Pi(D_1 - \mathbf{I}_{F_X,G}(D_1) \mid T_{nuis}(F_X)) \\ &\equiv D_1 - B_{1,F_X,G}(D_1). \end{aligned}$$

Thus $B_{F_X,G}^{-1}(f) = \mathbf{I}_{F_X,G}(I - B_{1,F_X,G})^{-1}(f)$. If $\mathbf{I}_{F_X,G} : L_0^2(F_X) \to L_0^2(F_X)$ is 1-1, then for all $D_1 \in L_0^2(F_X) \| B_{1,F_X,G}(D_1) \|_{F_X} < \| D_1 \|_{F_X}$. If $B_{1,F_X,G} : L_0^2(F_X) \to L_0^2(F_X)$ has operator norm strictly smaller than 1, for example (2.57) holds, then

$$(I - B_{1,F_X,G})^{-1} = \sum_{k=0}^\infty B_{1,F_X,G}^k$$

and $(I - B_{1,F_X,G})(D_1) = f$ can be solved by successive substitution:

$$D_1^{k+1} = f + B_{1,F_X,G}(D_1^k).$$

In many examples, it is possible to invert $B_{F_X,G} : T_{nuis}^{F,\perp}(F_X) \to T_{nuis}^{F,\perp}(F_X)$ explicitly. In other examples, solving $B_{F_X,G}(D) = D_{h_{eff}}$ results in integral equations for which particular algorithms are available. Lemma 2.7 above shows, in particular, that the operator $B_{F_X,G}$ is invertible. Therefore, another sensible strategy is to approximate $B'_{F_X,G} : \mathcal{H}^F \to \mathcal{H}^F$ (2.53) by a square matrix mapping index vectors (identifying the index h of the element in $T_{nuis}^\perp(F_X)$) into index vectors and invert this matrix using matrix inversion routines. The advantage of the general algorithm of Lemma 2.6 is that it never requires more than being able to apply and store one matrix identifying $I_{F_X,G}^*$. The same remark holds for the algorithm of Lemma 2.7. The algorithms for $\mathbf{I}_{F_X,G}\mathbf{I}_{F_X,G}^{*-}(D_{h_{eff}})$ and $B_{F_X,G}^{-1}(D_{h_{eff}})$ are of similar complexity so that there is little reason to prefer one above the other.

2.9 Estimation of the Optimal Index

Given the estimates $Q_n, G_n, \mu_n^0, \rho_n$, the best estimating function for μ is $IC(Y \mid Q_n, G_n, D_{h_{opt}(F_X,G)}(\cdot \mid \mu, \rho_n))$, where we provided representations of the optimal index $h_{opt}(F_X, G)$ in the preceding sections. In this section, we propose a representation of h_{opt} which naturally provides an estimator h_n of h_{opt}.

2.9. Estimation of the Optimal Index

In the previous section, we obtained representations h_{opt} of the form h_{ind,F_X} (the index mapping) applied to the optimal full data estimating function $D_{opt}(X \mid F_X, G)$ as a function of F_X and G. However, we know that $D_{opt}(X \mid F_X, G) = D_{h_{opt}(F_X,G)}(\cdot \mid \mu(F_X), \rho(F_X))$. Therefore, we are now concerned with establishing a parametrization of D_{opt} in terms of its index h and (μ, ρ) so that we can estimate it by substitution.

In general, an estimator h_n of h_{opt} proceeds as follows. Firstly, we construct an estimate $D_n(X)$ of the optimal full data function $D_{h_{opt}(F_X,G)}(X \mid \mu, \rho)$. If D_n is of the form $D_{h_n}(\cdot \mid \mu_n^0, \rho_n)$, then we also have obtained as estimate h_n of h_{opt}. However, if D_n is based on an implicit representation of D_{opt} involving an inverse B^{-1} or $\mathbf{I}^{*-}$, then estimation of this inverse using a truncated Neumann series representation can result in an estimate $D_n \notin \mathcal{D}(\mu_n^0, \rho_n)$. In that case we need, as discussed below, to project D_n into $\mathcal{D}(\mu_n^0, \rho_n)$ to obtain an estimate h_n of h_{opt}.

To be specific, let $\mathcal{L}(\mathcal{X})$ be a subspace of all pointwise well-defined functions of X with finite supremum norm. We call any function $h : \mathcal{L}(\mathcal{X}) \to \mathcal{H}^F$ an index mapping, and $h_{ind,F_X} : \mathcal{L}(\mathcal{X}) \to \mathcal{H}^F$ is the true index mapping defined by

$$D_{h_{ind,F_X}(D)}(\cdot \mid \mu(F_X), \rho(F_X)) = \Pi_{F_X}(D \mid T_{nuis}^{F,\perp}(F_X)).$$

Let $h_{ind,n}$ be an estimator of h_{ind,F_X}. Then, if $D_n \notin \mathcal{D}(\mu_n^0, \rho_n)$ we estimate $h_{ind,F_X}(D_n)$, and we denote the resulting estimator of h_{opt} with h_n:

$$h_n \equiv h_{ind,n}(D_n).$$

In the next subsections, we reparametrize the representations (2.51) and (2.53) of $D_{opt}(X \mid F_X, G)$ in terms of μ, ρ and the parameters identifying the optimal index h_{opt} and estimate h_{opt}, and D_{opt} accordingly.

2.9.1 Reparametrizing the representations of the optimal full data function

If we state an inverse of an operator applied to a function, then it will be implicitly assumed that this operator is $1-1$ and that this function is in the range of the operator. Firstly, consider the representation (2.51) of $D_{opt} = B_{F_X,G}^{-1}(S_{eff}^F)$. Recall the definition $\mathcal{D}(\mu, \rho) = \{D_h(\cdot \mid \mu, \rho) : h \in \mathcal{H}^F\}$. For each (h_{ind}, μ, ρ) (h_{ind} being an index mapping), let $\Pi_{h_{ind},\mu,\rho} : \mathcal{L}(\mathcal{X}) \to \mathcal{D}(\mu, \rho)$ be an operator such that for all $F_X \in \mathcal{M}^F$ and $D \in \mathcal{L}(\mathcal{X})$

$$\begin{aligned}\Pi_{h_{ind,F_X},\mu(F_X),\rho(F_X)}(D) &= \Pi(D \mid T_{nuis}^\perp(F_X)) \\ &= D_{h_{ind,F_X}(D)}(\cdot \mid \mu(F_X), \rho(F_X)).\end{aligned}$$

Thus $\Pi_{h,\mu,\rho}$ parametrizes the projection operator onto $T_{nuis}^{F,\perp}$ in terms of an index mapping h and the parameter values μ, ρ. Let $\mathbf{I}_{F_1,G_1} : \mathcal{L}(\mathcal{X}) \to \mathcal{L}(\mathcal{X})$

168   2. General Methodology

and denote its range with $R_\infty(\mathbf{I}_{F_1,G_1})$. For any $D \in R_\infty(\mathbf{I}_{F_1,G_1})$, define

$$B_{F_1,G_1,h_{ind},\mu,\rho}(D) = \Pi_{h_{ind},\mu,\rho}\mathbf{I}_{F_1,G_1}^{-1}(D).$$

Consider now the following representation of D_{opt}:

$$D_{opt}(F_1,G_1,h_{ind},h_{eff},\mu,\rho) \equiv B_{F_1,G_1,h_{ind},\mu,\rho}^{-1} D_{h_{eff}}(\cdot \mid \mu,\rho).$$

We can now show the following result.

Lemma 2.8 *Let* (μ,ρ), $(F_1,G_1), h_{ind}(\cdot)$ *be given. Assume* $\mathcal{D}(\mu,\rho) \subset R_\infty(\mathbf{I}_{F_1,G_1})$. *We have that* $B_{F_1,G_1,h_{ind},\mu,\rho} : \mathcal{D}(\mu,\rho) \to \mathcal{D}(\mu,\rho)$. *In particular, for any* $h_{eff} \in \mathcal{H}^F$

$$D_{opt}(F_1,G_1,h_{ind},h_{eff},\mu,\rho) \equiv B_{F_1,G_1,h_{ind},\mu,\rho}^{-1} D_{h_{eff}}(\cdot \mid \mu,\rho) \in \mathcal{D}(\mu,\rho). \tag{2.58}$$

This shows that given (μ,ρ) we end up in $\mathcal{D}(\mu,\rho)$ regardless of our choice of F_1, G_1, h_{ind}, and h_{eff}. Thus

$$D_{opt}(F_1,G_1,h_{ind},h_{eff},\mu,\rho) = D_{h_{opt}(F_1,G_1,h_{ind},h_{eff},\mu,\rho)}(\cdot \mid \mu,\rho)$$

for some mapping $(F_1,G_1,h_{ind},h_{eff},\mu,\rho) \to h_{opt}(F_1,G_1,h_{ind},h_{eff},\mu,\rho) \in \mathcal{H}^F$. Thus, estimation of F, G, h_{ind}, h_{eff} only affects the estimator $h_{opt,n}$ of the optimal index h_{opt} in $D_{h_{opt,n}}(\cdot \mid \mu_n^0, \rho_n)$. Since we prove a similar lemma for the representation (2.53) below, we will omit the proof of Lemma 2.8 here.

Consider now the representation (2.53) of $D_{opt}(F_X,G) = \mathbf{I}_{F_X,G}\{\Pi_{T^F}\mathbf{I}_{F_X,G}\}^{-1}(S_{eff}^F)$. Let us start by parametrizing the projection operator Π_{T^F} onto the full data tangent space. We have

$$\Pi_{F_X}(D \mid T^F(F_X)) = \Pi_{F_X}(D \mid < S_{eff}^F(\cdot \mid F_X) >) + D - \Pi_{F_X}(D \mid T_{nuis}^{F,\perp}(F_X)).$$

The first projection operator is given by

$$\Pi_{F_X}(D \mid < S_{eff}^F(\cdot \mid F_X) >) = c_{F_X}(D)D_{h_{eff}(F_X)}(\cdot \mid \mu(F_X),\rho(F_X)),$$

where $c_{F_X}(D) = \langle D, S_{eff}^{F\top}\rangle_{F_X}\langle S_{eff}^F, S_{eff}^{F\top}\rangle_{F_X}^{-1}$, and $S_{eff}^F = D_{h_{eff}}(\cdot \mid \mu(F_X),\rho(F_X))$. Above, we reparametrized the projection operator onto $T_{nuis}^{F,\perp}$ as $\Pi_{h_{ind},\mu,\rho}$ in terms of $(h_{ind,F_X},\mu(F_X),\rho(F_X))$. This suggests the following parametrization of the projection operator $\Pi_{F_X}(D \mid T^F(F_X))$: suppose that for every $(c,h_{ind},h_{eff},\mu,\rho) \in \{(c_{F_X},h_{ind,F_X},h_{eff}(F_X),\mu(F_X),\rho(F_X)) : F_X \in \mathcal{M}^F\}$

$$\Pi_{c,h_{ind},h_{eff},\mu,\rho}(D) \equiv c(D)D_{h_{eff}}(\cdot \mid \mu,\rho) + D - D_{h_{ind}(D)}(\cdot \mid \mu,\rho)$$

is a well-defined operator from $\mathcal{L}(\mathcal{X}) \to \mathcal{L}(\mathcal{X})$ satisfying

$$\Pi_{c_{F_X},h_{ind,F_X},h_{eff}(F_X),\mu(F_X),\rho(F_X)} = \Pi_{F_X}(\cdot \mid T^F(F_X)).$$

The unknown index mapping parameter h_{ind} ranges over all index mappings $h : \mathcal{L}(\mathcal{X}) \to \mathcal{H}^{\mathcal{F}}$.

2.9. Estimation of the Optimal Index   169

This suggests the following parametrization $D_{opt}(F_1, G_1, c, h_{ind}, h_{eff}, \mu, \rho)$ of $D_{opt}(F_X, G)$ (2.53):

$$\mathbf{I}_{F_1,G_1}\{\Pi_{c,h_{ind},h_{eff},\mu,\rho}\mathbf{I}_{F_1,G_1}\}^{-1}D_{h_{eff}}(\cdot \mid \mu, \rho).$$

Here, we implicitly assumed that this is an element of $\mathcal{L}(\mathcal{X})$. Notice that indeed $D_{opt}(F_X, G, c_{F_X}, h_{ind,F_X}, h_{eff}(F_X), \mu(F_X), \rho(F_X)) = D_{h_{opt}(F_X,G)}(\cdot \mid \mu(F_X), \rho(F_X))$.

We can now prove the following lemma.

Lemma 2.9 *For notational convenience, let* $\Pi_{1,\mu,\rho} = \Pi_{c,h_{ind},h_{eff},\mu,\rho}$. *Assume that* $h_{ind}: \mathcal{L}(\mathcal{X}) \to \mathcal{H}^\mathcal{F}$. *For any* F_1, G_1 *and* $h_{eff} \in \mathcal{H}^F$ *(so that* $D_{h_{eff}}(\cdot \mid \mu, \rho) \in \mathcal{D}(\mu, \rho)$) *satisfying* $\{\Pi_{1,\mu,\rho}\mathbf{I}_{F_1,G_1}\}^{-1}(D_{h_{eff}}) \in \mathcal{L}(\mathcal{X})$, *we have*

$$\mathbf{I}_{F_1,G_1}\{\Pi_{1,\mu,\rho}\mathbf{I}_{F_1,G_1}\}^{-1}D_{h_{eff}}(\cdot \mid \mu, \rho) \in \mathcal{D}(\mu, \rho). \quad (2.59)$$

Proof. We will show that for any possible value of the parameters we have $D_{opt}(F_1, G_1, c, h_{ind}, h_{eff}, \mu, \rho) \in \mathcal{D}(\mu, \rho)$. The proof is almost a direct consequence of the fact that for any $D \in \mathcal{L}(\mathcal{X})$ and $h_{eff} \in \mathcal{H}^F$

$$D - \Pi_{c,h_{ind},h_{eff},\mu,\rho}(D) = D_{h(D)}(\cdot \mid \mu, \rho) - c(D)D_{h_{eff}}(\cdot \mid \mu, \rho) \in \mathcal{D}(\mu, \rho) \quad (2.60)$$

and that

$$\Pi_{c,h_{ind},h_{eff},\mu,\rho}D_{opt}(F_1, G_1, c, h_{ind}, h_{eff}, \mu, \rho) = D_{h_{eff}}(\cdot \mid \mu, \rho). \quad (2.61)$$

Using short-hand notation $D_{opt} = D_{opt}(F_1, G_1, c, h_{ind}, h_{eff}, \mu, \rho)$, $\Pi_{1,\mu,\rho} = \Pi_{c,h_{ind},h_{eff},\mu,\rho}$, we have by (2.60) and (2.61)

$$\begin{aligned} D_{opt} &= \{D_{opt} - \Pi_{1,\mu,\rho}D_{opt}\} + \Pi_{1,\mu,\rho}D_{opt} \\ &= D_{h(D_{opt})}(\cdot \mid \mu, \rho) - c(D_{opt})D_{h_{eff}}(\cdot \mid \mu, \rho) + D_{h_{eff}}(\cdot \mid \mu, \rho). \end{aligned}$$

Since $D_{opt} \in \mathcal{L}(\mathcal{X})$ and $h: \mathcal{L}(\mathcal{X}) \to \mathcal{H}^\mathcal{F}$, this proves that $D_{opt} \in \mathcal{D}(\mu, \rho)$. □

2.9.2 Estimation of the optimal full data structure estimating function

Consider the representation (2.58) of the optimal full data structure function $D_{opt}(F_X, G)$. Estimation of this representation involves estimation of the components (F_X, G) identifying the nonparametric information operator, h_{ind,F_X} identifying the index mapping of the projection operator onto the orthogonal complement of the nuisance tangent space, and $h_{eff}(F_X)$ identifying the index of the full data canonical gradient $S_{eff}^F(\cdot \mid F_X)$ and $(\mu(F_X), \rho(F_X))$. Substitution of estimators for each of these components yields an estimator of D_{opt}:

$$\begin{aligned} D_n &= D_{opt}(F_n, G_n, h_n, h_{eff,n}, \mu_n^0, \rho_n) \\ &= \left\{\Pi_{h_n,\mu_n^0,\rho_n}\mathbf{I}_{F_n,G_n}^-\right\}^{-1}D_{h_{eff,n}}(\cdot \mid \mu_n^0, \rho_n). \end{aligned}$$

Similarly, an estimator based on representation (2.59) is given by

$$D_n = D_{opt}(F_n, G_n, c_n, h_n, h_{eff,n}, \mu_n^0, \rho_n)$$
$$= I_{F_n,G_n}\{\Pi_{c_n,h_n,h_{eff,n},\mu_n^0,\rho_n} I_{F_n,G_n}\}^- D_{h_{eff,n}}(\cdot \mid \mu_n^0, \rho_n).$$

Lemmas 2.8 and 2.9 show that the right-hand side is indeed an element of $\mathcal{D}(\mu_n^0, \rho_n)$ so that

$$D_n = D_{h_{opt,n}}(\cdot \mid \mu_n^0, \rho_n) \text{ for some } h_{opt,n} \in \mathcal{H}^F.$$

Thus $F_n, G_n, c_n, h_n, h_{eff,n}$ only affect the index estimate $h_{opt,n}$. If one uses approximations $\tilde{D}_n$ of these estimators D_n that are not necessarily elements of $\mathcal{D}(\mu_n^0, \rho_n)$, then, as mentioned in the previous subsection, one should use

$$h_{opt,n} = h_{ind,n}(\tilde{D}_n).$$

If in model $\mathcal{M}$ the full data working model $\mathcal{M}^w$ is such that it yields an (e.g., maximum likelihood) estimator F_n of the full data distribution F_X itself, then one could decide to use a substitution estimator for each of the full data distribution parameters:

$$D_n(\cdot \mid \mu_n^0, \rho_n) = I_{F_n,G_n} I_{F_n,G_n}^{*-1} D_{h_{eff}(F_n)}(\cdot \mid \mu_n^0, \rho_n), \quad (2.62)$$

where

$$I_{F_n,G_n}^{*-1} = \Pi_{c_{F_n}, h_{F_n}, h_{eff}(F_n), \mu_n^0, \rho_n} I_{F_n,G_n}.$$

2.10 Locally Efficient Estimation with Score-Operator Representation

Recall that at the true F_X, G

$$IC(\cdot \mid Q(F_X, G), G, D_h(\cdot \mid \mu, \rho)) = A_{F_X} I_{F_X,G}^- D_h(\cdot \mid \mu, \rho).$$

Suppose that we actually use this representation in terms of F_X, G to define our estimating function; that is, just parametrize IC in terms of F_X and G:

$$IC(\cdot \mid F_X, G, D_h(\cdot \mid \mu, \rho)) = A_{F_X} I_{F_X,G}^- D_h(\cdot \mid \mu, \rho).$$

Let F_n be an estimator of F_X according to the working model $\mathcal{M}^{F,w}$ and let G_n be an estimator of G according to the working model $\mathcal{G}$. In addition, assume that we estimate $D_{h_{opt}}$ with $D_{h_{opt,n}} = I_{F_n,G_n} I_{F_n,G_n}^{*-1} D_{h_{eff}(F_n)}(\cdot \mid \mu, \rho_n)$ as defined by (2.62) using F_n and G_n. Then, the resulting estimating function for μ is given by

$$IC(\cdot \mid F_n, G_n, D_{h_{opt,n}}(\cdot \mid \mu, \rho_n)) = A_{F_n} I_{F_n,G_n}^{*-} D_{h_{eff}(F_n)}(\cdot \mid \mu, \rho_n).$$

Since this is just a special application of the one-step estimator (2.35), we can apply Theorem 2.5, which shows, under regularity conditions, that

2.10. Locally Efficient Estimation with Score-Operator Representation 171

the resulting one-step estimator is consistent and asymptotically normal if either $\mathcal{M}^{F,w}$ is correctly specified or $\mathcal{G}$ is correctly specified and that it is efficient if both are correctly specified. The one-step estimator can be computed by inverting $\mathbf{I}^*_{F_n,G_n}$ with the successive substitution method of Lemma 2.6.

Note that, given estimators F_n, G_n, this provides us with a completely automated method for locally efficient estimation in any censored data model. Off course, here one also uses a substitution estimator $\rho_n = \rho(F_n, G_n)$.

3
Monotone Censored Data

3.1 Data Structure and Model

Let $\{X(t) : t \in \mathbb{R}_{\geq 0}\}$ be a multivariate stochastic process indexed by time t. Let T denote an endpoint of this stochastic process, and define $X(t) \equiv X(\min(t,T))$. Let $R(t) = I(T \leq t)$ be one of the components of $X(t)$. We define the full data as $X = \bar{X}(T) = (X(s) : s \leq T)$, where T is thus a function X.

Suppose that we observe the full data process $X(\cdot)$ up to the minimum of a univariate censoring variable C and T so that for the observed data we have:

$$Y = (\tilde{T} = \min(T,C), \Delta = I(T \leq \tilde{T}) = I(C \geq T), \bar{X}(\tilde{T})).$$

We will define $C = \infty$ if $C > T$ so that this data structure can be represented as

$$Y = (C, \bar{X}(C)).$$

In the next section, we provide several important examples of this monotone censored data structure.

Let $\mathcal{M}^F$ be a specified full data model for the distribution F_X of X, and let $\mu = \mu(F_X) \in \mathbb{R}^k$ be the full data parameter of interest. Let $G(\cdot \mid X)$ be the conditional distribution of C, given X, and it is assumed that G satisfies CAR (i.e., $G \in \mathcal{G}(CAR)$). Given working models $\mathcal{M}^{F,w} \subset \mathcal{M}^F$ and $\mathcal{G} \subset \mathcal{G}(CAR)$, we define the observed data model $\mathcal{M} = \{P_{F_X,G} : F_X \in \mathcal{M}^{F,w}\} \cup \{P_{F_X,G} : G \in \mathcal{G}\}$. We also define the observed data model

3.1. Data Structure and Model

$\mathcal{M}(\mathcal{G}) = \{P_{F_X,G} : F_X \in \mathcal{M}^F, G \in \mathcal{G}\}$. Candidates for the censoring model $\mathcal{G}$ are given below.

Let $g(c \mid X)$ be the conditional density of C, given X, either w.r.t. a Lebesgue density or counting measure, and let $\lambda_C(c \mid X)$ be the corresponding conditional hazard. Define $A(t) \equiv I(C \leq t)$. The conditional distribution G satisfies CAR if

$$E(dA(t) \mid X, \bar{A}(t-)) = E(dA(t) \mid \bar{A}(t-), \bar{X}(\min(t,C))).$$

In other words, the intensity of $A(t)$ w.r.t. the unobserved history $(X, \bar{A}(t-))$ should equal the intensity of $A(t)$ w.r.t the observed history $(\bar{A}(t-), \bar{X}(\min(t,C)))$. Equivalently, G satisfies CAR if for $c < T$

$$\lambda_C(c \mid X) = m(c, \bar{X}(c)) \text{ for some measurable function } m. \qquad (3.1)$$

If C is continuous, then a practical and useful submodel $\mathcal{G} \subset \mathcal{G}(CAR)$ (3.1) is the multiplicative intensity model w.r.t. the Lebesgue measure

$$E(dA(t) \mid \bar{A}(t-), \bar{X}(\min(t,C))) = I(\tilde{T} > t)\lambda_0(t) \exp\left(\alpha_0^\top W(t)\right),$$

where α_0 is a k-dimensional vector of coefficients, $W(t)$ is a k-dimensional time-dependent vector that is a function of $\bar{X}(t)$, and λ_0 is an unspecified baseline hazard. Note that

$$\lambda_C(t \mid X, T > t) \equiv \lambda_0(t) \exp\left(\alpha_0^\top W(t)\right)$$

denotes the Cox proportional hazards model for the conditional hazard λ_C.

If we knew that the censoring was independent of the survival time and the history, then, for $t < T$, this would reduce to

$$\lambda_C(t \mid X) = \lambda_0(t).$$

If C is discrete, then a natural model $\mathcal{G} \subset \mathcal{G}(CAR)$ is

$$E(dA(t) \mid \bar{A}(t-), \bar{X}(\min(t,C))) = I(\tilde{T} \geq t)\frac{1}{1 + \exp(-\{h_0(c) + \alpha_0^\top W(t)\})},$$

where h_0 could be left unspecified. This corresponds with assuming a logistic regression model for the conditional censoring hazard $\lambda_C(t \mid X) = P(C = t \mid X, C \geq t)$: for $t < T$

$$\log\left(\frac{\lambda_C(t \mid X)}{1 - \lambda_C(t \mid X)}\right) = h_0(t) + \alpha_0^\top W(t).$$

If the support of C gets finer and finer so that $P(C = t \mid X, C \geq t)$ approximates zero, then this model with h_0 unspecified converges to the Cox proportional hazards model with $\lambda_0 = \exp(h_0)$ and regression coefficients α_0 (see e.g., Kalbfleisch and Prentice, 1980).

Whatever CAR model for $\lambda_C(t \mid X)$ is used, the G part of the density of $P_{F_X,G}$ in terms of $\lambda_C(t \mid X)$ is given by the partial likelihood of $A(t) = I(C \leq t)$ w.r.t. history $\mathcal{F}(t) \equiv (\bar{A}(t-), \bar{X}(\min(t,C)))$ as defined in Andersen, Borgan, Gill and Keiding (1993) for the continuous case. Let

$\alpha(t) = E(dA(t) \mid \mathcal{F}(t)) = I(C \geq t, T \geq t)d\Lambda_C(t \mid X)$ be the intensity of $A(t)$ w.r.t. history $\mathcal{F}(t)$, where this can also denote a discrete probability in case C is discrete. Here $\Lambda_C(\cdot \mid X)$ is the cumulative of $\lambda_C(\cdot \mid X)$. The G part of the density of $P_{F_X,G}$ is given by

$$L(G) = \prod \alpha(t)^{dA(t)}(1 - \alpha(t))^{1-dA(t)}$$

$$= \left\{ \prod_{(0,\tilde{T}]} (1 - d\Lambda_C(t \mid X)) \right\}^{\Delta} \left\{ \prod_{(0,\tilde{T})} (1 - \lambda_C(t \mid X)) \times d\Lambda_C(\tilde{T} \mid X) \right\}^{1-\Delta}.$$

For the Cox proportional hazards model and logistic regression model for $\lambda_C(t \mid X)$, maximum likelihood estimation of G can be based on this likelihood and can be carried out with standard software. In particular, one can fit the Cox proportional hazards model with the S-plus function Coxph(). If we assume the logistic regression model for discrete C, then inspection of the likelihood $L(G)$ shows that one can obtain MLE by simply fitting the logistic regression model to a pooled sample. Here, a subject with observed censoring time $C = j$ (for simplicity, let the support of C be integer-valued) contributes j Bernoulli observations $(0, \ldots, 0, 1)$ with corresponding covariates $(1, W(1)), \ldots, (j, W(j))$, and a subject who fails between $C = j$ and $C = j + 1$ contributes j observations $(0, \ldots, 0)$ with corresponding covariates $(1, W(1)), \ldots, (j, W(j))$.

In Section 3.2 we will provide many challenging estimation problems that are applications of the general monotone censored data structure covered in this chapter. In Section 3.3 we define inverse probability of censoring weighted mappings $IC_0(Y \mid G, D)$ from full data estimating functions into observed data estimating functions and derive a closed-form representation of the influence curve of the corresponding estimators. We work out these estimators for the case where the full data model is a multiplicative intensity model for the intensity of a counting process $N(t) \subset X(t)$ w.r.t. a particular subset of $\bar{X}(t-)$. For example, one might be interested in estimating the causal effect of a randomized treatment arm on the intensity of survival or another counting process of interest. This implies that one does not want to adjust for other variables in the past except the past of the counting process and the treatment variable. Just fitting a Cox proportional hazards model only using the treatment as covariate is inconsistent if the hazard of censoring at time t conditional on X depends on more of $\bar{X}(t-)$ than the treatment variable. In addition, this method is highly inefficient if the data contain surrogates for survival or strong predictors of survival. In Section 3.4, we define the optimal mapping $IC(Y \mid Q, G, D) = IC_0(Y \mid G, D) - \Pi(IC_0 \mid T_{CAR})$ from full data estimating functions into observed data estimating functions indexed by nuisance parameters $Q = Q(F_X, G)$ and G. In Section 3.5, we discuss estimation of Q in detail. In Section 3.6, we study estimation of the optimal index h_{opt} and work out closed-form representations for the case where the full data model is the multivariate generalized linear regression model. In Section 3.7, we apply the methods to obtain a locally efficient estimator of the regression parameters in a multivariate generalized regression model (with outcome being a multivariate survival time) for the multivariate right-censored data structure when all failure times are subject to a common censoring time. In Section 3.8, we rigorously analyze a locally efficient estimator of the bivariate survival function based on a bivariate right-censored data structure by applying Theorem 2.4 of Chapter 2. Finally, in Section 3.9 we provide a general methodology for estimating optimal predictors of survival w.r.t. risk of a user supplied loss function based on our general right-censored data structure, thereby making significant improvements to the current literature on survival prediction. In the next subsection, we show that, without loss of optimality, the estimation methods can also be applied if censoring is cause-specific and the cause is observed.

3.1.1 Cause-specific censoring

In many applications, there exist various causes of censoring and the cause is typically known. In this situation, one observes (C, J), where C is the censoring time and J indexes the cause. For example, one cause might be the end of the study while another cause might be that the subject has severe side effects that made the doctor decide to stop treatment. In this case, one wants a model for the intensity $\alpha(t)$ that acknowledges that C is an outcome of competing censoring times that might follow Cox proportional hazards models using different subsets of covariates. In this case, we extend our data structure as

$$Y = (C, J, \bar{X}(C)),$$

where (C, J) now represents the joint censoring variable with conditional distribution G, given X. We can now identify the joint censoring variable by the random process $A(t) = (A_1(t), \ldots, A_J(t))$, where $A_j(t) = I(C \leq t, J = j)$, $j = 1, \ldots, J$. Thus, the G part of the density of $P_{F_X, G}$ is now given by $g(A \mid X)$, which can in the discrete case be represented as

$$g(A \mid X) = \prod_t \prod_j \alpha_j(t)^{dA_j(t)} (1 - \alpha_j(t))^{1 - dA_j(t)},$$

where $\alpha_j(t) = E(dA_j(t) \mid A_1(t), \ldots, A_{j-1}(t), \mathcal{F}(t))$, $j = 1, \ldots, J$. In the continuous case, this expression for $g(A \mid X)$ reduces to the partial likelihood of the multivariate counting process $A(t) = (A_1(t), \ldots, A_J(t))$ w.r.t. $\mathcal{F}(t)$ as defined in Andersen, Borgan, Gill, and Keiding (1993):

$$g(A \mid X) = \prod_t \prod_j \alpha_j(t)^{dA_j(t)} (1 - \alpha_j(t) dt)^{1 - dA_j(t)}.$$

Let $A.(t) = \sum_{j=1}^{J} A_j(t)$. Since the outcome of J does not affect the censoring of X and only affects the G part of the likelihood, it is not hard to show that the orthogonal complement of the nuisance tangent space for μ is identical to the orthogonal complement of the nuisance tangent space class of all estimating functions for μ for the reduced data structure $(C, \bar{X}(C))$, as presented in this chapter. The corresponding estimating functions only require an estimate of the intensity $\alpha(t) = E(dA.(t) \mid \mathcal{F}(t))$ (i.e., of the conditional distribution of C, given X) and, in particular, the survivor function

$$\bar{G}(t \mid X) \equiv P(C \geq t \mid X) = \exp\left(-\int_{[0,t)} \alpha(s)ds\right) \text{ of } C, \text{ given } X.$$

This censoring mechanism could be fit with the reduced data structure $(C, \bar{X}(C))$. However, if knowledge is available on the cause specific intensities of A_j, then a natural framework for fitting a continuous intensity α of A w.r.t. $\mathcal{F}(t)$ is to assume multiplicative intensity models

$$\alpha_j(t) \equiv E(dA_j(t) \mid \mathcal{F}(t)) = I(\tilde{T} \geq t)\lambda_{0j}(t)\exp(\alpha_j W_j(t))$$

and use $\alpha(t) = \sum_{j=1}^{J} \alpha_j(t)$. Again, one can use the S-plus function Coxph() to fit the intensities α_j, $j = 1, \ldots, J$ (Andersen, Borgan, Gill, and Keiding, 1993). Similarly, such a strategy could be applied if the censoring mechanism is discrete. In this case we note that $\bar{G}(t \mid X) = \prod_{[0,t)} \prod_{j=1}^{J}(1-\lambda_j(t))$, where $\lambda_j(t) \equiv E(dA_j(t) \mid A_1(t) = \ldots = A_{j-1}(t) = 0, C \geq t, \mathcal{F}(t))$. Thus, following Robins (1993a), we conclude that the methods presented in this chapter for single cause censoring can be applied by only using the additional data J to obtain an estimate G_n of $G(t \mid X)$ but further ignoring J.

3.2 Examples

3.2.1 Right-censored data on a survival time

Consider a longitudinal study in which the outcome of interest is the survival time T. We assume that each subject is regularly followed up and relevant time-dependent measurements are taken at each visit. Let $R(t) = I(T > t)$ be the survival status of the subject at time t. Let $L(t)$ be the time-dependent process representing these measurements at time t. We denote the history of $L(t)$ with $\bar{L}(t) = \{L(s) : s \leq t\}$. The time-independent baseline covariates are included in the vector $L(0)$. For full data on a subject we have $X = (T, \bar{L}(T)) = (\bar{R}(T), \bar{L}(T))$. Let C be the dropout time of the subject. We observe each subject up to the minimum of T and C. Thus we observe n i.i.d. observations $Y_1, \ldots, Y_n$ of

$$Y = \Phi(T, \bar{L}(T), C) \equiv (\tilde{T} = T \wedge C, \Delta = I(T \leq C), \bar{L}(\tilde{T})).$$

One can also represent this data structure as
$$Y = (\tilde{T}, \Delta, \bar{X}(\tilde{T}))$$
since $X(t) = (R(t), L(t))$. Thus, this data structure is of the type considered in this chapter. Important parameters might be 1) the marginal survival function of T, 2) regression parameters in a generalized linear regression model of $\log(T)$, onto some baseline covariates and/or treatment or regression parameters and 3) regression parameters of a Cox proportional hazards model for the hazard of T, adjusting for some baseline covariates, treatment, and possibly some of the time-dependent covariates.

Estimation with this data structure is a complicated and practically important problem. This data structure is an important extension of the marginal right censored data structure on T. For an extensive description of the literature on the marginal univariate right-censored data structure, we refer the reader to Andersen, Borgan, Gill and Keiding (1993). For maximum likelihood (or more general partial likelihood) estimation and inference with multiplicative intensity models such as the Cox proportional hazards model for this data structure, see Andersen, Borgan, Gill and Keiding (1993). Such models are of low enough dimension that the maximum likelihood estimator can be used. However, if one is interested in more marginal parameters, such as the marginal distribution of T or a regression model of T on a subset of the baseline and/or time-dependent covariates, then this literature does not provide an appropriate methodology.

Locally efficient estimation of regression parameters in Cox proportional hazards and accelerated failure time models for this data structure, allowing covariates outside the model, has been studied in Robins (1993a) and Robins and Rotnitzky (1992). The importance of assuming a CAR model in these real-life applications has been argued in detail in these papers. Locally efficient estimation of the marginal distribution of T has been studied and implemented with simulations in Hubbard, van der Laan and Robins (1999). Robins (1996) studies locally efficient estimation in the median regression model. Robins and Finkelstein (2000) apply the inverse probability of censoring weighted estimator of survival to analyze an AIDS clinical trial.

3.2.2 Right-censored data on quality-adjusted survival time

Consider a longitudinal study in which a quality adjusted survival time of a subject is the time variable of interest. Let T be the chronological survival time of the subject. Let $V(t)$ be the state of health of the subject at time t. Typically, one assumes that the state space is finite so that $V(t) \in \{1, \ldots, k\}$ for some k, but this is not necessary. We define the quality adjusted lifetime as $U \equiv \int_0^T Q(V(t))dt$, where Q is some given function. One sensible definition of quality-adjusted lifetime can be obtained by defining $V(t)$ as the quality of life at time t on a scale between 0 and 1 and $Q(t) = t$. In this case, one might define $V(t) = 1$ if the subject has a normal life at time t and $V(t) = 0$ if the subject is seriously suffering from the treatment (e.g., chemotherapy) at time t.

In many applications, one will observe additional information on the subject in terms of baseline covariates and time-dependent measurements (e.g., CD4 count in an AIDS application). Let $W(t) \in \mathbb{R}^k$, $t \in \mathbb{R}_{\geq 0}$ be a covariate process. We will denote the time-independent covariates with $W(0)$. Now, the full data process of interest is $X(t) = (R(t), V(t), W(t))$, where $R(t) = I(T \leq t)$ and the full data structure is $X = \bar{X}(T) = \{X(s) : s \leq t\}$. Note that observing X implies observing U. Therefore, if each subject is observed until death, then the natural nonparametric estimator of the quality-adjusted survival function $S_U(t) \equiv P(U > t) = 1 - F_U(t)$ is the empirical survival function based on $U_1, \ldots, U_n$. Due to limited follow-up time or other reasons, one will not always observe the process X up until time T; one observes the process X up until the minimum of a censoring time C and T, and one knows whether this minimum is either the censoring time or T. Thus, the observed data structure can be represented as

$$Y = (\tilde{T} \equiv C \wedge T, \Delta = I(\tilde{T} = T), \bar{X}(\tilde{T})), \qquad (3.2)$$

which thus corresponds with the data structure studied in this chapter. We observe n independent and identically distributed observations $Y_1, \ldots, Y_n$ of Y. As in the previous example, possible parameters of interest are the marginal distribution of U and regression parameters in Cox proportional hazards models or linear regression models with outcome $\log(U)$. Gelber, Goldhirsch, and Cavalli (1991) discuss quality-of-life data concerning operable breast cancer. The study compares a single cycle of adjuvant chemotherapy compared with longer-duration chemotherapy for premenopausal women or chemoendocrine therapy for postmenopausal women. To define the quality-adjusted lifetime, they considered three health states: time without systems and toxicity (TWiST), toxicity (TOX), and survival time after relapse (REL). They weighted the time spent in each category according to subjective judgments as to the quality of life in each state. Specifically, TWiST was weighted as 1, with the other states naturally having less weight. Their goal was to compare the efficacy of different treatment regimes on the weighted sum of the times, known as the quality-adjusted lifetime, and the parameter of interest to measure this was the mean quality-adjusted lifetime in each treatment group. In addition to Gelber, et al. (1991), many statistical analyses of lifetime data from clinical trials have been concerned with inference on the quality-adjusted lifetime distribution (e.g., Gelber, Gelman, and Holdhirsch, 1989; Gelber et al., 1992; Glasziou, Simes and Gelber, 1990; Goldhirsch et al., 1989; and Korn, 1993). In these studies, one observes for each subject a quality-of-life state process up to the minimum of chronological death, and censoring and weights are assigned to each of the states given a priori (an overview of this type of data is given by Cox et al., 1992). Zhao and Tsiatis (1997) proposed an ad hoc estimator of the quality-adjusted lifetime distribution itself for the marginal data structure.

Locally efficient estimators of treatment-specific marginal quality-adjusted survival functions have been developed and implemented in van der Laan and Hubbard (1999), analogous to the methods in this chapter (and Chapter 6).

3.2.3 Right-censored data on a survival time with reporting delay

Consider a study in which the survival time T of a subject is of interest. In most central data registries of certain types of patients (e.g., AIDS, cancer), data on a subject are reported with delay (e.g., Bachetti, 1996). This means that if a subject has not been reported dead at time t, then that might either mean that the subject is still alive or that the subject died before time t but that the death has not been reported yet.

Let $R(t) = I(T \leq t)$ represent the vital status of a subject at time t. Let V_1 report at time t until when the process R has been observed; If, at time t, R has been observed up to time $s \leq t$, then $V_1(t) = s$. In particular, if, at time t, T is already observed, then we have $V_1(t) = t$. Thus V_1 is an increasing function with $V_1(t) \leq t$.

One can describe V_1 in terms of monitoring times $U_1 < U_2 < \ldots < U_{k-1} < T$ and reporting times $A_1 < A_2 < \ldots < A_{k-1}$ of the subject under study. Here A_j is the time at which the vital status of the subject at time U_j is reported, $j = 1, \ldots, k-1$, and let A_k be the time at which T is reported, so at time A_j we know that $T > U_j$, $j = 1, \ldots, k-1$ and at time A_k we know that $T = t$ for some $t \leq A_k$. In the context of reporting delays as described above, we have

$$V_1(t) = \begin{cases} U_j & \text{if } t \in [A_j, A_{j+1}) \\ t & \text{if } t \geq A_k. \end{cases}$$

In longitudinal studies, one will typically also collect time-dependent covariates over time. Let $W(t)$, $t \in \mathbb{R}_{\geq 0}$, be a covariate process that is assumed to be subject to the same reporting delays as the vital status of T. The function V_1 provides us with a natural definition of the data observed on a subject up to time t. Consider the process

$$X(t) = (R(V_1(t)), V_1(t), W(V_1(t))). \tag{3.3}$$

Thus, observing the process X up to time t corresponds with observing the vital status process R, the ascertainment process V_1, and the covariate process W up to time $V_1(t)$. Let $\bar{X}(t) = \{X(s) : s \leq t\}$ represent the sample path of X up to time t. The data analyst observes this process $X(t)$ in the sense that at time t the computer contains the process X up to time t, assuming censoring occurs after t.

Let V be the time at which T is reported, so in the context above we have $V = A_k$. Note that at time V the computer contains the full data structure $X \equiv \bar{X}(V)$, which corresponds with observing T, $\bar{V}_1(T)$, and $\bar{W}(T)$. We assume that the reporting delay is finite; that is, if a subject dies, then it will eventually always be reported, which is a reasonable assumption for these central registries, although the reporting delay can be large. Let C represent the time at which the data analyst stops receiving information on the subject. For example, C might be the time at data analysis, but it could also be the time at which the subject switches treatment or leaves the study so that his/her true survival time can no longer be recovered. Living in the time scale of the data analyst, one observes the process X up to the minimum of C and V, and one knows whether this minimum is the censoring time or is the time V at which T is reported. If $C \geq V$, then the full data $\bar{X}(V)$ are observed, and if $C < V$, then the right censored data $\bar{X}(C)$ is observed. Thus, the observed data structure can be represented as

$$Y = (\tilde{T} \equiv C \wedge V(T), \Delta \equiv I(V(T) \leq C), \bar{X}(\tilde{T})), \quad (3.4)$$

which corresponds with the data structure studied in this chapter. We observe n independent and identically distributed observations $Y_1, \ldots, Y_n$ of Y. Note that CAR allows the probability of being censored at time c, given one is not censored yet, to depend on the reporting delay history and the observed covariate history. As in the previous examples, possible parameters of interest are the marginal distribution of T and regression parameters in Cox proportional hazard models or linear regression models with outcome $\log(T)$.

One should note that reporting delay causes bias in the naive Kaplan–Meier estimator of the distribution of T. For simplicity, let us assume that the U_j's are reported immediately (i.e., $A_j = U_j$) but that T is reported at a possibly delayed time A_k. Let C be the time at analysis, which is assumed to be independent of T. If death is reported before the censoring time C (i.e., $A_k < C$), then the censoring variable is simply C. Suppose now that at time C death has yet to be reported (i.e., $A_k > C$) and C is between $U_{j-1} = A_{j-1}$ and $U_j = A_j$. Then we cannot be sure that T did not happen between U_{j-1} and C since all we know is that $T > U_{j-1}$. It is common practice to set $C = U_{j-1}$ and thus let T be right-censored at U_{j-1}. The censoring variable is now a function of A_k and thus of T, which implies that censoring is no longer independent of T. This can lead to serious bias in the Kaplan–Meier estimator, as nicely illustrated in a simulation in Hu and Tsiatis (1996) and an analysis of the California AIDS Registry in Hubbard, van der Laan, Enaroria, and Colford (2000) earlier analyzed in Colford et al. (1997).

We already illustrated the applications of this data structure in studies in which data on a subject are reported with delay to the data analyst. The reporting delay data structure also appears naturally in the following interval-censored data type of application. Consider a T defined by an event that can only be detected at a monitoring time; for example, T might be the time of onset of a tumor or the time at which the CD4 count of an AIDS patient drops below a particular value. At the monitoring time, one can find out whether T happened, and if it happened one might be able to determine the precise value of T (or use an extrapolated approximation) between the last and current monitoring times. In this case, we have no reporting delay for the U_j's (i.e., $A_j = U_j$), $j = 1, \ldots, k-1$, but T is reported at the monitoring time A_k following T. If the precise value of T between two subsequent monitoring times can only be guessed, then in these kinds of applications it is also common practice to apply the Kaplan–Meier estimator to the guessed T's and be satisfied with estimation of their distribution. In both situations, the Kaplan–Meier estimator can be expected to be biased due to the "reporting delay" of T, while the data structure above will acknowledge this reporting delay phenomenon.

In van der Laan and Hubbard (1998), locally efficient estimators of the survival function have been developed and implemented analogously to the methods presented in this chapter.

3.2.4 Univariately right-censored multivariate failure time data

Consider a longitudinal study in which various time variables $\vec{T} = (T_1, \ldots, T_k)$ on the subject are of interest. For example, consider a study in which HIV-infected subjects have been randomized to treatment groups. In such a study, one might be concerned with comparing the multivariate treatment-specific survival functions of time from the beginning of the study until AIDS diagnosis, death, and time until particular AIDS-related events (e.g., types of opportunistic infections). As a second example, one might be interested in the bivariate survival function of time until recurrence of cancer (measured from extraction of tumor) and time until death. In this setting, the researcher could also have interest in the estimation of functions of the joint distribution, such as the distribution of the gap time $T_2 - T_1$ from recurrence to death. We will not require that time variables $T_1, \ldots, T_k$ be ordered. Let $L(t)$ represent a time-dependent covariate process that one measures on the subject over time. This process includes the baseline covariates $L(0)$. The full data on a subject is defined as $X = (\vec{T}, \bar{L}(T))$, where $T \equiv \max(T_1, \ldots, T_k)$.

Let C be the common right-censoring time, which could be the minimum of time until end of study or time until dropout of the subject. Each subject is observed until $\tilde{T} = \min(T, C)$. Let $\tilde{T}_j \equiv \min(T_j, C)$, $j = 1, \ldots, k$. Thus, the researcher observes, for each subject, the following data structure:

$$Y = (\tilde{T}_1, \ldots, \tilde{T}_k, \Delta_1 = (T_1 < C), \ldots, \Delta_k = (T_k \leq C), \bar{L}(\tilde{T})). \quad (3.5)$$

182   3. Monotone Censored Data

If we define the process $X(\cdot) = (I(T_1 > \cdot), \ldots, I(T_k > \cdot), \bar{L}(\cdot))$, then we can also represent the full data structure as $X = \bar{X}(T)$ and the observed data structure Y as

$$Y = (\tilde{T} = C \wedge T, \Delta = I(\tilde{T} = T), \bar{X}(\tilde{T})).$$

We refer to the latter general data structure as "univariately right-censored multivariate data". Note that CAR allows the hazard of censoring at c to be a function of $\bar{X}(c)$ and thus of the observed part (up until time c) of $(T_1, T_2, \ldots)$ and of time-dependent covariates $\bar{L}(c)$.

Possible parameters of interest are the multivariate failure time distribution and the distribution of waiting times if $T_1 < \ldots < T_k$. Note that such parameters can be defined as $\mu = EB$, where $B = b(X)$ is a function of X. If, for given $\vec{t} \in \mathbb{R}^k$, one takes $B = I(\vec{T} > \vec{t})$, then $\mu = S(\vec{t})$. Likewise, if, for given $t > 0$, $B = I(T_2 - T_1 > t)$, then $\mu = P(T_2 - T_1 > t)$. In addition, regression parameters in a generalized linear regression model of each survival time on baseline covariates and multiplicative intensity model involving the intensities of T_j w.r.t. a history including only a subset of the observed past are of great interest as well.

We will now review previous proposals for estimation of multivariate survival functions in the nonparametric full data model. All previous proposals based on CAR models have imposed the stronger assumption of independent censoring. Because the nonparametric maximum likelihood and self-consistency principles (Efron, 1967; Turnbull, 1976) do not lead to a consistent estimator for continuous survival data, most proposed estimators are explicit representations of the bivariate survival function in terms of distribution functions of the data (see Campbell and Földes, 1982; Tsai, Leurgans and Crowley, 1986; Dabrowska, 1988 and 1989; Burke, 1988; the so-called Volterra estimator of P.J. Bickel in Dabrowska, 1988; Prentice and Cai, 1992a and 1992b). These explicit estimators are generally inefficient, but because they are explicit, their influence curves can be explicitly calculated so asymptotic confidence intervals are easy to compute (see Gill, 1992; Gill, van der Laan and Wellner, 1995). In van der Laan (1996a), a modified NPMLE of the bivariate survival function, which requires a choice of a partition used to reduce the data, is proposed that is shown to be asymptotically efficient. The methods above allow but do not require that all failure times are censored by a common variable C. In contrast, Wang and Wells (1998) and Lin, Sun, and Ying (1999) assume that $T_1 < \ldots < T_k$ with probability 1 and, as in the present example, the failure times are all right-censored by the same censoring variable C. The Lin, Sun, and Ying (1999) estimator is an inverse of probability of censoring weighted (IPCW) estimator as proposed by Robins and Rotnitzky (1992) and defined for general CAR-censored data models in Gill, van der Laan, and Robins (1997). None of the explicit estimators are efficient. Further, none of the estimators incorporate data on prognostic covariates such as $L(t)$. As a consequence, all are inconsistent under informative right-censoring (i.e., when $\lambda_C(t \mid X)$ does actually depend on $\bar{X}(t)$). In van der Laan, Hubbard and Robins (2002), locally efficient estimators of the multivariate failure time distribution and waiting time distributions based on the general multivariate failure time data structure (3.5) are provided that are analogous to the methods presented in this chapter.

Finally, we remark that multiplicative intensity models for multivariate counting processes provide estimators of intensities for these data structures, but these methods are not appropriate (see Section 3.1) for estimating more marginal parameters. The literature on frailty models provides an extension of the multiplicative intensity model methodology for multivariate survival times by assuming that the time variables are independent given an unobserved time-independent frailty and the past (see e.g., Clayton and Cuzick, 1985; Hougaard, 1986; Oakes, 1989; Clayton, 1991; Klein, 1992; Costigan and Klein, 1993). In particular, this extension is implemented in S-plus as part of the Coxph function.

3.3 Inverse Probability Censoring Weighted (IPCW) Estimators

Let $\{D_h : h \in \mathcal{H}^F\}$ be a set of full data estimating functions $(\mu, \rho, X) \rightarrow D_h(X \mid \mu, \rho)$ for μ with nuisance parameter ρ indexed by $h \in \mathcal{H}^F$. Let $\mathcal{D} = \{D_h(\cdot \mid \mu, \rho) : h \in \mathcal{H}^F, \mu, \rho\}$ be the corresponding set of full data structure functions.

For $D(X) \in \mathcal{D}$, we define $\Delta(D) = I(D(X) \text{ is observed})$. There exists a real-valued random variable $V(D) \leq T$ so that $I(D(X) \text{ is observed}) = I(C \geq V(D))$. For $D \in \mathcal{D}$, define

$$IC_0(Y \mid G, D) = \frac{D(X)\Delta(D)}{P_G(\Delta(D) = 1 \mid X)} = \frac{D(X)\Delta(D)}{\bar{G}(V(D) \mid X)}, \quad (3.6)$$

where $\bar{G}(t \mid X) = P(C \geq t \mid X)$.

In model $\mathcal{M}(\mathcal{G})$, we can obtain an initial estimator of μ by solving

$$0 = \sum_{i=1}^{n} IC_0(Y_i \mid G_n, D_{h_n}(\cdot \mid \mu, \rho_n)),$$

where G_n is an estimator of G, and $h_n \in \mathcal{H}^F$ is a possibly data-dependent index specified by the user.

3.3.1 Identifiability condition

Let $\mathcal{D}(\rho_1, G)$ be defined (as in (2.13)) by

$$\begin{aligned}\mathcal{D}(\rho_1, G) &\equiv \{D \in \mathcal{D} : E_G(IC_0(Y \mid G, D) \mid X) = D(X) \ F_X\text{-a.e.}\} \\ &= \{D \in \mathcal{D} : \bar{G}(V(D) \mid X) > 0 \ F_X\text{-a.e.}\}. \quad (3.7)\end{aligned}$$

184   3. Monotone Censored Data

A fundamental condition in our asymptotics Theorem 2.4 for this estimator μ_n^0 of μ is that $D_h(X \mid \mu(F_X), \rho(F_X)) \in \mathcal{D}(\rho_1(F_X), G)$. This assumption can be a model assumption (e.g., one assumes that $P(Xobserved \mid X) > \delta > 0$, F_X-a.e., for some $\delta > 0$), but, if it is not a reasonable assumption for the particular application of interest, then it can be weakened by making this membership requirement an additional parameter of the full data estimating function in the manner described in Subsection 2.3.1 of Chapter 2, assuming that the set $\mathcal{D}(\rho_1, G)$ is not empty. Thus, one 1) identifies a subset $\mathcal{H}^F(\mu, \rho, \rho_1, G) \subset \mathcal{H}^F$ so that for all $h \in \mathcal{H}^F(\mu, \rho, \rho_1, G)$ $E_G(IC_0(Y \mid G, D_h(\cdot \mid \mu, \rho)) \mid X) = D_h(X \mid \mu, \rho)$ F_X-a.e. (for all possible μ, ρ, G) and 2) reparametrizes this restricted class of full data structure estimating functions $\{D_h : h \in \mathcal{H}^F(\mu, \rho, \rho_1, G)\}$ as $\{D_h^r : h \in \mathcal{H}^F\}$ by incorporating the extra nuisance parameter ρ_1, G (needed to map any $h \in \mathcal{H}^F$ into $\mathcal{H}^F(\mu, \rho, \rho_1, G)$) in the nuisance parameter of D_h^r. This reparametrization is specified in (2.14). Subsequently, we denote this reparametrized class of estimating functions with $\{D_h(\cdot \mid \mu, \rho) : h \in \mathcal{H}^F\}$ again, where ρ now includes the old ρ, ρ_1, and G. We showed this reparametrization in action in a right-censored data example covered in Examples 2.3, 2.4, and 2.5 in Chapter 2. We refer the reader to this worked-out example.

In the next subsection, we propose IPCW estimators of the regression parameters in a multiplicative intensity model and derive the confidence intervals by establishing a fundamental lemma establishing the projection on the tangent space of the censoring mechanism G under the Cox proportional hazards model $\mathcal{G}$. Subsequently, we complete this estimation problem by proposing locally efficient estimators according to our general methodology, as covered in the next section. We also show the extension of the estimators to the proportional rate models.

3.3.2 Estimation of a marginal multiplicative intensity model

Let $X(t) = (N(t), V_1(t), V_2(t))$ be a time-dependent process containing a counting process $N(t)$ and time-dependent covariates $V(t) = (V_1(t), V_2(t))$, where $V_1(t)$ represents covariates for which one wants to adjust in the multiplicative intensity model below. Let $Z(t) = (N(t), V_1(t))$. Suppose that for the full data of interest we have $\bar{X}(T)$ for some time variable (random or fixed) T. If T is random, then it is assumed that $R(t) = I(T \leq t)$ is a component of $Z(t)$. As the full data model, we consider a multiplicative intensity model

$$E(dN(t) \mid \bar{Z}(t-)) = Y(t)\lambda_0(t)\exp(\beta W(t)), \qquad (3.8)$$

where $Y(t)$ and $W(t)$ are functions of $\bar{Z}(t-)$, and $Y(t)$ is the indicator that $N(t)$ is at risk of jumping at time $t-$.

Suppose that for the observed data we have $Y = (C, \bar{X}(C))$ (recall that observed data $(\tilde{T} = \min(T, C), \Delta = I(T \leq C), \bar{X}(\tilde{T}))$ can always be rede-

3.3. Inverse Probability Censoring Weighted (IPCW) Estimators

fined as $(C, \bar{X}(C))$ by defining $C = \infty$ if $T < C$). Our parameter of interest is $\mu = \beta$.

This estimation problem covers a large class of important problems. For example, consider a trial in which subjects are randomized to a treatment arm Tr (e.g., Tr is a 1-0 variable), and suppose that the goal of this trial is to estimate the causal effect of treatment on the survival time T. In this case, let $N(t) = I(T \leq t)$ and $Z(t) = (N(t), Tr)$ so that

$$E(dN(t) \mid \bar{Z}(t-)) = I(T \geq t)\lambda(t \mid Tr)dt,$$

where $\lambda(t \mid Tr)dt = P(T \in dt \mid T \geq t, Tr)$ is the hazard of failure within treatment arm Tr. Assuming a multiplicative intensity model, in this case known as the Cox proportional hazards model (Andersen and Gill, 1982; Gill, 1984; Ritov and Wellner, 1988), corresponds with

$$\lambda(t \mid Tr) = \lambda_0(t) \exp(\beta Tr).$$

The (causal) parameter of interest is now the regression coefficient β in front of Tr. An ad hoc method for estimation of β would be to fit a Cox proportional hazards model for right-censored data on T ignoring the covariates beyond Tr. However, if C is not independent of T, given Tr, then this estimator will be inconsistent. For example, in this clinical trial, people might drop out of the treatment arm because of possible side effects or other severe complications measured by $X(t)$. In addition, this ad hoc method will be very inefficient, even when C is known to be independent of T, given Tr. In other words, there is a real need for a general methodology for estimation of a Cox proportional hazards model that does not adjust for all measured covariates of interest. Another example would be obtained by letting $N(t)$ be a counting process that repeatedly jumps. For example, $N(t)$ might jump each time a particular type of patient is admitted into the hospital. We refer to Pavlic, van der Laan, and Buttler (2001) for an application of the methods described in this subsection to estimate the intensity and rates of the lung exacerbations in cystic fibrosis patients.

Firstly, we need to know the orthogonal complement of the nuisance tangent space in the full data model in order to determine the class of full data estimating functions. Subsequently, we will map these into observed data estimating functions with our general mapping $IC_0(\cdot \mid G, D) - \Pi(IC_0(\cdot \mid G, D) \mid T_{CAR})$ for which we have a closed-form representation (Chapter 1, Theorem 1.1, and the next Section 3.4). Finally, we propose estimators of the nuisance parameters of this observed data estimating function for β.

In Lemma 2.2 in Chapter 2, we showed that all full data estimating functions are given by

$$\left\{ D_h(\cdot \mid \mu, \Lambda_0) = \int \{h(t, \bar{Z}(t-)) - g_\mu(h)\} dM_{\mu, \Lambda_0}(t) : h \right\}, \qquad (3.9)$$

where $dM(t) = dN(t) - E(dN(t) \mid \bar{Z}(t-))$ and

$$g(h)(t) = E(h(t, \bar{Z}(t-))Y(t)\exp(\beta W(t)))/E(Y(t)\exp(\beta W(t))).$$

186   3. Monotone Censored Data

In order to stress that dM depends on μ, Λ_0 and that $g(h)$ depends on μ, we will now and then denote these quantaties with dM_{μ,Λ_0} and g_μ, respectively. Here $\int g(h)(t)dM(t)$ equals the projection of $\int h(t,\bar{Z}(t-))dM(t)$ onto the tangent space $\{\int g(t)dM(t) : g\}$ of Λ_0. In other words, the full data estimating functions are of the form $\int h(t,\bar{Z}(t-))dM(t)$ for h chosen so that it is orthogonal to the tangent space of Λ_0. Thus, each h yields an estimating function for $\mu = \beta$ indexed by a nuisance parameter λ_0. The optimal estimating function in the full data model in which one observes n i.i.d. observations of X is obtained by selecting $h(t,\bar{Z}(t-)) = W(t)$, which corresponds with the full data efficient score $S^F_{eff}(X \mid F_X)$. Our general choice (3.6) $IC_0(Y \mid G, D_h)$ is given by

$$IC_{01}(Y \mid G, D_h(\cdot \mid \mu, \Lambda_0)) = D_h(X \mid \mu, \Lambda_0)\frac{\Delta}{\bar{G}(T \mid X)},$$

where $\Delta = I(C \geq T)$ and $\bar{G}(t \mid X) = P(C \geq t \mid X)$. Because D_h is an integral (sum) of unbiased estimating functions, an alternative choice of $IC_0(Y \mid G, D_h)$ is given by

$$IC_{02}(Y \mid G, D_h(\cdot \mid \mu, \Lambda_0)) = \int \{h(t,\bar{Z}(t-)) - g_\mu(h)(t)\}\frac{I(C \geq t)}{\bar{G}(t \mid X)}dM_{\mu,\Lambda_0}(t).$$

We have the following lemma (as in Robins, 1993a).

Lemma 3.1 *If $D(X)I(\bar{G}(T \mid X) > 0) = D(X)$ F_X-a.e., then*

$$E(IC_{01}(Y \mid G, D) \mid X) = D(X) \; F_X\text{-a.e.}$$

If $\int h(t,\bar{Z}(t-))I(\bar{G}(t \mid X) > 0)dM(t) = \int h(t,\bar{Z}(t-))dM(t)$ a.e., then

$$E(IC_{02}(Y \mid G, D) \mid X) = D(X) \; F_X\text{-a.e.}$$

Proof. We have

$$E\left(\frac{D(X)I(T \leq C)}{\bar{G}(T \mid X)} \mid X\right) = I(\bar{G}(T \mid X) > 0)D(X)$$

$$E(IC_{02}(Y \mid G, D) \mid X) = \int h(t,\bar{Z}(t-))I(\bar{G}(t \mid X) > 0)dM(t). \square$$

Let $IC_0(Y \mid G, D_h(\cdot \mid \mu, \Lambda_0))$ denote one of these two choices of estimating functions for μ with nuisance parameters Λ_0, G. Given estimators $G_n, \Lambda_{0,n}$ of G, Λ_0, each of these observed data estimating functions yields an estimating equation for $\mu = \beta$:

$$0 = \sum_{i=1}^{n} IC_0(Y_i \mid G_n, D_h(\cdot \mid \mu, \Lambda_{0,n})).$$

As discussed in Section 3.1, if we assume a multiplicative intensity model for $A(t) = I(C \leq t)$ w.r.t. $\mathcal{F}(t) = (\bar{A}(t), \bar{X}(\min(t,C)))$, then Coxph() can be used to obtain an estimate of G. We also need a reasonable estimator of Λ_0. Since our estimating function is orthogonal to the nuisance tangent

3.3. Inverse Probability Censoring Weighted (IPCW) Estimators

space in the observed data model $\mathcal{M}(G)$ with G known, which thus includes the tangent space generated by Λ_0, the influence curve of μ_n is not affected by the first-order behavior of $\Lambda_{0,n}$ (except that it needs to be consistent at an appropriate rate). Therefore, it suffices to construct an ad hoc estimator of Λ_0. Since $E(dN(t)) = EE(dN(t) \mid \bar{Z}(t-)) = \lambda_0(t)E(Y(t)\exp(\beta W(t)))$ it follows that

$$\Lambda_0(t) = \Lambda_0(t \mid \beta) \equiv \int_0^t \frac{E(dN(t))}{E(Y(t)\exp(\beta W(t)))}.$$

For general β, we denoted the right-hand side of the last equation with $\Lambda_0(t \mid \beta)$, while at the true β it equals $\Lambda_0(t)$. Now, note that

$$E(dN(t)) = E\left(dN(t)\frac{I(C > t)}{\bar{G}(t \mid X)}\right),$$

$$E(Y(t)\exp(\beta W(t))) = E\left(Y(t)\exp(\beta W(t))\frac{I(C > t)}{\bar{G}(t \mid X)}\right).$$

This suggests the following estimator of $\Lambda_0(t \mid \beta)$:

$$\Lambda_{0,n}(t \mid \beta) = \frac{1}{n}\sum_{i=1}^n \int \frac{dN_i(t)I(C_i > t)/\bar{G}_n(t \mid X_i)}{\frac{1}{n}\sum_{i=1}^n Y_i(t)\exp(\beta W_i(t))I(C_i > t)/\bar{G}_n(t \mid X_i)}.$$

Substitution of $\Lambda_{0,n}(t \mid \beta)$ for Λ_0 in our estimating function yields the following estimating equation for β:

$$0 = \sum_{i=1}^n IC_0(Y_i \mid G_n, D_h(\cdot \mid \beta, \Lambda_{0,n}(\cdot \mid \beta))). \tag{3.10}$$

We now reparametrize the full data estimating function so that it has a variation-independent nuisance parameter

$$D_h^r(X \mid \beta, \rho) = D_h(X \mid \beta, \Lambda_0(\beta)),$$

where ρ denotes the additional parameters beyond β identifying $\Lambda_0(\cdot \mid \beta)$. We denote this reparametrized class of full data structure estimating functions with $D_h(x \mid \beta, \rho)$ again.

We will now provide a sensible data-adaptive choice for the full data index h. If $\lambda_C(t \mid X) = \lambda_C(t \mid Z)$ so that censoring is explained by the covariates in our multiplicative intensity model, then a sensible estimating function is the one corresponding with the score of the partial likelihood for β and Λ_0 ignoring $V_2(t)$ which is given by (Andersen, Borgan, Gill, and Keiding, 1993)

$$\int \left\{W(t) - \frac{E(W(t)Y(t)I(C > t)\exp(\beta W(t)))}{E(Y(t)I(C > t)\exp(\beta W(t)))}\right\}I(C > t)dM(t). \tag{3.11}$$

Define

$$h^*(t, \bar{Z}(t-)) = \left\{ W(t) - \frac{E(W(t)Y(t)I(C > t)\frac{\bar{G}^*(t|Z)}{\bar{G}(t|Z)} \exp(\beta W(t)))}{E(Y(t)I(C > t)\frac{\bar{G}^*(t|Z)}{\bar{G}(t|Z)} \exp(\beta W(t)))} \right\} \bar{G}^*(t \mid Z),$$

where $\bar{G}^*(t \mid Z)$ is a conditional survivor function of C, given Z, corresponding with a hazard $\lambda_C(t \mid \bar{Z}(t-))$ approximating the true conditional survivor function $\bar{G}(t \mid X)$ but restricted to only depend on the covariates Z entering the full data multiplicative intensity model. Firstly, we note that $g(h^*) = 0$, which proves that $\int h^*(t, \bar{Z}(t-))dM(t)$ is an element of our class of full data estimating functions (3.9). Secondly, note that $IC_{02}(Y \mid G, D_{h^*}(\cdot \mid \mu, \rho))$ equals (3.11) if in truth $\bar{G}(t \mid X) = \bar{G}^*(t \mid Z)$ (i.e., our IPCW-estimating function reduces to the optimal estimating function under the assumption that $\lambda_C(t \mid X) = \lambda_C(t \mid Z)$). We propose to estimate h^* by substitution of estimators G_n^* of G^* and G_n of G, and by estimating the empirical expectations. One can base G_n^* on fitting a multiplicative intensity model for the censoring process $A(t)$ only using a past $(\bar{A}(t-), \bar{Z}(t-))$ while one can use the entire past for G_n. Let h_n^* be the resulting estimate of h^*. With this choice of h_n^*, the estimator β_n^0 is at least as efficient as the usual partial likelihood estimator if in truth $\lambda_C(t \mid X) = \lambda_C(t \mid Z)$ and remains consistent and asymptotically normal in model $\mathcal{M}(\mathcal{G})$. Therefore, this estimator is a true generalization of the usual partial likelihood estimator of β that ignores the observed covariates beyond $\bar{Z}(t)$. This estimator was analyzed by Robins (1993a) (for $N(t) = I(T \le t)$ being a failure time counting process), and used to analyze an AIDS trial in Robins and Finkelstein (2000). Pavlic, van der Laan, Buttler (2002) used this estimator in general multiplicative intensity models to analyze a recurrent event data set.

A nice fact is that β_n^0 can be implemented by using the weight option in the S-plus function Coxph() and assigning to each observation line (corresponding with a time-point t at which covariates change or events occur) of a subject the weight $w(t) \equiv I(C > t)\bar{G}_n^*(t \mid Z)/\bar{G}_n(t \mid X)$. The reason that the weighting still works for the baseline hazard is that at the true β

$$\lambda_0(t) = \lambda_0(t \mid \beta) = \frac{E(dN(t)w(t))}{E(Y(t)\exp(\beta W(t))w(t))}.$$

If $G_n = G$, then our general asymptotic Theorem 2.4 in Chapter 2 shows that, under regularity conditions, this estimator β_n^0 will be asymptotically linear with influence curve

$$c(\beta)^{-1}IC_0(Y \mid G, D_h(\cdot \mid \beta, \rho)), \qquad (3.12)$$

where $c(\beta) = -\frac{d}{d\beta}EIC_0(Y \mid G, D_h(\cdot \mid \beta, \rho))$ and h is the limit of h_n^*. If G is estimated according to a CAR model (such as the multiplicative intensity model for $A(t) = I(C \le t)$ w.r.t. $\mathcal{F}(t)$) whose unspecified parameters generate a tangent space $T_2(P_{F_X,G})$ in the observed data model, then Theorem

3.3. Inverse Probability Censoring Weighted (IPCW) Estimators

2.4 shows that β_n^0 will be asymptotically linear with influence curve equal to the projection of (3.12) onto the orthogonal complement of $T_2(P_{F_X,G})$. In particular, this means that one could use (3.12) as a "conservative" influence curve to construct conservative confidence intervals.

To find the correct influence curve of β_n^0, one has to calculate the projection operator onto $T_2(P_{F_X,G})$ that is provided in Lemma 3.2 in the next subsection for the Cox proportional hazards model for $\lambda_C(t \mid X)$. Application of Lemma 3.2 (i.e., (3.17)) teaches us that if $IC_0(Y \mid G, D_h) = D_h(X)\Delta/\bar{G}(T \mid X)$ and $\lambda_C(t \mid X)$ is modeled with the Cox proportional hazards model $\lambda_C(t \mid X) = \lambda_{0A}(t)\exp(\alpha W_A(t))$, then the influence curve $IC(Y)$ of β_n^0 is given by

$$IC(Y) = c(\beta)^{-1}\left\{IC_0(Y \mid G, D_h(\cdot \mid \beta, \rho)) - E(IC_0 S_\alpha^\top)E(S_\alpha^* S_\alpha^\top)^{-1}S_\alpha\right\}$$
$$c(\beta)^{-1}\left\{+\int \frac{E(D_h(X)I(T>t)\exp(\alpha W_A(t))}{E(Y_A(t)\exp(\alpha W_A(t))}dM_G(t)\right\},$$

where

$$dM_G(t) = dA(t) - E(dA(t) \mid \mathcal{F}(t)) = dA(t) - Y_A(t)\lambda_{0A}(t)\exp(\alpha W_A(t)),$$

and $S_\alpha = \int W_A(t)dM_G(t)$ is the partial likelihood score of α. Here $Y_A(t) = I(C \geq t, T \geq t)$ is the indicator of $A(t)$ being at risk of jumping at time t, given the observed past. The numerator can be estimated with inverse probability of censoring weighting by noticing that $E(D_h(X)I(T>t)\exp(\alpha W_A(t))) = E(D_h(X)I(T>t)\exp(\alpha W_A(t)I(C>T)/\bar{G}(T \mid X))$. Notice that it is straightforward to estimate $IC(Y)$. Let $\widehat{IC}(Y)$ be the estimated influence curve. We can now estimate the covariance matrix of the normal limiting distribution of $\sqrt{n}(\beta_n^0 - \beta)$ with

$$\hat{\Sigma} = \frac{1}{n}\sum_{i=1}^{n}\widehat{IC}(Y_i)\widehat{IC}(Y_i)^\top.$$

Similarly, we can apply Lemma 3.2 to compute the influence curve for the case where $IC_0(Y \mid G, D_h) = IC_{02}(Y \mid G, D_h)$ is given by $\int\{h(t,\bar{Z}(t-)) - g(h)(t)\}\frac{I(C>t)}{\bar{G}(t|X)}dM(t)$. In this case, the influence curve of β_n^0 is given by

$$IC(Y) = c(\beta)^{-1}\left\{IC_{02}(Y \mid G, D_h(\cdot \mid \beta, \rho)) - E(IC_{02}S_\alpha^\top)E(S_\alpha S_\alpha^\top)^{-1}S_\alpha\right\}$$
$$+c(\beta)^{-1}\int \frac{E\left\{\int_t^\infty h'(u)dM(u)\frac{I(T\geq t)\exp(\alpha W_A(t))\Delta}{\bar{G}(T|X)}\right\}}{E\{Y_A(t)\exp(\alpha W_A(t))\}}dM_G(t),$$

where $h'(u) \equiv h(u) - g(h)(u)$. This finishes the methodology for β_n^0 since we defined the estimator, and provided its influence curve and corresponding confidence interval.

The optimal mapping from full data estimating functions to observed data estimating functions is obtained by subtracting the projection of $IC_0(Y)$ onto T_{CAR} as given in the next section and Theorem 1.1 in Chapter

1,

$$IC(Y \mid Q, G, D_h(\cdot \mid \beta, \Lambda_0)) = IC_0(Y \mid G, D_h(\cdot \mid \beta, \Lambda_0)) - \int Q(u, \mathcal{F}(u)) dM_G(u),$$

where

$$Q = E(IC_0(Y) \mid C = u, \bar{X}(u)) - E(IC_0(Y) \mid C > u, \bar{X}(u)).$$

Note that $Q(u, \mathcal{F}(u))$ is the difference between the regression $E(IC_0(Y) \mid \bar{A}(u), \bar{X}(\min(C, u)))$ evaluated at $\bar{A}(u) = I(C = u)$ and $\bar{A}(u) = 0$, where we recall $A(u) = I(C \leq u)$. The latter suggests a simple estimation procedure for $Q(u, \mathcal{F}(u))$. If $IC_0 = IC_{01}$, then

$$Q(u, \mathcal{F}(u)) = -E(IC_{01}(Y \mid G, D_h) \mid C > u, \bar{X}(u)).$$

If $IC_0 = IC_{02}$, then it is straightforward to show that

$$Q(u, \mathcal{F}(u)) = E\left(\int_u^\infty \{h(t, \bar{Z}(t)) - g(h)(t)\} \frac{I(C > t)}{\bar{G}(t \mid X)} dM(t) \mid \bar{X}(u), C > u\right).$$

Given an initial consistent estimator β_n^0 and estimates G_n, $\Lambda_{0n}(\cdot \mid \beta_n^0)$, Q_n (the latter is discussed in Section 3.5), one can now define the one-step estimator

$$\beta_n^1 = \beta_n^0 + \frac{1}{n} \sum_{i=1}^n IC(Y_i \mid Q_n, G_n, D_{h_n^*}(\cdot \mid \beta_n^0, \rho_n)).$$

Even when $G(\cdot \mid X) = G(\cdot \mid Z)$, this estimator will generally improve on β_n^0. If we implement the c_{nu} extension (Chapter 2, Section 2.3), then we can guarantee that this estimator improves on β_n^0. Finally, if h_n converges to h_{opt} (see Section 2.6 or Chapter 2), then it is efficient, but for computational ease we would usually recommend our simple choice h_n^*. Robins (1993a), however, shows h_{opt} is the solution to a Fredholm type 2 integral equation and describes how to construct a locally efficient estimator of β by numerically solving that integral equation to obtain an estimate h_n of h_{opt}.

Remark.

Robins and Rotnitzky (1992) show that if we replace CAR by the weaker, also non-identifiable, assumption that the cause specific hazard of C at t given $\bar{X}(t-)$ and $\{N(u); u \geq t\}$ does not depend on $\{N(u); u \geq t\}$ for each t, then the model for the observed data Y is identical to the model $M(CAR)$. Thus both the theory and methodology developed under the assumption of CAR actually hold under this weaker assumption.

3.3.3 Extension to proportional rate models.

As the full data model, we now consider a proportional rate model

$$E(dN(t) \mid \bar{Z}^*(t-)) = Y(t)\lambda_0(t)\exp(\beta W(t)), \qquad (3.13)$$

where $\bar{Z}^*(t-)$ is a covariate process not including the past $\bar{N}(t)$ of the counting process itself and $Y(t), W(t)$ are functions of $\bar{Z}^*(t-)$. Proportional rate models avoid the need to model the effect of $\bar{N}(t-)$ on $dN(t)$. These models have been considered by Pepe and Cai (1993), Lawless (1995), Lawless and Nadeau (1995), Lawless, Nadeau, and Cook (1997), and Lin, Wei, Yang and Ying (2000), .

These authors propose to use the analog of the Andersen–Gill partial likelihood estimating functions to obtain parameter estimates for the proportional rate model. The estimates obtained are only consistent and asymptotically normally distributed under the assumption that censoring only depends on the covariates entering the proportional rate model; that is, $\lambda_C(t \mid \bar{X}(t)) = \lambda_C(t \mid \bar{Z}^*(t))$. This assumption becomes more questionable as the conditioning set $\bar{Z}^*(t)$ decreases, which is what the use of proportional rate models encourages. In particular, in recurrent event applications the past of the counting process is often a predictor of censoring; for example, the number of asthma attacks or hospital admissions might predict the censoring time (e.g., dropout time by change of treatment) of a subject. In addition, these estimates are inefficient, in general, even if the full data structure is observed. The reason for this is that partial likelihood is not the correct likelihood in the proportional rate model.

Our methods described in the previous subsection are readily applicable to the proportional rate model as well. As the class of full data estimating functions, one can use $D_h = \int h(t, \bar{Z}^*(t-))dM_r(t)$, where $dM_r(t) \equiv dN(t) - E(dN(t) \mid \bar{Z}^*(t-))$ and h is arbitrary. As in the full data intensity models, the orthogonal complement of the nuisance tangent space in the full data model is a subset of these estimating functions. We will not aim to specify this precise subset but instead just accept using full data estimating functions that are not necessarily orthogonal to Λ_0. We can map these full data estimating functions into a class of observed data estimating functions with the same mappings $IC(Y \mid Q, G, D_h)$, presented above. In particular, our proposed choices for the index h of the full data estimating function can still be applied. This yields simple-to-implement estimators that are at least as efficient as the "partial-likelihood"-based estimating functions used in Lin, Wei, Yang, and Ying (2000) and remain consistent if $\lambda_C(t \mid \bar{X}(t)) \neq \lambda_C(t \mid \bar{Z}^*(t))$. If we do not enforce D_h to be orthogonal to the nuisance tangent space of the baseline hazard in the full data model, then our confidence intervals based on the observed data estimating function itself are not necessarily conservative anymore. Therefore, obtaining a meaningful estimate of variance requires either calculating the projection onto the nuisance tangent space of the baseline hazard (in

192   3. Monotone Censored Data

the full data model) so that we can enforce $D_h \in T_{nuis}^{F,\perp}$ or just using the bootstrap. We recommend the latter.

3.3.4 Projecting on the tangent space of the Cox proportional hazards model of the censoring mechanism

Let $H(P_{F_X,G}) \subset T_{CAR}(P_{F_X,G})$ be a subspace of $T_{CAR}(P_{F_X,G})$ and $(Q_1, G) \to IC_{nu}(\cdot \mid Q_1, G)$ be a mapping from $Q_1 \times \mathcal{G}$ to pointwise-defined functions of Y so that $\{IC_{nu}(\cdot \mid Q_1, G) : Q_1 \in Q_1\} \subset H(P_{F_X,G})$ for all $G \in \mathcal{G}$. As in Chapter 2, we define a more efficient choice of IC_0 as

$$IC_0(Y \mid Q_1, G, D) = \frac{D(X)\Delta(D)}{\bar{G}(V(D) \mid X)} - IC_{nu}(\cdot \mid Q_1, G, D),$$

where the true parameter value of Q_1 is $Q_1(F_X, G)$ defined by

$$IC_{nu}(\cdot \mid Q_1(F_X, G), G, D) = \Pi_{F_X, G}\left(\frac{D(X)\Delta(D)}{\bar{G}(V(D) \mid X)} \mid H(P_{F_X,G})\right).$$

The following lemma establishes this projection IC_{nu} for the case where $H(P_{F_X,G})$ is the tangent space of G under the Cox proportional hazards model.

Lemma 3.2 *Consider the partial likelihood of the counting process $A(t) = I(C \leq t)$ w.r.t. observed history $\mathcal{F}(t) = (\bar{A}(t-), \bar{X}_A(\min(t-, C)))$ for a multiplicative intensity model $\alpha_A(t)dt \equiv E(dA(t) \mid \mathcal{F}(t)) = Y_A(t)\lambda_{0A}(t)\exp(\beta_A W(t))dt$,*

$$L(\beta_A, \Lambda_{0A}) = \prod_t \alpha_A(t)^{dA(t)}(1 - \alpha_A(t)dt)^{1-dA(t)},$$

where $\prod$ denotes the product integral (Gill and Johansen, 1990; Andersen, Borgan, Gill, and Keiding, 1993). Let $dM_G(t) \equiv dA(t) - \alpha_A(t)dt$. The score for the regression parameter β_A is given by

$$S_{\beta_A} = \int W(t)dM_G(t).$$

The tangent space $T_{\Lambda_{0A}}$ is given by

$$T_{\Lambda_{0A}} = \overline{\left\{\int g(t)dM_G(t) : g\right\}}.$$

Thus the tangent space $T_{\Lambda_{0A},\beta_A}(P_{F_X,G})$ generated by the censoring mechanism parameters (Λ_{0A}, β_A) is given by

$$T_{\Lambda_{0A},\beta_A}(P_{F_X,G}) = \langle \int W(t)dM_G(t)\rangle + \overline{\left\{\int g(t)dM_G(t) : g\right\}}.$$

We have

$$\Pi\left(\int H(t, \mathcal{F}(t))dM_G(t) \mid T_{\Lambda_{0A}}\right) = \int g(H)(t)dM_G(t) \qquad (3.14)$$

3.3. Inverse Probability Censoring Weighted (IPCW) Estimators

$$\equiv \int \frac{E\{H(t, \mathcal{F}(t))Y_A(t)\exp(\beta_A W(t))\}}{E\{Y_A(t)\exp(\beta_A W(t))\}} dM_G(t).$$

Thus, the efficient score of β_A is given by

$$\begin{aligned} S^*_{\beta_A} &= S_{\beta_A} - \Pi(S_{\beta_A} \mid T_{\Lambda_{0A}}) \\ &= \int \left\{ W(t) - \frac{E\{W(t)Y_A(t)\exp(\beta_A W(t))\}}{E\{Y_A(t)\exp(\beta_A W(t))\}} \right\} dM_G(t) \end{aligned}$$

and

$$T_{\Lambda_{0A},\beta_A}(P_{F_X,G}) = \langle S^*_{\beta_A} \rangle \oplus \overline{\left\{ \int g(t) dM_G(t) : g \right\}}. \quad (3.15)$$

Consider now the special case where $A(t)$ is discrete on a fine grid $t_1 < \ldots < t_k$ so that the assumed multiplicative intensity model $\alpha_A(t_j) = E(dA(t_j) \mid \mathcal{F}(t_j)) = Y_A(t_j)\lambda_{0A}(t_j)\exp(\beta_A W(t_j))$, $j = 1,\ldots,k$, is appropriate: note that $\alpha_A(t_j)$ are now conditional probabilities. Given any function $V(Y) \in L^2(P_{F_X,G})$, we have $\Pi(V \mid T_{CAR}) = \int H_V(t, \mathcal{F}(t)) dM_G(t)$, where $H_V(t, \mathcal{F}(t)) = H_{V,1}(t, \bar{X}(t)) - H_{V,2}(t, \bar{X}(t))$ with $H_{V,1} = E(V(Y) \mid C = t, \bar{X}(t))$ and $H_{V,2} = E(V(Y) \mid C > t, \bar{X}(t))$. Thus, given any function $V(Y)$, we have

$$\Pi(V \mid T_{\Lambda_{0A}}) = \int g(H_V)(t) dM_G(t).$$

Thus, given any function $V(Y)$, we have that $\Pi(V \mid T_{\Lambda_{0A},\beta_A})$ is given by

$$E(V S^{*\top}_{\beta_A}) E(S^*_{\beta_A} S^{*\top}_{\beta_A})^{-1} S^*_{\beta_A} + \int \{g(H_{V,1}) - g(H_{V,2})\}(t) dM_G(t). \quad (3.16)$$

Consider the case where $Y_A(t) = I(C \geq t, T > t)$. We have for any $V = V(X, C)$ (thus, in particular, for $V = V(Y)$)

$$g(H_{V,1})(t) = \frac{E\left\{V(X,t) I(T \geq t) \bar{G}(t \mid X) \exp(\beta_A W(t)) \frac{I(C \geq \min(t,T))}{\bar{G}(\min(t,T) \mid X)}\right\}}{E\{Y_A(t)\exp(\beta_A W(t))\}}$$

and

$$g(H_{V,2})(t) = \frac{E\{Q_{V,2}(\bar{X}(t)) I(C \geq \min(t,T))/\bar{G}(\min(t,T) \mid X)\}}{E\{Y_A(t)\exp(\beta_A W(t))\}},$$

where $Q_{V,2}(\bar{X}(t)) = E\{V(X,C) I(T \geq t) \bar{G}(t \mid X) \exp(\beta_A W(t)) \mid C > t, \bar{X}(t)\}$ and $\bar{G}(t \mid X) \equiv P(C \geq t \mid X)$. (Note that we can set $I(C \geq \min(t,T))/\bar{G}(\min(t,T) \mid X)$ equal to 1 as well in both formulas, but the inclusion of this term shows how one can estimate it from the observed data).

In particular, if $U_G(D_h)(Y) = D_h(X)\Delta/\bar{G}(T \mid X)$, then

$$\Pi(U_G(D_h) \mid T_{\Lambda_{0A},\beta_A}) = E(U_G(D_h) S^{*\top}_{\beta_A}) E(S^*_{\beta_A} S^{*\top}_{\beta_A})^{-1} S^*_{\beta_A}$$

$$-\int \frac{E\left\{D_h(X)I(T \geq t)\exp(\beta_A W(t))\frac{I(C \geq t)}{\bar{G}(t|X)}\right\}}{E\{Y_A(t)\exp(\beta_A W(t))\}} dM_G(t) \quad (3.17)$$

(Note that we can set $\Delta/\bar{G}(T \mid X)$ to 1 in this formula again).

As remarked earlier, since C can be discrete on an arbitrarily fine grid, the projection (3.16) for the *discrete* multiplicative intensity model also holds for the continuous multiplicative intensity model under appropriate measurability conditions. For a formal treatment of the continuous case, see van der Vaart (2001). In Chapter 6 we state an immediate generalization (Lemma 6.1) of this lemma to multiplicative intensity models for a general counting process $A(t)$.

Proof. The statements up to and including (3.15) were proved in Section 2.2 of Chapter 2. For the projection onto T_{CAR}, we refer to Theorem 1.1, which was only formally proved for the case where C is discrete. Thus, we only need to show the last projection result (3.17) and the general formulas $g(H_{V,1})(t)$ and $g(H_{V,2})(t)$. In this proof, we will now and then suppress the index A that we used for the parameters of the censoring intensity $E(dA(t) \mid \mathcal{F}(t))$. Firstly, consider the special case $V(C, X) = U_G(D_h)(Y) = D_h(X)I(C > T)/\bar{G}(T \mid X)$. Since $H_{V,1} = 0$, we have

$$H_V(t, \mathcal{F}(t)) = -E(D_h(X)\Delta/\bar{G}(T \mid X) \mid C > t, \bar{X}(t)).$$

Let us denote the expectation with $f(\bar{X}(t))$. Thus, the numerator of $-g(H_V)(t)$ is given by $E(E(D_h(X)\Delta/\bar{G}(T \mid X) \mid C > t, \bar{X}(t))Y_A(t)\exp(\alpha W(t)))$. We have $E(f(\bar{X}(t))Y_A(t)\exp(\alpha W(t))) = E(f(\bar{X}(t))I(T \geq t)\bar{G}(t \mid X)\exp(\alpha W(t)))$, where we use $Y_A(t) = I(C \geq t, T \geq t)$. We can move $I(T \geq t)\bar{G}(t \mid X)\exp(\alpha W(t))$ inside the conditional expectation of $f(\bar{X}(t))$. The resulting term can now be rewritten as follows:

$$E(E(D_h(X)\Delta \bar{G}(t \mid X)I(T \geq t)\exp(\alpha W(t))/\bar{G}(T \mid X) \mid C > t, \bar{X}(t)))$$

$$= E(E(D_h(X)I(T \geq t)\exp(\alpha W(t)) \mid C > t, \bar{X}(t)))$$

$$= E(E(D_h(X)I(T \geq t)\exp(\alpha W(t)) \mid \bar{X}(t)))$$

$$= E(D_h(X)I(T \geq t)\exp(\alpha W(t))).$$

At the first equality, we conditioned on X and $C > t$ and used that $E(\Delta \mid C > t, X) = \bar{G}(T \mid X)/\bar{G}(t \mid X)$, and at the second equality we use that, by CAR, for any function $V(X)$ $E(V(X) \mid C > t, \bar{X}(t)) = E(V(X) \mid \bar{X}(t))$. Finally, for the purpose of estimation of this last expectation we note that

$$E(D_h(X)I(T \geq t)\exp(\alpha W(t))) = E(D_h(X)\exp(\alpha W(t))\Delta/\bar{G}(T \mid X)),$$

which proves (3.17).

For a general choice of $V = V(X, C)$ we have $g(H_V) = g(H_{V,1}) - g(H_{V,2})$, where $H_{V,1} = E(V(X,C) \mid C = t, \bar{X}(t))$ and $H_{V,2} = E(V(X,C) \mid C > t, \bar{X}(t))$. The numerator $E(E(V(X,C) \mid C > t, \bar{X}(t))Y_A(t)\exp(\alpha W(t)))$ of $g(H_{V,2})$ is given by

$$E(E(V(X,C)I(T \geq t)\bar{G}(t \mid X)\exp(\alpha W(t)) \mid C > t, \bar{X}(t))),$$

Let $Q_{V,2}(\bar{X}(t)) = E(V(X,C)I(T \geq t)\bar{G}(t \mid X)\exp(\alpha W(t)) \mid C > t, \bar{X}(t))$. Then the last term is given by

$$E(Q_{V,2}(\bar{X}(t))I(C \geq \min(t,T))/\bar{G}(\min(t,T) \mid X)).$$

The numerator $E(E(V(X,C) \mid C = t, \bar{X}(t))Y_A(t)\exp(\alpha W(t)))$ of $g(H_{V,1})$ is given by

$$EQ_{V,2}(\bar{X}(t)) = E(E(V(X,t)\bar{G}(t \mid X)I(T \geq t)\exp(\alpha W(t)) \mid C = t, \bar{X}(t))).$$

By CAR, we have for any function $D(X)$ that $E(D(X) \mid C = t, \bar{X}(t)) = E(D(X) \mid \bar{X}(t))$. Thus, the numerator $E(V(X,t)\bar{G}(t \mid X)I(T \geq t)\exp(\alpha W(t)))$ of $g(H_{V,2})$ is actually given by

$$E(V(X,t)\bar{G}(t \mid X)I(T \geq t)\exp(\alpha W(t))I(C \geq \min(t,T))/\bar{G}(\min(t,T) \mid X)).$$

□

3.4 Optimal Mapping into Estimating Functions

The mapping from D_h into observed data estimating functions is a sum of two mappings IC_0 and IC_{CAR}, where IC_0 is an initial mapping satisfying $E_G(IC_0(Y \mid G, G) \mid X) = D(X)$ F_X-a.e. for D in a non empty subset $\mathcal{D}(\rho_1(F_X), G) \subset \mathcal{D}$ and IC_{CAR} is the projection of IC_0 onto the tangent space $T_{CAR}(P_{F_X,G})$. By Theorem 1.1, we have

$$T_{CAR}(P_{F_X,G}) = \overline{\left\{\int Q(u, \bar{X}(u))dM_G(u) : Q\right\}} \subset L_0^2(P_{F_X,G}),$$

where

$$dM_G(u) = I(\tilde{T} \in du, \Delta = 0) - I(\tilde{T} \geq u)\Lambda_C(du \mid X)$$

is the martingale of $A(\cdot) = I(C \leq \cdot)$ w.r.t. history $\mathcal{F}(t) = \sigma(\bar{A}(t-), \bar{X}(\min(C, t-)))$. Here $Q(u, \bar{X}(u))$ ranges over all functions for which $\int Q(u, \bar{X}(u))dM_G(u)$ has finite variance so that it is an element of $L_0^2(P_{F_X,G})$. By Theorem 1.1 (for the discrete case) and van der Vaart (2001) (for the continuous case), we also have for any $D \in \mathcal{D}$

$$IC_{CAR}(Y \mid Q(F_X,G), G, D) = \int Q(F_X, G)(u, \bar{X}(u))dM_G(u),$$

where

$$Q(F_X,G)(u,\bar{X}(u)) = E(IC_0(Y) \mid C=u,\bar{X}(u)) - E(IC_0(Y) \mid C>u,\bar{X}(u)). \tag{3.18}$$

If $IC_0(Y \mid G, D) = D(X)\Delta(D)/\bar{G}(V(D) \mid X)$, then

$$\begin{aligned} Q(F_X,G)(u,\bar{X}(u)) &\equiv -E_{F_X,G}\left(IC_0(Y \mid G, D) \mid \bar{X}(u), C>u\right) \quad (3.19) \\ &= -\frac{1}{\bar{G}(u \mid X)} E_{F_X}(D(X) \mid \bar{X}(u), T \geq u). \end{aligned}$$

Given a full data estimating function $D_h(\cdot \mid \mu, \rho)$ for μ, we now define the corresponding observed data estimating function $IC(Y \mid Q(F_X,G), G, D_h(\cdot \mid \mu, \rho))$ by

$$IC_0(Y \mid G, D_h(\cdot \mid \mu, \rho)) - IC_{CAR}(Y \mid Q(F_X,G), G, D_h(\cdot \mid \mu, \rho)).$$

Note that $(Q, G, D) \to IC(\cdot \mid Q, G, D)$ is a well-defined mapping from $\mathcal{Q} \times \mathcal{G} \times \mathcal{D}$ to pointwise well-defined functions of Y, where $\mathcal{Q} = \{(u, X) \to Q(u, \bar{X}(u))\}$ is the parameter space for Q.

Given a data dependent index $h_n \in \mathcal{H}^F$, an estimator ρ_n of ρ, an estimator G_n of the censoring distribution G, and an estimator Q_n of $Q(F_X, G)$, we estimate μ with the solution of the following estimating equation:

$$0 = \sum_{i=1}^n IC(Y_i \mid Q_n, G_n, D_{h_n}(\cdot \mid \mu, \rho_n)).$$

If an initial CAN estimator μ_n^0 is available, then it suffices to use the one-step estimator.

3.5 Estimation of Q

In this section, we provide various estimators Q_n of $Q(F_X, G)$. If the model for G is correct so that G_n converges to the true G, then the estimator μ_n remains CAN if Q_n is inconsistent. On the other hand, if G is misspecified so that $G_n \to G^1 \neq G$, then μ_n will still remain CAN if $Q_n \to Q(F_X, G^1)$. In the latter case, we call μ_n a doubly robust estimator. This double robustness of μ_n (under regularity conditions of Theorem 2.5) is a consequence of the identity $E_{F_X,G}IC(Y \mid Q(F_1, G_1), G_1, D) = 0$ if either $F_1 = F_X$ or $G_1 = G$, (see (2.30) and (2.31)) for any $D \in \mathcal{D}(\rho_1(F_X), G_1)$ with $E_{F_X}D(X) = 0$. Here, it is assumed that at misspecified G_1 we have that $G(\cdot \mid X)$ is dominated by $G_1(\cdot \mid X)$, F_X-a.e, or that $E(IC(Y \mid Q(F_X, G_1), G_1, D) \mid X) \in R(I_{F_X,G_1})$ (see Section 1.6, Theorems 1.6 and 1.7): the latter would hold, if $\bar{G}_1(\cdot \mid X) > \delta > 0$, F_X-a.e. In Subsection 3.5.1, we use inverse weighting (by G) to estimate Q in conjunction with standard regression. However, such estimators Q_n will not yield robustness of μ_n w.r.t. misspecification of the model for G. In the Subsection 3.5.2, we provide likelihood-based methods assuming full data models $\mathcal{M}^{F,w}$ for F_X resulting in a substitution estimator $Q(F_n, G_n)$ of Q so that μ_n is CAN if either $\mathcal{M}^{F,w}$ or $\mathcal{G}$ is correctly specified. This method is a special case of the general method provided in Section 1.6. Finally, in Subsection 3.5.3, we derive a representation of $Q = Q(\theta(F_X), G)$ (due to Robins, 2000, and Tchetgen, and Robins, 2002), where θ corresponds with a set of regressions. Estimation of these regressions θ according to user-supplied regression models does not correspond with a substitution estimator $Q(\theta(F_n), G_n)$, but still yields the desired double robustness for practical purposes.

3.5.1 Regression approach: Assuming that the censoring mechanism is correctly specified

Firstly, consider the case where $IC_0(D) = D(X)\Delta/\bar{G}(V \mid X)$. In that case, $Q(F_X, G)$ is given by (3.19). For notational convenience, define $\Delta_h = \Delta(D_h(\cdot \mid \mu, \rho))$, and let $V_h = V(D_h(\cdot \mid \mu, \rho))$. The regression formula (3.19) suggests estimating $Q(F_X, G)$ by regressing observations

$$O_{i,n} \equiv D_{h_n}(X_i \mid \mu_n^0, \rho_n) \Delta_{h_n, i} \frac{\bar{G}_n(u \mid X_i)}{\bar{G}_n(V_{h_n, i} \mid X_i)}$$

against covariates extracted from $\bar{X}_i(u)$, only using the subjects with $\tilde{T}_i \geq u$.

For example, at each censoring time u, one could use the S-plus function GLM to fit a generalized logistic regression with outcomes $O_{i,n}$ and covariates $W_i(u) \equiv (W_{i1}(u), \ldots, W_{im}(u))$ extracted from $\bar{X}_i(u)$:

$$E(O_n \mid W_1(u), \ldots, W_m(u)) = \frac{\exp(\beta(u)^\top W(u))}{1 + \exp(\beta(u)^\top W(u))}. \tag{3.20}$$

These regressions are only based on the $n(u)$ observations for which $\tilde{T}_i > u$. Let $\hat{\beta}(u)$ be the resulting estimate. It makes sense to average $\hat{\beta}_j(u)$ over neighborhoods of u to obtain a smooth estimate $u \to \tilde{\beta}_j(u)$, $j = 1, \ldots, m$. Since $\hat{\beta}(u)$ is an estimate based on only $n(u)$ observations, the averages should be weighted averages, where the estimate $\hat{\beta}_j(u)$ has weight $1/n(u)$. In this manner, the resulting estimate $\tilde{\beta}_j(u)$ for u far into the tail of the empirical distribution of $\tilde{T}$ will be based on extrapolation.

Let us now consider estimation based on the general representation (3.18) of $Q(F_X, G)$. We propose to assume a multivariate GLM $E(IC_0(Y) \mid (\bar{A}(t), \bar{X}(\min(t, C))) = g_t(W(t) \mid \beta)$, where the regression model needs to satisfy $g_t = 0$ for $t > \min(T, C)$. Estimation in these regression models has been considered in Example 1.1 and Lemma 2.1. In other words, we regress the observed $\widehat{IC}_0(Y_i)$ onto time t and covariates $W(t)$ extracted from $(\bar{A}(t), \bar{X}(\min(t, C)))$. Note that each subject contributes an observation to each time point before $\tilde{T}$. Such a regression can be fit by applying the S-plus function GLM() to the pooled sample. Subsequently, one evaluates this fit at a history $C = u, \bar{X}(u)$ and a history $C > u, \bar{X}(u)$ so that the difference of these two fits is an estimate of $Q(F_X, G)(u, \bar{X}(u))$.

3.5.2 Maximum likelihood estimation according to a multiplicative intensity model: Doubly robust

Since the parameter $Q(F_X, G)$ is a function of F_X and G one can also use a substitution estimator $Q_n = Q(F_n, G_n)$ for some estimate F_n of F_X and G_n of G. For example, consider the representation (3.19). An estimator of $E(D(X) \mid \bar{X}(u), T \geq u)$ in conjunction with G_n also yields an estimator of $Q(F_X, G)$. An estimator of F_X itself provides us, in particular, with an estimator of $E(D(X) \mid \bar{X}(u), T \geq u)$. By the representation (3.19) of $Q(F_X, G)$, we have that $Q(F_X, G)$ is a simple function of $E(IC_0(Y) \mid \bar{A}(t), \bar{X}(\min(C, t)))$, where $A(t) = I(C \leq t)$. As proposed in Section 1.6, we can view $Q(F_n, G_n)$ as a conditional expectation under P_{F_n, G_n} of an observed random variable $IC_0(Y)$, given an observed past, and estimate this conditional expectation with Monte-Carlo simulation. Given an estimator F_n of F_X, evaluation of $E_{F_n}(D(X) \mid \bar{X}(u), T > u)$ can be carried out with Monte-Carlo simulation as well. Namely, we just generate many observations $\bar{X}$ from $f_{F_n}(\bar{X} \mid \bar{X}(u), T > u) = f_{F_n}(\bar{X}(T))/f_{F_n}(\bar{X}(u))$, where we specified above the densities $f_F(\bar{X}(t))$. Subsequently, we simply take the empirical average of the corresponding observations of $D(X)$. This is analogous to the Monte-Carlo simulation method presented in Section 1.6. Therefore, an important route for estimation of $Q(F_X, G)$ is to estimate F_X with maximum likelihood estimation according to some guessed working model $\mathcal{M}^{F,w}$. Of course, if there are many times u and many histories $\bar{X}(u)$ at which such expectations must be evaluated, them computational burden can be prohibitive and the methods described in Section 3.5.4 will be required.

We have for the observed data $\bar{X}(\tilde{T})$, where the process X includes $N_0(t) = I(T \leq t)$. By CAR, the F_X part of the likelihood of $Y = (\tilde{T}, \Delta, \bar{X}(\tilde{T}))$ under $P_{F_X, G}$ is the density $f_X(\bar{X}(t))\big|_{t=\tilde{T}}$ of observing $\bar{X}(\tilde{T})$, viewing $\tilde{T}$ as a fixed non-random number. Thus, if $\Delta = 1$ with $T = t$, then it is the likelihood of $\bar{X}(t)$, where $X(t)$ includes the event $T = t$, and if $\Delta = 0$ with $C = c$, then it is the likelihood of $\bar{X}(c)$. Thus, we just need to develop a likelihood for observing $\bar{X}(t)$ for given t. We have

$$f_X(\bar{X}(t)) = \prod_{s \in (0,t]} f_X(X(s) \mid \bar{X}(s-)) = \prod_{s \in (0,t]} f_X(X(ds) \mid \bar{X}(s-)).$$

Therefore, a sensible strategy to build up a likelihood for F_X is to model the conditional density $f(X(s) \mid \bar{X}(s-))$ of $X(s)$ or $f(X(ds) \mid \bar{X}(s-))$, given the full data history $\bar{X}(s-)$, where $\bar{X}(s-)$ always includes the event $T \geq s$.

3.5. Estimation of Q

To be specific, let us consider the situation where $X(s) = (N_0(s), N_1(s), \ldots, N_K(s))$, where $N_j(s)$ are counting processes, $j = 1, \ldots, K$. As in Andersen, Borgan, Gill, and Keiding (1993), let us also assume that no two counting processes jump at the same time. In that case, we can model $f_X(X(ds) \mid \bar{X}(s-))$ with a multiplicative intensity model for the multivariate counting process $X(s)$ w.r.t. the history $\mathcal{F}(s) = \{\bar{X}(u) : u < s\}$ as done in Andersen, Borgan, Gill, and Keiding (1993). Let

$$\lambda_j(s \mid \bar{X}(s-))ds = E(N_j(ds) \mid \mathcal{F}(s-)), \quad j = 0, \ldots, K,$$

and consider the multiplicative intensity models

$$\lambda_j(s \mid \bar{X}(s-)) = I(\tilde{T} \geq s)\lambda_{0,j}(s) \exp(\alpha^\top W_j(s)),$$

where $W_j(s)$ is a vector function of $\bar{X}(s)$. The F_X part of the likelihood of Y can be represented in terms of these intensities as follows:

$$f_X(\bar{X}(\tilde{T})) = \prod_{s \in (0,\tilde{T}]} \prod_{j=0}^{K} (1 - \Lambda_j(ds \mid \bar{X}(s-)))^{1-dN_j(s)} \Lambda_j(ds \mid \bar{X}(s-))^{dN_j(s)},$$

where $\Lambda_j(t \mid \bar{X}(t-)) = \int_0^t \lambda_j(s \mid \bar{X}(s-))ds$ denotes the cumulative intensity. This can be written as

$$f_X(\bar{X}(\tilde{T})) = \exp\left(-\int_0^{\tilde{T}} \Lambda_.(ds \mid \bar{X}(s-))\right) \prod_{j=0}^{K} \prod_{\{s : dN_j(s)=1\}} (1 - \Lambda_j(ds \mid \bar{X}(s-))), \quad (3.21)$$

where $\Lambda_. = \sum_{j=0}^{K} \Lambda_j$ is the cumulative intensity of $N_. = \sum_{j=0}^{K} N_j$. As in Andersen, Borgan, Gill, and Keiding (1993), it can be explicitly maximized w.r.t. the baseline hazards $\lambda_{0,j}$, given α, resulting in a closed-form profile likelihood for α. Estimation and inference are implemented in the S-plus function Coxph. Since we parametrized the full data distribution $f_X(\bar{X}(s))$ in terms of the intensities λ_j, estimates of these intensities also yield an estimate of the full data distribution.

Suppose now that with each counting process N_j there is associated a marker process M_j that changes value at s if and only if $N_j(ds) = 1$, $j = 1, \ldots, k$, so that the full data process is given by $\bar{X}(s) = (\bar{N}_1(s), \bar{W}_1(s), \ldots, \bar{N}_k(s), \bar{M}_k(s))$. Then, the F_X part of the likelihood of Y is given by

$$f_X(\bar{X}(\tilde{T})) = \prod_{s \in (0,\tilde{T}]} \prod_{j=0}^{K} (1 - \Lambda_j(ds \mid \bar{X}(s-)))^{1-dN_j(s)} \times$$

$$\prod_{s \in (0,\tilde{T}]} \prod_{j=0}^{K} \{P(M_j(ds) \mid dN_j(s) = 1, \bar{X}(s-))\Lambda_j(ds \mid \bar{X}(s-))\}^{dN_j(s)},$$

which can be written as

$$\exp\left\{-\int_0^{\tilde{T}} \Lambda.(ds \mid \bar{X}(s-))\right\} \prod_{j=0}^{K} \prod_{\{s:dN_j(s)=1\}} (1 - \Lambda_j(ds \mid \bar{X}(s-)))$$

$$\prod_{j=0}^{K} \prod_{\{s:dN_j(s)=1\}} P(dM_j(s) \mid dN_j(s) = 1, \bar{X}(s-)).$$

Thus, if one models the conditional marker distribution separately from the counting process intensities, then one obtains the maximum likelihood estimator of the intensities by maximizing the product of (3.21) over the i.i.d. subjects, ignoring the conditional marker distribution, and the maximum likelihood estimator of the conditional marker distribution is obtained by maximizing the product over the i.i.d. subjects of

$$\prod_{j=0}^{K} \prod_{\{s:dN_j(s)=1\}} P(dM_j(s) \mid dN_j(s) = 1, \bar{X}(s-)).$$

3.5.3 Maximum likelihood estimation for discrete models: Doubly robust

Suppose that $\bar{X}(t) = (X(0), \ldots, X(t))$, $t \in \{0, 1, \ldots, T\}$, is a discrete process and $X(s) = (X_1(s), \ldots, X_m(s))$ is a k-dimensional vector with discrete components. Assume that either T is fixed or that T is a discrete random variable with outcome space $\{1, \ldots, m\}$ included in the X process (e.g., $X_1(s) = I(T \leq s)$). We have

$$f_X(X(s) \mid \bar{X}(s-1)) = \prod_{j=1}^{m} f(X_j(s) \mid (X_1, \ldots, X_{j-1})(s), \bar{X}(s-1)).$$

One could model $f(X_j(s) \mid (X_1, \ldots, X_{j-1})(s), \bar{X}(s-1))$ with a multinomial logistic regression model $f_{\theta_j}(X_j(s) \mid (X_1, \ldots, X_{j-1})(s), \bar{X}(s-1))$, $j = 1, \ldots, m$. This gives the following parametrization:

$$\begin{aligned}f_X(\bar{X}(t)) &= \prod_{s=0}^{t} \prod_{j=1}^{m} f_{\theta_j}(X_j(s) \mid (X_1, \ldots, X_{j-1})(s), \bar{X}(s-1)) \\ &= \prod_{j=1}^{m} \prod_{s=0}^{t} f_{\theta_j}(X_j(s) \mid (X_1, \ldots, X_{j-1})(s), \bar{X}(s-1)).\end{aligned}$$

If one models these m multinomial conditional distributions separately, then for each $j \in \{1, \ldots, m\}$ one obtains the maximum likelihood estimator of θ_j by maximizing the multinomial likelihood

$$L_j(\bar{X}(\tilde{T}) \mid \theta_j) = \prod_{s=0}^{\tilde{T}} f_{\theta_j}(X_j(s) \mid (X_1, \ldots, X_{j-1})(s), \bar{X}(s-1)).$$

3.5.4 Regression approach: Doubly robust

We have seen that $Q(F_X, G)$ is a simple function of $E(IC_0(Y) \mid \bar{A}(t), \bar{X}(\min(C, t)))$, where $A(t) = I(C \leq t)$. The next theorem (based on Robins, 2000, and Tchetgen, and Robins, 2002) provides a representation of $E(IC_0(Y) \mid \bar{A}(t), \bar{X}(\min(C, t)))$ in terms of time t-specific F_X parameters and G, where each t-specific F_X-parameter is simply a regression (expectation) of an observed random variable (that is neither a function of G or G_n), given the observed past. Estimation of each of these regressions according to user-supplied working regression models plus our usual estimator G_n of G yields an estimator Q_n of $Q(F_X, G)$. Since each time-t specific F_X-parameter is separately modeled, the resulting estimator Q_n of $Q(F_X, G)$ cannot necessarily be represented as $Q(F_n, G_n)$ for some full data structure distribution F_n; since the functional form of the user supplied time-t specific regression models might be incompatible with any joint distribution, this approach does not correspond with posing a proper working model for F_X. Nonetheless, the estimator Q_n does estimate the F_X and G components in the $Q(F_X, G)$ separately and therefore exploits the protection property (i.e., $E_{F_X, G} IC(Y \mid Q(F_X, G_1), G_1, D)) = 0$ for all $G_1 \in \mathcal{G}(CAR)$ with $G_1 \equiv G$ and D being a mean zero function in $\mathcal{D}(\rho_1(F_X), G_1))$. Thus from a practical perspective, if one does a good job in modeling the regressions defining the F_X parameters, then the estimator μ_n will be robust against misspecification of the model for G in the sense that the bias of the estimator of μ will be small even if the user-supplied regression models are incompatible. See Robins and Rotnitzky (2002) for a general discussion of such "generalized" doubly robust estimators.

Theorem 3.1 *Let $A(t) = I(C \leq t)$, $X(t) = (R(t), L(t))$, $R(t) = I(T \leq t)$, and let $X = (\bar{X}(T))$ be the full data structure. As observed data structure we have $Y = (C, \bar{X}(C)) \sim P_{F_X, G}$, where $G \in \mathcal{G}(CAR)$ (i.e., $E(dA(t) \mid \bar{A}(t-), X) = E(dA(t) \mid \bar{A}(t-), \bar{X}(\min(t, C))))$. Suppose that $\mathcal{F}(t) \equiv (\bar{A}(t), \bar{X}(\min(C, t)))$ only changes at time points $t_1 < \ldots < t_m$ labeled with $j = 1, \ldots, m$. Thus, in particular, we also assume that T is discrete. Let $D(X, t) = f(\bar{X}(t))$ for some function f. Suppose that $D(X, T)$ is only a function of the full data structure $X = \bar{X}(T)$ through $\bar{X}(V)$ for a random variable $V = V(D)$, which satisfies that $V \leq T$ with probability 1. In other words, $D(X, t)$ is constant for $t \geq V$. Let $IC_0(Y \mid G, D) = D(X, V)\Delta(D)/\bar{G}(V(D) \mid X)$ as defined in (3.6), where $\Delta(D) = I(C \geq V(D))$, and $\bar{G}(t \mid X) = P(C \geq t \mid X)$. For notational convenience, let $V = V(D)$ and $\Delta = \Delta(D)$. Let $R^*(u) \equiv I(V \leq u)$. We have (note $dR^*(u) = I(V = u)$)*

$$E(IC_0(Y) \mid \mathcal{F}(t)) = \frac{I(V \leq t)}{\bar{G}(V \mid X)} I(T \leq t) D(X, V)$$
$$+ \int_{\{u: u > t\}} E\left(\frac{I(C \geq \min(V, u))}{\bar{G}(\min(V, u) \mid X)} D(X, u) dR^*(u) \mid \mathcal{F}(t)\right).$$

202   3. Monotone Censored Data

Define

$$g(u,t) \equiv E\left(\frac{I(C \geq \min(V,u))}{\bar{G}(\min(V,u) \mid X)}D(X,u)dR^*(u) \mid \mathcal{F}(t)\right).$$

We have for $u > t$

$$g(u,t=j) = \frac{I(C \geq \min(V,j))}{\bar{G}(\min(V,j) \mid X)}\left(\phi_j \circ \ldots \circ \phi_{u-1}\left(D(X,u)dR^*(u)\right)\right),$$

where for any function $B(X)$

$$\phi_j(B) \equiv E(B \mid \bar{A}(j) = 0, \bar{X}(j)), \; j = 1,\ldots,m.$$

We note that

$$\phi_{u-1}(D(X,u)dR^*(u)) = E(D(X,u)d\Lambda_V(u) \mid \bar{A}(u-1) = 0, \bar{X}(u-1)),$$

where

$$d\Lambda_V(u) \equiv E(dR^*(u) \mid \bar{A}(u-1) = 0, \bar{X}(u-1), L^*(u)),$$

where $L^*(u)$ *is the remaining (beyond* $R^*(u)$*) data collected at time* u*, so that* $X(u) = (R^*(u), L^*(u))$.

Proof. Let $R^*(u) = I(V \leq u)$. We have

$$\begin{aligned}
IC_0(Y) &= D(X,V)\frac{I(C \geq V)}{\bar{G}(V \mid X)} \\
&= \sum_u D(X,u)\frac{I(C \geq \min(V,u))}{\bar{G}(\min(V,u) \mid X)}dR^*(u) \\
&= \sum_{u \leq t} D(X,u)\frac{I(C \geq \min(V,u))}{\bar{G}(\min(V,u) \mid X)}dR^*(u) \\
&\quad + \sum_{u > t} D(X,u)\frac{I(C \geq \min(V,u))}{\bar{G}(\min(V,u) \mid X)}dR^*(u).
\end{aligned}$$

Thus

$$E(IC_0(Y) \mid \mathcal{F}(t)) = I(V \leq t)\frac{I(C \geq V)}{\bar{G}(V \mid X)}D(X,V) + \sum_{u>t} g(u,t).$$

Application of Lemma 3.3 with $B = \frac{I(C \geq \min(V,u))}{\bar{G}(\min(V,u)\mid X)}D(X,u)dR^*(u)$ and $D_u(\bar{X}(u)) = D(X,u)dR^*(u)$ yields the iterative representation of $g(u,t = j)$. □

Lemma 3.3 *Consider the setting and definitions of Theorem 3.1. Let* $u \in \{1,\ldots,m\}$ *be given. If* $E(B \mid \mathcal{F}(u)) = \frac{I(C \geq \min(V,u))}{\bar{G}(\min(V,u)\mid X)}D_u(\bar{X}(u))$ *for some function* D_u *of* $\bar{X}(u)$*, then*

$$E(B \mid \mathcal{F}(u-1)) = \frac{I(C \geq \min(V,u-1))}{\bar{G}(\min(V,u-1) \mid X)}D_{u-1}(\bar{X}(u-1)),$$

where
$$D_{u-1}(\bar{X}(u-1)) = E(D_u(\bar{X}(u)) \mid \bar{A}(u-1) = 0, \bar{X}(u-1)).$$
Thus, iteration of this result shows that for any $j \in \{1, \ldots, u-1\}$
$$E(B \mid \mathcal{F}(j)) = \frac{I(C \geq \min(V, j))}{\bar{G}(\min(V, j) \mid X)} D_j(\bar{X}(j)),$$
where
$$D_j(\bar{X}(j)) = \phi_j \circ \ldots \circ \phi_{u-1}(D_u).$$

Proof. For notational convenience, define $X_A(u) = X(\min(u, C))$. Define $w(u) \equiv I(C \geq \min(V, u))/\bar{G}(\min(V, u) \mid X)$, and note that, by CAR, $\bar{G}(u \mid X)$ is only a function of $\bar{X}(u-1)$. We have

$$E(B \mid \mathcal{F}(u-1)) = E\left(E\left(B \mid \mathcal{F}(u)\right) \mid \mathcal{F}(u-1)\right)$$
$$= E\left(w(u) D_u(\bar{X}(u)) \mid \bar{A}(u-1), \bar{X}_A(u-1)\right)$$
$$= E\left(w(u) E\left(D_u(\bar{X}(u)) \mid \bar{A}(u), \bar{X}_A(u-1)\right) \mid \bar{A}(u-1), \bar{X}_A(u-1)\right)$$
$$= E\left(w(u) E\left(D_u(\bar{X}(u)) \mid \bar{A}(u-1), \bar{X}_A(u-1)\right) \mid \bar{A}(u-1), \bar{X}_A(u-1)\right)$$
$$= w(u-1) E\left(D_u(\bar{X}(u)) \mid \bar{A}(u-1) = 0, \bar{X}_A(u-1)\right).$$

The first equality uses the iterative conditional expectation property $E(X \mid Y) = E(E(X \mid Y, Z) \mid Y)$, the second equality holds by assumption, the third equality holds by CAR since $\bar{G}(t \mid X) = P(C \geq t \mid X)$ is only a function of $\bar{X}(t-1)$, the fourth equality uses $I(C \geq u) = 0$ if $\bar{A}(u-1) \neq 0$ and that by CAR $E\left(D_u(\bar{X}(u)) \mid \bar{A}(u-1) = 0, A(u), \bar{X}(u-1)\right) = E\left(D_u(\bar{X}(u)) \mid \bar{A}(u-1) = 0, \bar{X}(u-1)\right)$, and the last equality follows by noting that $\bar{G}$ and the conditional expectation of D_u are fixed, given $\bar{X}(u-1)$, and thus that it just remains to integrate out $A(u)$. This completes the proof. □

Let's first discuss estimation of the first term $\phi_{u-1}(D(X, u) d\Lambda_V(u))$ of the recursive representation defining $g(u, t = j)$. We note that
$$d\Lambda_V(u) = E(I(V \in du, C > u) \mid C > u, \bar{X}(u-1), L^*(u)).$$
Thus $d\Lambda_V(t) I(C > t) = E(dN(t) \mid \mathcal{F}_1(t))$ is an intensity of a counting process $N(\cdot) \equiv I(V \leq \cdot, \Delta = 1)$, $\Delta = I(V < C)$, w.r.t. an observed past $\mathcal{F}_1(t) \equiv (\bar{X}(\min(t-1, C)), \bar{A}(t), L^*(\min(t, C)))$. Given a model for this intensity, the unknown parameters can be estimated by maximizing the partial likelihood
$$\prod_{i=1}^{n} \prod_{t} (d\Lambda_{Vi}(t))^{dN_i(t)} (1 - d\Lambda_{Vi}(t))^{1 - dN_i(t)},$$

where $N_i(\cdot) = I(V_i \leq \cdot, \Delta_i = 1)$ and $d\Lambda_i(t) = E(dN_i(t) \mid \mathcal{F}_{1i}(t))$. An estimate of $d\Lambda_V(u)$ also yields an estimate of $E(I(V \geq u) \mid \mathcal{F}_1(u)) = 1 - d\Lambda_V(u)$. Given an estimate $d\hat{\Lambda}_V$, the term $E(D(X, u)d\hat{\Lambda}_V(u) \mid C \geq u, V \geq u, \bar{X}(u-1))$ can be estimated by regressing $D(X, u)d\hat{\Lambda}_V(u)$ on $\bar{X}(u-1)$ among subjects with $V \geq u, C \geq u$.

Given an estimate of the ϕ_l-term, the ϕ_{l-1} term is a regression of the ϕ_l-term on $(\bar{A}(j) = 0, \bar{X}(j))$, which can thus be estimated with standard multivariate regression methodology, $l = u - 1, \ldots, j$. For further details on the implementation of this estimation procedure, we refer to Tchetgen, and Robins (2002).

3.6 Estimation of the Optimal Index

Our estimating function $IC(Y \mid Q, G, D_h)$ requires a choice h of full data estimating function. Representation (2.58) of the optimal index h_{opt} involves the inverse of the nonparametric information operator $\mathbf{I}_{F_X,G} : L_0^2(F_X) \to L_0^2(F_X)$. The following lemma yields a closed-form expression for the inverse of the nonparametric information operator for the monotone censored data structure studied in this chapter that was proved in Robins and Rotnitzky (1992).

Lemma 3.4 *The inverse of the nonparametric information operator* $\mathbf{I}_{F_X,G} : L_0^2(F_X) \to L_0^2(F_X)$ *is given by:*

$$\mathbf{I}_{F_X,G}^{-1}(D) = \frac{D(X)}{\bar{G}(T \mid X)} - \int_0^T Q(F_X, G)(u, \bar{X}(u))\Lambda_C(du \mid X).$$

Proof. By Theorem 1.3, we have

$$A_{F_X}\mathbf{I}_{F_X,G}^{-1}(D) = \frac{D(X)\Delta}{\bar{G}(\tilde{T} \mid X)} + \int Q(F_X, G)(u, \bar{X}(u))dM_G(u)$$

$$= \Delta\frac{D(X)}{\bar{G}(T \mid X)} + Q(F_X, G)(\tilde{T}, \bar{X}(\tilde{T}))(1 - \Delta)$$

$$- \int_0^{\tilde{T}} Q(F_X, G)(u, \bar{X}(u))\Lambda_C(du \mid X).$$

We also know that

$$A_{F_X}(h)(\tilde{T}, \Delta, \bar{X}(\tilde{T})) = \Delta h(X) + (1 - \Delta)A_{F_X}(h)(\tilde{T}, 0, \bar{L}(\tilde{T})).$$

Thus

$$\mathbf{I}_{F_X,G}^{-1}(D) = A_{F_X}\mathbf{I}_{F_X,G}^{-1}(D)\Delta$$

$$= \frac{D(X)}{\bar{G}(T \mid X)} - \int_0^T Q_{X,C}(D)(u, \bar{X}(u))\Lambda_C(du \mid X). \square$$

This result gives us a firm grip on handling the representation (2.58) of the optimal full data estimating function. In order to illustrate this, we consider in the next subsection the multivariate generalized linear regression full data model.

3.6.1 The multivariate generalized regression model

Consider the generalized linear regression model $Z = g(X^* \mid \beta) + \epsilon$, where $(Z, X^*) \subset \bar{X}(T)$ and $E(K(\epsilon) \mid X^*) = 0$ for a known monotone function K. Here Z, g, and ϵ are allowed to be multivariate, and we denote their dimension by p. This allows, in particular, that Z and X^* are time-dependent and subject to right-censoring. For example, $Z(t) = \beta_0 + \beta_1 t + \beta_2 X^*(t) + \epsilon_t$ with $t = 1, \ldots, p$, as in the repeated measures Example (over time) 1.2 in Chapter 1. Let $\beta \in \mathbb{R}^q$.

By Lemma 2.1 we have $T_{nuis}^{F,\perp} = \{D_h(X \mid \beta) = h(X^*)K(\epsilon(\beta)) : h\}$, and the projection operator onto this space is given by $\Pi_{F_X}(D \mid T_{nuis}^{F,\perp}) = h_{F_X}(D)(X^*)K(\epsilon)$, where the explicit index mapping $h_{F_X} : L_0^2(F_X)^q \to \mathcal{H}^F(F_X)$ is given by

$$h_{F_X}(D) = E(\{D(X) - E(D \mid X^*)\}K(\epsilon)^\top \mid X^*) E(K(\epsilon)K(\epsilon)^\top \mid X^*)^{-1}.$$

Note that the index mapping h_{F_X} maps an r-dimensional function D into an $r \times p$ matrix function of X^*. In addition, Lemma 2.1 tells us that the index of the efficient score in the full data model is given by

$$h_{eff}(X^*) = \frac{d}{d\beta} g(X^* \mid \beta)_{q \times p}^\top \mathrm{diag} E(K'(\epsilon) \mid X^*)_{p \times p} E(K(\epsilon)K(\epsilon)^\top \mid X^*)^{-1}.$$

We propose as observed data estimating function for β $IC(Y \mid Q_n, G_n, D_{h_n}(\cdot \mid \beta))$, where h_n is a locally consistent estimator of h_{opt}. Under the regularity conditions of Theorem 2.4, the resulting estimate will be efficient if Q_n, G_n are consistent and $h_n \to h_{opt}$, and it remains CAN if G_n is consistent.

By Theorem 2.7, we have that h_{opt} is the solution in $q \times p$ matrix functions h of

$$B'(h) \equiv h_{F_X} \mathbf{I}_{F_X,G}^{-1} D_h = h_{eff}.$$

Lemma 3.4 above now gives us a closed-form representation of the mapping $B' : \mathcal{H}^F(F_X) \to \mathcal{H}^F(F_X)$. This shows that h_{opt} is the solution in h of

$$h_{eff} = h_{F_X}\left(\frac{h(X^*)K(\epsilon)}{\bar{G}(T \mid X)}\right) - h_{F_X}\left(\int_0^T Q(F_X, G, D_h)(u, \bar{X}(u))\Lambda_C(du \mid X)\right). \tag{3.22}$$

Thus, the optimal index $h_{opt}(X^*)$ is a solution of an integral equation for the $q \times p$ matrix function h given by

$$h(X^*)_{q \times p} c(X^*)_{p \times p} - C(D_h)(X^*)_{q \times p} = h_{eff}(X^*)_{q \times p}, \tag{3.23}$$

where
$$c()_{p\times p} \equiv h_{F_X}\left(\frac{K(\epsilon)}{\bar{G}(T\mid X)}\right),$$
$$C(D_h)_{q\times p} \equiv h_{F_X}\left(\int_0^T Q(F_X, G, D_h)(u, \bar{X}(u))\Lambda_C(du\mid X)\right).$$

In the definition of $c()$, h_{F_X} is applied to a p-dimensional function so that $c()$ is here a $p\times p$ matrix function of X^*. Similarly, since D_h is a q-dimensional estimating function, $C(D_h)$ is a $q\times p$ matrix function of X^*. Substitution of the available estimates $Q_n(D)$, G_n, β_n^0, $h_{eff,n}$ results in estimators $C_n(h)$ and c_n of $C(h)$ and c, respectively. We propose to estimate h_{opt} with the solution h_n of
$$h(X^*)c_n(X^*) - C_n(D_h)(X^*) = h_{eff,n}(X^*). \tag{3.24}$$

As an example, consider the univariate regression case so that $p=1$ and $c_n(X^*)$ is a scalar. If X^* is k-variate, then (3.24) is an integral equation for k-variate real valued functions. By discretizing the functions, this equation can be reduced to a matrix inversion problem. In some cases, $C_n(h)$ happens to have a nice (e.g., upper-diagonal) structure so that the corresponding matrix is easy to invert.

3.6.2 The multivariate generalized regression model when covariates are always observed

We want to highlight the closed-form solution of (3.23) in the very important special case $X^* \subset X(0)$ so that X^* is always observed. In this case, $C(D_h) = h(X^*)C(K)$, where $C(K)$ is a $p\times p$ matrix function of X^*. This reduces (3.23) to
$$h(X^*)\{c(X^*) - C(K)(X^*)\} = h_{eff}(X^*).$$

Suppose that the $p\times p$ matrix $\{c(X^*) - C(K)(X^*)\}$ is invertible at almost every X^*. We are now in the fortunate situation of having a closed-form solution of the optimal index,
$$h_{opt}(X^*) = h_{eff}(X^*)\{c(X^*) - C(K)(X^*)\}^{-1},$$
where $c(X^*) - C(K)(X^*)$ actually equals the $p\times p$ matrix $h(\mathbf{I}^{-1}_{F_X,G}(K))$. We can estimate h_{opt} explicitly with
$$h_n(X^*) = h_{eff,n}(X^*)\{c_n(X^*) - h_n(C_n(K_n))(X^*)\}^{-1}. \tag{3.25}$$
Here K_n estimates $K(\epsilon(\beta))$ with $K(\epsilon(\beta_n^0))$.

We could also immediately apply Theorem 2.8 which says that $h_{opt}(X^*)$ is given by
$$h_{eff}(X^*)E(IC(Y\mid Q,G,K)IC(Y\mid Q,G,K)^\top\mid X^*)E(K(\epsilon)K(\epsilon)^\top\mid X^*)^{-1}. \tag{3.26}$$

This representation of h_{opt} suggests the following estimate h_n. To construct our estimation function, we already needed to estimate $IC(Y \mid Q, G, D)$ which thus also results in an estimate $IC(Y \mid Q_n, G_n, K_n)$. For every $(k, l) \in \{1, \ldots, p\}^2$, we can now construct the n observations

$$O_{kl,i} \equiv IC(Y_i \mid Q_n, G_n, K_{k,n}) IC(Y_i \mid Q_n, G_n, K_{l,n}).$$

Given a maximum likelihood estimator P_{F_n, G_n} of the data generating distribution, as in section 1.6, one can estimate the conditional expectations with Monte-Carlo simulation. Alternatively, one can assume a regression model for $E(O_{k,l} \mid X^*)$ and estimate it by regressing $O_{kl,i}$ onto X^*, $(k, l) \in \{1, \ldots, p\}^2$. The latter estimator h_n is easy to implement.

Note that the condition $X^* \subset X(0)$ includes the repeated measures regression model of time-dependent measurements (outcomes) on baseline covariates X^*. We conclude that if X^* is time-dependent (so that we only observe $\bar{X}^*(C)$), then one will need to solve the integral equation (3.24), and if X^* consists of baseline covariates only, then one can use the explicit estimator (3.25).

Estimation of the full data index mapping

Estimation of the optimal index involves, in particular, estimation of $h_{eff} = h_{F_X}(S^F_{eff})$. In this subsection we consider estimation of the index mapping $h_{F_X}(D)$ for a given function $D \in \mathcal{L}(\mathcal{X})$. We will illustrate such an estimator for the multivariate generalized linear regression model in which $h_{F_X}(D) = E(DK(\epsilon)^\top \mid X^*) E(K(\epsilon) K(\epsilon)^\top \mid X^*)^{-1}$. Again, there are two approaches. Firstly, if one has an estimator $F_{X,n}$ of F_X according to a working model $\mathcal{M}^{F,w}$, then it makes sense to estimate $h_{F_X}(D)$ with the substitution estimator $h_{F_{X,n}}(D)$. Secondly, one can model the conditional expectations in $h_{F_X}(D)$ as parametric or semiparametric regressions using the inverse weighting approach: for any function $D(X)$,

$$E(D(X) \mid X^*) = E\left(D(X) \frac{\Delta(D)}{\bar{G}(V(D) \mid X)} \mid X^* \right). \qquad (3.27)$$

Define $Y^* \equiv D(X) \Delta(D) / \bar{G}(V(D) \mid X)$, and assume a generalized linear regression model $E(Y^* \mid X^*) = g(X^* \mid \beta)$. In general, estimation of $E(D(X) \mid X^*)$ (and thus β) is now reduced to a regression of an always observed outcome Y^* onto covariates X^*. If X^* are observed baseline covariates, then one can estimate this regression directly. If X^* is time-dependent so that we only observe $\bar{X}^*(C)$, then estimation of β is an example of the problem studied in this chapter. Specifically, we can estimate β by the IPCW estimator that corresponds with using as the estimating function $IC_0(Y \mid G, D_h)$ (3.6), or we can use the optimal $IC(Y \mid Q, G, D_h)$, where D_h is a full data estimating function $D_h = h(X^*)(Y^* - g(X^* \mid \beta))$ for the model $E(Y^* \mid X^*) = g(X^* \mid \beta)$. The IPCW estimator β_n can be computed with the S-plus function GLM() for fitting $E(Y^* \mid X^*) = g(X^* \mid \beta)$ by weighting the i-th observation by $\Delta_i / \bar{G}_n(T_i \mid X_i)$, $i = 1, \ldots, n$.

3.7 Multivariate failure time regression model

In this section, we apply the estimating function methodology presented in the previous sections to construct a locally efficient estimator of regression parameters in a multivariate failure time regression model.

Recall the previously defined univariate right-censored multivariate failure time data structure. In other words, let $X(\cdot) = (I(T_1 > \cdot), \ldots, I(T_k > \cdot), \bar{L}(\cdot))$ include observing a multivariate failure time $\vec{T} = (T_1, \ldots, T_k)$, and let the observed data structure Y be given by

$$Y = (\tilde{T} = C \wedge T, \Delta = I(\tilde{T} = T), \bar{X}(\tilde{T})).$$

Here $T = \max_j T_j$. For notational convenience, we assume that the timescale has been log-transformed so that T_j denotes the log of the true survival time, $\bar{X}(t)$ denotes observing the process X up until the log of the time t, and C denotes the log of the censoring time.

For example, consider a longitudinal study in which subjects at entry are randomized to a treatment arm Tr. Suppose that we are interested in determining the treatment effect of Tr on the multivariate survival time $\vec{T}$, possibly adjusted for a particular baseline covariate V. In that case, one might want to assume a multivariate generalized regression model

$$\vec{T} = g(X^* \mid \beta) + \epsilon,$$

where $X^* = (Tr, V)$, $g(X^* \mid \beta)^\top = (g_1(X^* \mid \beta), \ldots, g_k(X^* \mid \beta))$, $\beta \in \mathbb{R}^q$ and $\epsilon^\top = (\epsilon_1, \ldots, \epsilon_k)$. It is assumed that $E(K(\epsilon) \mid X^*) = 0$ for some specified choice of monotone function K. The full data estimating functions are given by $\{D_h(X) = h(X^*)\epsilon(\beta) : h\}$, where h varies over $q \times k$ matrix functions of X^*.

The optimal mapping $D_h \to IC(Y \mid Q(F_X, G), G, D_h(\cdot \mid \beta))$ from full data estimating functions to observed data estimating functions is given by

$$IC(Y \mid D_h) = D_h(X \mid \beta) \frac{I(C > T)}{\bar{G}(T \mid X)} + \int Q(F_X, G)(u, \bar{X}(u)) dM_G(u),$$

where

$$Q(F_X, G)(u, \bar{X}(u)) \equiv E_{F_X, G}\left(D_h(X \mid \beta) \frac{I(C > T)}{\bar{G}(T \mid X)} \mid \bar{X}(u), T \geq u \right).$$

In order to use this as an estimating function for β, we need an estimate of its nuisance parameters $Q(F_X, G), G$ and need an estimate h_n of the optimal choice h_{opt}. Given estimators Q_n, G_n, h_n, we estimate β by solving the corresponding estimating equation

$$0 = \frac{1}{n} \sum_{i=1}^{n} IC(Y_i \mid Q_n, G_n, D_{h_n}(\cdot \mid \beta)).$$

As mentioned in Chapter 1, we could solve this estimating equation by minimizing its Euclidean norm as a function of β using the S-plus function nlminb(). We assume the Cox proportional hazards model for G and let G_n be the corresponding partial likelihood estimator. It remains to discuss estimation of Q and h_{opt}.

Estimation of Q

To start with we refer to the maximum likelihood method presented in section 1.6, which requires a full parametrization of the likelihood of the (ordered) observed data. Here, we will discuss some ad hoc simple to implement estimation methods based on the representation $Q(u, \bar{X}(u)) = E(D_h(X) \mid \bar{X}(u), T > u)/\bar{G}(u \mid X)$. If L is time-dependent, then one could estimate Q with the regression approach provided in Section 3.5.1. For the purpose of selecting a summary measure, $W_j(u), j = 1, \ldots, k$, it is useful to note that $(\bar{X}(u), \tilde{T} \geq u)$ is equivalent with $(\Delta_1(u), \ldots, \Delta_k(u), \Delta_1(u)T_1, \ldots, \Delta_k(u)T_k, \bar{L}(u))$, where $\Delta_j(u) \equiv I(T_j \leq u), j = 1, \ldots, k$.

We will now discuss a few model based methods for estimation of Q when L is time-independent. For notational convenience, let $k = 2$. If L is time-independent, then IC depends on F_X only through a multivariate conditional distribution of $\vec{T}$, given L. In particular, estimation of Q only requires an estimate of the bivariate conditional distribution of (T_1, T_2), given L. One could model this conditional survival function with the bivariate survival model based on the copula family (Genest and MacKay, 1986; Genest and Rivest, 1993; Joe, 1993). Frailty models (Clayton, 1978; Clayton and Cuzick, 1985; Hougaard, 1986, 1987; Clayton, 1991; Klein, 1992; Costigan and Klein, 1993) assume that the two components of $\vec{T}$ are conditionally independent given the covariates W and an unobserved frailty Z, where the frailty distribution has mean 1 and supposed to be known up until its variance σ. The bivariate distributions generated by frailty models are a subclass of the (Archimedean) copula family (Oakes, 1989). A particular copula family, corresponding with a gamma frailty, is given by

$$S(t_1, t_2 \mid W) = (S_1(t_1 \mid W)^{-\sigma} + S_2(t_2 \mid W)^{-\sigma} - 1)^{-1/\sigma}, \quad (3.28)$$

where S_1, S_2 denote the conditional marginal survival functions. This model is equivalent with assuming that the two components of $\vec{T}$ are conditionally independent given the covariates W and an unobserved frailty Z, where the frailty distribution is known to have mean 1 and variance σ (Oakes, 1989). Under this assumption, the conditional distribution of $\vec{T}$, given W, is parametrized by σ and the univariate conditional distributions of T_j, given the frailty Z and W, $j = 1, 2$. It is now common to assume also that each of the univariate hazards of T_j, given the frailty Z and covariates W, equal the frailty Z times a Cox proportional hazards model with covariates W:

$$\lambda_{T_j}(t \mid W, Z) = Z \lambda_{0,j}(t) \exp(\beta_j^\top W), \ j = 1, 2.$$

This model can be fit with the S-plus function COXPH() activating the gamma frailty option, where one uses a stratum variable indicating for each line in the data file which of the two failure-time components it represents.

For the burn victim data, van der Laan, Hubbard, and Robins (2002) fit a full (additive) model with all of the variables and allowed the coefficients of the Cox model to differ by the time variable (excision versus infection). Only two baseline covariates were found to be significantly related to either of the failure times: treatment and gender. The S-plus syntax for the final model was

$$coxph(\mathrm{Surv}(t, d) \sim \mathrm{strata}(\mathrm{time}) + L1 + L2 + \mathrm{frailty}(\mathrm{id})) \quad (3.29)$$

For smaller sample sizes, one could choose a parametric survival regression model and assume independence of the time variables, conditional on the covariates. For example, van der Laan, Hubbard, and Robins (2002) assume that the conditional log hazards of both T_1 and T_2 are a linear function of treatment and gender and fit two exponential models using the SurvReg procedure in S-plus:

$$\mathrm{survReg}(\mathrm{Surv}(t1, d1) \sim L1 + L2, \mathrm{dist} = \text{``exponential''}),$$
$$\mathrm{survReg}(\mathrm{Surv}(t2, d2) \sim L1 + L2, \mathrm{dist} = \text{``exponential''}).$$

Now, $Q(u)$ will be a reasonably simple function of u, $\bar{X}(u)$ and the coefficients returned by these regression procedures. Van der Laan, Hubbard, and Robins (2002) provide an example of S-plus code used to get both the IPCW estimator and the one-step locally efficient estimator using Cox regression for censoring and exponential survival regression for the conditional failure times.

Finally, when no covariate process $\bar{L}(\tilde{T})$ has been recorded for data analysis, the following method is available. By CAR, we have

$$P(T_1 > t_1 \mid T_2) = P(T_1 > t_1 \mid T_2, C > T_2) = P(T_1 > t_2 \mid \tilde{T}_2, \Delta_2 = 1),$$

so we can nonparametrically estimate this conditional distribution at $T_2 = u_2$ with the Kaplan–Meier estimator based on the observations with an observed T_2 close to u_2. Similarly, we can nonparametrically estimate $P(T_2 < t_2 \mid T_1)$. However, due to the curse of dimensionality, this method should not be used when the sample size is moderate and the dimension k of $\vec{T}$ is larger than 2 or so.

Estimation of the optimal index for the full data estimating function

Here, we refer to the method discussed in the previous section. Recall the representation (3.26) of h_{opt} with

$$h_{eff}(X^*) = \frac{d}{d\beta}g(X^* \mid \beta)_{q \times p}^\top E(K'(\epsilon) \mid X^*)_{p \times p} E(K(\epsilon)K(\epsilon)^\top \mid X^*)^{-1}.$$

We estimate h_{eff} by using $E(D(X) \mid X^*) = E(D(X)\Delta/\bar{G}(T \mid X) \mid X^*)$ and assuming a regression model. Similarly, we estimate $E(IC(Y \mid Q, G, K)IC(Y \mid Q, G, K)^\top \mid X^*)$ by regressing $IC(Y_i \mid Q_n, G_n, K_\beta)IC(Y_i \mid Q_n, G_n, K_\beta)^\top$ onto X^*.

In general, under regularity conditions of Theorem 2.4, the resulting estimate β_n will be consistent and asymptotically linear if the Cox proportional hazards model for G is correctly specified. In addition, if Q_n and h_n are consistent, then we will be fully efficient. If we estimate Q with a substitution estimator $Q_n = Q(F_n, G_n)$, where F_n is an estimate of F_X according to some working model $\mathcal{M}^{F,w}$ and we also estimate $h_{opt}(F_X, G)$ with the substitution estimator $h_{opt}(F_n, G_n)$, then, under the conditions of the asymptotics Theorem 2.5, the resulting estimator β_n will be consistent and asymptotically linear if either the Cox proportional hazards model for G or the working model $\mathcal{M}^{F,w}$ is correctly specified, and it will be fully efficient if both models are correctly specified.

3.8 Simulation and data analysis for the nonparametric full data model

Consider the multivariate right-censored data structure with baseline covariates and let the full data model be nonparametric. Suppose that the parameter of interest is $\mu = P(T_1 > t_1, T_2 > t_2)$ or its marginals. We describe here a summary of a simulation study and data analysis carried out in van der Laan, Hubbard, and Robins (2002).
Simulation study. A simulation study was performed to examine the relative performance of a smoothed NPMLE ignoring the baseline covariates, the IPCW (μ_n^0), and the locally efficient one-step estimators (μ_n^1). In all simulations, the failure times are bivariate, censoring is independent of the failure times, and the Cox regression model with all available covariates included as regressors was used to estimate the censoring distribution for both μ_n^0 and μ_n^1. We used two methods to estimate $Q(u)$ (used in the one-step estimator): 1) the known values derived analytically from the data-generating distributions (subsequently referred to as μ_n^1) and 2) linear regression of O_G against time-independent covariates, W, as described in Subsection 3.5.1 (subsequently referred to as $\mu_n^{1,REG}$). We wish to compare the performance of the one-step estimators under different models for $Q(u)$. Using the true function $Q(u)$ in μ_n^1 is essentially equivalent

to a low-dimensional correctly specified parametric model. Thus, in our simulations, μ_n^1 will be fully efficient. On the other hand, since under the distributions chosen for our simulations the true regression $Q(u)$ of O_G on the aforementioned covariates is nonlinear, μ_n^{1REG} will be somewhat inefficient owing to misspecification of the model for $Q(u)$. The ratio of the mean squared errors (MSE), based on the 1000 trials of each simulation, is used to compare the efficiency of the competing estimators. In addition, we report the percentage of iterations in which a conservative 95% confidence interval (based on (2.38)) includes the true value μ. All simulations have a sample size of 500.

Unordered T_1, T_2

Simulation 1. The parameter μ is $S_{T_2}(t_2) = P(T_2 > t_2)$. Both C and T_1 are $U(5, 10)$ random variables and $T_2 = T_1 + e$, where e is logistically distributed with mean 0 and standard deviation 0.4. (The logistic distribution was chosen because it allows one to determine Q analytically.) The only covariate available is $W = T_1$, which contains important information about T_2.

The results given in Table 3.1 show significant improvement of the IPCW and one-step estimators relative to the Kaplan–Meier estimator (in this case, the NPMLE with no covariates). As expected, the estimator μ_n^1 performs best. Misspecification of the model for $Q(u)$ results in an estimator μ_n^{1REG} that does not always improve upon the IPCW estimator but also does not have performance worse than μ_n^0. Finally, in all of the simulations, our confidence intervals for both μ_n^1 and μ_n^{1REG} perform well. Note that, as predicted by theory, t this is true even when the model for $Q(u)$ is misspecified.

Ordered T_1, T_2

Simulation 2. In these simulations, $T_1 \sim U(5,7)$, $C \sim U(5, 13.5)$, and $T_2 = T_1 + L(0) + e$, where $L(0) \sim U(0,5)$ and $e \sim U(0, 0.5)$. Both T_1 and $L(0)$ serve as the covariates $W = (T_1, L(0))$ for μ_n^0, μ_n^1, and μ_n^{1REG}. The parameter μ of interest is $P(T_2 - T_1 > t)$. In addition to μ_n^0 and μ_n^1, we also calculated both the NPMLE based on discretization of the data and ignoring the covariate W (see van der Laan, Hubbard, and Robins, 2002) and the IPCW estimator of Lin, Sun, and Ying (1999). In this setting, the NPMLE estimates the marginal distribution of T_1 with the Kaplan-Meier estimator, it groups the uncensored observations ($\tilde{T}_1, \Delta_1 = 1$) into p equal-sized groups with $\tilde{T}_1 \in (a_j, a_{j+1}]$, $j = 1, \ldots, p$, and it estimates the conditional distribution of T_2, given $T_1 = t$ with $t \in (a_j, a_{j+1}]$, with the Kaplan–Meier estimator based on the observations with an uncensored $\tilde{T}_1 \in (a_j, a_{j+1}]$. The smaller the number of groups, p, the greater the smoothing. In this simulation, we found the optimal number of groups to be 8, which was used in the simulations.

3.8. Simulation and data analysis for the nonparametric full data model

Table 3.1. Simulation 1. SE^1 is MSE ($\times 100$) Kaplan–Meier, SE^2 is MSE ($\times 100$) μ_n^0, SE^3 is MSE ($\times 100$) μ_n^1, SE^4 is MSE ($\times 100$) $\mu_n^{1,REG}$, $RSE^1 = MSE^1/MSE^2$, $RSE^2 = MSE^1/MSE^3$, $RSE^3 = MSE^1/MSE^4$ and CI^1 is the percentage of iterations in which the μ_n^1 (and similar results were obtained for $\mu_n^{1,REG}$) confidence intervals contain the true $S_2(t)$.

t	S_2	SE^1	SE^2	SE^3	SE^4	RSE^1	RSE^2	RSE^3	CI^1
5.7	0.86	2.5	2.5	2.5	2.5	1.0	1.0	1.0	95
6.0	0.81	3.3	3.2	3.2	3.2	1.0	1.0	1.0	95
6.2	0.76	4.3	4.0	3.9	4.0	1.1	1.1	1.1	94
6.4	0.71	4.8	4.4	4.3	4.4	1.1	1.1	1.1	95
6.7	0.67	5.7	5.0	4.9	5.0	1.1	1.2	1.1	94
6.9	0.62	6.6	5.5	5.3	5.6	1.2	1.2	1.2	94
7.1	0.57	6.9	5.7	5.4	5.7	1.2	1.3	1.2	95
7.4	0.52	7.4	6.1	5.7	6.0	1.2	1.3	1.2	96
7.6	0.48	8.1	6.4	6.0	6.3	1.3	1.3	1.3	95
7.9	0.43	8.9	6.7	6.2	6.6	1.3	1.4	1.3	94
8.1	0.38	9.3	6.9	6.1	6.6	1.3	1.5	1.4	95
8.3	0.33	9.1	6.7	5.8	6.4	1.4	1.6	1.4	95
8.6	0.29	9.6	7.0	6.0	6.6	1.4	1.6	1.4	95

Table 3.2. Simulation 2. SE^1 is the MSE ($\times 100$) Lin, Sun, and Ying's (1999) estimator, SE^2 is MSE ($\times 100$) the NPMLE, SE^3 is MSE ($\times 100$) μ_n^0, SE^4 is MSE ($\times 100$) μ_n^1, SE^5 is MSE ($\times 100$) $\mu_n^{1,REG}$, $RSE^1 = MSE^1/MSE^2$, $RSE^2 = MSE^1/MSE^3$, $RSE^3 = MSE^1/MSE^4$, and $RSE^4 = MSE^1/MSE^5$. These MSE's are reported at time points 0.7, 1.1, 1.5, 1.9, 2.3, 2.6, 3.0, 3.4, and 3.8.

S	SE^1	SE^2	SE^3	SE^4	SE^5	RSE^1	RSE^2	RSE^3	RSE^4
0.90	2.3	2.3	2.2	2.1	2.3	1.0	1.0	1.1	1.0
0.80	4.1	4.1	3.7	3.3	3.8	1.0	1.1	1.2	1.1
0.70	5.6	5.6	4.8	4.4	4.7	1.0	1.2	1.3	1.2
0.60	6.7	6.7	5.5	5.0	5.5	1.0	1.2	1.3	1.2
0.50	7.2	7.2	5.9	5.4	5.9	1.0	1.2	1.3	1.2
0.40	7.2	7.2	5.7	5.1	5.7	1.0	1.3	1.4	1.3
0.30	6.9	6.8	5.5	4.5	5.5	1.0	1.2	1.5	1.3
0.20	5.8	5.8	5.0	4.0	5.0	1.0	1.2	1.5	1.3
0.10	3.7	3.8	3.5	2.5	3.5	1.0	1.1	1.5	1.2

The results (Table 3.2) show an equivalent performance for both Lin, Sun, and Ying's estimator and the NPMLE. However, μ_n^0, μ_n^1, and $\mu_n^{1,REG}$ have substantially increased performance by utilizing the covariate information. We also computed in simulation 2 the percentage of iterations in which the μ_n^1 and the $\mu_n^{1,REG}$ confidence intervals contain the true $S(t) \equiv P(T_2 - T_1 > t)$, respectively. These percentages were almost identical for the two estimators, and for $\mu_n^{1,REG}$ they are given by 94, 96, 95, 94, 95, 95, 95, 94, 95.

Table 3.3. Simulation 3. SE^1 is MSE ($\times 100$) μ_n^0, SE^2 is MSE ($\times 100$) NPMLE, SE^3 is MSE ($\times 100$) μ_n^1, SE^4 is MSE ($\times 100$) μ_n^{1REG}, $RSE^1 = MSE^1/MSE^2$, $RSE^2 = MSE^1/MSE^3$, and $RSE^3 = MSE^1/MSE^4$.

t_1	t_2	S	SE^1	SE^2	SE^3	SE^4	RSE^1	RSE^2	RSE^3
6.6	5.5	0.70	4.7	4.6	4.3	4.7	1.0	1.1	1.0
7.8	5.5	0.52	6.1	6.3	5.3	6.1	1.0	1.1	1.0
7.1	6.0	0.45	5.4	5.5	5.1	5.5	1.0	1.1	1.0
8.2	6.0	0.31	5.5	5.6	4.8	5.4	1.0	1.1	1.0
8.9	5.5	0.30	5.6	6.2	4.8	5.4	0.9	1.2	1.0
7.6	6.5	0.21	4.0	3.8	3.4	4.0	1.0	1.2	1.0
9.4	6.0	0.17	4.4	4.5	3.2	4.0	1.0	1.4	1.1
8.8	6.5	0.14	3.4	3.1	2.5	3.2	1.1	1.3	1.0
9.9	6.5	0.07	2.5	2.2	1.4	2.2	1.2	1.8	1.1

Simulation 3. In this simulation, we estimated the joint distribution, $P(T_2 > t_2, T_1 > t_1)$, using the data-generating distributions and covariates as in simulation 2. In addition to μ_n^0 and μ_n^1, the NPMLE described in simulation 2 is computed.

The results (Table 3.3) suggest that the NPMLE and μ_n^0 perform equivalently. As in the simulations above, the one-step estimator, μ_n^1, has high relative efficiency, whereas μ_n^{1REG} gains little over the IPCW estimator. Van der Laan, Hubbard, and Robins (2002) show the true $Q(u)$ (for a fixed u and T_1) and the best linear fit versus W that makes clear that a simple linear model does not fit well. This is the reason that μ_n^{1REG} is not as efficient as μ_n^1. Thus, to maximize the efficiency of the one-step estimator, one should explore different possible models for $Q(u)$. However, even in the case where the model is poorly chosen, there appears to be little risk in trying to improve over the IPCW estimator. As shown in Chapter 2, the one-step estimator can be modified (c_{nu} adjustment) to be guaranteed more efficient than a given initial estimator.

Data analysis of burn victim data

We report here a data analysis carried out in van der Laan, Hubbard, and Robins (2002). Klein and Moeschberger (1997) and Ichida, Wassell, and Keller (1993) consider estimation of the joint distribution of time to wound excision and time to wound infection in a population of burn victims. We apply our methodology to this burn victim data on time to wound excision (T_1) and time to *Straphylocous areaus* wound infection (T_2) among 154 burn victims. Note that the times are not necessarily ordered.

In preliminary exponential and Cox regressions, only two of the ten available covariates were found to be significantly associated with T_1 or T_2: cleansing treatment (1=body cleansing, 0=routine bathing) and gender (0=male, 1=female). Henceforth, we shall ignore data on other baseline covariates. In Table 3.5, we provide results for five different estimators.

3.8. Simulation and data analysis for the nonparametric full data model   215

Table 3.4. Results of estimation of $P(T_1 > t_1, T_2 > t_2)$ using 1) IPCW estimators using both the Kaplan–Meier ($u^0_{n,KM}$) and Cox regression ($u^0_{n,COX}$) estimators of censoring, and 2) the one-step estimators using exponential regression ($u^1_{n,EXP}$). The standard errors are in parentheses (bootstrap/explicit).

t_1, t_2	$u^0_{n,KM}$	$u^0_{n,COX}$	$u^1_{n,EXP}$
8.3, 15	0.52 (0.05/0.07)	0.52 (0.05/0.07)	0.51 (0.05/0.05)
16.6, 15	0.22 (0.04/0.05)	0.22 (0.04/0.05)	0.22 (0.04/0.04)
25, 15	0.10 (0.04/0.06)	0.11 (0.04/0.06)	0.11 (0.04/0.04)
8.3, 30	0.35 (0.06/0.07)	0.36 (0.07/0.07)	0.36 (0.06/0.07)
16.6, 30	0.20 (0.05/0.07)	0.22 (0.06/0.08)	0.22 (0.05/0.06)
25, 30	0.07 (0.04/0.04)	0.08 (0.04/0.04)	0.08 (0.04/0.04)
8.3, 45	0.22 (0.08/0.08)	0.22 (0.09/0.09)	0.22 (0.09/0.10)
16.6, 45	0.13 (0.07/0.08)	0.14 (0.08/0.09)	0.14 (0.08/0.08)

The first two are the IPCW estimators $u^0_{n,KM}$ and $u^0_{n,COX}$, the next two are the one-step estimators $u^1_{n,EXP}$ and $u^1_{n,COX}$, and the final estimator is Dabrowska's estimator, $u_{n,DAB}$. For $u^0_{n,KM}$, the censoring distribution was estimated ignoring all covariates a priori, which could only be legitimate if censoring and failure were known to be independent. For $u^0_{n,COX}$ and the two one step estimators, the censoring distribution was estimated by partial likelihood assuming the Cox model with covariates gender and cleansing treatment. For $u^1_{n,COX}$ and $u^1_{n,EXP}$, $Q(u)$ was estimated conditionally on the time-independent covariates sex and cleansing treatment by the conditionally independent Cox and exponential regression models, respectively. We started out fitting the frailty model, but the estimate of the variance of the latent frailty was found to be nearly 0 (implying conditional independence of T_1 and T_2). Therefore, our final estimate of $Q(u)$ was based on fitting a simple Cox regression model for each of the two time variables separately. With the exception of Dabrowska's estimator, for which we only calculated the bootstrap estimator of the standard error, all estimators had standard errors calculated using the nonparametric bootstrap and using an explicit representation of their influence curves. For the IPCW estimators, these standard errors were calculated using the explicit representation provided in Lemma 3.2 of the influence curve based on a Cox regression model of the censoring distribution. For the locally efficient estimators, the conservative standard errors were calculated based on the estimating function itself.

The results are listed in Tables 3.4 and 3.5. First, the IPCW estimators are very similar, implying that utilizing the covariate information using the IPCW estimator, at least as done here, does not improve the efficiency of the estimator. Likewise, $u^1_{n,EXP}$ also has similar standard errors and so does not appear to benefit significantly from utilizing the covariate information. On the other hand, the one-step estimator, $u^1_{n,COX}$, appears to result in a significant improvement over the IPCW estimators and the one-

216   3. Monotone Censored Data

Table 3.5. Results of estimation of $P(T_1 > t_1, T_2 > t_2)$ for the one-step estimators using Cox regression $(u_{n,COX}^1)$ for estimating $Q(u)$, and Dabrowska's estimator, $(u_{n,DAB})$. The standard errors in parentheses (bootstrap/explicit) - Dabrowska's estimator has only bootstrap standard errors.

t_1, t_2	$u_{n,COX}^1$	$u_{n,DAB}$
8.3, 15	0.49(0.04/0.04)	0.46(0.04)
16.6, 15	0.28(0.04/0.04)	0.25(0.04)
25, 15	0.14(0.04/0.03)	0.10(0.04)
8.3, 30	0.42(0.04/0.04)	0.37(0.05)
16.6, 30	0.24(0.04/0.04)	0.23(0.04)
25, 30	0.12(0.04/0.03)	0.09(0.04)
8.3, 45	0.40(0.04/0.05)	0.37(0.14)
16.6, 45	0.24(0.04/0.04)	0.23(0.09)

step estimator using exponential regression. In addition, it appears to have significantly higher efficiency than $u_{n,DAB}$ at the larger quantiles of T_2.

For the burn data, exponential regression is a poor model for $Q(u)$, which suggests that $u_{n,COX}^1$ is a better estimator than $u_{n,EXP}^1$. For instance, the exponential model assumes a constant hazard in time, whereas the Cox regression models used to estimate $u_{n,COX}^1$ suggest that, for both T_1 and T_2, the baseline hazards increase significantly with time. There are many ways of evaluating the relative fit of competing models for $Q(u)$. However, one of the by-products of the one-step estimator is the estimated projection constant c_n as defined in Subsection 2.5.1 in Chapter 2, and this constant lends itself to selecting a good fit for $Q(u)$. Specifically, c_n close to 1 strongly suggests that the estimated influence curve is close to the efficient influence curve and thus that the estimated $Q(u)$ is close to the true $Q(u)$. Thus, the c_n can be used as a model selection measure, where a c_n relatively closer to 1 corresponds with a better estimate of $Q(u)$. In Table 3.6 below, we report the c_n's for all of the quantiles using both the exponential and Cox model estimates of $Q(u)$. As expected, the c_n's are almost always closer to 1 for the Cox model relative to the exponential model, providing more evidence that the Cox model is a better choice to estimate $Q(u)$.

Dependent censoring was not a factor for these burn data. However, dependent censoring can be a major problem in other substantive settings. For example, Robins and Finkelstein (2000) demonstrated the importance of dependent censoring attributable to strong time-dependent prognostic factors in their analysis of the effect of bactrim versus aerosolized pentamidine on the survival of AIDS patients in ACTG trial 021. They showed that adding strong prognostic factors to a Cox model for censoring not only helped correct the bias due to dependent censoring but also greatly improved efficiency. Presumably, a reanalysis of the same data but now with a bivariate survival outcome (say, time to PCP and time to death) would demonstrate an even greater advantage of our one-step estimator.

Table 3.6. c_n's for using both exponential (EXP) and Cox regressions to estimate $Q(u)$ in the one-step estimators.

t_1	t_2	EXP	COX
8.33	15.00	1.9	0.9
16.67	15.00	2.4	0.7
25.00	15.00	0.9	0.8
8.33	30.00	-0.7	0.8
16.67	30.00	0.9	0.8
25.00	30.00	0.1	0.5
8.33	45.00	0.4	0.9
16.67	45.00	2.8	0.9

3.9 Rigorous Analysis of a Bivariate Survival Estimate

In this section, we provide a rigorous analysis of our locally efficient estimator of the marginal bivariate survival function based on bivariate right-censored data when the two failure times are subject to a common censoring variable and no other covariates are available.

Given a bivariate survival time $\vec{T} = (T_1, T_2) \sim F$, define the process $X(\cdot) = (I(T_1 > \cdot), I(T_2 > \cdot))$. Suppose that both time variables are subject to a common right-censoring variable C. Let $T = \max(T_1, T_2)$. Then, the observed data structure Y is given by

$$Y = (\tilde{T} = C \wedge T, \Delta = I(\tilde{T} = T), \bar{X}(\tilde{T})).$$

Let the full data model for F be nonparametric. In addition, we will assume that C is independent of (T_1, T_2). Suppose that we are concerned with estimation of $\mu \equiv \bar{F}(t_1, t_2) = P(T_1 > t_1, T_2 > t_2)$. Let $t = (t_1, t_2)$.

The only full data estimating function is given by $I(\vec{T} > t) - \bar{F}(t)$. We estimate $G(\cdot) = P(C < \cdot)$ efficiently with the Kaplan–Meier estimator G_n based on the right-censored (by $T = T_1 \vee T_2$) C_i's. As the initial estimator of $\bar{F}(t)$, we use the IPCW estimator

$$\bar{F}_n^0(t) = \frac{1}{n} \sum_{i=1}^n \frac{I(\vec{T}_i > \vec{t})\Delta_i}{\bar{G}_n(T_i)},$$

which corresponds with using the IPCW estimating function $IC_0(Y \mid G, \mu) = I(\vec{T} > \vec{t})\Delta/\bar{G}(T) - \mu$.

The projection of IC_0 onto T_{CAR} is given by $IC_{CAR}(Y \mid F, G) \equiv -\int Q(F, G)(u, \bar{X}(u)) dM_G(u)$, where

$$Q(F, G)(u, \bar{X}(u)) = \frac{1}{\bar{G}(u)} \bar{F}(t \mid \bar{X}(u), T \geq u)$$

and $dM_G(u) = I(\tilde{T} \in du, \Delta = 0) - I(\tilde{T} \geq u)dG(u)/\bar{G}(u-)$. We can express $\bar{F}(t \mid \bar{X}(u), \tilde{T} > u)$ in terms of the conditional distribution of T_1, given T_2, the conditional distribution of T_2, given T_1, and the bivariate survival function of (T_1, T_2). In other words, $\bar{F}(t \mid \bar{X}(u))$ is a parameter of the bivariate distribution F of $\vec{T}$. Let $IC(Y \mid F, G, \mu) \equiv IC_0(Y \mid G, \mu) - IC_{CAR}(Y \mid F, G)$, which equals the efficient influence curve for estimation of $\mu = \bar{F}(t)$.

The one-step estimator requires specification of an initial estimator $\bar{F}_n^0(t)$, an estimator G_n of the cumulative distribution G and an estimate F_n of the bivariate distribution F:

$$\bar{F}_n^1(t) = \bar{F}_n^0(t) + \frac{1}{n}\sum_{i=1}^n IC(Y_i \mid F_n, G_n, F_n^0(t)).$$

It remains to discuss estimation of $\bar{F}(t \mid \bar{X}(u), \tilde{T} > u)$ which depends on conditional cumulative distributions of T_1, given T_2, and T_2, given T_1. Notice that by independence of C and T_1, given T_2, we have

$$P(T_1 > t_1 \mid T_2) = P(T_1 > t_1 \mid T_2, C > T_2) = P(T_1 > t_2 \mid \tilde{T}_2, \Delta_2 = 1),$$

so we can nonparametrically estimate this conditional distribution at $T_2 = u_2$ with the Kaplan–Meier estimator based on the observations with an observed T_2 close to u_2. Similarly, we can nonparametrically estimate $P(T_2 < t_2 \mid T_1)$. Alternatively, one can estimate these conditional distributions using kernel density estimators as in van der Laan (1994). Under smoothness conditions it will be possible to verify the conditions of the asymptotic Theorem 2.4 for the resulting one-step estimator, which proves that it is globally efficient.

In spite of the fact that the curse of dimensionality of this problem is not as dramatic as in the right-censored data example with a covariate process, so that it is actually possible to construct a globally efficient estimator under additional smoothness assumptions, the practical performance of this globally efficient estimator at moderate sample sizes might seriously suffer from the smoothing. Therefore, even in this marginal bivariate estimation problem, it is still useful that our one-step estimation method allows estimation of F according to some lower-dimensional working model for the bivariate distribution F. The user is free to specify the submodel. Above, we discussed estimation of F with a copula family or equivalently with frailty models.

In this section, we consider the case where F is estimated under the working model for the bivariate distribution F, which assumes that T_1 is independent of T_2. If T_1 and T_2 are independent, then

$$\bar{F}(\vec{t} \mid \bar{X}(u), \tilde{T} > u) = \begin{cases} I(T_1 > t_1, T_2 > t_2) & \text{if } \Delta_u = (1,1). \\ I(T_1 > t_1)\frac{\bar{F}_2(t_2 \vee u)}{\bar{F}_2(u)} & \text{if } \Delta_u = (1,0). \\ I(T_2 > t_2)\frac{\bar{F}_1(t_1 \vee u)}{\bar{F}_1(u)} & \text{if } \Delta_u = (0,1). \\ \frac{\bar{F}_1(t_1 \vee u)}{\bar{F}_1(u)}\frac{\bar{F}_2(t_2 \vee u)}{\bar{F}_2(u)} & \text{if } \Delta_u = (0,0). \end{cases}$$

We estimate $\bar{F}(t \mid \bar{X}(u), \tilde{T} > u)$ by substituting the marginal Kaplan–Meier estimators for F_1, F_2. In other words, we estimate the bivariate distribution $F(x_1, x_2)$ with $F_{1,KM}(x_1)F_{2,KM}(x_2)$ with the product of Kaplan-Meier estimators. Theorem 3.2 below proves that the corresponding one-step estimator $\bar{F}_n^1(t)$ is efficient if T_1 and T_2 happen to be independent and it remains consistent and asymptotically linear otherwise.

Theorem 3.2 Let $t = (t_1, t_2)$ be given. Suppose that $\bar{G}(t_1 \vee t_2 + \epsilon) > 0$ and $\bar{F}_T(t_1 \vee t_2 + \epsilon) > 0$ for some $\epsilon > 0$, where $\bar{F}_T$ is the survival function of $T = T_1 \vee T_2$. Let F^1 be the bivariate cumulative distribution defined by $F^1(x_1, x_2) = F_1(x_1)F_2(x_2)$; that is, F^1 is the product of the two true marginal cumulative distributions.

Then $\bar{F}_n^1(t)$ is a consistent and asymptotically linear estimator of $\bar{F}(t)$ with influence curve

$$IC(Y \mid F^1, G, F(t)) - IC_{nu}(Y),$$

where

$$IC_{nu}(Y) = -\int \frac{E(I(\vec{T} > t)\Delta/\bar{G}(T \mid X))}{E(I(\tilde{T} > u))} dM_G(u)$$
$$+ \int \frac{E\left\{\bar{F}^1(u \mid \bar{X}(u), T > u)I(T > u)\right\}}{E(I(\tilde{T} > u))} dM_G(u).$$

If T_1 and T_2 are independent, then $\bar{F}_n^1(t)$ is an asymptotically efficient estimator of $\bar{F}(t)$ ($IC_{nu} = 0$).

We will prove this theorem by applying the general asymptotics theorem (Theorem 2.4). Firstly, we make the following practical observation. The next lemma proves that we can artificially make each observation with $\tilde{T} > t_1 \vee t_2$ equal to $\tilde{T} = t_1 \vee t_2 + \epsilon$ for some $\epsilon > 0$ without losing any information. In other words, for estimation of $\bar{F}(t)$ there is no information in observing $\bar{X}(u), u > t_1 \vee t_2$, which is not surprising since observing $\bar{X}(t_1 \vee t_2)$ already implies observing $I(T_1 \leq t_1, T_2 \leq t_2)$. This insight will be important in proving the asymptotics since it shows that the quantities $\bar{F}(\vec{t} \mid \bar{X}(u), \tilde{T} > u)$ and $\bar{G}(u)$ only need to be estimated on the interval $[0, t_1 \vee t_2 + \epsilon]$ for some arbitrarily small $\epsilon > 0$.

Lemma 3.5 Define the following reduction of Y: $Y_r \equiv Y = (\tilde{T}, \Delta, \bar{X}(\tilde{T}))$ if $\tilde{T} \leq t_1 \vee t_2$, and let $Y_r \equiv (t_1 \vee t_2 + \epsilon, \Delta, \bar{X}(t_1 \vee t_2 + \epsilon))$ for an arbitrarily *small given $\epsilon > 0$ otherwise.* We have

$$IC(Y \mid F, G, F(t)) = IC(Y_r \mid F, G, F(t)).$$

Proof. Firstly, if $\tilde{T} \leq t_1 \vee t_2$, then $Y_r = Y$ so that we have nothing to verify. Suppose now that $\tilde{T} > t_1 \vee t_2$. Note that the projection term IC_{CAR} only integrates $\bar{F}(t \mid \bar{X}(u), \tilde{T} > u)$ over $u \leq \tilde{T} = (T_1 \vee T_2) \wedge C$. Since $I(\tilde{T} \in du, \Delta = 0) = 0$ for $u \leq t_1 \vee t_2$, we have that $\int_0^{t_1 \vee t_2} \bar{F}(t \mid \bar{X}(u), \tilde{T} > u) dM(u)/\bar{G}(u)$ is only a function of Y_r. For u with $t_1 \vee t_2 < u < T_1 \vee T_2$, we have

$$\begin{aligned}
\bar{F}(t \mid \bar{X}(u), \tilde{T} > u) &= I(t_1 < T_1 < u, T_2 > u) + I(T_1 > u, t_2 < T_2 < u) \\
&\quad + I(T_1 > u, T_2 > u) \\
&= I(T_1 > t_2, T_2 > t_2) I(T_1 \vee T_2 > u) \\
&= I(T_1 > t_1, T_2 > t_2).
\end{aligned}$$

Let $D(\vec{T}) = I(T_1 > t_1, T_2 > t_2)$. Thus

$$\begin{aligned}
\int_{t_1 \vee t_2}^{\infty} \bar{F}(t \mid \bar{X}(u), \tilde{T} > u) \frac{dM(u)}{\bar{G}(u)} &= D(\vec{T}) \left\{ \frac{1 - \Delta}{\bar{G}(\tilde{T})} - \int_{t_1 \vee t_2}^{\tilde{T}} \frac{dG(u)}{\bar{G}^2(u)} \right\} \\
&= -\frac{D(\vec{T}) \Delta}{\bar{G}(\tilde{T})} + \frac{D(\vec{T})}{\bar{G}(t_1 \vee t_2)}.
\end{aligned}$$

The first term, which depends on $\tilde{T}$ itself through $\bar{G}(\tilde{T})$, cancels with the $IC_0(Y \mid G, \mu) = D(\vec{T})\Delta/\bar{G}(T) - \mu$ term. The second term only depends on $\bar{X}(t_1 \vee t_2)$. We conclude that the efficient influence curve $IC(Y \mid F, G, F(t))$ only depends on Y through Y_r. □

Since the efficient influence curve $IC(Y \mid F, G, F(t))$ only depends on Y through Y_r we propose to truncate in the sense that we replace each observation Y_i by $Y_{i,r}$, $i = 1, \ldots, n$ before estimating $\bar{F}(t \mid \bar{X}(u), \tilde{T} > u)$. This modification happens to have no effect for our special one-step estimator $\bar{F}_n^1(t)$ using the product of two Kaplan–Meier estimators as an estimator of F, because our untruncated estimator $\bar{F}_n(t \mid \bar{X}(u), \tilde{T} > u)$ still satisfies (just as $\bar{F}(t \mid \bar{X}(u), \tilde{T} > u)$ does)

$$\bar{F}_n(t \mid \bar{X}(u), \tilde{T} > u) = I(T_1 > t_2, T_2 > t_2) \text{ if } t_1 \vee t_2 < u \leq \tilde{T}.$$

As a consequence, by imitating the proof of Lemma 3.5, one can prove that

$$IC(Y \mid F_n, G_n, F_n^0(t)) = IC(Y_r \mid F_n, G_n, F_n^0(t))$$

so that, in fact, the substitution $Y_{i,r}$ for Y_i, $i = 1, \ldots, n$, has no effect for our particular one-step estimator $\bar{F}_n^1(t)$.

3.9. Rigorous Analysis of a Bivariate Survival Estimate   221

3.9.1 Proof of Theorem 3.2

We will first prove a lemma that establishes all of the needed consistency results for the plug-in estimators in IC.

Lemma 3.6 *Suppose that $\bar{G}(t_1 \vee t_2 + \epsilon) > 0$ for some $\epsilon > 0$. Moreover, assume that $\bar{F}_T(t_1 \vee t_2 + \epsilon) > 0$ for some $\epsilon > 0$, where $\bar{F}_T$ is the survival function of $T = T_1 \vee T_2$.*

Then $F_{1n}, F_{2n}, \bar{G}_n$ are uniformly consistent on $[0, t_1 \vee t_2]$, and $\bar{F}_n^0(t_1 \vee t_2)$ is consistent. Moreover, $IC(Y \mid F_n = (F_{1n}, F_{2n}), G_n, \bar{F}_n^0(t))$ converges to $IC(Y \mid F^1 = (F_1, F_2), G, F(t))$ in $L^2(P_{F,G})$.

Furthermore, $(\sqrt{n}(F_{1,n} - F_1), \sqrt{n}(F_{2,n} - F_2), \sqrt{n}(G_n - G))$ converges weakly as a random element of the cadlag function space $(D[0, t_1 \vee t_2 + \epsilon])^3$ endowed with the supremum norm and the Borel sigma algebra (van der Vaart and Wellner, 1996) to a Gaussian process.

Proof. If $\bar{G}(t_1 \vee t_2 + \epsilon) > 0$ (the censoring distribution for T_1, T_2), then the Kaplan–Meier estimators $F_{1,n}, F_{2,n}$ are uniformly consistent on $[0, t_1 \vee t_2]$ and their standardized versions converge weakly as random elements of the cadlag function space endowed with the supremum norm and the Borel sigma algebra (Andersen, Borgan, Gill and Keiding, 1993).

Similarly, if $\bar{F}_T(t_1 \vee t_2 + \epsilon) > 0$ (the censoring distribution for G), then the Kaplan–Meier estimator G_n of G is uniformly consistent on $[0, t_1 \vee t_2]$, and its standardized version converges weakly as random elements of the cadlag function space endowed with the supremum norm and the Borel sigma algebra (Andersen, Borgan, Gill, and Keiding, 1993). The latter proves that $\bar{F}_n^0(\vec{t})$ is a consistent estimator of $\bar{F}(\vec{t})$. It is now straightforward to prove the lemma. □

Proof of Theorem 3.2. We will prove the theorem by applying Theorem 2.4. In order to apply this theorem, it is convenient to express $IC(Y \mid Q_n, G_n, F_n^0(\vec{t}))$ as a function of $(\tilde{T}_1, \tilde{T}_2, \Delta_1, \Delta_2)$. Firstly, note that

$$\bar{F}(t \mid \bar{X}(u), T > u) = I(t_1 < T_1 \le u, T_2 > u)\frac{\bar{F}_2(t_2 \vee u)}{\bar{F}_2(u)}$$

$$+ I(T_1 > u, t_2 < T_2 \le u)\frac{\bar{F}_1(t_1 \vee u)}{\bar{F}_1(u)}$$

$$+ I(T_1 > u, T_2 > u)\frac{\bar{F}_1(t_1 \vee u)}{\bar{F}_1(u)}\frac{\bar{F}_2(t_2 \vee u)}{\bar{F}_2(u)} - \bar{F}(t_1, t_2).\quad(3.30)$$

It is now straightforward to show that $IC(Y \mid (F_1, F_2), G, F(t))$ is given by

$$IC(\tilde{T}_1, \tilde{T}_2, \vec{\Delta}) = \frac{I(\tilde{T}_1 > t_1, \tilde{T}_2 > t_2)\Delta}{\bar{G}(\tilde{T})}$$

$$+ \frac{1-\Delta}{\bar{G}(\tilde{T})}\left\{I(\tilde{T}_1 > t_1)\frac{\bar{F}_2(t_2 \vee \tilde{T})}{\bar{F}_2(\tilde{T})}\vec{\Delta} = (1,0) + I(\tilde{T}_2 > t_2)\frac{\bar{F}_1(t_1 \vee \tilde{T})}{\bar{F}_1(\tilde{T})}\vec{\Delta} = (0,1)\right\}$$

$$+\frac{1-\Delta}{\bar{G}(\tilde{T})}\left\{\frac{\bar{F}_1(t_1\vee\tilde{T})}{\bar{F}_1(\tilde{T})}\frac{\bar{F}_2(t_2\vee\tilde{T})}{\bar{F}_2(\tilde{T})}\vec{\Delta}=(0,0)-\bar{F}(\vec{t})\right\}$$

$$-\int_0^{\tilde{T}}I(t_1<\tilde{T}_1<u,\tilde{T}_2>u)\frac{\bar{F}_2(t_2\vee u)}{\bar{F}_2(u)}\frac{dG(u)}{\bar{G}^2(u)}$$

$$-\int_0^{\tilde{T}}I(\tilde{T}_1>u,t_2<\tilde{T}_2<u)\frac{\bar{F}_1(t_1\vee u)}{\bar{F}_1(u)}\frac{dG(u)}{\bar{G}^2(u)}$$

$$-\int_0^{\tilde{T}}I(\tilde{T}_1>u,\tilde{T}_2>u)\frac{\bar{F}_1(t_1\vee u)}{\bar{F}_1(u)}\frac{\bar{F}_2(t_2\vee u)}{\bar{F}_2(u)}\frac{dG(u)}{\bar{G}^2(u)}+\bar{F}(\vec{t})\int_0^{\tilde{T}}\frac{dG(u)}{\bar{G}^2(u)}.$$

Recall that by Lemma 3.5 and the remark under this lemma that we can do as if $\tilde{T}_1, \tilde{T}_2$ only lives on $[0, t_1 \vee t_2 + \epsilon)$. Moreover, note that $\bar{F}_T > \delta > 0$ implies that $\bar{F}_1 > \delta > 0$ and $\bar{F}_2 > \delta > 0$. Thus, the assumptions in the theorem and Lemma 3.6 imply that all denominators are bounded away from $\delta > 0$ with probability tending to 1. We are now ready to verify the conditions of Theorem 2.4.

Condition (i). We need to prove that $IC(\cdot \mid F_n, G_n, F_n^0(t))$ falls in a Donsker class with probability tending to 1. The class of bivariate real-valued functions with a uniform sectional variation norm $\|\cdot\|_{v,*}$, as defined in Gill, van der Laan, and Wellner (1995) smaller than a universal $M < \infty$ is a Donsker class (see also van der Laan, 1996b, Chapter 1). Therefore, it suffices to prove that $I(\vec{\Delta} = (\delta_1, \delta_2))IC(\cdot \mid F_n, G_n, F_n^0(t))$ is a Donsker class for each of the four possible combinations of $(\delta_1, \delta_2) \in \{(1,1), (0,0), (1,0), (0,1)\}$. This proof is similar to the ones given in Gill, van der Laan, and Wellner (1995) and van der Laan (1996b). Firstly, we have that indicators such as $I(\tilde{T}_1 < u, \tilde{T}_2 > u)$ have a uniform sectional variation norm bounded by 4. Secondly, $\bar{G}_n$ converges to $\bar{G}$ in probability and $\bar{G} > \delta > 0$ on $[0, t_1 \vee t_2 + \epsilon)$. Moreover, $(\tilde{T}_1, \tilde{T}_2) \to \bar{G}(\tilde{T})$ is uniformly (in n) bounded w.r.t. the uniform sectional variation norm as well since $\bar{G}$ is a survival (thus monotone and bounded) function. Furthermore, the uniform sectional variation norm of a function $1/f$, $f > \delta > 0$, can be bounded by a constant only depending on δ times the uniform sectional variation norm of f (Gill, 1993). It is now a straightforward exercise to prove that $I(\vec{\Delta} = (\delta_1, \delta_2))IC(\cdot \mid F_n, G_n, F_n^0(t))$ has a uniform sectional variation norm bounded by $M < \infty$ with probability tending to 1.

Condition (ii). This is a direct consequence of Lemma 3.6.

Condition (iii). In order to prove this condition we need to prove that the term $P_{F,G} \int (\bar{F}_n - \bar{F}^1)(t \mid \bar{X}(u), T > u) \frac{1}{\bar{G}_n(u)} (dM_{G_n} - dM_G) = o_P(1/\sqrt{n})$. This term consists of a sum of terms of the type

$$\int_0^{t_1 \vee t_2} f(u) \left\{ \frac{\bar{F}_{2,n}(t_2 \vee u)}{\bar{F}_{2,n}(u)} - \frac{\bar{F}_2(t_2 \vee u)}{\bar{F}_2(u)} \right\} \left\{ \frac{dG_n(u)}{\bar{G}_n(u)} - \frac{dG(u)}{\bar{G}(u)} \right\},$$

where we exchanged integration over u and Y (defining the expectation w.r.t. $P_{F,G}$). This term can be shown to be $o_P(1/\sqrt{n})$ by applying the

3.9. Rigorous Analysis of a Bivariate Survival Estimate

Helly–Bray lemma of Gill, van der Laan, and Wellner (1995), which proves that terms $\int Z_n d(F_n - F) \to 0$ in probability when Z_n converges weakly in $(D[0,\tau], \|\cdot\|_\infty)$ to a function Z, $\| F_n - F \|_\infty$ converge in supremum norm to zero with probability tending to 1, $\| F_n \|_{v,*} < M < \infty$ with probability tending to 1, and $\| F \|_{v,*} < \infty$. Note that the supremum norm convergence requirements of this lemma follow directly form Lemma 3.6. Moreover, the bounded variation requirements have been proved by condition (i) above.

Condition (iv) It is straightforward to show that $\sqrt{n}(\Phi(G_n) - \Phi(G))$ minus its linearization in $\sqrt{n}(G_n - G)$ converges to zero if $\sqrt{n}(G_n - G) \to Z$ in supremum norm over $[0, t_1 \vee t_2 + \epsilon]$. In other words, $G \to \Phi(G)$ is compactly differentiable in the sense of Gill (1989). A compactly differentiable functional of an efficient estimator is efficient as well (van der Vaart, 1991). Since G_n (the Kaplan–Meier estimator of G) is an efficient estimator of G under the independent censoring model, this proves that $\Phi(G_n)$ is an efficient estimator of $\Phi(G)$ and thereby proves condition (iv).

Application of Theorem 2.4 now proves that $F_n^1(\vec{t})$ is asymptotically linear with influence curve given by

$$\Pi(IC(\cdot \mid F^1 = (F_1, F_2), G, F(t)) \mid T_2(P_{F,G})^\perp),$$

where $T_2(P_{F,G})$ is the tangent space of G at the true data-generating distribution $P_{F,G}$ in the model with F nonparametric and C independent of $X = \vec{T}$.

Note that this tangent space $T_2(P_{F,G})$ corresponds exactly with the tangent space $T_{\Lambda_0} = \{\int g(t) dM_G(t) : g\}$ of the baseline hazard in the Cox proportional hazards model when assuming $\alpha = 0$ (i.e., no covariates). Therefore, we can apply Lemma 3.2, which yields the required projections onto T_{Λ_0}. Firstly, recall the representation $IC = IC_0 - IC_{CAR}$, where $IC_0(Y) = D(X)\Delta/\bar{G}(T) - \mu$, $D(X) = I(\vec{T} > t)$, and $\mu = \bar{F}(t)$. Application of Lemma 3.2 (3.17) gives

$$\Pi(IC_0(Y) \mid T_{\Lambda_0}) = -\int \frac{E(I(\vec{T} > t)\Delta/\bar{G}(T \mid X))}{E(I(\tilde{T} > u))} dM_G(u). \quad (3.31)$$

We have that $IC_{CAR} = -\int H(u, \bar{X}(u)) dM_G(u)$, where $H(u, \bar{X}(u)) = \bar{F}^1(t \mid \bar{X}(u))/\bar{G}(u)$. Application of Lemma 3.2 (3.14) provides the projection $\Pi(\int H dM_G \mid T_{\Lambda_0}) = \int g(H) dM_G$,

$$\Pi\left(\int H dM_G \mid T_{\Lambda_0}\right) = -\int \frac{E\left\{H(u, \bar{X}(u))I(\tilde{T} > u)\right\}}{EI(\tilde{T} > u)} dM_G(u)$$

$$= -\int \frac{E\{\bar{F}^1(u \mid \bar{X}(u), T > u) I(T > u)\}}{EI(\tilde{T} > u)} dM_G(u),$$

so we conclude that

$$IC_{nu}(Y) = -\int \frac{E(I(\vec{T} > t)\Delta/\bar{G}(T \mid X))}{EI(\tilde{T} > u)} dM_G(u)$$

$$+ \int \frac{E\left\{\bar{F}^1(u \mid \bar{X}(u), T > u)I(T > u)\right\}}{EI(\tilde{T} > u)} dM_G(u).$$

Finally, note that if $F^1(u \mid \bar{X}(u), T > u)$ equals the true distribution $F(u \mid \bar{X}(u), T > u)$, then the last integral equals (3.31) so that IC_{nu} equals zero or equivalently $\Pi(IC(\cdot \mid F^1 = (F_1, F_2), G, F(t)) \mid T_2(P_{F,G})^\perp) = IC(\cdot \mid F, G, F(t))$ is the efficient influence curve. This proves the last statement of the theorem. $\square$

3.10 Prediction of Survival

There have been a number of proposals for nonparametric regression methods for survival outcomes. In essence, all these methods propose a sequence of regression models of increasing complexity. The final choice of model is determined through a model selection criterion. One refers to such a sequence of models as a sieve.

Kooperberg, Stone, and Truong (1995) propose a sieve of multiplicative intensity models for the hazard of survival which allows interaction effects between covariates and with time, and they use model selection techniques (AIC, BIC) to data-adaptively select the model. Their implementation is called HARE. Hastie and Tibshirani (1990a,b) fit additive Cox-proportional hazards models wherein covariate effects are modeled via sums of univariate smooth functions. There are also many modifications of classification and regression trees, CART, (Breiman, Friedman, Olshen, Stone, 1984) that are specific to censored survival data. These are sometimes referred as survival trees and can roughly be divided into two categories. Methods in the first category use a within node homogeneity measure. Examples of such approaches include Gordon and Olshen (1985), Davis and Anderson (1989), and Leblanc and Crowley (1992). To be more specific, Davis and Andersen (1989) use the negative log-likelihood of an exponential model for each node as a measure of split homogeneity and the squared difference of the parent node log-likelihood and a weighted sum of child node log-likelihoods as the split function. Methods in the second category due to Segal (1988) use a between node homogeneity measure with the split function determined by the two sample log rank test statistic. In essence, all of these methods are attempting to replace the least squares split functions utilized by CART for uncensored continuous observations with alternatives suitable for a censored survival outcome.

Suppose, with complete (i.e., uncensored) data, one would calculate a "complete data survival predictor" by first applying a particular data-driven model selection criterion to select a single model out of L candidate models and then report the efficient survival predictor computed under the selected model. In that case we believe that a methodology for building a predictor and assessing its performance based on censored data should satisfy the following two properties. First, when applied to uncensored data, the censored data methodology should predict the same survival as the "complete data survival predictor". The CART implementations (Segal, 1988, and Davis, and Andersen, 1989) for censored survival data seem to lack this logic since, when applied to the complete (i.e., uncensored), data, these CART implementations do not reduce to a prefered complete data methodology. (e.g., CART where the split function and model selection criterion aim at minimizing the risk of the squared prediction error loss function, as proposed by Breiman, Friedman, Olshen, Stone, 1984). In other words, the exponential and log-rank split functions and the associated model criterion seem to be choices which are convenient for handling censored data, but do not reduce to the choices suggested for uncensored data. In general, the literature on prediction of survival based on right censored data does not seem to propose performance assessments of predictors which estimate the risk of the predictor w.r.t. a user supplied loss function, while this is standard practice in the prediction literature for uncensored data: for example, it is common practice to estimate the risk of a predictor with the empirical mean of the corresponding loss function over an (independent) test sample. Secondly, none of the methods proposed in the literature incorporate external (to the predictor) covariate processes to allow for informative censoring and gain in efficiency. For example, consistent estimation of the parameters in a particular Cox-proportional hazards model relies on C and T being independent, given the covariates in the model. Consequently, the meaning of this assumption depends on the complexity of the model. Clearly, this fact can lead to serious bias.

In the next subsections, we exploit the methodology developed in this chapter to present a general framework for building survival predictors, which satisfies both properties. This methodology can be applied to any sieve. In particular, we illustrate its applicability to the CART-sieve (rectangular partitions of the feature space) and to generalized linear regression. See Keles, van der Laan, Dudoit (2002), and Molinaro, van der Laan, Dudoit (2002) for details.

3.10.1 General methodology

Suppose that we observe n i.i.d. observations on a right-censored data structure $Y = (C, \bar{X}(C))$, where $X(t) = (R(t), L(t))$, $R(t) = I(T \leq t)$, T is a survival time, and $\bar{X}(T)$ is the full-data structure. Recall our convention that $C = \infty$ if T occurs before right censoring. Let $W = L(1)$ denote a p-dimensional vector of time-independent covariates. Suppose that the goal is to build a so called prediction of log-survival $Z = \log(T)$ based on the time-independent covariates W, which could then be used to predict the log survival time of a new incoming subject. We will denote such a predictor with $C(W)$.

The performance of a prediction applied to a particular observation (Z, W) is measured by a loss function $L(Z, C(W))$. Particular examples of loss functions are

$$L_2(Z, W) \equiv (Z - C(W))^2$$
$$L_1(Z, W) \equiv |Z - C(W)|.$$

The performance of a predictor on a population is typically measured by the so called average loss or risk

$$R(C(\cdot)) = E_{P_{F_X}, G} L(Z, C(W)).$$

One can now define an optimal predictor as the predictor minimizing the risk $C(\cdot) \to R(C(\cdot))$ over all possible predictors:

$$C_{opt} = \max_{C(\cdot)}^{-1} R(C(\cdot)).$$

For example, the optimal predictors w.r.t. loss functions L_2 and L_1 are given by

$$C_{opt,2}(W) = E(Z \mid W)$$
$$C_{opt,1}(W) = \text{Median}(Z \mid W),$$

respectively. Here, $\text{Median}(Z \mid W)$ denotes the median of the conditional distribution of Z, given W.

In the remainder of this section we will address model based estimation of $C_{opt}(W)$ for a given model, estimation of the risk of the predictor based on a test sample, and model/feature selection.

Model based estimation of the optimal predictor

Given a regression model $Z = m(W \mid \beta) + \epsilon$ with $E(K(\epsilon) \mid W) = 0$ for a given monotone function K, define $C_n(W) = m(W \mid \beta_n)$, where β_n is an estimator of the unknown parameter vector β. To obtain an estimate of $C_{opt,2}$ and $C_{opt,1}$ one uses $K(\epsilon) = \epsilon$ (i.e, mean regression) and $K(\epsilon) = I(\epsilon > 0) - 1/2$ (i.e., median regression), respectively. In this chapter we provided a closed form locally efficient estimator β_n of β based on observing $(C_i, \bar{X}(C_i))$, $i = 1, \ldots, n$. In particular, we provided simple to compute inverse probability of censoring weighted estimators which rely on correct specification of the censoring mechanism $\bar{G}(t \mid X) \equiv P(C \geq t \mid X)$. Specifically, given estimators G_n and Q_n of the censoring mechanism G and a conditional regression Q, respectively, we defined β_n as the solution of the estimating equation

$$0 = \sum_{i=1}^n IC_0(Y_i \mid G_n, D_{h_n}(\cdot \mid \beta))$$
$$+ \sum_{i=1}^n \int Q_n(u, \bar{X}_i(u)) dM_{G_n,i}(u),$$

where

$$Q_n(u, \bar{X}(u)) \equiv \hat{E}\left(IC_0(Y \mid G_n, D_{h_n}(\cdot \mid \beta)) \mid \bar{X}(u), C > u\right),$$

$$IC_0(Y \mid G, D_h(\cdot \mid \beta)) = \frac{\Delta_i}{\bar{G}(T_i \mid X_i)} D_h(X_i \mid \beta)$$

is the inverse probability of censoring weighted estimating function of the full data estimating function $D_h(X \mid \beta) = h(W)K(\epsilon(\beta))$, and $dM_G(u) = dG(u \mid X)/\bar{G}(u \mid X)$. Here h_n is (say) either the least squares choice $h_n(W) = d/d\beta m(W \mid \beta_n^0)$ (for some initial estimator β_n^0) or the closed form estimator of the optimal index h_{opt} as provided in this chapter. We proposed a variety of methods for estimation of the regression of $IC_0(Y)$ onto $\bar{X}(u), C > u$. The inverse probability of censoring weighted estimator is defined as the solution β_n^0 of

$$\begin{aligned}0 &= \sum_{i=1}^n IC_0(Y_i \mid G_n, D_{h_n}(\cdot \mid \beta)) \\ &= \sum_{i=1}^n \frac{\Delta_i}{\bar{G}_n(T_i \mid X_i)} h_n(W_i) K(\epsilon_i(\beta)).\end{aligned}$$

If we use $h_n(W) = d/d\beta m(W \mid \beta)$ and $K(\epsilon) = \epsilon$, then this estimator corresponds with minimizing the weighted sum of squared residuals $\sum_i w_i \epsilon_i(\beta)^2$ with weights $w_i = \Delta_i/\bar{G}_n(T_i \mid X_i)$, $i = 1, \ldots, n$, which can thus be computed with standard regression software.

The above methodology can also be applied to a multiplicative intensity model $\lambda_T(t \mid W) = \lambda_0(t) \exp(m(W, t \mid \beta))$ for the conditional hazard of T, given W, whose corresponding conditional survival function can be mapped into a mean or median prediction. The class of estimating functions for β and corresponding estimators were provided in Section 3.3.

Estimating the performance of a given predictor

To evaluate the performance of an estimated predictor one sets aside part of the original sample as a test sample. The remainder of the sample of n observations is called a learning sample (where a learning sample can be further split up in a trainings and validation sample for the purpose of model selection: see next subsection) and the estimated predictor $C_n(W)$ should only be based on the learning sample. One uses the test sample to estimate the risk of a given predictor C_n. To do so we estimate the unknown conditional parameter

$$\theta(C) = EL(Z, C(W))$$

based on the n_{test} test sample observations and then evaluate our estimate at $C = C_n$. In the case of uncensored data it is common practice to estimate $\theta(C)$ by the empirical mean $1/n_{Test} \sum_{i \in Test} L(Z_i, C(W_i))$. With censored data, we will estimate $\theta(C)$ by a locally efficient estimator assuming a a nonparametric full-data model. We believe that this estimator will be approximately efficient for $\theta(C)$ under our semiparametric full data regression model since the regression model provides little information concerning $\theta(C)$. Specifically, our estimator is given by

$$\hat{\theta}(C \mid Test) = \frac{1}{n_{Test}} \sum_{i \in Test} IC_0(Y_i \mid G_n, L(\cdot)) \qquad (3.32)$$

$$+ \frac{1}{n_{Test}} \sum_{i \in Test} \int \hat{E}\left(IC_0(Y \mid G_n, L(\cdot)) \mid \bar{X}_i(u), C_i > u\right) dM_{G_n,i}(u)$$

By definition of the inverse probability of censoring weighted mapping $D \to IC_0(\cdot \mid G, D)$, we have

$$IC_0(Y_i \mid G, L(\cdot)) = \frac{\Delta_i}{\bar{G}(T_i \mid X_i)} L(Z_i, C(W_i)).$$

A less efficient simple inverse probability of censoring weighted estimator $\hat{\theta}^0(C \mid Test)$ is given by:

$$\hat{\theta}^0(C \mid Test) = \frac{1}{n_{Test}} \sum_{i \in Test} \frac{\Delta_i}{\bar{G}_n(T_i \mid X_i)} L(Z_i, C(W_i)). \qquad (3.33)$$

Model/Feature selection

The above method for estimation of the optimal predictor based on n i.i.d. observations (the learning sample) assumes a prespecified regression model for Z, given W. If W is very high dimensional relative to sample size, then one would want to consider a large collection of subsets of the covariate vector W and evaluate the performance of the corresponding subset-specific regression models with a model selection criterion. To carry out such a model selection method we split the sample into trainings and validation samples J times, and we index each particular sample split by $j = 1, \ldots, J$. Let $W^l \subset W$ represent a subset of covariates in W, $l = 1, \ldots, L$, where one might have that the size of W^l increases with l, although one might allow $(W^l : l = 1, \ldots, L)$ to include subsets of the same size. In order to select a particular sequence of subsets, a common method is to run a forward selection method on the sample. Let p be the dimension of W, and let $m(W \mid \beta)$ be a regression model with $p+1$-dimensional parameter vector β, one parameter for each covariate. Now, $m_l(W \mid \beta)$ is defined as the restricted regression model in which each coefficient in front of a covariate in W/W^l is set equal to zero. In this manner, the set of covariates W^l defines the model and $m_l(W \mid \beta)$ now defines a sieve.

Consider a given sample split j and model choice l. Let $\hat{\beta}_{j,l}$ be the IPCW-estimator or the locally efficient estimator of β, as proposed above, based on the training sample j under the model $m_l(W \mid \beta)$. Let $\hat{C}_{j,l}(W) = m(W^l \mid \hat{\beta}_{j,l})$ be the corresponding predictor. Let $\hat{\theta}_{j,l}$ be the IPCW-estimator or the locally efficient estimator of the conditional risk θ of the given predictor $\hat{C}_{j,l}(\cdot)$ based on the *validation sample j*. As remarked in Section 1.7, an important version of this method uses common (to each sample j) estimates *based on the whole sample of size n* of the nuisance parameters G and (the regression) Q which appear in the estimating functions defining the estimators of the regression coefficients and the conditional risk.

Let

$$l^* = \min_l{}^{-1} \sum_{j=1}^{J} \hat{\theta}_{j,l}$$

be the model choice l that minimizes the average (across the J splits) of the j-specific risk estimates. Let $\hat{\beta}_{l^*}$ be our proposed estimator based on the whole sample of size n, assuming the model $m(W^{l^*} \mid \beta)$. Our proposed predictor is now $m(W^{l^*} \mid \hat{\beta}_{l^*})$.

Another common method is to let the actual selection of the subsets W^l be determined with forward(/backward) selection based on the training samples. Then $W^l = W_j^l$ is indexed by the trainings samples indexed by j. Now, W_j^l varies across j, but the dimension of W_j^l (say l) does not vary with j. As a consequence, l^* does not correspond with selecting a particular set of covariates, but with selecting an optimal dimension.

Remark on proportion for sample splitting

We note that it is important to choose the training sample large relative to the validation sample since one is interested in finding the model which would result in an optimal trade off between variance and bias for the predictor based on the *whole sample* of size n. As an extreme one can consider leave-one out cross-validation. For example, if we use the IPCW-estimator of the risk, then leave-one out cross-validation gives us

$$l^* = \min_l{}^{-1} \sum_{j=1}^{n} \frac{\Delta_j}{\bar{G}_n(T_j \mid X_j)} L(Z_j, \hat{C}_{-j}(W_j)),$$

where the expectation of the criterion $1/n \sum_{j=1}^{n} \frac{\Delta_j}{\bar{G}(T_j|X_j)} L(Z_j, \hat{C}_{-j}(W_j))$ indeed equals the conditional risk $EL(Z, \hat{C}_{n-1}(W))$ of the predictor $\hat{C}_{n-1}$, regarding $\hat{C}_{n-1}$ as fixed in taking the expectation. In spite of the fact that the leave-one out cross-validation results in an criterion which is essentially unbiased for the conditional risk $EL(Z, \hat{C}_n(W))$, given $\hat{C}_n$, the criterion's conditional variance is reduced by increasing the size of the validation sample. Consequently, finding the optimal proportion for the sample splitting is itself a selection problem involving the trade-off between bias and variance.

Remark

In this remark we explain the logic behind the model selection procedure. For the sake of presentation, let the loss function be the L_2-loss function.

The model selection criterion, say $l \to c_n(l)$, $l = 1, \ldots, L$, provides a value for each l-specific estimate $\hat{C}_{np,l}$ based on np observations. Ignoring the second order bias in $c_n(\cdot)$, the criterion has the property that its expectation is given by

$$l \to E c_n(l) \approx E(Z - \hat{C}_{np,l}(W))^2,$$

where the expectation is now taken over (Z, W) (test sample) and the independent set of np observations (Z_i, W_i) (trainings sample). Here the expectation is exact under no censoring. The right-hand side can be rewritten (up till a constant independent of l) as

$$l \to E(C_{opt,2}(W) - \hat{C}_{np,l}(W))^2.$$

In other words, ignoring second order bias, the minimum l^* of $l \to E c_n(l)$ identifies the classifyer $\hat{C}_{np,l^*}$ which has the smallest mean squared error w.r.t. optimal classifyer $C_{opt,2}$ among the L classifyers $\hat{C}_{np,l}$, $l = 1, \ldots, L$. Thus our final estimator $\hat{C}_{n,l^*}$ based on the learning sample has been fully aimed at estimating $C_{opt,2}$ through 1) the choice of model and 2) the locally efficient estimator, given the model choice.

It should be noted that the variance of the corresponding estimator of this minimum l^* is affected by the number L of models considered and the L-variate distribution of $(c_n(1), \ldots, c_n(L))$. We refer to our remark in Section 1.7 regarding potential improvements by incorporating in the model selection procedure an estimate of the L-variate covariance matrix of $(c_n(1), \ldots, c_n(L))$.

3.10.2 Prediction of survival with Regression Trees

The methodology described above can also be applied to the particular sieve defined by regression trees. The algorithm of Breiman, Friedman, Olshen, and Stone (1984) for regression trees relies on a split criterion. Given a group of elements representing a node in the tree, one considers, for each covariate W_j and constant C, splitting the group by $W_j < C$ and $W_j > C$, and the performance of such a split is evaluated by the split criterion. One chooses the split which minimizes the split criterion across covariates W_j and the splitting constant C. The split criterion for splitting a node N into two nodes N_1, N_2 (thus $N = N_1 \cup N_2$), proposed by Breiman, Friedman, Olshen, and Stone (1984) for continuous (uncensored) outcomes is given by

$$R_N(C) - (R_{N_1}(C) + R_{N_2}(C)),$$

where, for a given node N one defines $R_N(C) = \sum_{i \in N} L_2(Y_i, C(X_i))$, where we note that prediction $C(X_i)$ for a given regression tree is defined as $1/|N(X_i)| \sum_{i \in N(X_i)} Y_i$, where $N(X_i)$ denotes the terminal node of the tree containing X_i. One can also represent this split criterion as the difference of the average loss of the predictor defined by the tree before the split of node N and the average loss of the predictor defined by the tree defined by the split of this node N in two children nodes N_1 and N_2: thus, the split criterion simply compares the average loss over the sample of two predictors. Therefore, given a regression tree with a number of nodes, the algorithm looks for the split of one of the terminal nodes in this tree which results in a one node extended regression tree with minimal average loss across the sample. Analogous to the methodology proposed above, our proposal is to replace this difference of average losses of the two predictors by their locally efficient or inverse probability of censoring weighted estimator of the expectation of the loss. Since the two regression trees only differ in their prediction of the elements in the node N, this is equivalent to the following. For each of the three nodes $N^* \in \{N, N_1, N_2\}$, one replaces $R_{N^*}(C)$ in the split criterion by the corresponding inverse probability of treatment weighted estimator (see (3.33))

$$\hat{\theta}^0(C \mid N^*) = \frac{1}{\mid N^* \mid} \sum_{i \in N^*} L_2(Y_i, C(X_i)) \frac{\Delta_i}{\bar{G}(Y_i \mid X_i)}$$

based on the sample defined by the node N^*, or the locally efficient estimator $\hat{\theta}(C \mid N^*)$ defined by (3.32).

As above, to evaluate the performance of the predictor $C(\cdot)$ defined by a regression tree trained on a learning sample (or the J trainings samples), we estimate its conditional risk $\theta(C)$ with the inverse probability of treatment weighted estimator $\hat{\theta}^0(C \mid S)$ or locally efficient estimator $\hat{\theta}(C \mid S)$ of the risk $\theta(C)$ based on a test sample S (or validation samples S_j, $j = 1, \ldots, J$).

4
Cross-Sectional Data and Right-Censored Data Combined

4.1 Model and General Data Structure

Consider the following general data structure. Let $X_1(t), X_2(t)$ be two time-dependent processes, and let $X(t) = (X_1(t), X_2(t))$. Let $R(t) = I(T \leq t)$ be included in $X_2(t)$, where T marks an endpoint such as death or a fixed potential follow-up time. The full data structure is defined as $X = \bar{X}(T) = (\bar{X}_1(T), \bar{X}_2(T))$, which includes observing T itself. Here $\bar{X}(t) = (X(s) : s \leq t)$. Suppose that the observed data structure is given by

$$Y = (C, X_1(C), \bar{X}_2(C)), \qquad (4.1)$$

where we define $C \equiv \infty$ if $C > T$, and $X_1(\infty)$ is set to an arbitrary constant, so that the observation $X_1(\infty)$ contains no information. In other words, if $C < T$, then we observe the process X_1 at time C and observe the process X_2 up to time C, while if $C > T$, then we observe $Y = (T, \bar{X}_2(T))$. Given a particular full data model $\mathcal{M}^F$ such as the generalized linear regression model, multiplicative intensity model, or nonparametric model, let $\mu = \mu(F_X)$ be a parameter of interest defined on this full data model.

Example 4.1 (Cross-sectional data on competing failure times) A special example of this general data structure naturally occurs in a cross-sectional study in which one is interested in observing two competing failure times. Let U be the age at menopause, and let $J = 1$ if the menopause is natural and $J = 2$ if the menopause is surgically induced. Let C be the age at which the woman is interviewed. In order to obtain reliable data in such studies one might decide to determine only whether the woman has reached menopause and the type of menopause, and if the menopause was caused by an operation, then one determines the exact age at menopause. In this example, the full data structure is given by (U, J) and the observed data structure by $(C, I(U \leq C, J = 1), I(U \leq C, J = 2)U)$. By defining the processes $X_1(t) = I(U \leq t, J = 1)$ and $X_2(t) = I(U \leq t, J = 2)$, one can also represent this data structure as $Y = (C, X_1(C), \bar{X}_2(C))$. □

Example 4.2 (Multivariate current status data with a covariate process up until the monitoring time) The general data structure (4.1) occurs in a cross-sectional study in which one obtains at the monitoring time current status data on a number of events and possibly right censored data on directly observable events. In this case, $X_1(t) = (I(T_1 \leq t), \ldots, I(T_k \leq t))$ for some event time variables $T_1, \ldots, T_k$, and $X_2(t)$ represents the directly observable data. For example, T_j might be the time until onset of tumor j, $j = 1, \ldots, k$. The observed data structure is $(C, X_1(C), \bar{X}_2(C))$. The data structure $(C, X_1(C))$ is called multivariate current status data. □

Example 4.3 (Current status data on a counting process with a surrogate process) Consider a cross-sectional study in which one asks randomly selected subjects the number of sexual partners they have had. Let C be the age of the subject at the interview. Let $X_1(t)$ be the number of sexual partners the subject has had up until age t. Suppose that one also asks the subject to give the dates to their best recollection. Let $X_2(0)$ denote the baseline covariates and $X_2(t)$ denote a counting process jumping at the guessed dates. Then, one observes on each subject $(C, X_1(C), \bar{X}_2(C))$. The parameters of interest are the distribution of the times to jth sexual partner and are thus parameters of the distribution of $X_1(t)$. Here $\bar{X}_2(C)$ represents a surrogate process that can be used to increase efficiency and possibly explain informative monitoring. Another class of examples is obtained by letting $X_1(t)$ be a counting process jumping when the subject moves into the next state of a disease process. □

The data-generating distribution of Y (4.1) is indexed by the full data distribution $F_X \in \mathcal{M}^F$ and the conditional cumulative distribution $G(\cdot \mid X)$ of C, given X, which we call the censoring mechanism or monitoring mechanism. Our estimation methods require an estimate of G according to some submodel of CAR. Let $A(t) = I(C \leq t)$. The conditional density of C, given X, w.r.t. a counting measure on a grid or Lebesgue measure is given by

$$g(C \mid X) = g(\bar{A} \mid X) = \prod_t g(A(t) \mid \bar{A}(t-), X). \tag{4.2}$$

We will assume that

$$E(dA(t) \mid X, \bar{A}(t-)) = E(dA(t) \mid \bar{A}(t-), \bar{X}_2(\min(t, C))), \tag{4.3}$$

which implies that G satisfies CAR. For example, in the discrete case, this is equivalent with assuming that for $t < T$

$$\lambda_C(t \mid X) \equiv P(C = t \mid X, C \geq t) = P(C = t \mid \bar{X}_2(t), C \geq t).$$

Van der Laan and Jewell (2002) prove results for the current status data structure $(C, X_1(C))$ that strongly suggest that at most data-generating distributions of interest (4.3) is locally equivalent with CAR. Under the assumption (4.3), we can represent the censoring mechanism (4.2) by the partial likelihood of the counting process A w.r.t. history $\mathcal{F}(t) \equiv (\bar{X}_2(\min(t,C)), \bar{A}(t-))$,

$$g(\bar{A} \mid X) = \prod_t (\alpha(t \mid \mathcal{F}(t))^{dA(t)}(1 - \alpha(t \mid \mathcal{F}(t)))^{1-dA(t)},$$

where $\alpha(t \mid \mathcal{F}(t)) \equiv E(dA(t) \mid \mathcal{F}(t))$ is the intensity of $A(t)$ w.r.t. history $\mathcal{F}(t)$. Given a model for the intensity $\alpha()$, the maximum likelihood estimator of $\alpha()$ is obtained by maximizing the likelihood

$$L(\alpha()) \equiv \prod_{i=1}^n g(\bar{A}_i \mid X_i) = \prod_{i=1}^n \prod_t \alpha(t \mid \mathcal{F}_i(t))^{dA_i(t)} \{1 - \alpha(t \mid \mathcal{F}_i(t))\}^{1-dA_i(t)}.$$

We refer to Section 3.1 of Chapter 3 for a detailed discussion of estimation of α under discrete or continuous censoring schemes using logistic regression or Cox proportional hazards models. If C is continuous and one uses the Cox proportional hazards model, then the discrete baseline hazard estimator Λ_{0n} must be smoothed since we will need an estimate of the actual Lebesgue density $g(c \mid X)$. For example, one can smooth Λ_{0n} by convolving it with a kernel:

$$\tilde{\Lambda}_{0n}(t) \equiv \int K(x - t/h) d\Lambda_{0n}(x).$$

This smoothing method is theoretically investigated in Andersen, Borgan, Gill, and Keiding (1993).

4.2 Cause Specific Monitoring Schemes

In some applications, the full data are monitored at the minimum of two competing monitoring times coming from different monitoring mechanisms. For example, in a carcinogenicity experiment, a mouse is monitored at one of the planned sacrificing times (highly discrete) or at natural death (continuous). In this situation, one observes (C, J), where C is the monitoring time and J indexes the cause. One now needs a model for the monitoring intensity $\alpha(t)$ that acknowledges that C is an outcome of competing monitoring times that might follow (e.g.) Cox proportional hazards models using different subsets of covariates. For that purpose, one should extend

our data structure to
$$Y = (C, J, X_1(C), \bar{X}_2(C)),$$
where (C, J) now represents the joint censoring variable with conditional distribution G, given X. We can identify the joint censoring variable by the random process $A(t) = (A_1(t), \ldots, A_J(t))$, where $A_j(t) = I(C \leq t, J = j)$, $j = 1, \ldots, J$.

Since the outcome of J does not affect the censoring of $X = (X_1, X_2)$ and only affects the G part of the likelihood, it follows that the class of all estimating functions for μ is identical to the class of estimating functions for μ for the reduced data structure $(C, X_1(C), \bar{X}_2(C))$ as presented in this chapter. The estimating functions only require an estimate of conditional density of C, given X, that could be fit with the reduced data structure $(C, \bar{X}(C))$. However, if knowledge is available on the cause-specific intensities of A_j, then the following modeling strategy is sensible.

Under CAR, the G part of the density of $P_{F_X,G}$ is in the discrete case given by:
$$g(A \mid X) = \prod_t \prod_j \alpha_j(t)^{dA_j(t)} (1 - \alpha_j(t))^{1-dA_j(t)},$$
where $\alpha_j(t) = E(dA_j(t) \mid \mathcal{F}_j(t))$, $\mathcal{F}_j(t) \equiv (A_1(t), \ldots, A_{j-1}(t), \mathcal{F}(t))$, $j = 1, \ldots, J$, and $\mathcal{F}(t) = (\bar{A}(t-), \bar{X}_2(\min(C, t)))$. In the continuous case, this expression for $g(A \mid X)$ reduces to the partial likelihood of the multivariate counting process $A(t) = (A_1(t), \ldots, A_J(t))$ w.r.t. $\mathcal{F}(t)$ as defined in Andersen, Borgan, Gill, and Keiding (1993),
$$g(A \mid X) = \prod_t \prod_j \alpha_j(t)^{dA_j(t)} (1 - \alpha_j(t)dt)^{1-dA_j(t)},$$
where $\alpha_j(t) = E(dA_j(t) \mid \mathcal{F}(t))$ is the intensity of $A_j(t)$ w.r.t. history $\mathcal{F}(t)$. This now implies a model and method of estimation of the intensity of $A_\cdot(t) \equiv I(C \leq t) = \sum_{j=1}^J A_j(t)$; that is, the intensity of the monitoring time $C = \min(C_1, \ldots, C_J)$ and thereby of its conditional density $g(C \mid X)$.

4.2.1 Overview

In this chapter, we apply the general methodology presented in Chapter 2. Firstly, in Section 4.2 we define the optimal mapping from full data estimating functions into observed data estimating functions and provide the corresponding estimating function methods. If the full data model is nonparametric then there is only one full data estimating function so the method in Section 4.2 yields locally efficient estimators of μ without further work. However, for non saturated full data models, locally efficient estimation requires estimation of the optimal choice of the full data estimating function. In Section 4.3, we study estimation of the optimal index

236   4. Cross-Sectional Data and Right-Censored Data Combined

of the full data estimating function in a multivariate generalized linear regression model, thereby providing us with locally efficient estimators for this class of full data models. Section 4.4 and 4.5 apply the methods to two special cases. In Section 4.4, we apply the methods to obtain a locally efficient estimator of regression parameters when observing current status data of a failure time T and time-dependent covariates observed up until the monitoring time. In Section 4.5, we provide the locally efficient estimation methodology for current status data when subjects can die before being monitored.

4.3 The Optimal Mapping into Observed Data Estimating Functions

Let $\{D_h(\cdot \mid \mu, \rho) : h \in \mathcal{H}^F\}$ be a class of full data estimating functions for μ that are orthogonal to the nuisance tangent space in the sense that they satisfy $D_h(X \mid \mu(F_X), \rho(F_X)) \in T_{nuis}^{F,\perp}(F_X)$ for all $h \in \mathcal{H}^F$ and all $F_X \in \mathcal{M}^F$.

Let $IC_0(Y \mid G, D_h)$ be a given mapping from full data estimating functions into observed data estimating functions satisfying $E(IC_0(Y \mid G, D_h) \mid X) = D_h(X)$ F_X-a.e. for full data estimating functions D_h in a non-empty set $\mathcal{D}(\rho_1(F_X), G)$, where $\mathcal{D}(\rho_1, G)$ is defined in (2.13). One now identifies a subset $\mathcal{H}^F(\mu, \rho, \rho_1, G) \subset \mathcal{H}^F$ so that for all $h \in \mathcal{H}^F(\mu, \rho, \rho_1, G)$ $E_G(IC_0(Y \mid G, D_h(\cdot \mid \mu, \rho) \mid X) = D_h(X \mid \mu, \rho)$ F_X-a.e. (for all possible μ, ρ, G). As mentioned in Chapter 2, we now reparametrize the full data structure estimating functions as $D_h^r(\cdot \mid \mu, (\rho, \rho_1, G)) \equiv D_{\Pi(h \mid \mathcal{H}(\mu, \rho, \rho_1, G))}(\cdot \mid \mu, \rho)$, where $\Pi(\cdot \mid \mathcal{H}(\mu, \rho, \rho_1, G))$ is a user-supplied mapping into $\mathcal{H}^F(\mu, \rho, \rho_1, G)$, which is the identity mapping on $h \in \mathcal{H}^F(\mu, \rho, \rho_1, G)$. In other words, $h \in \mathcal{H}^F(\mu, \rho, \rho_1, G)$ guarantees that $D_h(X \mid \mu, \rho) \in \mathcal{D}(\rho_1, G)$. Subsequently, for notational convenience, we denote this reparametrized class of estimating functions with $D_h(\cdot \mid \mu, \rho)$ again, where ρ is now the old ρ augmented with ρ_1 and G. The only purpose of this reparametrization is to define a class of estimating functions D_h indexed by a common index set $\mathcal{H}^F$ whose elements are a member of $T_{nuis}^{F,\perp}(F_X)$ and $\mathcal{D}(\rho_1(F_X), G)$ when evaluated at the true parameter values. In the next subsection, we show this for regression with current status data.

Given this class of full data estimating functions, we propose as mapping from full data estimating functions to observed data estimating functions $D_h \rightarrow IC(\cdot \mid Q, G, D_h) \equiv IC_0(\cdot \mid G, D_h) - \Pi(IC_0(\cdot \mid G, D_h) \mid T_{CAR})$, where T_{CAR} is defined as the tangent space of G at $P_{F_X,G}$ under the sole assumption (4.3). This space T_{CAR} equals the tangent space under CAR given by $\{V(Y) : E(V(Y) \mid X) = 0\}$ if (4.3) is equivalent with assuming CAR. This condition holds at many data-generating distributions (van der Laan, and Jewell, 2002). If it holds, then this mapping corresponds with

4.3. The Optimal Mapping into Observed Data Estimating Functions

the optimal mapping into observed data estimating functions (Chapter 2). Thus, strictly speaking, we should use a notation different from T_{CAR} for this space. We note that, if the condition does not hold at a particular data-generating distribution, then our closed-form optimal estimating function is not truly the efficient influence curve so that our resulting estimators are not fully efficient. Since in that case an efficient estimator will not be computationally feasible in the presence of time-dependent covariates, we still propose our mapping as the practical way to obtain high-quality estimators.

To avoid technical measurability conditions in establishing the projection onto T_{CAR}, we will assume that C is discrete. By making C discrete on an arbitrarily fine grid, all resulting formulas can be used for the continuous case as well. For a formal proof of the continuous case, see van der Vaart (2001). Arguing as in the proof of Theorem 1.1, we have

$$T_{CAR} = \overline{\left\{ \int H(t, \mathcal{F}(t)) dM_G(t) : H \right\}},$$

where $dM_G(t) = dA(t) - \alpha(t \mid \mathcal{F}(t))$. Since C is censored by a random T, we have $dM_G(t) = I(C \in dt, C < T) - I(\min(C,T) \geq t)\Lambda_{C|X}(dt \mid X)$. If T is a fixed endpoint with $P(C \leq T) = 1$ so that C is always observed, then we have $dM(t) = I(C \in dt) - I(C \geq t)\Lambda_{C|X}(dt \mid X)$. By Theorem 1.1, we have that the projection $\Pi(V \mid T_{CAR})$ is given by

$$\int \{E(V(Y) \mid A(t) = 1, \mathcal{F}(t)) - E(V(Y) \mid A(t) = 0, \mathcal{F}(t))\} dM_G(t)$$

$$= \int \{E(V(Y) \mid C = t, \bar{X}_2(t)) - E(V(Y) \mid C > t, \bar{X}_2(t))\} dM_G(t).$$

Note that these representations of the projections are also applicable if C is continuous. An alternative representation of this projection (for discrete C) is simply

$$\sum_{\{j:t_j \leq C\}} E(V(Y) \mid \bar{A}(t_j-), A(t_j), \bar{X}_2(t_j)) - E(V(Y) \mid \bar{A}(t_j-), \bar{X}_2(t_j)).$$
(4.4)

Given a choice for the full data estimating function $D_h(\cdot \mid \mu, \rho)$, we use as the estimating function for μ

$$IC(Y \mid Q(F_X, G), G, D_h(\cdot \mid \mu, \rho)) = IC_0(Y \mid G, D_h) - IC_{CAR}(Y \mid Q, G),$$
(4.5)

where

$$IC_{CAR}(Y \mid Q(F_X, G), G) = \int Q(F_X, G)(t, \bar{X}_2(t)) dM(t),$$
(4.6)

and $Q(F_X, G)$ is given by

$$E_{P_{F_X, G}} \{IC_0(Y \mid G, D_h) \mid C = t, \bar{X}_2(t)) - IC_0(Y \mid G, D_h) \mid C > t, \bar{X}_2(t))\}.$$

Given estimators Q_n, G_n, h_n and ρ_n, one estimates μ with the solution μ_n of the corresponding estimating equation,

$$0 = \frac{1}{n}\sum_{i=1}^{n} IC(Y_i \mid Q_n, G_n, D_{h_n}(\cdot \mid \mu, \rho_n)).$$

We will now discuss estimation of Q. The first method is directly motivated by the representation (4.4). Let μ_n^0 be an initial estimator of μ. In absolute generality, we can estimate these two conditional expectations defining Q (semi)parametrically by regressing $IC_0(Y \mid G_n, D_{h_n}(Y \mid \mu_n^0, \rho_n))$ onto t and covariates extracted from the past $(\bar{A}(t-), A(t), \bar{X}_2(\min(t,C)))$ and subsequently evaluating the fitted regression at each t by substituting for $\bar{A}(t-), A(t)$ values $\bar{A}(t-) = 0, A(t) = 1$, and $\bar{A}(t) = 0$, respectively. Here, one assumes a regression model that acknowledges that for $t > \min(T, C)$ the regression is known (either zero or the outcome itself): For example, $E(IC_0(Y) \mid \bar{A}(t), \bar{X}_2(\min(t,C))) = I(\min(T,C) > t) g_t(W(t) \mid \beta)$, where $W(t)$ are covariates extracted from $(\bar{A}(t), \bar{X}_2(\min(t,C)))$. Then, each subject contributes multiple observations $(\widehat{IC_0}(Y), t = j, \bar{A}(j), \bar{X}_2(j))$, $t_j \leq \min(C,T)$. Note that this estimation procedure is equivalent with directly fitting (4.4).

Another method would be to regress an estimate $IC_0(Y \mid G_n, D_{h_n}(\cdot \mid \mu_n^0, \rho_n))$ onto covariates extracted from $\bar{X}_2(t)$ among observations with $C \approx t$ (smoothing) and $C > t$, respectively, and subsequently smooth all of these t-specific regressions over t taking into account the variance of each of these t-specific regression estimates by (e.g.) weighting them by 1 over the number of observations used to fit the regression.

Finally, one can fully parametrize the likelihood of the observed data structure Y as in Section 1.6 and estimate $P_{F_X,G}$ with a maximum likelihood estimator P_{F_n,G_n}. The observed data structure Y can be represented as sequential data collected in the following ordering $X_2(1), A(1), X_{1,A(1)}(1), \ldots, X_{2,\bar{A}(k-1)}(k), A(k), X_{1,\bar{A}(k)}(k))$, where we define $A(j) = I(C = j)$, $X_{2,\bar{A}(j-1)}(j) = \bar{X}_2(\min(j,C))$ and $X_{1,\bar{A}(j)}(j) = X_1(j)I(C = j)$. Note that $A(j)$ appears before $X_{1,\bar{A}(j)}(j)$. One can now simply apply the corresponding likelihood parametrization as presented in Section 1.6. In particular, the conditional expectations defining $Q(F_n, G_n)$ can now be evaluated with the Monte-Carlo simulation method described in detail in Section 1.6. To be specific, a parametrization of the likelihood of the observed data structure $Y = (C, X_1(C), \bar{X}_2(C))$ is given by

$$\prod_{t \in [0,C]} P(X_2(t) \mid \bar{X}_2(t-), C \geq t)\, P(X_1(t) \mid \bar{X}_2(t), C = t)\big|_{t=C}.$$

Thus one needs to pose models for $P(X_2(t) \mid \bar{X}_2(t-)) = P(X_2(t) \mid \bar{X}_2(t-), C \geq t)$ and $P(X_1(t) \mid \bar{X}_2(t)) = P(X_1(t) \mid \bar{X}_2(t), C = t)$ and estimate the unknown parameters by maximizing the likelihood of $Y_1, \ldots, Y_n$.

4.3. The Optimal Mapping into Observed Data Estimating Functions

4.3.1 Identifiability condition

A fundamental condition in our asymptotic Theorem 2.4 for the estimator μ_n of μ is that $\mathcal{D}(\rho_1(F_X), G_1)$ is non empty so that the reparametrized full data estimating functions satisfy that $D_h(X \mid \mu(F_X), \rho(F_X, G_1)) \in \mathcal{D}(\rho_1(F_X), G_1) \cap T_{nuis}^{F, \perp}(F_X)$. This set of allowed full data functions $\mathcal{D}(\rho_1(F_X), G)$ is defined in (2.13) as the set of full data structure estimating functions D for which $E(IC_0(Y \mid G, D) \mid X) = D(X)$ F_X-a.e. If

$$1 > E(dA(t) \mid C \geq t, T \geq t, \bar{X}_2(t)) > 0 \text{ a.e.,} \qquad (4.7)$$

then this will hold for each possible full data structure estimating function. This condition is needed to have nonparametric identifiability of F_X: it says that, at any point in time t at which the subject is not yet monitored, the decision to be monitored needs to be non deterministic, whatever the observed past might have been. The assumption (4.7) can be a model assumption, but if it is not a reasonable assumption for the particular application of interest, then it can typically be weakened by doing the reparametrization in the manner described above and in Subsection 2.3.1 of Chapter 2. This is only possible if the set $\mathcal{D}(\rho_1(F_X), G)$ is not empty. Otherwise, our particular parameter of interest is simply not estimable based on $IC_0(Y \mid G, D)$. We showed this reparametrization in action in a right-censored data example covered in Examples 2.3, 2.4, and 2.5 in Chapter 2. We refer the reader to this worked-out example. In the next example, we illustrate it for estimation of a regression parameter with current status data on the outcome.

Example 4.4 (Regression with current status data) Suppose that we observe $Y = (C, I(T_1 \leq C), \bar{L}(C))$, where T_1 is the time variable of interest. Consider a regression model $T_1 = Z^\top \beta + \epsilon$ of T_1 on observed baseline covariates $Z \in L(0)$, where $E(K(\epsilon(\beta) \mid Z) = 0$ for a given monotone function K with support $[-\tau, \tau]$. The full data estimating functions are $D_h(T_1, Z \mid \beta) = h(Z) K_\beta(T_1, Z)$, where $h \in \mathcal{H}^F = \{h(Z) : \| h \|_\infty < \infty\}$ and $K_\beta(T_1, Z) = K(T_1 - Z^\top \beta)$. In Chapter 2, we derived the IPCW mapping for current status data structures

$$IC_0(Y \mid G, D_h) \equiv \frac{D'_h(C, Z)\bar{\Delta}}{g(C \mid X)} + D_h(\alpha_X, Z)$$

$$= h(Z) \left(\frac{K'_\beta(C, Z)\bar{\Delta}}{g(C \mid X)} + K_\beta(\alpha_X, Z) \right), \qquad (4.8)$$

where D' is the derivative of D with respect to the first argument, $K'_\beta(t, Z)$ is the derivative with respect to t of $K(t - Z^\top \beta)$, α_X is the left endpoint in the support of $g(\cdot \mid X)$, and $\bar{\Delta} = 1 - \Delta$. If $g(\cdot \mid X)$ is centered at $Z^\top \beta$, then one would expect to have $K_\beta(\alpha_X, Z) = K(-\tau)$ is known, but, in general, one might need to estimate α_X from the data.

We will now derive an index set $\mathcal{H}(\beta, G)$ so that for $h \in \mathcal{H}(\beta, G)$ $E(IC_0(Y \mid G, D_h(\cdot \mid \beta)) \mid X) = D_h(X \mid \beta)$ and subsequently do the reparametrization of our restricted class of estimating functions.

Theorem 4.1 *(Andrews, van der Laan, and Robins, 2002) We assume that (i) K is selected to be constant outside $[-\tau, \tau]$ and to be strictly increasing with two continuous derivatives on $[-\tau, \tau]$, (ii) $Pr(-\tau < \epsilon < \tau \mid Z) > \delta_1 > 0$ with probability 1 for some $\delta_1 > 0$, (iii) the support of $g(\cdot \mid X)$ is an open interval (α_W, α^Y) with $W = (Z, L(0))$ being the baseline covariates, and (iv) $Pr(Z \in \mathcal{Z}(\beta, G)) > \delta_2 > 0$ for some $\delta_2 > 0$, where*

$$\mathcal{Z}(\beta, G) \equiv \{z : \alpha^Y - \beta z > \min(T_1 - \beta z, \tau), \alpha_W - \beta z < \max(T_1 - \beta z, -\tau)\}, \tag{4.9}$$

where the inequalities need to hold $F_{X \mid Z=z}$ a.e. Assume that $\mathcal{Z}(\beta, G)$ is non empty. We define

$$\mathcal{H}^F(\beta, G) = \{h(Z)I(Z \in \mathcal{Z}(\beta, G)) : \sup_z \mid h(z) \mid < \infty\}.$$

If $h \in \mathcal{H}^F(\beta, G)$, then $E(IC_0(Y \mid G, D_h(\cdot \mid \beta)) \mid X) = D_h(X \mid \beta)$.

Therefore, under the conditions of theorem 4.1, we have that

$$\mathcal{D}(\rho_1(F_X), G) \supset \mathcal{D}(\beta, G) = \{D_h(\cdot \mid \beta) : h \in \mathcal{H}^F(\beta, G)\}.$$

Proof of theorem. Condition (ii) teaches us that the estimating function is not zero with probability one. Using short-hand notation $\mathcal{Z} = \mathcal{Z}(\beta, G)$, the conditional expectation is given by (by (iii))

$$I(Z \in \mathcal{Z})h(Z) \int_{\alpha_W}^{\max(\min(T_1, \alpha^Y), \alpha_W)} K'_\beta(c, Z) dc + K_\beta(\alpha_W, Z).$$

This can be rewritten as

$$I(Z \in \mathcal{Z})h(Z)K_\beta(\max(\min(T_1, \alpha^Y), \alpha_W), Z)$$

$$= I(Z \in \mathcal{Z})h(Z)K(\max(\min(\epsilon, \alpha^Y - \beta Z), \alpha_W - \beta Z))$$

$$= I(Z \in \mathcal{Z})h(Z)K(\max(\min(\epsilon, \alpha^Y - \beta Z), -\tau)) \text{ by (i), (iv) and (4.9)}$$

$$= I(Z \in \mathcal{Z})h(Z)K(\min(\epsilon, \alpha^Y - \beta Z)) \text{ by (i)}$$

$$= I(Z \in \mathcal{Z})h(Z)K(\min(\epsilon, \tau)) \text{ by (iv) and (4.9)}$$

$$= I(Z \in \mathcal{Z})h(Z)K(\epsilon) \text{ by (i)}.$$

This proves the theorem. □

Thus, our reparametrized class of full data estimating functions is given by

$$\{D_h(X \mid \beta, \rho = G) \equiv h(Z)I(Z \in \mathcal{Z}(\beta, G))K(\epsilon(\beta)) : h \in \mathcal{H}^F\}.$$

4.3. The Optimal Mapping into Observed Data Estimating Functions   241

The IPCW estimating functions $IC_0(Y \mid G, D_h(\cdot \mid \beta, \rho))$ are given by

$$IC_0(Y) = \frac{h(Z)I(Z \in \mathcal{Z}(\beta, G))K(\epsilon(\beta))\overline{\Delta}}{g(C \mid X)} + D_h(\alpha_X, Z)$$

$$= h(Z)I(Z \in \mathcal{Z}(\beta, G))\left(\frac{K'_\beta(C, Z)\overline{\Delta}}{g(C \mid X)} + K_\beta(\alpha_X, Z)\right) \quad (4.10)$$

Under regularity conditions, it can be shown that the asymptotics of the estimator β_n defined by the solution of the corresponding estimating equation is asymptotically equivalent with the estimator setting (β, G) equal to the truth in $\mathcal{Z}(\beta, G)$ (as if it is known to the user). This is shown in the same way as carried out for the right-censored data structure in Examples 2.3, 2.4, and 2.5 in Chapter 2. □

4.3.2 Estimation of a parameter on which we have current status data

Suppose that $X_1(t) = N(t) = \sum_{j=1}^{k} I(T_j \leq t)$ is a counting process with jumps at random times $T_1 < T_2 < \ldots < T_k$ or $X_1(t) = (I(T_1 \leq t), \ldots, I(T_k \leq t))$ is a multivariate failure time process. Assume also that the parameter of interest is either a smooth functional such as $\mu = \int r(t)(1 - F_j(t))dt$ of the marginal distribution F_j of T_j or a regression parameter of a generalized regression model with outcome T_j and covariates extracted from the baseline covariates $X_2(0)$. If one assumes a saturated full data model or this generalized regression full data model, then the full data estimating functions are $D(T_j \mid \mu) = R(T_j) - \mu$ with $R(T_j) = \int_0^{T_j} r(s)ds$ or $\{h(Z)(T_j - m(\beta \mid Z)) : h\}$, respectively. Consequently, these estimating functions are only functions of T_j and Z. In general, if the full data model has variation-independent parameters for the distribution of (T_j, Z) and X, given (T_j, Z), then the full data estimating functions for a parameter μ of the distribution of (T_j, Z) will only be a function of (T_j, Z). Consider such a full data estimating function $D(T_j, Z \mid \mu)$, where we suppress the possible dependence on a nuisance parameter ρ. Consider

$$IC_0(Y \mid G, D) = D'(C, Z \mid \mu)\frac{I(T_j > C)}{g(C \mid X)} + D(a, Z \mid \mu), \quad (4.11)$$

where $D'(t, Z) \equiv d/dt D(t, Z)$ if C is continuous, and if C is discrete on a grid $t_1 < t_2 < \ldots < t_K$, then $D'(t, Z) = D(t_{j+1}, Z) - D(t_j, Z)$, $t \in [t_j, t_{j+1})$. Here a is the left-support point of $g(\cdot \mid X)$, which can thus be a function of $X_2(0)$. Indeed, if C is continuous and for all c, $I(c < T_j)D'(c, Z)/g(c \mid X) < \infty$ F_X-a.e., then we have

$$E(IC_0(Y \mid G, D) \mid X) = \int_a^{T_j} D'(c, Z)dc + D(a, Z \mid \mu)$$
$$= D(T_j, Z).$$

Similarly, this holds if C is discrete and $D'(t, Z)$ is defined accordingly.

Let us now consider the projection formula (4.6) in more detail for this choice of $V = IC_0(Y)$. Firstly, note that $D(a, Z \mid \mu)$ cancels out. Secondly, notice that

$$E(IC_0(Y) \mid G, D) \mid C = t, \bar{X}_2(t)) = \frac{D'(t, Z \mid \mu)}{g(t \mid X)} \bar{F}_j(t \mid \bar{X}_2(t)) + D(a, Z \mid \mu),$$

where $\bar{F}_j(t \mid \bar{X}_2(t)) = P(T_j > t \mid \bar{X}_2(t))$. Let $g(c \mid X)$ be the density w.r.t. λ, where λ is either the Lebesgue measure (g is continuous) or the counting measure on a set of grid points (g is discrete), so $d\lambda(c) = dc$ or $d\lambda(c) = \delta_c$, where δ_c is 1 if c is one of the grid points and zero otherwise. By first conditioning on $X, C > t$ and noting that $g(c \mid X, C > t) = I(C > t)g(c \mid X)/\bar{G}(t \mid X)$, one obtains that $E(IC_0(Y) \mid C > t, \bar{X}_2(t)) - D(a, Z \mid \mu)$ can be expressed as

$$E\left(\frac{1}{\bar{G}(t \mid X)} \int_{(t,\infty)} D'(c, Z \mid \mu) I(T_j > c) d\lambda(c) \mid C > t, \bar{X}_2(t)\right)$$
$$= \frac{1}{\bar{G}(t \mid X)} \int_{(t,\infty)} D'(c, Z \mid \mu) \bar{F}_j(c \mid \bar{X}_2(t)) d\lambda(c).$$

This proves the following representation of the class (4.5) of observed data estimating functions:

$$IC(Y \mid F_X, G, D_h) = D'(C, Z \mid \mu) \frac{I(T_j > C)}{g(C \mid X)} + D(a, Z \mid \mu) \quad (4.12)$$
$$- \int \left\{ \frac{D'(t, Z \mid \mu)}{g(t \mid X)} \bar{F}_j(t \mid \bar{X}_2(t)) \right\} dM(t)$$
$$+ \int \left\{ \frac{1}{\bar{G}(t \mid X)} \int_{(t,\infty)} D'(c, Z \mid \mu) \bar{F}_j(c \mid \bar{X}_2(t)) d\lambda(c) \right\} dM(t).$$

For the purpose of estimation of the nuisance parameters in these estimating functions, one could parametrize the likelihood of Y as explained in section 4.2 and estimate $F_j(c \mid \bar{X}_2(t))$ with the corresponding maximum likelihood estimator. Recall that the likelihood is parametrized by $P(N(t) = m \mid \bar{X}_2(t), C = t)$ while, by noting that $T_j < t$ is equivalent with $N(t) > j$, $F_j(c \mid \bar{X}_2(t)) = P(N(t) > j \mid \bar{X}_2(t), C = t)$. Alternatively, one can still use the representation $IC(Y \mid F_X, G, D_h) = IC(Y \mid Q(F_X, G), G, D_h)$ in terms of the observed data conditional expectations defining Q and estimate them in the manner explained above. Direct estimation of $F_j(c \mid \bar{X}_2(t))$ using inverse weighting as in IC_0 is discussed in Section 4.4. We estimate μ with the solution μ_n corresponding with the estimating equation $0 = \sum_i IC(Y_i \mid F_n, G_n, D_{h_n}(\cdot \mid \mu))$. An initial estimator μ_n^0 can be defined as a solution of the estimating equation $\sum_i IC_0(Y_i \mid G_n, D_{h_n}(\cdot \mid \mu)) = 0$.

4.3. The Optimal Mapping into Observed Data Estimating Functions   243

Example 4.5 (Continuation of Example 4.1) Let us consider the menopause example in which $X_j(t) = I(J = j, T \leq t)$ $j = 1, 2$, with T now the age at menopause. Let $F_j(t) = P(T \leq t, J = j)$, $j = 1, 2$. Suppose that the full data model is nonparametric. Formula (4.12) is not directly applicable because of the inclusion of J in the full data processes $X_j(t)$, $j = 1, 2$. However, the derivation is completely analogous.

Let us represent a full data structure estimating function as $D(T, J, Z)$. As general initial mapping, we can choose the following analogue of (4.11):

$$IC_0(Y \mid G, D) = -D'(C, J, Z)\frac{I(T \leq C)}{g(C \mid X)} + D(\infty, J, Z \mid \mu).$$

Note that, given an estimating function $D(T, J, Z \mid \mu)$, indeed $E(IC_0(Y \mid G, D) \mid X) = D(T, J, Z \mid \mu)$. In addition, note that, if $T \leq C$, then J is always observed so that the first term is indeed a function of the observed data. Here we assume that $D(\infty, J, Z \mid \mu)$ reduces to a function of the observed data as well. For example, suppose that C is continuous and that the parameter of interest is a smooth functional $\mu = \int r(t)F_1(t)dt$ of F_1. In this case, the only full data estimating function is $D(X_1 \mid \mu) = \int r(t)I(J = 1, T \leq t)dt - \mu$ so that

$$IC_0(Y \mid G, D) = r(C)I(J = 1)\frac{I(T \leq C)}{g(C \mid X)} - \mu.$$

The projection IC_{CAR} of IC_0 onto T_{CAR} is given by $\int \{E(IC_0(Y) \mid C = t, \bar{X}_2(t)) - E(IC_0(Y) \mid C > t, \bar{X}_2(t))dM_G(t)$, which provides us with the efficient influence function $IC(Y \mid Q(F_X, G), G, D)$ for this parameter μ. □

4.3.3 Estimation of a parameter on which we have right-censored data

If the parameter of interest is a component of the distribution of X_2, then the full data estimating functions are functions of X_2 so that for any $D(X_2)$ we can define

$$IC_0(Y \mid G, D) = D(X_2)\frac{I(C \geq T)}{\bar{G}(T \mid X)}.$$

In this case, we have that (4.5) reduces to the optimal mapping given in Chapter 3 for the right-censored data structure $(C, \bar{X}_2(C))$ ignoring the current status data on X_1:

$$\begin{aligned}IC(Y \mid Q, G, D) &= IC_0(Y \mid G, D) \\ &+ \int E(IC_0(Y \mid G, D) \mid \bar{X}_2(t), C > t)dM_G(t).\end{aligned} \quad (4.13)$$

Estimation of $Q(t, \mathcal{F}(t)) = -E(IC_0(Y \mid G, D) \mid \bar{X}_2(t), C > t)$ can be carried out as discussed above and in Chapter 3.

Example 4.6 (Continuation of Example 4.1) Let us consider the menopause example in which $X_j(t) = I(J = j, T \leq t)$ $j = 1, 2$. Let $F_j(t) = P(T \leq t, J = j)$, $j = 1, 2$. Suppose that the full data model is nonparametric. If the parameter of interest is $\mu = F_2(t)$, then the full data estimating function is $D(T, J) = I(T \leq t, J = 2) - F_2(t)$, and we can set

$$IC_0(Y \mid G, D) = (I(T \leq t, J = 2) - \mu) \frac{I(C \geq T)}{\bar{G}(T \mid X)}.$$

The optimal estimating function is (4.13) with this choice of IC_0. □

4.3.4 Estimation of a joint-distribution parameter on which we have current status data and right-censored data

Consider now the special case where $X_1(t) = (I(T_1 \leq t), L_1(t))$ and $X_2(t) = (I(T_2 \leq t), L_2(t))$ for some unordered time variables T_1, T_2 and that parameters of the joint distribution of (T_1, T_2) are of interest. In this case, it is actually possible to identify the joint distribution of (T_1, T_2) from the observed data and, in particular, to obtain estimating functions for smooth functionals of this joint distribution; namely, consider a full data estimating function $D_1(T_1)D_2(T_2)$, where D_1 is differentiable in T_1 with derivative d_1. Suppose that the parameter of interest is $\mu = ED_1(T_1)D_2(T_2)$. Note that the bivariate distribution of (T_1, T_2) is identified by the expected value of a countable collection $D_{1j}(T_1)D_{2j}(T_2)$, $j = 1, \ldots$, of basis functions. In other words, the class of estimating functions $\{D_1(T_1)D_2(T_2) : D_1, D_2\}$, D_1, D_2 ranging over smooth functions, identifies enough smooth functionals of the bivariate distribution so that the whole bivariate distribution is identified. Alternatively, if we set $D_1(T_1) = K((T_1 - t_1)/h)/h$ equal to a kernel K centered at t_1 with bandwidth h and $D_2(T_2) = I(T_2 \leq t_2)$, then $ED_1(T_1)D_2(T_2)$ approximates $d/dt_1 F(t_1, t_2)$ for $h \to 0$. Thus, for fixed h, this expectation μ defines a regular root-n-estimable parameter to which we can apply our methodology.

Consider the following mapping applied to such full data estimating functions $D(T_1, T_2) = D_1(T_1)D_2(T_2)$:

$$IC_0(Y \mid G, D) = \frac{d_1(C)D_2(T_2)I(T_2 < C < T_1)}{g(C \mid X)} + \frac{D_1(T_2)D_2(T_2)I(T_2 < C)}{\bar{G}(T_2 \mid X)}.$$

It is easily verified that, under the conditions 1) $D(T_1, T_2)I(\bar{G}(T_2 \mid X) > 0) = D(T_1, T_2)$ F_X-a.e. and 2) $\sup_c d_1(c)D_2(T_2)I(T_2 < c < T_1)/g(c \mid X) < \infty$ F_X-a.e., we indeed have $E(IC_0(Y \mid G, D) \mid X) = D_1(T_1)D_2(T_2)$ F_X-a.e. Using this estimating function with $D(T_1, T_2) = K((T_1 - t_1)/h)/hI(T_2 \leq t_2)$ yields an estimate of a smooth approximation of the irregular parameter $d/dt_1 P(T_1 \leq t_1, T_2 \leq t_2)$ at (t_1, t_2). The projection IC_{CAR} of IC_0 onto T_{CAR} is given by the formula (4.6). Thus the optimal estimating function for $\mu = ED(T_1, T_2)$ in the nonparametric full data model is

$$IC_0(Y \mid G, D) - \mu$$
$$- \int \{E(IC_0(Y) \mid C = u, \bar{X}_2(u)) - E(IC_0(Y) \mid C > u, \bar{X}_2(u))\} dM_G(u).$$

The above approach can be generalized to derive the class of estimating functions for parameters of the bivariate distribution of (T_1, T_2), given a set of baseline covariates, under a particular full data model such as the multivariate generalized linear regression model. In the next section, we study estimation of the optimal index h_{opt} if the full data model is a multivariate generalized linear regression model.

4.4 Estimation of the Optimal Index in the MGLM

Consider the case where $X_1(t) = N(t) = \sum_{j=1}^{p} I(T_j \leq t)$ is a counting process with jumps at random times $T_1 < T_2 < \ldots < T_p$. Let us assume the multivariate generalized linear regression model $\vec{T} = g(X^* \mid \beta) + \epsilon$, where, for a known monotone function K, $E(K(\epsilon) \mid X^*) = 0$ and $X^* \subset X_2(0)$ are always observed baseline covariates. Here $g(X^* \mid \beta)$ and ϵ are p-dimensional vectors, and let $\beta \in \mathbb{R}^q$ be q-dimensional. By Lemma 2.1, we have $\Pi_{F_X}(D \mid T_{nuis}^{F\perp}) = h_{F_X}(D)(X^*) K(\epsilon)$ for a specified explicit mapping $h_{F_X} : L_0^2(F_X)^q \to \mathcal{H}^F(F_X)$ given by

$$h_{F_X}(D) = E(\{D(X) - E(D \mid X^*)\} K(\epsilon)^\top \mid X^*) E(K(\epsilon) K(\epsilon)^\top \mid X^*)^{-1}.$$

Note that h_{F_X} maps an r-dimensional function D into an $r \times p$ matrix function of X^*.

To obtain the optimal index h_{opt}, we apply Theorem 2.8, which says that

$$h_{opt\ p \times p} = h_{eff\ q \times p} h_{F_X}(I^{-1}(K))_{p \times p}^{-1},$$

where the $q \times p$ matrix $h_{eff}(F_X)(X^*)$ identifying the efficient score $h_{eff}(F_X)(X^*) K(\epsilon)$ (see Lemma 2.1) is given by

$$h_{eff}(F_X) = d/d\beta g(X^* \mid \beta)_{q \times p}^\top \text{diag}(E(K'(\epsilon) \mid X^*)) E(K(\epsilon) K(\epsilon)^\top \mid X^*)^{-1},$$

(the last two factors are $p \times p$-matrices) $I^{-1}(K) = I_{F_X,G}^{-1}(K)$ is the inverse of the nonparametric information operator applied to K, and

$$h_{F_X}(I^{-1}(K)) = E(I^{-1}(K)(X) K(\epsilon)^\top \mid X^*) E(K(\epsilon) K(\epsilon)^\top \mid X^*)^{-1}.$$

We consider two approaches for estimation of h_{opt}. Firstly, if one carries out maximum likelihood estimation according to a fully parametrized likelihood of the observed data, then one can estimate h_{opt} with the substitution estimator $h_{opt}(F_{X,n}, G_n)$: see the end of section 4.2. However, an easy method is the following. Theorem 2.8 expresses h_{opt} as

$$h_{opt} = h_{eff}(X^*)E(IC(Y \mid K)IC(Y \mid K)^\top \mid X^*)E(K(\epsilon)K(\epsilon)^\top \mid X^*)^{-1}, \quad (4.14)$$

where we used shorthand notation $IC(Y \mid K) = IC(Y \mid Q, G, K)$. This representation (4.14) is now ready to be estimated. To construct our estimation function, we already needed to estimate $IC(Y \mid Q, G, D)$. For every $(k, l) \in \{1, \ldots, p\}^2$, we can now construct the n observations

$$O_{kl,i} \equiv IC(Y_i \mid Q_n, G_n, K_{k,n})IC(Y_i \mid Q_n, G_n, K_{l,n}).$$

Subsequently, we assume a regression model for $E(O_{k,l} \mid X^*)$ and estimate it by regressing $O_{kl,i}$ onto X^* accordingly: $(k, l) \in \{1, \ldots, p\}^2$. This yields an estimate of $E(IC(Y \mid Q, G, K)IC(Y \mid Q, G, K)^\top \mid X^*)$. In this way, we obtain an easy-to-compute estimator of h_{opt}.

Estimation of the optimal index involves estimation of $h_{F_X}(D) = E(DK(\epsilon)^\top \mid X^*)E(K(\epsilon)K(\epsilon)^\top \mid X^*)^{-1}$ for a given function $D \in \mathcal{L}(\mathcal{X})$. One can represent the conditional expectations in $h_{F_X}(D)$ with regressions using our inverse weighting mapping $IC_0(Y \mid G, D)$: for any function $D(X)$,

$$E(D(X) \mid X^*) = E(IC_0(Y \mid G, D) \mid X^*). \quad (4.15)$$

Thus, we can estimate $E(D(X) \mid X^*)$ by regressing $\widehat{IC}_0(Y)$ onto the baseline covariates X^* according to some guessed regression model.

4.5 Example: Current Status Data with Time-Dependent Covariates

Consider a study in which the time variable of interest T is the onset of a disease or tumor or an infection time that cannot be directly observed. Let $R(t) = I(T \leq t)$. Let C be a monitoring time at which one observes $R(C) = I(T \leq C)$; that is, whether the onset occurred or not. Let $L(t)$ represent measurements taken on the subject at time t. The full data structure is $X = (T, \bar{L}(\tau)) \sim F_X$, where τ is the endpoint of the support of T. The observed data structure is

$$Y = (C, R(C), \bar{L}(C)).$$

Let $\mu = \mu(F_X)$ be the parameter of interest, and we will assume CAR on the conditional distribution of C, given X.

We first review previous work on current status data (C, Δ) when covariate data are absent. Previous work and examples of pure current status data (i.e., without covariates) can be found in Diamond, McDonald, and Shah (1986), Portier (1986), Portier and Dinse (1987), Jewell and Shiboski (1990), Diamond and McDonald (1991), Keiding (1991), and Sun and Kalbfleish (1993), among several others. In its nonparametric setting, it is also known as interval censoring, case I (Groeneboom, 1991; Groeneboom

4.5. Example: Current Status Data with Time-Dependent Covariates

and Wellner, 1992). Current status data commonly arise in epidemiological investigations of the natural history of disease and in animal tumorigenicity experiments. Jewell, Malani, and Vittinghoff (1994) give two examples that arise from studies of human immunodeficiency virus (HIV) disease, one of which we will reconsider in Section 4.5.12. In van der Laan, Bickel, and Jewell (1997), a regularized NPMLE is considered that allows using standard smoothing methods for densities or nonparametric regression.

In each of the aforementioned papers, inferences on the distribution of T were made under the assumptions that (i) T and C are independently distributed, (ii) no data are available on additional time-independent or time-dependent covariates, and (iii) no assumptions are made about the distribution, F_T, of T. The nonparametric maximum likelihood estimator (NPMLE) of F_T is the pooled adjacent violators estimator for the estimation of the monotone regression $F_T(t) = E(\Delta \mid C = t)$ of Barlow, Bartholomew, Bremner, and Brunk (1972), where $\Delta = I(T \leq C)$ is the current status indicator at time C. The asymptotic distribution of this estimator has been analyzed by Groeneboom and Wellner (1992), and efficiency of the NPMLE of smooth functionals of F_T (such as its mean and variance) has been proved by Groeneboom and Wellner (1992), van de Geer (1994), and Huang and Wellner (1995).

Notice that the data structure $Y = (C, \bar{R}(C), \bar{L}(C))$ is a special case of our general data structure (4.1) with $X_1(t) = R(t)$ and $X_2(t) = L(t)$. Therefore, we can apply the optimal estimating function $IC(Y \mid F_X, G, D_{h_{opt}}(\cdot \mid \mu))$ (4.12) given in Sections 4.2 and 4.3 for the nonparametric full data structure model and generalized regression model of T onto baseline covariates. For example, suppose that the parameter of interest is $\mu = \int r(t)(1 - F_T(t))dt$ for a given r and that the full data model is nonparametric. In this example, the optimal estimating function is $IC(Y \mid F_X, G, D_{opt}(\cdot \mid \mu))$ with $D_{opt}(T \mid \mu) = R(T) - \mu$, where $R(t) = \int_0^t r(s)ds$. In van der Laan and Robins (1998), this estimating function is used to construct a locally efficient one-step estimator of μ. We refer to van der Laan and Robins (1998) for a detailed treatment of this case including simulations, data analysis, and asymptotic theorems. By incorporating information on the surrogate marker process, $\bar{L}(C)$, these estimators are guaranteed to be both more efficient than the NPMLE that ignores data on $\bar{L}(C)$, and to remain consistent and asymptotically normal, whatever the joint distribution of $(T, \bar{L})$. The NPMLE that incorporates data on $\bar{L}(C)$ fails to attain these goals because of the curse of dimensionality (Robins and Ritov, 1997).

In the remainder of this section we will discuss the locally efficient estimator for the generalized regression model in detail. This work is based on Andrews, van der Laan and Robins (2002).

4.5.1 Regression with current status data

Our goal is to estimate the parameter vector β of the regression model $T = Z^\top \beta + \epsilon$, where Z is a vector of time-independent covariates, and the conditional distribution of the error ϵ, given Z, has location parameter equal to zero but has an otherwise non restricted conditional distribution. In addition to data on Z, data on additional time-independent and dependent covariate processes up to time C, denoted by $\bar{L}(C) = \{L(s) : s \leq C\}$, may be available that explain any dependence between the time T and the monitoring time C and might be used to improve estimation of β.

A more classical setting of this estimation problem would be to say that we observe current status data $(C_1, I(T_1 \leq C_1), Z, \bar{L}_1(C_1))$ on a chronological time variable T_1, while we are willing to assume that the regression model holds for $T \equiv m(T_1)$, where m is a given monotone transformation. For example, if $m(x) = \ln(x)$, then this regression model includes the accelerated failure time model $\ln T_1 = \beta^\top Z + \epsilon$, ϵ independent of Z, as a submodel. This setting is transformed to our setting by simply replacing the observed data $(C_1, I(T_1 \leq C_1), Z, \bar{L}_1(C_1))$ by the equivalent $(C \equiv m(C_1), I(T \leq C), Z, \bar{L}(C))$, where $L(s) \equiv L_1(m(s))$.

Note that we do not specify a parametric family for the error distribution. Furthermore, we do not assume that the error ϵ is independent of Z. Rather, we only assume that the conditional distribution of ϵ, given Z, has a specified location parameter equal to zero; that is, in order to make β identifiable, we assume

$$E[K(\epsilon) \mid Z] = E[K(T - Z^\top \beta) \mid Z] = 0, \qquad (4.16)$$

where $K(\cdot)$ is a known monotone function. If $K(\epsilon) = \epsilon$, then (4.16) implies that the conditional mean, given Z, of the error distribution is zero. However, estimation of the mean is quite difficult with current status data because the distribution of the monitoring mechanism must extend as far as the tails of the distribution of T. Thus, other measures of the center may be advantageous or necessary.

The conditional median model is obtained when $K(\epsilon) = I(\epsilon < 0) - 1/2$. Estimation of β requires a smoother $K(\cdot)$ than this because the median is not $\sqrt{n}$-estimable. In fact, our proof of the asymptotic properties of our estimators requires that K is twice differentiable a.e. (w.r.t. support of $C - Z^\top \beta$). A convenient family is $K(\cdot) = 2\Phi(\cdot) - 1$, where Φ is a (typically symmetric, mean zero) continuous distribution function. If the mass of Φ is concentrated near zero, we have a "smoothed median"; if Φ has large variance, we have a trimmed mean. We propose to choose a K with compact support $[-\tau, \tau]$ for some user supplied τ.

Consider the following ideal mouse tumorigenicity experiment designed to investigate the relationship between the time, T, until the development of liver adenoma and the dose level, Z, of a suspected tumorigen. Suppose that study mice are randomly allocated to dose groups and that liver adenomas

4.5. Example: Current Status Data with Time-Dependent Covariates

are never, in themselves, the primary cause of an animal's death. Therefore, each mouse is sacrificed (monitored) at a random time C; at autopsy, it is determined whether a tumor has developed before C. In such studies, it is easy to collect daily measurements of the weight of each mouse prior to sacrifice. Let $L(u)$ be the weight at time u, and let $\bar{L} = L(\cdot)$ be the entire weight process. Only the weight process up to time C is observed: $\bar{L}(C) = \{L(u) : 0 < u < C\}$. Thus, for each individual, $Y = (C, \Delta = I(T \leq C), Z, \bar{L}(C))$ is observed, which we consider as a censored observation of the full data structure $X = (T, Z, \bar{L})$. Because mice with liver adenomas tend to lose weight, $\bar{L}(C)$ and T are associated.

One reasonable monitoring scheme is to increase the hazard of monitoring shortly after a mouse begins to lose weight. If the time of sacrifice can be made closer to the time of tumor onset, then more efficient estimation is possible. This monitoring scheme introduces dependence between C and T, and estimators that ignore this dependence will be biased. Collecting information on a surrogate process and allowing the censoring time to depend on it is a design superior to carcinogenicity experiments that require independent censoring.

In the mouse experiment, the dependence between C and T is only through the observed covariates; that is, the Lebesgue hazard of censoring at time t, given the full (unobserved) data $X = (T, Z, \bar{L})$, is only a function of Z and the observed portion of the covariate process, $\bar{L}(t)$:

$$\lambda_C(t \mid X) = \lambda_C(t \mid Z, \bar{L}(t)). \quad (4.17)$$

This implies that $G(\cdot \mid X)$, the conditional distribution function of C, satisfies coarsening at random (4.3).

Our proposed locally efficient estimator based on (4.12) (and Section 4.3 on the optimal index) of β is consistent and asymptotically normal if we succeed in consistently estimating $\lambda_C(\cdot \mid X)$ at a suitable rate under the assumption (4.17). One such case is the idealized experiment described above, where $\lambda_C(t \mid Z, \bar{L}(t))$ is known by design because it is under the control of the investigator (so estimation of $\lambda_C(t \mid Z, \bar{L}(t))$ is not even necessary). In general, a correctly specified semiparametric model that admits a consistent estimator for $\lambda_C(t \mid Z, \bar{L}(t))$ can be used. Here, we emphasize modeling $\lambda_C(t \mid Z, \bar{L}(t))$ by a time-dependent Cox proportional hazards model:

$$\lambda_C(t \mid Z, \bar{L}(t)) = \lambda_0(t) \exp(\alpha^\top W(t)), \quad (4.18)$$

where $W(t)$ is a function of $(Z, \bar{L}(t))$. Our model for the observed data distribution is now specified since the observed data distribution $P_{F_X, G}$ of Y is indexed by the full data structure distribution F_X which needs to satisfy the regression model (4.16), and the conditional distribution $G(\cdot \mid X)$, which needs to satisfy a semiparametric model such as (4.18).

Our locally efficient estimator also uses an estimator of $F(t \mid Z, \bar{L}(u)) = P(T \leq t \mid Z, \bar{L}(u))$ for various u's and t. By the curse of dimensionality one will need to specify a lower-dimensional working model for this conditional distribution and estimate it accordingly. The resulting one-step estimator is locally efficient in the sense that it is asymptotically efficient for our model if the working model contains the truth and it remains consistent and asymptotically normal otherwise. Thus, our estimator uses time-dependent covariate information, such as the weight history of the mouse up to time u, to predict the time T until onset, thereby recovering information lost due to censoring. To illustrate the potential gain possible, if the weight process perfectly predicts T, then our estimator is asymptotically equivalent with the Kaplan–Meier estimator if we specify a correct model for $F(t \mid Z, \bar{L}(u))$.

Current practice is to sacrifice the mice at one point in time. Since our methodology shows that sophisticated mouse experiments can be nicely analyzed, we hope that experiments of the type above will be carried out in the future. In Andrews, van der Laan, and Robins (2002), we analyze a cross sectional study to estimate the time until transmission distribution in a previously analyzed HIV-partner study. In this data analysis, we estimate the effects of history of sexually transmitted disease and condom use in a model $\log(T) = \beta Z + \epsilon$, which thus includes the accelerated failure time model as a submodel, while using covariates outside the model to allow for informative censoring and to improve efficiency. It is important to note that such an analysis is not possible with any of the existing methods since these methods assume that there are no relevant covariates outside the regression model (see the next subsection).

4.5.2 Previous work and comparison with our results

Several authors have investigated estimation of regression parameters using current status data, (C, Δ), together with a time-independent covariate, Z (Rabinowitz, Tsiatis, and Aregon, 1995; Rossini and Tsiatis, 1996; Huang, 1996; Shen, 2000). Rabinowitz, Tsiatis, and Aregon (1995) fit an accelerated failure time model $\ln T_1 = \beta^\top Z + \epsilon$ (for a failure time T_1) that requires error ϵ to be independent of the covariates Z. Huang (1996) derives an efficient estimator of the regression parameters of the proportional hazards model. Rossini and Tsiatis (1996) assume a semiparametric proportional odds regression model and carry out sieve maximum likelihood estimation. In each case the monitoring time may depend on the covariates of the model, Z, but not on additional covariates. Thus, all covariates that explain the dependence between C and T must be included in the model for T. Because the models are for time-independent covariates only, no time-dependent covariates can be used to explain the dependence between C and T. Similar remarks apply to the linear regression with current status data considered by Shen (2000). None of these limitations apply to our approach.

We would like to stress the implication of our results for the accelerated failure time model as studied by Rabinowitz, Tsiatis, and Aregon (1995).

4.5. Example: Current Status Data with Time-Dependent Covariates

Consider our model with the additional restriction on the regression model that ϵ is independent of Z. By working on the log scale, it follows that this restricted model generalizes the problem of estimation of β in the accelerated failure time model of Rabinowitz, Tsiatis, and Aragon (1995) based on current status data, namely by allowing the presence of additional time-dependent and time-independent covariates. The literature does not provide an estimator in this estimation problem. However, since this restricted model is a submodel of our model, our locally efficient one-step estimator (e.g., using as working model the accelerated failure time model) yields a closed-form consistent and asymptotically normally distributed estimator of the regression parameters in the accelerated failure time model. This one-step estimator will be highly efficient in the accelerated failure time model and will remain consistent and asymptotically normal when the monitoring mechanism depends on the additional (time-dependent) covariates. Furthermore, it will still be consistent if the error distribution is not independent of Z but $E(K(\epsilon) \mid Z) = 0$.

4.5.3 An initial estimator

Suppose that we have n independent observations, $Y_i = (C_i, \Delta_i = I(T_i \leq C_i), Z_i, \overline{L}_i(C_i))$. The component Z_i is a vector, and the component $\overline{L}_i(C_i)$ may itself have several components, each of which may be a time-dependent process or a time-independent covariate. If none of the components of $\overline{L}$ is time-dependent, we will indicate this by using W_i rather than $\overline{L}_i(C_i)$.

The full data estimating functions are of the form $D(T, Z) = h(Z)K_\beta(T, Z)$ for some $h(Z)$, where $K_\beta(T, Z) = K(T - Z^T\beta)$. The IPCW mapping (4.8) $IC_0(Y \mid G, D_h)$ is given by

$$\frac{D'_h(C, Z)\overline{\Delta}}{g(C \mid X)} + D_h(\alpha_X, Z) = h(Z)\left(\frac{K'_\beta(C, Z)\overline{\Delta}}{g(C \mid X)} + K_\beta(\alpha_X, Z)\right), \quad (4.19)$$

where D' is the derivative of D with respect to the first argument, $K'_\beta(t, Z)$ is the derivative with respect to t of $K(t - Z^T\beta)$, α_X is the left endpoint in the support of $g(\cdot \mid X)$, and $\overline{\Delta} = 1 - \Delta$. For a given $D(T, Z) = h(Z)K_\beta(T, Z)$ and given consistent estimator $g_n(\cdot \mid X)$, we can use $IC_0(Y \mid G_n, D_h)$ as an estimating function for β.

Under the assumption that $\mathcal{D}(\beta, G)$ is non empty (see Subsection 4.3.1 and Theorem 4.1), there exist choices $h(Z) = h(Z)I(Z \in \mathcal{Z}(\beta, G))$ for which the estimating function (4.19) is unbiased. If $\max_c K'_\beta(c, Z)/g(c \mid X) < \infty$, F_X-a.e., then one can use as initial estimator of the k-vector regression parameter β, the solution, β_n^0, of the estimating equation corresponding with $h(Z) = Z$

$$\frac{1}{n}\sum_{i=1}^{n} Z_i \left(\frac{K'_{\beta_n^0}(C_i, Z_i)\overline{\Delta}_i}{g_n(C_i \mid X_i)} + K_{\beta_n^0}(\alpha_{X_i}, Z_i)\right) = 0. \quad (4.20)$$

Formal conditions for existence and $\sqrt{n}$-consistency of β_n^0 are proved in Andrews, van der Laan, and Robins (2002).

4.5.4 The locally efficient one-step estimator

The full data structure estimating functions are given by $\{D_h(X \mid \beta, G) = h(Z)I(Z \in \mathcal{Z}(\beta, G))K_\beta(T, Z) :\| h \|_\infty < \infty\}$ (see Theorem 4.1). The optimal mapping $IC(Y \mid F_X, G, D) = IC_0(Y \mid G, D) - IC_{CAR}(Y \mid F_X, G, D)$ from full data structure estimating functions to observed data estimating functions is given by (4.12), namely

$$IC_{CAR}(Y \mid F, G, D) \equiv \int \frac{D'(u, Z)\overline{F}(u \mid Z, \overline{L}(u))}{g(u \mid X)} dM(u) \quad (4.21)$$
$$- \int \frac{1}{\overline{G}(u \mid X)} \int_u^\infty D'(t, Z)\overline{F}(t \mid Z, \overline{L}(u)) dt\, dM(u),$$

where $F(\cdot \mid Z, \bar{L}(u))$ is the conditional cumulative distribution of T, given $(Z, \bar{L}(u))$ and $dM(u) = I(C \in du) - \Lambda_C(du \mid X)I(C > u)$. For convenience, we used shorthand F in $IC_{CAR}(Y \mid F, G, D)$ for $F(\cdot \mid Z, \bar{L}(u))$ for various u.

If $\bar{L} = W$ is time-independent, then

$$IC_{CAR}(Y \mid F, G, D)$$
$$= \frac{D'(C, Z)\overline{F}(C \mid Z, W)}{g(C \mid X)} - \int_0^\infty D'(u, Z)\overline{F}(u \mid Z, W) du, \quad (4.22)$$

in which case

$$IC(Y \mid F, G, D) = \frac{D'(C, Z)}{g(C \mid X)}(F(C \mid Z, W) - \Delta) + E[D(T, Z) \mid Z, W].$$

The efficient influence curve for estimation of β in the observed model equals $IC(Y \mid F, G, D_{opt})$, where the optimal $D_{h_{opt}}$ is given in Section 4.3 up to a standardization. We have $D_{opt}(T, Z) \equiv h_{opt}(Z)K_\beta(T, Z)$, where

$$IC(Y \mid F, G, D_{h_{opt}}) = h_{opt}(Z)IC(Y \mid F_X, G, K_\beta)$$
$$= \frac{ZE(K'_\beta \mid Z)}{\phi(Z)} IC(Y \mid F_X, G, K_\beta), \quad (4.23)$$

and $h_{opt}(Z) = (ZE(K'_\beta \mid Z))/\phi(Z)$ with

$$\phi(Z) = E(IC(Y \mid F, G, K_\beta)^2 \mid Z). \quad (4.24)$$

Note that, if, conditional on $Z = z$, $\epsilon(\beta)$ has zero probability to fall in the support $[-\tau, \tau]$ of $K(\cdot)$, then $h_{opt}(z) = 0$, which reflects that the optimal choice h_{opt} aims to only use observations that provide information about

4.5. Example: Current Status Data with Time-Dependent Covariates

β. If $\overline{L} = W$ is time-independent, then ϕ simplifies to the expression

$$\phi(Z) = E\left(E(K_\beta \mid Z, W)^2 + \int \frac{F(t \mid Z, W)\overline{F}(t \mid Z, W)K_\beta'^{\,2}(t, Z)}{g(t \mid X)} dt \,\bigg|\, Z \right), \quad (4.25)$$

and if $(Z, \overline{L}) = Z$, then it simplifies further to

$$\phi(Z) = \int \frac{F(t \mid Z)\overline{F}(t \mid Z)K_\beta'^{\,2}(t, Z)}{g(t \mid X)} dt. \quad (4.26)$$

Given estimators F_n, G_n, h_n of F, G, h_{opt}, we propose as the estimator of β the solution of the estimating equation:

$$0 = \frac{1}{n}\sum_{i=1}^{n} IC(Y_i \mid F_n, G_n, D_{h_n}(\cdot \mid \beta, G_n)). \quad (4.27)$$

Let

$$c_n = -\frac{1}{n}\sum_{i=1}^{n} IC_0(Y_i \mid G_n, d/d\beta D_{h_n}(\cdot \mid \beta, G_n))|_{\beta=\beta_n^0}.$$

be the derivative matrix of the estimating equation (4.27) in β as needed in the first step of the Newton–Raphson algorithm. Here, we used that the derivative w.r.t. β in IC_{CAR} is in truth equal to zero and should thus not be included in the estimate either. Then, the one-step estimator (the first step of Newton–Raphson algorithm) is given by

$$\beta_n^1 = \beta_n^0 + \frac{1}{n}\sum_{i=1}^{n} IC(Y_i \mid F_n, G_n, c_n^{-1} D_{h_n}(\cdot \mid \beta_n^0, G_n)).$$

4.5.5 Implementation issues

The following estimation method can always be used to compute the one-step estimator. Estimation of the efficient influence curve (4.23) involves estimation of (F, G, h_{opt}, β). The initial estimate of β and the estimate of the censoring density g were discussed above. We now discuss each of the three others in turn and how to compute the one-step estimator β_n^1.

F_n **for time-independent case.** If $\overline{L} = W$ is time-independent, then IC_{CAR} is given by (4.22). To estimate $F(\cdot \mid Z, W)$, we can use the identity

$$F(t \mid Z, W) = E[I(T \leq t) \mid Z, W] = E[\Delta \mid C = t, Z, W], \quad (4.28)$$

where $\Delta = I(T \leq C)$. The second equality follows from CAR.

The proposed submodel can be chosen to be a highly parametric model or a flexible semiparametric model. The former leads to an efficient estimator in fewer circumstances. Nonetheless, the finite sample performance of a parametric model is comparable if not superior to a semiparametric model because it recognizes the main effects of the covariates and is more stable where the data are sparse. This comparison is made in the second example in the simulation section.

One possible semiparametric model for $F(\cdot \mid Z, W)$ is a logistic generalized additive model.

$$\begin{aligned} F(t \mid Z, W) &= E[\Delta \mid C = t, Z = (Z_1, \ldots, Z_k), W = (W_1, \ldots, W_l)] \\ &= \frac{\exp(f_C(t) + f_{Z_1}(Z_1) + \cdots + f_{W_l}(W_l))}{1 + \exp(f_C(t) + f_{Z_1}(Z_1) + \cdots + f_{W_l}(W_l))}. \end{aligned} \quad (4.29)$$

The S-plus function `gam` with `family=binomial(link=logit)` produces an F_n based on the observed data $\{Y_i\}_{i=1}^n$. Of course, the probit model (`family=binomial(link=probit)`) can also be used. Furthermore, some or all of the general functions $f_C, f_{Z_1}, \ldots, f_{W_l}$, can be replaced by more parametric polynomials.

The factor $IC(Y_i \mid F, G, K_\beta)$ in (4.23) can now be estimated for each Y_i using the expressions for $IC_0(Y_i \mid G_n, K_{\beta_n^0})$ and $IC_{CAR}(Y_i \mid F_n, G_n, K_{\beta_n^0})$ given in (4.19) and (4.22). If $K'_{\beta_n^0}(\cdot, Z_i)$ is zero except on the interval $(Z_i^\top \beta_n^0 - \tau, Z_i^\top \beta_n^0 + \tau)$, the integral in (4.22) is easily approximated (e.g., the trapezoidal rule).

F_n for time-dependent case. If $\overline{L}$ is time-dependent, IC_{CAR} must be estimated directly from (4.21). It is necessary to estimate $F(t \mid Z, \overline{L}(u))$ for a given (t, u) with $t \geq u$. First, consider the case where the density of C depends only on the time-independent covariates (even though $F(t \mid Z, \overline{L}(u))$ may depend on the time-dependent covariates). Then, we proceed using the CAR identity

$$F(t \mid Z, \overline{L}(u)) = E(\Delta \mid C = t, Z, \overline{L}(u), C \geq u). \quad (4.30)$$

To avoid the curse of dimensionality, for each u we replace $\overline{L}(u)$ by a vector of summary measures, $W_u(\overline{L}(u))$, which hopefully captures the most relevant information for predicting T. Now, for each u, we can estimate $F(\cdot \mid Z, \overline{L}(u)) \approx F(\cdot \mid Z, W_u)$ by the GAM in (4.29). The model is fit using data Y_i for which $C_i \geq u$ (i.e., those observations for which $\overline{L}(u)$ is observed), and we typically smooth the u-specific regression parameters w.r.t. μ weighting each u-specific regression by $1/n(u)$, where $n(u) = \sum_i I(C_i \geq u)$.

For the general case where the censoring mechanism also depends on the time-dependent covariate, the identity (4.30) is not guaranteed by CAR. One can now decide to use the representation of $IC(Y \mid F, G, D)$ in terms of $IC(Y \mid Q, G, D)$ and estimate the conditional observed data expectations defining Q as proposed in Section 4.2 (including the maximum likelihood estimation method). Alternatively, one similarly proceeds in estimating $F(t \mid Z, \overline{L}(u))$ in two stages by using the CAR relationship given in van der Laan and Robins (1998),

$$F(t \mid Z, \overline{L}(u)) = E\left(\xi(u, t) \mid Z, \overline{L}(u), C \geq u\right), \quad (4.31)$$

4.5. Example: Current Status Data with Time-Dependent Covariates

where

$$\xi(u,t) = \frac{\overline{G}(u \mid X)}{\overline{G}(t \mid X)} I(C \geq t) F(t \mid Z, \overline{L}(t), C \geq t). \tag{4.32}$$

We can estimate $F(\cdot \mid Z, \overline{L}(t), C \geq t)$ for each t from those individuals for which $C_i \geq t$ just as above (see (4.30), but now t plays the role of u). Note that from the fitted model we only need the function evaluated at the left endpoint, $F_n(t \mid Z, \overline{L}(t), C \geq t)$. From F_n and G_n, we can calculate $\widehat{\xi}_i(u,t)$ for each individual from (4.32). Now, for each u, regress $\widehat{\xi}_i(u,t)$ on t, Z, and $W_u(\overline{L}(u))$ using individuals for which $C_i \geq u$. The S-plus function GAM() with "family=quasi(link=logit, variance=constant)" can be used to fit a logistic GAM model. This is our estimate $F_n(t \mid Z, \overline{L}(u))$, the final piece needed to estimate IC_{nu} in the most general case (4.21).

h_{opt}. The vector-valued function $h_{opt}(Z)$ is proportional to Z. The constant of proportionality is the ratio of

$$E(K'_\beta \mid Z) = E\left(\frac{K''(C - \beta^\top Z)(1 - \Delta)}{g(C \mid X)} \mid Z\right) + K'(\alpha_X - \beta^\top Z) \tag{4.33}$$

and $\phi(Z)$. Using β_n^0 and $g_n(\cdot \mid X)$ to obtain an observed outcome, (4.33) can be estimated by regressing an observed outcome on Z. The function $\phi(Z)$ can be estimated in several ways depending on the number and type of covariates available. In general, $\phi(Z)$ is the conditional expectation, given Z, of $IC^2(Y \mid \beta, F, G, K_\beta)$. An estimate of IC has already been computed, and its square can be regressed on Z by fitting a parametric or semiparametric model (e.g., splines, gam, running medians).

Although this regression method can always be used, in some cases $\phi(Z)$ has other expressions with more structure that can be exploited. In particular, if there are no covariates other than Z, then ϕ is given by (4.26) and can be estimated by substitution of an estimator of $F(t \mid Z) = E(\Delta \mid C = t, Z)$.

If $\overline{L} = W$ is time independent, $\phi(Z)$ is given by (4.25) which can thus be estimated by substitution of an estimator of $F(t \mid Z, W) = E(\Delta \mid C = t, Z, W)$. Equation (4.25) will be more accurate than (4.24) but potentially more computationally intensive.

4.5.6 Construction of confidence intervals

Under regularity conditions stated in Andrews, van der Laan, and Robins (2002) (corresponding with the conditions of Theorem 2.4 in Chapter 2), μ_n^1 is asymptotically linear with influence curve given by $IC - \Pi(IC \mid T_G)$, where T_G is the tangent space of G under the assumed Cox proportional hazards model for the monitoring mechanism $g(c \mid X)$, and $IC = IC(Y \mid F_1, G, D_h(\cdot \mid \beta))$ denotes the limit of the estimated efficient influence curve $\widehat{\ell}^*_{eff}(Y) \equiv IC(Y \mid F_n, G_n, D_{h_n}(\cdot \mid \beta_n^0))$ for $n \to \infty$. Thus, a confidence region for the parameter vector β or individual confidence intervals for each regression parameter can be constructed by estimating the covariance matrix $\Sigma = E(\ell^*_{eff}(Y)\ell^*_{eff}(Y)^\top)$ of the efficient influence function, ℓ^*_{eff}. If the model for $F(t \mid Z, \overline{L}(u))$ is correctly specified, the vector $\sqrt{n}(\beta_n^1 - \beta)$ is asymptotically distributed $N(0, \Sigma)$ because the projection term $\Pi(IC \mid T_G) = 0$ in this case. Thus, an asymptotic 95% confidence region for β is

$$\left\{ \beta \in \mathbb{R}^k \mid (\beta_n^1 - \beta)^\top \widehat{\Sigma}^{-1}(\beta_n^1 - \beta) \leq \frac{k}{n} \chi^2_{0.95, k, \infty} \right\}$$

(e.g., Morrison, 1990), where $\widehat{\Sigma}$ is the empirical variance of the estimated efficient influence function,

$$\widehat{\Sigma} = \frac{1}{n} \sum_{i=1}^{n} \left(\widehat{\ell^*_{eff}}(Y_i) - \frac{1}{n} \sum_{i'=1}^{n} \widehat{\ell^*_{eff}}(Y_{i'}) \right) \left(\widehat{\ell^*_{eff}}(Y_i) - \frac{1}{n} \sum_{i'=1}^{n} \widehat{\ell^*_{eff}}(Y_{i'}) \right)^\top.$$

A 95% confidence interval for a single parameter is $\beta_n^1 \pm 1.96\widehat{\sigma}/\sqrt{n}$, where $\widehat{\sigma}$ is the appropriate diagonal element of $\widehat{\Sigma}$.

If the model for $F(t \mid Z, \overline{L}(u))$ is misspecified, the confidence intervals above are conservative. The projection operator onto T_G exists in closed form and is provided in Lemma 3.2 in Chapter 3. However, unless F is very poorly specified, the conservative intervals will be fairly accurate.

4.5.7 A doubly robust estimator

Consider the reparametrized class of full data estimating functions satisfying $D_h(\cdot \mid \beta, G) \in T_{nuis}^{F, \perp}(F_X) \cap \mathcal{D}(\rho_1(F_X), G)$ at its true parameter values β, G. Given estimates F_n, G_n of the nuisance parameters F, G and a choice h_n for the full data structure estimating function, consider the estimator β_n solving

$$0 = \frac{1}{n} \sum_{i=1}^{n} IC(Y_i \mid F_n, G_n, D_{h_n}(\cdot \mid \beta, G_n)).$$

Recall that our one-step estimator is just the first step of the Newton–Raphson algorithm for solving this estimating equation for β, where we chose β_n^0 as initial estimator. As proved in general in Chapter 2 (see (2.30) and (2.31)), due to the orthogonality of $IC(Y \mid F, G, D_h(\cdot \mid \beta, G))$ w.r.t. G, we actually have the double robustness property w.r.t. the nuisance parameters F, G of this estimating function $IC(Y \mid F, G, D_h(\cdot \mid \beta, G))$; that is, for $D_h(\cdot \mid \beta, G_1) \in \mathcal{D}(\rho_1(F_X), G_1)$

$$EIC(Y \mid F_1, G_1, D_h(\cdot \mid \beta, G_1)) = 0 \text{ if either } F_1 = F \text{ or } G_1 = G$$

and $dG/dG_1 = g/g_1 < \infty$. (As shown in Section 1.6, the latter condition can be deleted for our T_{CAR}-orthogonalized estimating function if we enforce a condition on g_1 so that $\mathcal{D}(\rho_1(F_X), G_1)$ is contained in the range of the nonparametric information operator $I_{F_X, G_1} : L^2_0(F_X) \to L^2_0(F_X)$, such

4.5. Example: Current Status Data with Time-Dependent Covariates 257

as $\inf_c g_1(c \mid X) > \delta > 0$, F_X-a.e.) We like to stress once more that this result shows that, at a correctly specified F, one only needs the identifiability condition to hold at the estimated G_n. Therefore, it is important to use a G_n for which the identifiability condition (e.g., $\max_c K'(c, Z)/g_n(c \mid X) < \infty$, F_X-a.e.). This means that, in fact, under regularity conditions, β_n will be consistent and asymptotically linear if either $F(t \mid Z, \bar{L}(t))$ is correctly estimated, or G is correctly estimated and the identifiability condition holds at the true G (see Theorem 2.5). This requires direct estimators of $F(t \mid Z, \bar{L}(t))$ that do not depend on correct specification of the model for G, such as estimators based on maximum likelihood estimation or the regression representation (4.30). We expect that it will also be possible to develop representations of $E(IC_0(Y) \mid \bar{A}(t), Z, \bar{L}(t))$ separating g and F_X in the same manner as shown in theorems 3.1 and 6.2.

If one wants to obtain a confidence region for β based on β_n in this model $\mathcal{M}$ that is more nonparametric than $\mathcal{M}(\mathcal{G})$, then we recommend using the nonparametric bootstrap. This double robustness property of β_n implies that, in practice, a minor misspecification of the model for G can be corrected by doing a good job in estimation of $F(t \mid Z, \bar{L}(t))$ and vice versa.

4.5.8 Data-adaptive selection of the location parameter

The regression parameter β represents the effect of Z on the location parameter identified by K. Thus, the choice of location parameter affects immediately the interpretation of β and should therefore be subject-matter-driven. However, one might also decide to choose the location parameter that can be estimated with best precision. Suppose that we choose a family of monotone functions K_τ with compact support $[-\tau, \tau]$ that (e.g.) approximates the median function $K(x) = I(x > 0) - 0.5$ for $\tau \to 0$ and approximates the mean function $K(x) = x$ for $\tau \to \infty$. In that case, one can calculate an estimate of the conditional variance $\widehat{\Sigma}(z)$ of the prediction $z^\top \beta_n$, given $Z = z$, for a range of τ's. Suppose now that one selects the τ that minimizes the average variance $1/n \sum_{i=1}^n \widehat{\Sigma}(Z_i)$. This corresponds with choosing the location parameter that results in a predicted location parameter for the conditional distribution of T, given Z, which has minimal variance. This seems to be a particularly attractive procedure in the situation that one believes that ϵ is independent of Z and has a symmetric distribution centered at zero.

4.5.9 Simulations

Two simulation studies are presented to illustrate the applicability and efficiency of these methods. Example 1 demonstrates that the asymptotic properties of the one-step estimator apply to a data set of moderate size.

258   4. Cross-Sectional Data and Right-Censored Data Combined

The superiority of the one-step estimator over the initial estimator is also shown. The effects of an additional time-independent covariate, W, and the submodel selected for $F(\cdot \mid Z, W)$ are considered in Example 2.

The function K used in these simulations is a smoothed truncated mean given by

$$K(t) = \begin{cases} -\tau & t < -\tau \\ t + \frac{\tau}{\pi}\sin(\frac{\pi t}{\tau}) & -\tau \le t \le \tau \\ \tau & \tau < t \end{cases}. \tag{4.34}$$

with $\tau = 3$. K has two continuous derivatives, both of which are zero outside the interval $(-\tau, \tau)$.

4.5.10   Example 1: No unmodeled covariate

The data-generating distribution has $\beta = (\beta_0, \beta_1) = (0, 1)$, $Z_0 \equiv 1$ (intercept), $Z_1 \sim N(0, 1)$, $T \mid Z \sim N(Z_1, 1)$, and $C \mid Z \sim N(Z_1, 1)$. We have for observed data (C, Δ, Z). The general method of estimation described in Subsection 4.5.5 was used with the following specifics. The censoring distribution was estimated via linear regression of C on Z with independent normal error. The distribution of $T \mid Z$ was estimated using (4.28) and a generalized linear model with probit link. h_{opt} was computed after approximating the integrals $E(K_{\beta_n^0}(T, Z) \mid Z) = -\int K'_{\beta_n^0}(t, Z) F(t \mid Z) dt$ and the expression (4.26) for $\phi(Z)$ by Simpson's Rule with 20 intervals. The results in Table 4.1 are based on 1000 repetitions.

The one-step estimator is efficient in this example because the submodel chosen for F is correct. In finite samples, we estimate the efficiency by comparing the variance of the estimator with the variance of the efficient influence curve. Similarly we estimate the efficiency of the one-step estimator relative to the initial estimator. Results for the parameter β_1 at three sample sizes are given in Table 4.1 (similar patterns are seen for β_0). The results show that for n large, the variance of the one-step estimator of β approximates the optimal asymptotic variance defined by the variance of the efficient influence curve.

4.5.11   Example 2: Unmodeled covariate

Suppose that in addition to Z, another covariate, W, has been collected that is associated with T. Our method uses the information contained in the covariate to improve the estimate of β. The strength of the relationship between T and W is one factor that determines how much our one-step estimator can improve the initial estimator that does not use W. In this example, we consider three covariates: $W_1 = T$, $W_2 = T + \text{small error}$, and $W_3 = T + \text{large error}$. The first corresponds with a perfect surrogate for T, the second with a good predictor of T, and the third with a poor predictor of T.

4.5. Example: Current Status Data with Time-Dependent Covariates 259

Table 4.1. Comparison of initial and one-step estimators for the simple linear regression example. The one-step estimator is asymptotically efficient and appears to be fully efficient even for moderate sample sizes.

Estimator	Sample Size	Asymptotic Relative Efficiency	Relative Efficiency (baseline=Initial)
Initial ($\beta_{n,1}^0$)	250	0.53	1
	500	0.76	1
	1000	0.81	1
One-step ($\beta_{n,1}^1$)	250	0.67	1.2
	500	1.05	1.3
	1000	1.05	1.3

The degree to which we will be able to exploit the information in W also depends on the submodel that we select for $F(\cdot \mid Z, W)$. It is frequently wise to be optimistic and select a small submodel; for example, a generalized linear model often outperforms a generalized additive model if linearity is at all reasonable. In this example, we consider two one-step estimators. The first estimator is the generic method described in Section 4.5.5. The assumed model for $F(\cdot \mid Z, W)$ is correct for each of the three covariates. Thus β_n^1 is asymptotically efficient in each case.

The second one-step estimator assumes that W is a perfect surrogate for T. This is correct in the first scenario because $W_1 = T$ but not correct for the second or third cases. Under the assumption $W = T$, one could directly estimate β by linear regression: $W = Z^\top \beta + \epsilon$. This direct linear regression method is optimal in case 1 where $W_1 = T$. However, in the two other cases, this estimator is inconsistent. On the other hand, our estimator is consistent in each of the three cases and is asymptotically equivalent with this direct linear regression method if $W = T$.

The simulation results are presented in Table 4.2. The initial estimator is exactly the estimator in the previous example. It does not use the information provided by the covariate W and thus is not nearly efficient. If W is very informative, as in the first two cases, the variance bound is less than half the variance of the initial estimator.

The generic one-step estimator is efficient, but for samples with $N = 1000$ the variance bound is about 10% smaller than the variance of the estimator. The special one-step estimator that assumes $W = T$ reaches the efficiency bound (and then some) when W is very informative. When W is a poor predictor of T, the performance of this estimator suffers, as should be expected, because the assumption $W = T$ is bad. The variance of the special estimator is larger than the generic estimator in this case.

Details. The data-generating distribution has $Z_0 \equiv 1$ (intercept), $Z_1 \sim N(0,1)$, $T \mid Z \sim N(Z_1, 1)$, $W_1 \mid T, Z = T$, $W_2 \mid T, Z \sim N(T, 0.1^2)$, $W_3 \mid T, Z \sim N(T, 1.0^2)$, and $C \mid Z, W \sim N(Z_1, 1)$. The general method of

Table 4.2. Comparison of (the variances of) the initial estimator and two one-step estimators. The generic one-step estimator is efficient in each case. The special one-step estimator assumes $W = T$ and is therefore efficient only in case 1. The generic one-step estimator has not reached the (asymptotic) efficiency bound in this simulation ($N = 1000$), but the special one-step estimator has done so in the first two cases in which W is a perfect or good predictor of T.

Est.	Avail. Cov.	Asymp. Rel. Eff.	Rel. Eff. Init.	Rel. Eff. Gen.
Initial ($\beta^0_{n,1}$)	$W_1 = T$	0.40	1	
	W_2	0.44	1	
	W_3	0.78	1	
Generic ($\beta^1_{n,1}$)	$W_1 = T$	0.90	2.20	1
	W_2	0.93	2.12	1
	W_3	0.94	1.19	1
Special ($\beta^{1*}_{n,1}$)	$W_1 = T$	1.03	2.32	1.15
	W_2	1.08	2.48	1.08
	W_3	0.90	1.15	0.96

estimation described in Section 4.5.5 was used with the following specifics to compute the generic one-step estimator. The censoring distribution was estimated via linear regression of C on Z with independent normal error. The distribution of $T \mid Z, W$ was estimated using (4.28) and a generalized linear model with probit link. From the data model, it can be shown that $f_{W|Z}$ can be estimated consistently with a linear regression with normal errors in each of the three cases. This estimate can be used to more accurately estimate $\phi(Z)$ as defined in (4.25).

The special one-step estimator based on the assumption $W = T$ is easier to compute because the assumption implies $F(t \mid Z, W) = I(t > W)$, $E(K'_{\beta^0_n} \mid Z, W) = K'_{\beta^0_n}(W, Z)$, and

$$\phi(Z) = \int f_{W|Z}(w \mid Z) K_{\beta^0_n}(w, Z)^2 dw.$$

Results in Table 4.2 are based on 1000 repetitions.

4.5.12 Data Analysis: California Partners' Study

The methods described in this paper were applied to a data set extracted from the California Partners' Study. Each case consists of a monogamous heterosexual couple in which the male is HIV-positive due to a prior sexual contact. The "failure time variable" on which current status data are available is the time (in months) until infection of the female partner. Several time-independent covariates are available, including an indicator of condom use (never=1, ever=0), an indicator of bleeding (ever=1, never=0),

4.5. Example: Current Status Data with Time-Dependent Covariates

an indicator of a sexually transmitted disease (STD) history in the female (ever=1, never=0), an estimate of the rate of sexual contact (contacts per month), and the age of the female (years). There are 87 subjects with complete information on these five covariates. More detailed descriptions of the data are available in Padian, et al. (1987), Jewell and Shiboski (1990), Shiboski and Jewell (1992), and Padian, Shiboski, Glass, and Vittinghoff (1997).

Our ultimate goal is to estimate the regression parameters in the model $T = Z^\top \beta + \epsilon$, where T is the log of the transmission time. Define the following notation: $Z_0 \equiv 1$ is the intercept, $Z_1 = I(\text{no condom use})$, $Z_2 = I(\text{STD history})$, $Z_3 = Z_1 Z_2$. We expect the coefficients of Z_1 and Z_2 to be negative, indicating that these risk factors lower the expected time until transmission of the disease. We include the interaction term because the effect of STD history may not be observed if condoms are used.

Before estimating β, we must model the censoring mechanism. The distribution of C may be dependent on the covariates in the model and on covariates external to the regression model. Several classes of models for the conditional distribution of C given covariates are feasible, including simple linear regression and Cox proportional hazards. In each of these classes, the only significant dependence is between the monitoring time and Z_1. By the asymptotic theory (i.e., a larger censoring model implies a gain in efficiency), it may be safer to include more rather than fewer covariates and to specify a semiparametric rather than parametric model to protect against dependence between T and C as much as possible. With that in mind, we chose to use the Cox proportional hazards model and to include all five covariates mentioned in the paragraph describing the data set.

With a model for the censoring mechanism in hand, we proceed to compute an initial estimate of β based on (4.20). The length of the support window of K' can be varied (as can the functional form of K) to obtain results for a range of estimators from smoothed median regression to trimmed mean regression. Table 4.3 displays how the initial and one-step estimates depend on the selection of the window length. For the analysis of log transmission time, the estimates do not change substantially with τ. In a similar analysis of the untransformed transmission time, the estimates changed due to the right skewness of the distribution. For example, the intercept, which represents the time until infection in pairs with neither risk factor, was largest for large τ and smallest for small τ. A wide window indicates that the tail of the distribution will have an effect, while a small window indicates that only the center of the data is measured.

For $\tau = 0.25$, the initial estimator is $\beta_n^0 = (4.44, -0.54, -0.31, 0.24)$; that is, the conditional log time until infection is centered at $T = 4.44 - 0.54 Z_1 - 0.31 Z_2 + 0.24 Z_3$.

The remaining item is to compute the one-step estimator. The covariates in this data set are time-independent so equation (4.22) applies. The cumulative distribution function $F(t|Z, W)$ was estimated using the generalized

Table 4.3. Dependence of estimates on window length. K' is zero outside $Z^\top\beta\pm\tau$. If τ is larger than 0.3, this window extends beyond the support of g_n. If τ is smaller then 0.15, the initial estimator has numerous solutions.

τ	Parameter	β_n^0	β_n^1
0.17	Z_0	4.43	4.42
	Z_1	-0.52	-0.49
	Z_2	-0.27	-0.26
	Z_3	0.15	0.26
0.21	Z_0	4.43	4.43
	Z_1	-0.53	-0.50
	Z_2	-0.29	-0.26
	Z_3	0.17	0.30
0.25	Z_0	4.44	4.43
	Z_1	-0.54	-0.50
	Z_2	-0.31	-0.27
	Z_3	0.20	0.42
0.29	Z_0	4.45	4.44
	Z_1	-0.56	-0.51
	Z_2	-0.33	-0.28
	Z_3	0.24	0.45

additive model as in (4.29) with $Z = (Z_0, Z_1, Z_2, Z_3)$ and logit link function. The indicator of bleeding and the age of the female were used as covariates outside the regression model (that is, W). Adjusting for these covariates is not possible with any other technique in the literature. The one-step estimator is $\beta_n^1 = (4.43, -0.50, -0.27, 0.42)$; that is, the conditional log time until infection is centered at $T = 4.43 - 0.50Z_1 - 0.27Z_2 + 0.42Z_3$.

The individual standard errors of the coefficients of the two main effect indicator variables are 0.19 and 0.11, respectively. Thus, the indicators of no condom use and of STD history are significant ($0.01 < p < 0.02$) factors in predicting the log time until transmission. The coefficient of the interaction is not statistically significant.

4.6 Example: Current Status Data on a Process Until Death

Consider a carcinogenicity experiment in which $T_1, \ldots, T_{k-1}$ are ordered time points of interest and T_k is time until death of the mouse. For example suppose the chemical under test produces liver tumors that do not metatasize . Then T_1 is time of onset of a tumor, $T_2, ..., T_{k-1}$ are the times at which the tumor mass has replaced prespecified increasing fractions of the liver tissue, T_k is the time of death due to nearly complete replacement

4.6. Example: Current Status Data on a Process Until Death

of the liver by tumor, and C is time of death due to any other cause. Thus $T_1 < \ldots < T_k$. Let $N(t) = \sum_{j=1}^{k} I(T_j \leq t)$. In addition, let $L(t)$ be a time-dependent covariate process measured on the mouse over time. We have for the full data $X = (\vec{T} = (T_1, \ldots, T_k), \bar{L}(T_k))$, and the observed data structure is

$$Y = (\tilde{T}_k = \min(C, T_k), \Delta_k = I(T_k \leq C), \bar{L}(\tilde{T}_k), N(\tilde{T}_k)), \qquad (4.35)$$

where C is the monitoring time at which the current status of the mouse is determined (if T_k did not happen yet) w.r.t. the k events corresponding with $T_1, \ldots, T_k$.

This data structure is a special case of our general data structure (4.1) with $X_1(t) = N(t)$ and $X_2(t) = (R(t), L(t))$, where $R(t) = I(T_k \leq t)$. In other words, the full data structure is defined as $X = (\bar{X}_1(T_k), \bar{X}_2(T_k))$, and the observed data structure (4.35) is equivalent with

$$Y = (C, X_1(C), \bar{X}_2(C)),$$

where we redefined C by setting $C \equiv \infty$ if $C > T_k$.

Let $g(c \mid X)$ be the conditional density of C, given X, w.r.t. the Lebesgue measure or w.r.t. a counting measure. We have that the monitoring mechanism $G(\cdot \mid X)$ satisfies CAR if for $c < T_k$

$$\lambda_C(c \mid X) = \lambda_C(c \mid \bar{L}(c)). \qquad (4.36)$$

Parameters of interest are, in particular, the marginal distributions F_j, $j = 1, \ldots, k$, of $T_1, \ldots, T_k$, respectively, and regression parameters in generalized regression models of T_j, given baseline covariates.

The bivariate marginal version (i.e., $L(t)$ is empty) of this problem with $T_1 < T_2$ has received attention in the literature. Kodell, Shaw, and Johnson (1982) studied the nonparametric maximum likelihood estimator under the additional assumption that S_1/S_2 is a survival function. Dinse and Lagakos (1982) proposed to estimate F_2 with the Kaplan–Meier estimator $F_{2,KM}$ and to estimate F_1 with the maximizer of the likelihood $F_1 \to L(F_1, F_{2,KM})$ under the constraint that $F_1 \leq F_{2,KM}$. They questioned the efficiency of the Kaplan–Meier estimator. Turnbull and Mitchell (1984) studied the actual NPMLE of (F_1, F_2) and computed it with the EM-algorithm. Van der Laan, Jewell, and Peterson (1997) provide a simple-to-compute estimator for F_1 and prove that this estimator and the Kaplan–Meier estimator for F_2 are efficient under a weak assumption on F_1, F_2. As pointed out by Piet Groeneboom, the simulation study in van der Laan, Jewell, Peterson (1997) wrongly implements the NPMLE so that we refer the reader to future work of Groeneboom for a practical comparison of the NPMLE with these ad hoc (but efficient for smooth functionals) estimators. There is no literature on this data structure extended with time-dependent covariates $L(t)$.

We consider two estimation problems. In the first problem the full data structure model is nonparametric and the parameter of interest is a smooth functional $\int r(t)(1 - F_j(t))dt$ of the marginal distribution of

T_j. In the second problem, the full data structure model is a generalized regression model $T_j = g(X^* \mid \beta) + \epsilon$, $E(K(\epsilon) \mid X^*) = 0$, with outcome T_j and covariates extracted from the baseline-covariates $X_2(0)$, $j = 1, \ldots, k-1$, and the parameter of interest is β. In the nonparametric full data structure model, the only full data estimating function is $D(T_j \mid \mu) = R(T_j) - \mu$ and in the regression model the estimating functions are given by $\{D_h(T_j, X^* \mid \mu) = h(X^*)K(\epsilon) : h\}$. Consider such a full data estimating function $D(T_j, Z \mid \mu)$. In Section 4.2 we provided the initial mapping (4.11)

$$IC_0(Y \mid G, D) = D'(C, Z \mid \mu)\frac{I(T_j > C)}{g(C \mid X)} + D(a, Z \mid \mu)$$

and the optimal mapping $IC(Y \mid F_X, G, D_h)$ (4.12), where now $dM_G(t) = I(C \in dt, C < T_k) - I(\tilde{T}_k \geq t)\Lambda_{C|X}(dt \mid X)$. Recall that $D'(t,Z) \equiv d/dt D(t,Z)$ and a is the left support point of $g(\cdot \mid X)$, which can be a function of $X_2(0)$. The optimal choice $D_{h_{opt}}$ in the regression models is provided in Section 4.3 (4.14), and alternative representations are provided in Section 4.4 (just set $T = T_j$). Locally efficient estimation of μ and β now proceeds precisely as in Section 4.2, where again the optimal index h_{opt} is provided in closed form in Section 4.3.

Let us now consider estimation of T_k-related parameters. Again, consider two estimation problems. In the first problem, the full data structure model is nonparametric and the parameter of interest is $\mu = F_k(t) = P(T_k \leq t)$ at a given point t. In the second problem, the full data structure model is a generalized regression model $T_k = g(X^* \mid \beta) + \epsilon$, $E(K(\epsilon) \mid X^*) = 0$, with outcome T_k and covariates extracted from the baseline covariates $X_2(0)$, $j = 1, \ldots, k-1$, and the parameter of interest is β. In the nonparametric full data structure model, the only full data structure estimating function is $D(T_k \mid \mu) = I(T_k \leq t) - \mu$, and in the regression model, the full data structure estimating functions are given by $\{D_h(T_k, X^* \mid \mu) = h(X^*)K(\epsilon) : h\}$. We now use as IPCW mapping for any function $D(X_2)$

$$IC_0(Y \mid G, D) = D(X_2)\frac{I(C > T_k)}{\bar{G}(T_k \mid X)}.$$

In Section 4.2 we provided the optimal mapping $IC(Y \mid F_X, G, D_h)$ (4.13)

$$IC_0(Y \mid G, D) + \int E(IC_0(Y \mid G, D) \mid \bar{X}_2(u), \tilde{T}_k > u)dM_G(u).$$

Notice that this is precisely the same mapping as given in Chapter 3 for the reduced data structure $(C, \bar{X}_2(C))$. In other words, for the purpose of estimating T_k related parameters, one can reduce the data to $(C, \bar{X}_2(C))$ without loss of (asymptotic) information under the assumption that (4.3) is equivalent with assuming CAR on the censoring mechanism. Thus, the optimal index h_{opt} is provided in Chapter 3 for the generalized regression

4.6. Example: Current Status Data on a Process Until Death

model. Locally efficient estimation of μ and β now proceeds precisely as in Chapter 3.

Finally, another full data structure model of interest is the Cox proportional hazards model for the hazard of T_k given some covariates extracted from X_2. We covered estimation on multiplicative intensity models such as the Cox proportional hazards model for a failure time T_k in detail in Section 3.3 of Chapter 3. In particular, one optimal mapping involves just applying $IC(Y \mid F_X, G, D_h)$ to the full data estimating functions for this full data model as provided in Chapter 3, while another one is based on inverse weighting within the integral defining the full data estimating function. In Section 3.3 of Chapter 3, we propose locally optimal indexes h_{opt}^* and corresponding estimators. One can also use the results of Chapter 3 to characterize the optimal index h_{opt}, as in Robins (1993a) and Robins and Rotnitzky (1992).

5
Multivariate Right-Censored Multivariate Data

5.1 General Data Structure

Consider a time-dependent process $X(t) = (X_1(t), X_2(t))$, where $X_k(t)$ includes as a component $R_k(t) = I(T_k \leq t)$, $k = 1, 2$. Let the full data be $X = (\bar{X}_1(T_1), \bar{X}_2(T_2)) \sim F_X \in \mathcal{M}^F$, where $\bar{X}_k(t) = \{X_k(s) : s \in [0, t]\}$. Let $T = \max(T_1, T_2)$ so that we can also represent the full data structure by $\bar{X}(T)$.

Let C_1, C_2 be two censoring variables. Define $\tilde{T}_k = \min(T_k, C_k)$ and $\Delta_k = I(C_k > T_k)$, $k = 1, 2$. We have for observed data

$$Y = (\tilde{T}_1, \Delta_1, \bar{X}_1(\tilde{T}_1), \tilde{T}_2, \Delta_2, \bar{X}_2(\tilde{T}_2)). \tag{5.1}$$

In other words, one observes two processes, $X_1(t \wedge T_1)$ and $X_2(t \wedge T_2)$, over time t that are subject to their own right-censoring times C_1 and C_2, respectively.

For example, consider a study in which a multivariate survival time on a unit consisting of two related subjects (such as twins or child/parent) is of interest. Contrary to the univariate right-censored data structure studied in Chapter 3, we do not assume that each of the subjects is subject to the same censoring mechanism. For example, we could let time begin on a particular calendar date prior to the birth of either subject in the pair. We could then let I_k denote the time until the birth of subject k, and T_k the time until the death of subject k, $k = 1, 2$. The process $X_k(t)$ should include as components $I(I_k \leq t), I(T_k \leq t)$ beyond other data $L_k(t)$ that one collects on subject k, $k = 1, 2$. The time variable of interest might be the time $T'_k = T_k - I_k$ between the two events. In that case the bivariate survival function $\mu = P(T'_1 > t_1, T'_2 > t_2)$ might be the parameter of interest. In other settings, one might be concerned with the estimation of

$$\mu = S(t_1, t_2) = P(T_1 > t_1, T_2 > t_2)$$

based on n i.i.d. $Y_1, \ldots, Y_n$ copies of Y.

The current literature provides no methods for estimation of such marginal parameters μ from multivariate right-censored data in the presence of time-varying covariate processes that predict both censoring and failure. The following example shows that multivariate censoring can also occur for different components on a single subject.

Example 5.1 We consider an NIH-funded longitudinal study (Prof. Tager and Prof. Satariano, Department of Epidemiology, UC Berkeley), which follows up an elderly cohort in Sonoma County for 8 years, where entry times are random. This data set is analyzed in Chapter 6. Each subject is monitored intensively every 2 years. At these monitoring times, one collects data on activity and health, among other variables. One of the purposes of this study is to estimate the causal effect of activity on time T until death. A proportion of the subjects drop out of the study before the end of the study and before death. However, if the person dies, then information on time of death will always be available. Let the origin $t = 0$ be the entry time of the subject. Define $X_1(t) = I(T \leq t)$, and let $X_2(t)$ be the time-dependent process including activity and health information. Let $X_k(t) = X_k(\min(t,T))$, $k = 1, 2$. we have for full data $X = (\bar{X}_1(T), \bar{X}_2(T)) = (T, \bar{X}_2(T))$. Let C_1 be the difference between the time at entry and the time the study ends. Let C_2 be the dropout time. We have that T is right-censored by C_1, while the process $X_2(t)$ is right-censored by C_2. Thus, the observed data structure on each subject is given by $Y = (C_1, \bar{X}_1(C_1), C_2, \bar{X}_2(C_2))$. □

The distribution of the observed data Y of equation (5.1) is indexed by the full data distribution F_X and the conditional bivariate distribution $G(\cdot \mid X)$ of (C_1, C_2). We will consider three types of full data models: nonparametric, multivariate generalized linear regression, and the multiplicative intensity. The first model is relevant for the nonparametric estimation of the marginal bivariate survival function $S(t_1, t_2)$. On the other hand, if one is concerned with understanding the effect of covariates on a marginal location parameter of the bivariate distribution of (T_1, T_2), then the bivariate generalized linear regression model $\log(T_j) = m_j(\beta \mid Z) + \epsilon_j$, $E(K(\epsilon_j(\beta)) \mid Z) = 0, j = 1, 2$, will be appropriate. As possible choices of K, we might recommend $I(\epsilon < 0) - 1/2$ (median regression), $I(\epsilon < 0) - p$ (pth quantile regression), a smooth approximation of $I(\epsilon < 0) - 1/2$ (smooth median regression), or $K(\epsilon) = \min(\epsilon, \tau)$ for $\epsilon > 0$ and $K(\epsilon) = \max(\epsilon, -\tau)$ for $\epsilon < 0$ (truncated mean regression). Such robust location parameters are needed because there will be insufficient data in the tail of the distribution to identify location parameters such as the mean that depend on the whole distribution. Finally, if one wishes to study the effect of covariates on the time T to death (or on the intensity of a general counting process) one might assume a multiplicative intensity model $E(dN(t) \mid \mathcal{F}(t)) = Y(t)\lambda_0(t)\exp(\beta W(t))dt$, where $N(t)$ is a counting process of interest contained in $X(t)$ such as $N(t) = I(T \leq t)$, and $\mathcal{F}(t)$ is a history that can be any function of $\bar{X}(t-)$ that includes $\bar{N}(t-)$. For each of these three models, we previously derived the class of full data structure estimating functions $\{D_h(\cdot \mid \mu, \rho) : h\}$ in Section 2.2 of Chapter 2.

5.1.1 Modeling the censoring mechanism

In order to establish practical and effective modeling techniques for the bivariate conditional censoring mechanism G under CAR, we will represent the bivariate censoring variable as a bivariate time-dependent process. Let $A_k(t) = I(C_k \leq t)$, $k = 1, 2$, and we define $C_k = \infty$ if $C_k \geq T_k$, $k = 1, 2$. For a given $A = (A_1, A_2)$, we define $X_A = (\bar{X}_1(C_1), \bar{X}_2(C_2))$. We define $\bar{X}_A(t) = (\bar{X}_1(C_1 \wedge t), \bar{X}_2(C_2 \wedge t))$ as the part of X_A that is observed by time t. Note $\bar{X}_A(t)$ only depends on A through $\bar{A}(t)$. Now, we can define the observed data as

$$Y = (A, X_A), \tag{5.2}$$

which corresponds with observing $\bar{Y}(t) = (\bar{A}(t), \bar{X}_A(t))$ through time t. The distribution of the observed data Y is thus indexed by the distribution of X and the conditional distribution of A, given X.

Let us now consider modeling and estimation of the conditional distribution $g(A \mid X)$ in both the discrete and continuous cases. Firstly, we will assume that $A_k(t)$, $k = 1, 2$, only change value at time points $j = 1, \ldots, p$ (indicating the actual times).

We are in a setting where we can assume the SRA: for all $j \in \{1, \ldots, p\}$,

$$g(A(j) \mid \bar{A}(j-1), X) = g(A(j) \mid \bar{A}(j-1), \bar{X}_A(j)). \tag{5.3}$$

Then

$$g(\bar{A} \mid X) = \prod_{j=1}^{p} g(A(j) \mid \bar{A}(j-1), X) \tag{5.4}$$

$$= \prod_{j=1}^{p} g_1(A_1(j) \mid \mathcal{F}_1(j)) \prod_{j=1}^{p} g_2(A_2(j) \mid \mathcal{F}_2(j)), \tag{5.5}$$

where $\mathcal{F}_1(j) = (A_2(j), \bar{A}(j-1), \bar{X}_A(j))$ and $\mathcal{F}_2(j) = (\bar{A}(j-1), \bar{X}_A(j))$. Let $\lambda_k(j \mid \mathcal{F}_k(j)) = P(C_k = j \mid C_k \geq j, \mathcal{F}_k(j))$ be the conditional hazard of C_k w.r.t history $\mathcal{F}_k$, $k = 1, 2$. Then

$$\alpha_k(j \mid \mathcal{F}_k(j)) \equiv P(A_k(j) = 1 \mid \mathcal{F}_k(j)) = Y_k(j)\lambda_k(j \mid \mathcal{F}_k(j))$$

and
$$g_k(A_k(j) \mid \mathcal{F}_k(j)) = \alpha_k(j)^{A_k(j)}(1 - \alpha_k(j))^{1-A_k(j)}, \; k = 1, 2.$$

Here $Y_k(j)$ is the indicator that C_k is still at risk of occurring at time j. If C_k is always observed, then one will typically have $Y_k(j) = I(C_k \geq j)$, or if C_k is censored by T_k and set equal to ∞ if $T_k \leq C_k$, then one will typically have $Y_k(j) = I(C_k \geq j, T_k > j)$. However, in the setting described above, where different subjects have different starting points I_k we would have $Y_k(t) = I(C_k \geq t, T_k > t, I_k < t)$, $k = 1, 2$.

We propose to model the discrete intensities α_k, $k = 1, 2$, with separate models. For example, we could assume a logistic regression model

$$\lambda_k(j \mid \mathcal{F}_k(j)) = \frac{1}{1 + \exp(m(j, W_k(j) \mid \gamma_k))}, \tag{5.6}$$

where $W_k(j)$ are functions of the observed past $\mathcal{F}_k(j)$, and $m(j, W_k(j) \mid \gamma_k)$ is a known function of $j, W_k(j)$ and the unknown regression parameters γ_k. In particular, we propose to model the effect of time j to be as nonparametric as possible so that this model contains, in particular, the independent censoring model that assumes that (C_1, C_2) is independent of X. If the grid is fine, then we can use the multiplicative intensity model $\lambda_k(j \mid \mathcal{F}_k(j)) = \lambda_0(t) \exp(\gamma W_k(j))$, $k = 1, 2$.

By factorization of the likelihood $P_{F_X,G}(dy)$ in F_X and G parts, the maximum likelihood estimator of $\gamma = (\gamma_1, \gamma_2)$ is defined by

$$\gamma_n = \max_{\gamma}^{-1} \prod_{i=1}^{n} \prod_{j=1}^{C_i} g_{1,\gamma_1}(A_{1i}(j) \mid \mathcal{F}_{1i}(j)) g_{2,\gamma_2}(A_{2i}(j) \mid \mathcal{F}_{2i}(j)).$$

If the models for g_1 and g_2 have no common parameters, then

$$\gamma_{1n} = \max_{\gamma_1}^{-1} \prod_{i=1}^{n} \prod_{j=1}^{C_i} \alpha_{1,\gamma_1}(j \mid \mathcal{F}_{1i}(j))^{dA_1(j)} \{1 - \alpha_{1,\gamma_1}(j \mid \mathcal{F}_{1i}(j))\}^{1-dA_1(j)}$$

and

$$\gamma_{2n} = \max_{\gamma_2}^{-1} \prod_{i=1}^{n} \prod_{j=1}^{C_i} \alpha_{2,\gamma_2}(j \mid \mathcal{F}_{2i}(j))^{dA_2(j)} \{1 - \alpha_{\gamma_2}(j \mid \mathcal{F}_{2i}(j))\}^{1-dA_2(j)}.$$

If we assume the logistic regression model (5.6), then γ_{kn} can be obtained by applying the S-plus functions GLM() or GAM() with logit link to the pooled sample $(A_{ki}(j), j, W_{ki}(j))$, $i = 1, \ldots, n$, $j = 1, \ldots, m_{ki} \equiv \min(C_{2i}, T_{2i})$, treating it as $N_k = \sum_i m_{ki}$ i.i.d. observations on a Bernoulli random variable A_k with covariates time t and W.

If $A(t)$ is *continuous*, then one can define $g(\bar{A} \mid X)$ formally as the partial likelihood of the bivariate counting process $A = (A_1, A_2)$ w.r.t. observed history $\mathcal{F}(t) = \sigma(\bar{Y}(t-))$ (Andersen, Borgan, Gill, and Keiding, 1993)

$$g(\bar{A} \mid X) = \prod_{t,k} \alpha_k(t)^{\Delta A_k(t)} \prod_t (1 - \alpha.(t)dt)^{1-\Delta A.(t)}, \tag{5.7}$$

where

$$\alpha_k(t) = E(dA_k(t) \mid \mathcal{F}(t))$$

is the intensity of A_k w.r.t. $\mathcal{F}(t)$ and $\alpha.(t) = \sum_{k=1}^{2} \alpha_k(t)$ is the intensity of $A. = A_1 + A_2$. To estimate $g(\bar{A} \mid X)$ one could assume a multiplicative intensity model (Andersen, Borgan, Gill, and Keiding, 1993)

$$\alpha_k(t) = Y_k(t)\lambda_k(t \mid \mathcal{F}_k(t)) \equiv Y_k(t)\lambda_{0k}(t)\exp(\gamma W_k(t)),$$

where $Y_k(t)$ is the indicator that A_k is at risk of jumping at time t.

To summarize, by treating the bivariate censoring variable (C_1, C_2) as a bivariate time-dependent process (A_1, A_2) indexed by the same time t as the full data and assuming the SRA, we have succeeded in presenting a flexible modeling framework allowing us to use standard software.

5.1.2 Overview

The general theory of Chapter 2 teaches us that one obtains an optimal mapping from full data estimating functions to observed data estimating functions by making an initial mapping $D_h \to IC_0(Y \mid D_h)$ orthogonal to T_{CAR}. For the univariate right-censored data structure studied in Chapter 3 (i.e., $C_1 = C_2$ with probability one), CAR is equivalent with SRA. However, for the multivariate right censored data structure, CAR does not have a nice intuitive description. For example, contrary to the univariate right-censored data structure, if $X_j(t) = I(T_j \leq t)$, $j = 1, \ldots, k$, then CAR is (significantly) weaker than assuming that $(C_1, \ldots, C_k)$ is independent of $(T_1, \ldots, T_k)$. Due to the complexity of CAR, the projection operator onto T_{CAR} does not exist in closed form and is, in general, very computer intensive to implement. For the marginal data structure (i.e., $X_j(\cdot) = I(T_j \leq \cdot)$, $j = 1, \ldots, k$), implementation of the projection operator onto T_{CAR} is practically possible and is carried out in Section 5.3 of this chapter for the case $k = 2$. This work is a slight generalization of Quale, van der Laan, and Robins (2001) which provides the complete methodology and implementation for the nonparametric full data structure model. For the general data structure (5.1) or equivalently (5.2) we recommend projecting onto $T_{SRA} \subset T_{CAR}$ instead, where T_{SRA} is the observed data tangent space of G under the sole assumption SRA (5.3). This methodology is carried out in the next section in Keles, van der Laan, and Robins (2002), it is implemented and studied in detail for the special case where the full data model is saturated and $\mu = S(t_1, t_2)$ is a bivariate survival function.

5.2 Mapping into Observed Data Estimating Functions

We refer to Section 5.1 for the representation $Y = (A_1, A_2, X_{1,A_1}, X_{2,A_2})$ of the observed data structure, where $A_k(t) = I(C_k \leq t)$, $X_{k,A_k}(t) = X_k(\min(t, C_k, T_k))$, and C_k is set to ∞ if $C_k \geq T_k$, $k = 1, 2$. We also refer to Section 5.1 for the modeling of the censoring mechanism $g(\bar{A} \mid X)$ under the assumption SRA (5.3). Let $\mu = \mu(F_X)$ be the parameter of interest. To avoid dealing with technical and measurability conditions in establishing the projection onto the tangent space T_{SRA}, we will assume that $A_k(t)$ only change value at time points $j = 1, \ldots, p$. In other words, we assume that C_1, C_2 are discrete on a grid $\{1, \ldots, p\}^2$. Since the time points can be chosen to be the grid points of an arbitrarily fine partition, this assumption can be made without loss of *practical* applicability.

In this section, we will first discuss the construction of an initial mapping and/or estimating function from full data structure estimating functions to observed data estimating functions. We illustrate it for the case where the full data structure model is nonparametric and the parameter of interest μ is a bivariate survival function at a given point in the plane. It results in a new estimator of the bivariate survival function that allows informative censoring and is always at least as efficient as Dabrowska's estimator. We will refer to this estimator as the generalized Dabrowska's estimator. We illustrate its practical performance with some simulations. Subsequently, we provide the general SRA-orthogonalized initial estimating functions and define the corresponding estimators of μ. Finally, we provide a closed-form formula of the optimal choice of full data structure function for the multivariate generalized regression model on always observed covariates.

5.2.1 The initial mapping into observed estimating data functions

Let $D_h \to IC_0(Y \mid Q_0, G, D_h)$ be an initial mapping from full data estimating functions into observed data estimating functions. Suppose that we have reparametrized (if needed) the class of full data estimating functions so that $D_h(\cdot \mid \mu(F_X), \rho(F_X, G)) \in T_{nuis}^{F,\perp}(F_X) \cap \mathcal{D}(\rho_1(F_X), G)$, $h \in \mathcal{H}^F$ for all $P_{F_X,G} \in \mathcal{M}(\mathcal{G})$. We refer to Section 2.3 and Subsection 3.3.1 for the reparametrization that is specified in (2.14). The set of full data structure estimating functions $\mathcal{D}(\rho_1(F_X), G)$ satisfying $E_G(IC_0(Y \mid Q_0, G, D) \mid X) = D(X)$ F_X-a.e. for all possible Q_0 (see definition 2.13) needs to be nonempty in order to do this reparametrization. Under strong assumptions on G, one will typically have that $\mathcal{D}(\rho_1(F_X), G)$ equals the set $\mathcal{D} = (D_h(\cdot \mid \mu(F_X), \rho(F_X)) : \mu, \rho, h \in \mathcal{H}^F)$ of all possible full data functions. In the latter case, the reparametrization is not necessary. For notational convenience, we denote the reparametrized class of full data structure estimating functions with $\{D_h(\cdot \mid \mu, \rho) : h \in \mathcal{H}^F\}$ again, where ρ now possibly also includes G as a component.

A possible choice for the initial mapping is $IC_0(Y \mid G, D) = D(X)\Delta/\bar{G}(T_1, T_2 \mid X)$, where $\Delta = I(C_1 = \infty, C_2 = \infty)$ and $\bar{G}$ is the bivariate conditional survivor function of the underlying (i.e., uncensored) (C_1, C_2). If $\bar{G}(T_1, T_2 \mid X) > 0$ F_X-a.e., then the set of allowed full data structure estimating functions $\mathcal{D}(\rho_1(F_X), G)$ equals all possible full data structure estimating functions $\mathcal{D}$. Alternatively, $IC_0(Y \mid G, D) = D(X)\Delta(D)/P(\Delta(D) = 1 \mid X)$, where $\Delta(D) = I(D(X)$ observed). For example, consider the case where $\mu = S(t_1, t_2) = P(T_1 > t_1, T_2 > t_2)$, and let the full data model be nonparametric so that $D(X) = I(T_1 > t_1, T_2 > t_2) - \mu$. Then, we can choose $IC_0(Y \mid G, D) = I(T_1 > t_1, T_2 > t_2)I(C_1 > t_1, C_2 > t_2)/\bar{G}(t_1, t_2 \mid X) - \mu$.

Instead of specifying a mapping, one can also construct one initial estimating function $IC_0(Y \mid Q_0, G, D(. \mid \mu))$ for μ by choosing it such that $IC_0(Y \mid Q_0(F_X, G), G, D(. \mid \mu(F_X)))$ equals an influence curve of a regular asymptotically linear estimator of μ in the observed data model with G known or G modeled with some submodel of CAR.

It is important to note that the choice of $IC_0(Y \mid Q_0, G, D(. \mid \mu))$ is potentially very relevant for the asymptotic efficiency of our proposed mapping $IC_0(Y \mid Q_0, G, D(. \mid \mu)) - \Pi(IC_0(Y \mid Q_0, G, D(. \mid \mu)) \mid T_{SRA})$ even when the full data model is nonparametric. (Recall that if the full data model is nonparametric, then $IC_0(Y \mid Q_0, G, D(. \mid \mu)) - \Pi(IC_0(Y \mid Q_0, G, D(. \mid \mu)) \mid T_{CAR})$ equals the efficient influence curve for each choice of $IC_0(Y \mid Q_0, G, D(. \mid \mu))$ and thus does not depend on $IC_0(Y \mid Q_0, G, D(. \mid \mu))$.) Off course, if the projection of $IC_0(Y \mid Q_0, G, D(. \mid \mu))$ onto T_{CAR} equals the projection onto T_{SRA}, then we would actually have the optimal mapping $IC_0(Y \mid Q_0, G, D(. \mid \mu)) - \Pi(IC_0(Y \mid Q_0, G, D(. \mid \mu)) \mid T_{CAR})$. However, under bivariate censoring (i.e, we do not have that $C_1 = C_2$ with probability 1) such choices IC_0 will generally not exist in closed form since the projection operator onto T_{CAR} involves a Neumann series for which we have no closed form expression. Consequently, the only real guarantee that we have is that this mapping leads to estimators with a better influence curve than $IC_0(Y \mid Q_0, G, D(. \mid \mu))$.

Therefore, it is particularly important here to explain, given an RAL estimator of μ, how one can obtain a mapping $D_h \to IC_0(Y \mid Q_0, G, D_h)$ from full data estimating functions into observed data estimating functions so that for a particular choice D_h of full data estimating function it provides an estimator that is asymptotically equivalent with the given RAL estimator. This explanation was given in Subsection 2.3.2 in Chapter 2 and is repeated here for the purpose of making this chapter self-contained.

Let μ_n be a given RAL estimator, and let $IC(Y \mid F_X, G)$ be its influence curve. Since $IC(Y \mid F_X, G)$ is a gradient of the pathwise derivative of μ, we have that $E_G(IC(Y \mid F, G) \mid X) \in T_{nuis}^{F,\perp}(F_X)$ for all $F \in \mathcal{M}^F$. Let $h^* \equiv h_{F_X}(E_G(IC(Y \mid F_X, G) \mid X))$ be the corresponding index

$$D_{h^*}(X \mid \mu(F_X), \rho(F_X)) = E_G(IC(Y \mid F_X, G) \mid X).$$

Note that h^* is typically a function of (F_X, G); though this is not true if the full-data model is nonparametric in which case there is only one full-data estimating function. Let $D_h \to IC_0(Y \mid Q_0, G, D_h)$ be an initial mapping from full data estimating functions into observed data estimating functions satisfying $E(IC_0(Y \mid Q_0, G, D_h(\cdot \mid \mu, \rho)) \mid X) = D_h(X \mid \mu, \rho)$ F_X-a.e. for all Q_0. We now define $IC_{CAR}(Y \mid Q_0, F_X, G)$ as

$$IC(Y \mid F_X, G) - IC_0(Y \mid Q_0, G, D_{h^*(F_X, G)}(\cdot \mid \mu(F_X), \rho(F_X))).$$

Note that $E_G(IC_{CAR}(Y \mid Q_0, F, G) \mid X) = 0$ for all $F \in \mathcal{M}^F$ and Q_0. We now define as mapping from full data estimating functions into observed data estimating functions

$$IC(Y \mid Q_0, F_X, G, D_h) = IC_0(Y \mid Q_0, G, D_h) + IC_{CAR}(Y \mid Q_0, F_X, G). \tag{5.8}$$

This mapping is now an example of an initial mapping $IC_0(Y \mid Q_0, G, D(\cdot \mid \mu))$ and satisfies $E_G(IC(Y \mid (Q_0, F), G, D_h) \mid X) = D_h(X)$ F_X-a.e. for all possible (Q_0, F). If $h = h^*$, then it provides an estimating function for μ that yields an estimator asymptotically equivalent with μ_n. Note also that other choices of D_h might result in even more efficient estimators.

5.2.2 Generalized Dabrowska estimator of the survival function in the nonparametric full data model

Consider the data structure and model described in Section 5.1, where the full data model is nonparametric and $\mu = S(t_1, t_2) = P(T_1 > t_1, T_2 > t_2)$ is the parameter of interest. The only full data estimating function is $D(X \mid \mu) = I(T_1 > t_1, T_2 > t_2) - \mu$. We first apply the method described in the previous subsection to the independent censoring model $\mathcal{G}^*$, and subsequently we extend the estimating function to all $G \in \mathcal{G}(CAR)$; see Section 2.3 in Chapter 2 for the treatment of this general method for obtaining estimating functions.

A well-known estimator of $\mu = S(t_1, t_2)$ based on marginal bivariate right-censored data in the independent censoring model $\mathcal{G}^*$ for G is the Dabrowska estimator (Dabrowska, 1988,1989). The influence curve $IC_{Dab}(Y \mid F, G, (t_1, t_2)) \equiv IC_{Dab}(Y)$ of Dabrowska's estimator is derived in Gill, van der Laan, and Wellner (1995) and van der Laan (1990) and is given by

$$IC_{Dab}(Y) = \bar{F}(t_1, t_2) \left\{ -\int_0^{t_1} \frac{I(\tilde{T}_1 \in du, \Delta_1 = 1) - I(\tilde{T}_1 \geq u)\Lambda_1(du)}{P_{F,G}(\tilde{T}_1 \geq u)} \right.$$

$$-\int_0^{t_2} \frac{I(\tilde{T}_2 \in du, \Delta_2 = 1) - I(\tilde{T}_2 \geq u)\Lambda_2(du)}{P_{F,G}(\tilde{T}_2 \geq u)}$$

$$+\int_0^{t_1}\int_0^{t_2} \frac{I(\tilde{T}_1 \in du, \tilde{T}_2 \in dv, \Delta_1 = 1, \Delta_2 = 1)}{P_{F,G}(\tilde{T}_1 \geq u, \tilde{T}_2 \geq v)}$$

$$-\int_0^{t_1}\int_0^{t_2} \frac{I(\tilde{T}_1 \geq u, \tilde{T}_2 \geq v)\Lambda_{11}(du, dv)}{P_{F,G}(\tilde{T}_1 \geq u, \tilde{T}_2 \geq v)}$$

$$-\int_0^{t_1}\int_0^{t_2} \frac{I(\tilde{T}_1 \in du, \tilde{T}_2 \geq v, \Delta_1 = 1)\Lambda_{01}(dv, u)}{P_{F,G}(\tilde{T}_1 \geq u, \tilde{T}_2 \geq v)}$$

$$+\int_0^{t_1}\int_0^{t_2} \frac{I(\tilde{T}_1 \geq u, \tilde{T}_2 \geq v)\Lambda_{10}(du, v)\Lambda_{01}(dv, u)}{P_{F,G}(\tilde{T}_1 \geq u, \tilde{T}_2 \geq v)}$$

$$-\int_0^{t_1}\int_0^{t_2} \frac{I(\tilde{T}_1 \geq u, \tilde{T}_2 \in dv, \Delta_2 = 1)\Lambda_{10}(du, v)}{P_{F,G}(\tilde{T}_1 \geq u, \tilde{T}_2 \geq v)}$$

$$+\int_0^{t_1}\int_0^{t_2} \frac{I(\tilde{T}_1 \geq u, \tilde{T}_2 \geq v)\Lambda_{10}(du, v)\Lambda_{01}(dv, u)}{P_{F,G}(\tilde{T}_1 \geq u, \tilde{T}_2 \geq v)}\Bigg\},$$

where $\Lambda_j(du) = P(T_j \in du \mid T_j \geq u)$, $j = 1, 2$, $\Lambda_{10}(du \mid v) = P(T_1 \in du \mid T_1 \geq u, T_2 \geq v)$, $\Lambda_{01}(dv, u) = P(T_2 \in dv \mid T_1 \geq u, T_2 \geq v)$ and $\Lambda_{11}(du, dv) = P(T_1 \in du, T_2 \in dv \mid T_1 \geq u, T_2 \geq v)$.

Here $P_{F,G}(\tilde{T}_1 > s, \tilde{T}_2 > t) = S(s,t)\bar{G}(s,t)$. Firstly, we note that it is straightforward to verify that $E_{P_{F_X,G}}(IC_{Dab}(Y \mid F, G, (t_1, t_2)) \mid X) = D(X \mid \mu)$ for all independent censoring distributions $G \in \mathcal{G}^*$ satisfying $\bar{G}(t_1, t_2) > 0$. In addition, as predicted, if we replace G in this influence curve by any G satisfying CAR and $\bar{G}(t_1, t_2 \mid X) > 0$ F_X-a.e., then we still have:

$$E_{P_{F_X,G}}(IC_{Dab}(Y \mid F, G, (t_1, t_2)) \mid X) = I(T_1 > t_1, T_2 > t_2) - \mu \quad (5.9)$$

for all bivariate distributions F.

Let $IC_0(Y \mid G, D) = D(X)\Delta/\bar{G}(T_1, T_2 \mid X)$. We now define

$$IC_{CAR}(Y \mid F, G) \equiv IC_{Dab}(Y \mid F, G) - IC_0(Y \mid G, D(\cdot \mid \mu(F))).$$

By (5.9), $E_G(IC_{CAR}(Y \mid F, G) \mid X) = 0$ for all $G \in \mathcal{G}(CAR)$ and bivariate distributions F.

We now define an observed data estimating function for μ indexed by the true censoring mechanism G and a bivariate distribution F as

$$IC(Y \mid F, G, D(\cdot \mid \mu)) = IC_0(Y \mid G, D(\cdot \mid \mu)) + IC_{CAR}(Y \mid F, G).$$

Note that this estimating function for μ satisfies (5.9), and it reduces to Dabrowska's influence curve at the true μ and F. Given consistent estimators F_n of F and G_n of G, let μ_n be the solution of

$$0 = \frac{1}{n}\sum_{i=1}^n IC(Y_i \mid F_n, G_n, D(\cdot \mid \mu)).$$

We will refer to μ_n as the generalized Dabrowska estimator. Under regularity conditions similar to those in Theorem 2.4, μ_n is asymptotically linear with influence curve $IC(Y) \equiv \Pi(IC(\cdot \mid F, G, D(\cdot \mid \mu)) \mid T_2^\perp(P_{F_X,G}))$, where $T_2(P_{F_X,G}) \subset T_{CAR}$ is the observed data tangent space of G under the posed model $\mathcal{G}$. Since $IC(Y \mid F, G, D(\cdot \mid \mu))$ is already orthogonal to the tangent space T_{indep} for the independent censoring model $\mathcal{G}^*$, we have two important results. Firstly, if the posed model $\mathcal{G}$ is the independent censoring model, then $IC(Y \mid F, G, D(. \mid \mu))$ equals $IC_{Dabr}(Y)$. Secondly, if the tangent space $T_2(P_{F_X,G})$ contains scores that are not in T_{indep}, then this proposed estimating function will result in an estimator more efficient than Dabrowska's estimator if T_1 or T_2 depend on the available covariates used in the censoring model $\mathcal{G}$, even when (C_1, C_2) is independent of X.

Remark

It is of interest to note here that we have shown that the CAR-component $IC_{CAR}(Y \mid F, G)$ of Dabrowska's influence curve is not an element of $T_{SRA}(P_{F_X,G})$ at data generating distributions in bivariate frailty models, excluding the complete independence case (i.e., $T_1 \perp T_2 \perp C_1 \perp C_2$ independent) under which Dabrowska's influence curve equals the efficient influence curve and $IC_{CAR} \in T_{SRA}$. This explains why $IC_{Dab}(Y \mid F, G) - \Pi(IC_{Dab} \mid T_{SRA})$ does not equal $IC_0(Y \mid G, D) - \Pi(IC_0(Y \mid G, D) \mid T_{SRA})$ and thus that the choice of estimating function can affect the efficiency of the T_{SRA}-orthogonalized estimating function (contrary to the T_{CAR}-orthogonalized estmating functions). In fact, we have seen that the T_{SRA}-orthogonalized estimating function of IC_0 was typically outperformed by Dabrowska's estimator, which motivated us to consider T_{SRA}-orthogonalized estimating function corresponding with Dabrowska's influence curve, as implemented in Sunduz, van der Laan, Robins (2002), and, in general, defined in the next section.

5.2.3 Simulation study of the generalized Dabrowka estimator.

We performed a simulation study to compare performances of the generalized Dabrowska estimator μ_n with Dabrowska's estimator μ_n^{Dab} for estimating the parameter $\mu = S(t_1, t_2)$ in the general right-censored data structure. In the simulations below, we used frailty models (Clayton and Cusick, 1985) with and without covariates to generate survival and censoring times. We have two main simulation setups.

- Simulation I (Informative censoring): We generated binary baseline covariates $Z1, Z2 \sim$ Bernoulli(p) for each pair of subjects. Consecutively, both censoring and survival times were made dependent on these baseline covariates to enforce informative censoring. Survival times T_1 and T_2 are generated from a gamma frailty model with truncated baseline hazard. This assumes a proportional hazards model of the type

$$\lambda_i(t \mid W = w, Z_i = z_i) = \lambda_0(t) w e^{\beta_t z_i}, \qquad i = 1, 2,$$

where w represents a realization from the hidden gamma random variable. A truncated exponential baseline hazard was chosen to ensure that $\bar{G}(t_1, t_2 \mid X) > 0 \ \forall t_1, t_2$ in the support of F_X. Similarly, C_1, C_2 were generated from a gamma frailty model with covariate Z using a constant baseline hazard, where the frailty in this model is independent of the frailty w used in the model for (T_1, T_2). Through the coefficients in front of the Z's (β_t for (T_1, T_2) and β_c for (C_1, C_2)), we adjusted the amount of dependence between survival and censoring times.

- Simulation II (Independent censoring): We generated survival times as in simulation setup I, but generated censoring times independent of T_1, T_2. This corresponds to setting $\beta_c = 0$ in conditional hazards of C_1, C_2.

We first report the mean squared error ratios for μ_{Dab} and μ_n from a simulation study of setup I for moderate informative censoring in Table 5.1. The two estimators are evaluated on a 4×4 grid. We see that μ_n outperforms μ_n^{Dab} at all grid points. This result indicates that our generalization of Dabrowska's estimator is truly accounting for informative censoring.

In Table 5.2, we report the relative performance of the two estimators when censoring times are independent of the failure times (i.e., $G(. \mid X) = G(.)$ (generating from setup II)). In this particular case, μ_n still estimates $G(. \mid X)$ by a bivariate frailty model with covariates (i.e., ignoring independence). We observe from Table 5.2 that both estimators perform about the same under this scenario, though the generalized Dabrowska estimator performs slightly better (as predicted by theory). This particular simulation implies that even in the case where censoring is independent of survival times, we get an estimator that is as good as or better than Dabrowska's estimator by estimating $\bar{G}(. \mid X)$ from a model that includes independent censoring as a sub-model.

5.2.4 The proposed mapping into observed data estimating functions

Let T_{SRA} be the tangent space of G under the sole assumption SRA. For notational convenience, we will sometimes use shorthand notation IC_0 for the initial observed data estimating function $IC_0(. \mid Q_0, G, D_h(\cdot \mid \mu, \rho))$. In order to improve the efficiency of our estimating function IC_0 and to obtain the double robustness property, we orthogonalize IC_0 with respect to T_{SRA} and thus define as new estimating function $IC_0 - \Pi(IC_0 \mid T_{SRA})$. Theorem 5.1 (which is a copy of Theorem 1.2 in Chapter 1) below provides

5.2. Mapping into Observed Data Estimating Functions   277

Table 5.1. **Simulation I:** $MSE_{\mu_n}/MSE_{\mu_{Dab}}$ for simulations of 250 subjects over 200 iterations. F and G are both generated from frailties with covariate $Z \sim$ Bernoulli (0.5). $G(. \mid X)$ is estimated using a bivariate frailty model with covariates. Correlations between T_1 and C_1 and T_2 and C_2 are approximately 0.4. $P(T_1 < C_1) = 0.65$ and $P(T_2 < C_2) = 0.65$.

	$t_1 = 0.1$	$t_1 = 1$	$t_1 = 4$	$t_1 = 10$
$t_2 = 0.1$	0.9615430	0.8015517	0.2000056	0.2023185
$t_2 = 1$	0.9222071	0.6194325	0.2619613	0.2579991
$t_2 = 4$	0.1769921	0.3169093	0.1994758	0.2131806
$t_2 = 10$	0.2335622	0.3569389	0.2638717	0.2433467

Table 5.2. **Simulation II:** $MSE_{\mu_n}/MSE_{\mu_{Dab}}$ for simulations of 250 subjects over 200 iterations. F is generated from frailties with covariate $Z \sim$ Bernoulli (0.5). $G(. \mid X)$ is from a bivariate frailty model. T and C are independent. $G(. \mid X)$ is estimated using a bivariate frailty with covariates Z. Correlations between T_1 and C_1 and T_2 and C_2 are approximately 0. $P(T_1 < C_1) = 0.70$ and $P(T_2 < C_2) = 0.70$.

	$t_1 = 0.05$	$t_1 = 0.2$	$t_1 = 3$	$t_1 = 8$
$t_2 = 0.05$	0.9990788	0.9985483	0.9702160	0.9813311
$t_2 = 0.2$	0.9924038	0.9946938	0.9650496	0.9741110
$t_2 = 3$	0.9814260	0.9789798	0.9504253	0.9650510
$t_2 = 8$	0.9806082	0.9821724	0.9665981	0.9789226

the following representation of this projection $\Pi(IC_0 \mid T_{SRA})$:

$$\sum_{k=1}^{2} \sum_{t=0}^{C_k} \{E(IC_0(Y) \mid A_k(t), \mathcal{F}_k(t)) - E\left[E(IC_0(Y) \mid A_k(t), \mathcal{F}_k(t)) \mid \mathcal{F}_k(t)\right]\}.$$

An equivalent representation is given by

$$\Pi(IC_0 \mid T_{SRA}(P_{F_X,G})) = \sum_{k=1}^{2} \int H_k(u, \mathcal{F}_k(u)) dM_{G,k}(u),$$

where

$$H_k(u, \mathcal{F}_k(u)) = E(IC_0(Y) \mid C_k = u, \mathcal{F}_k(u)) - E(IC_0(Y) \mid C_k > u, \mathcal{F}_k(u))$$

and

$$dM_{G,k}(u) = I(C_k = u) - I(C_k \geq u, T_k > u)\lambda_k(u \mid \mathcal{F}_k(u)), k = 1, 2.$$

Recall that we redefined $C_k = \infty$ if T_k was smaller or equal than its censoring time. We will now introduce some reparametrizations to clarify the nuisance parameter components in the representation of projections onto T_{SRA}.

Define
$$Q_k(F_X, G)(A_k(t), \mathcal{F}_k(t)) \equiv E(IC_0(Y) \mid A_k(t), \mathcal{F}_k(t)), \quad k=1,2.$$
Then
$$E(Q_k(F_X, G)(A_k(t), \mathcal{F}_k(t)) \mid \mathcal{F}_k(t)) \equiv E\left[E(IC_0(Y) \mid A_k(t), \mathcal{F}_k(t)) \mid \mathcal{F}_k(t)\right].$$
Now, the projection $\Pi(IC_0 \mid T_{SRA})$ can be represented as
$$IC_{SRA}(Y \mid Q_1, Q_2) \equiv \sum_{k=1}^{2} \sum_{t} Q_k(F_X, G)(A_k(t), \mathcal{F}_k(t))$$
$$- \sum_{k=1}^{2} \sum_{\delta \in \{0,1\}} Q_k(F_X, G)(\delta, \mathcal{F}_k(t)) \lambda_k(t \mid \mathcal{F}_k(t))^\delta (1 - \lambda_k(t \mid \mathcal{F}_k(t)))^{1-\delta}.$$

Here δ represents the outcome of $A_k(t)$. Note that $Q_k(F_X, G)(1, \mathcal{F}_k(t)) = E(IC_0(Y) \mid C_k = t, \mathcal{F}_k(t))$ and $Q_k(F_X, G)(0, \mathcal{F}_k(t)) = E(IC_0(Y) \mid C_k > t, \mathcal{F}_k(t))$. Let $Q = (Q_0, Q_1, Q_2)$ so that we can denote the proposed estimating function with

$$IC(Y \mid Q, G, D) = IC_0(Y \mid Q_0, G, D) - IC_{SRA}(Y \mid (Q_1, Q_2), G, D).$$

Since $D_h(\cdot \mid \mu(F_X), \rho(F_X, G)) \in T_{nuis}^{F, \perp}(F_X) \cap \mathcal{D}(\rho_1(F_X), G)$, application of Lemma 1.9 teaches us that this estimating function has the double robustness property: if $G_1, G \in \mathcal{G}(SRA)$ and $dG/dG_1 < \infty$, then

$$E_{P_{F_X, G}} IC(Y \mid Q(F_1, G_1), G_1, D_h(\cdot \mid \mu(F_X), \rho(F_X, G_1))) = 0$$

if $F_1 = F_X$ or $G_1 = G$.

Given a possibly data-adaptive choice for the full data estimating function $D_{h_n}(\cdot \mid \mu, \rho)$ and estimates G_n, Q_n, ρ_n, we estimate μ by solving

$$0 = \sum_{i=1}^{n} IC(Y_i \mid Q_n, G_n, D_{h_n}(\cdot \mid \mu, \rho_n)).$$

If we use the notation $\widehat{IC}(Y \mid \mu_n) \equiv IC(Y \mid Q_n, G_n, D_h(\cdot \mid \mu_n, \rho_n))$, then this estimating equation can also be represented as

$$0 = \sum_{i=1}^{n} \widehat{IC}(Y_i \mid \mu).$$

In absolute generality, we can estimate the conditional expectations $E(IC_0(Y) \mid C_k = t, \mathcal{F}_k(t))$ and $E(IC_0(Y) \mid C_k > t, \mathcal{F}_k(t))$ (semi) parametrically by regressing an estimate of $IC_0(Y)$ onto t and covariates extracted from the past $(A_k(t), \mathcal{F}_k(t))$ and subsequently evaluating the fitted regression at each t by substituting for $\bar{A}_k(t)$ values $A_k(t) = 1$, $\bar{A}_k(t-1) = 0$ and $\bar{A}_k(t) = 0$, respectively. Here, one assumes a regression model $E(IC_0(Y) \mid (t, A_k(t), \mathcal{F}_k(t))) = g_t(W(t) \mid \beta)$ with $g_t(W(t) \mid \beta)$ known (0 or $IC_0(Y)$

itself) for $t \geq \tilde{T} = \min(\max(T_1, T_2), \max(C_1, C_2))$. Here each subject contributes $\tilde{T}$ observations $(t = j, A_k(j), \mathcal{F}_k(j)), j = 1, \ldots, \tilde{T}$. Another method would be to regress an estimate of $IC_0(Y)$ onto covariates extracted from $\mathcal{F}_k(t)$ among observations with $C_k \approx t$ (smoothing) and $C_k > t$, respectively, and subsequently smooth all of these t-specific regression estimates over t, taking into account the variance of each (e.g., by weighting them by 1 over the number of observations used to fit the regression). The above methods to estimate $Q(F_X, G)$ do not result in a doubly robust estimator μ_n. In order to obtain a doubly robust estimator, we refer to Section 1.6 for the maximum likelihood method for estimation of the conditional expectations, where the conditional expectations under the maximum likelihood estimator P_{F_n, G_n} are evaluated with Monte-Carlo simulation (see also Sunduz, van der Laan, Robins, 2002, for worked out details on this algorithm), and to Section 6.4 for a method based on a representation of $Q(F_X, G)$ which allows separate estimation of F_X-regressions and G, based on Robins (2000), and Tchetgen, Robins (2002).

Let $IC(Y \mid \mu) = IC(Y \mid Q, G, D_h(\cdot \mid \mu, \rho))$ denote the limit of $\widehat{IC}(Y \mid \mu)$ for $n \to \infty$. For obtaining a Wald-type confidence interval for μ, it is convenient to assume that the model for G is correctly specified (i.e., our observed data structure model is $\mathcal{M}(\mathcal{G})$). Let $T_G \subset T_{SRA}$ be the tangent space of the chosen model for G. In that case, application of Theorem 2.4 of Chapter 2 teaches us that, under the specified regularity conditions of Theorem 2.4, μ_n is asymptotically linear with influence curve $c^{-1}\{IC(Y \mid \mu) - \Pi(IC \mid T_G)\}$, where $c = d/d\mu P_{F_X, G} IC(Y \mid \mu) = d/d\mu P_{F_X, G} IC_0(Y \mid \mu)$. Thus, a conservative confidence band for μ can be based on the conservative estimate of the covariance matrix of the normal limit distribution of $\sqrt{n}(\mu_n - \mu)$,

$$\widehat{\Sigma} = c_n^{-1} \left\{ \frac{1}{n} \sum_{i=1}^{n} \widehat{IC}(Y_i) \widehat{IC}(Y_i)^\top \right\} c_n^{-1\top},$$

where c_n is the empirical estimate of the derivative matrix c. To obtain a confidence interval in $\mathcal{M}$, we propose to use the bootstrap.

We refer to Chapter 2 for the minor modification $IC_0 - c^* IC_{SRA}$ of IC involving a c^* defining the projection of IC_0 onto the one-dimensional space $\langle IC_{SRA} \rangle$, which guarantees that μ_n is asymptotically linear with an influence curve that is more efficient than $IC_0(Y)$. Thus, by setting IC_0 equal to the influence curve of an initial estimator μ_n^0, the resulting estimate μ_n will be guaranteed more efficient than μ_n^0 even when Q_n is heavily misspecified. Here $c^* = \langle IC_0, IC_{SRA}^\top \rangle \langle IC_{SRA}, IC_{SRA}^\top \rangle^{-1}$ so that $c^* IC_{SRA} = \Pi(IC_0 \mid \langle IC_{SRA} \rangle)$ is the projection of IC_0 onto the one-dimensional space spanned by the components of IC_{SRA}. Note that c^* can be estimated with empirical covariances of $\widehat{IC}_0, \widehat{IC}_{SRA}$, and recall that $c_n^* \approx I$ if $\widehat{IC}_{SRA} \approx IC_{SRA} = \Pi(IC_0 \mid T_{SRA})$. Therefore, c_n^* can also be used in selecting a good fit Q_n.

280   5. Multivariate Right-Censored Multivariate Data

Theorem 5.1 *Recall the setting of Section 5.1.1 in which C_k, $k = 1,2$, are discrete on time points $j = 1, \ldots, p$ and always observed (infinity if failure T_k is observed). The nuisance tangent space of G at $P_{F_X,G}$ under the sole assumption SRA (5.3) is given by*

$$T_{SRA}(P_{F_X,G}) = T_{SRA,1}(P_{F_X,G}) \oplus T_{SRA,2}(P_{F_X,G}),$$

where

$$T_{SRA,k}(P_{F_X,G}) = \overline{\left\{ \int H(u, \mathcal{F}_k(u)) dM_{G,k}(u) : H \right\}} \cap L_0^2(P_{F_X,G})$$

and

$$dM_{G,k}(u) = I(C_k = u) - \lambda_k(u \mid \mathcal{F}_k(u))I(C_k \geq u, T_k > u), \quad k = 1,2.$$

The projection of any function $V(Y) \in L_0^2(P_{F_X,G})$ onto $T_{SRA}(P_{F_X,G})$ is given by

$$\Pi(V \mid T_{SRA}(P_{F_X,G})) = \sum_{k=1}^{2} \int H_k(u, \mathcal{F}_k(u)) dM_{G,k}(u),$$

where

$$H_k(u, \mathcal{F}_k(u)) = E(V(Y) \mid C_k = u, \mathcal{F}_k(u)) - E(V(Y) \mid C_k > u, \mathcal{F}_k(u)).$$

An alternative representation of this projection is given by:

$$\Pi(V \mid T_{SRA}) = \sum_{k=1}^{2} \sum_{t=1}^{p} E(V(Y) \mid A_k(t), \mathcal{F}_k(t)) - E(V(Y) \mid \mathcal{F}_k(t)),$$

where $E(V(Y) \mid \mathcal{F}_k(t)) \equiv E(E(V(Y) \mid A_k(t), \mathcal{F}_k(t)) \mid \mathcal{F}_k(t))$.

Note that the latter summation over t runs between 1 and C_k since the difference between the two conditional expectations equals 0 for $t > C_k$.

Proof. Firstly, we will derive the tangent space T_{SRA} for $g(\bar{A} \mid X)$ under the sole assumption (5.3). By factorization of $g(\bar{A} \mid X)$ in the two products, we have that $T_{SRA} = T_{SRA,1} \oplus T_{SRA,2}$, where $T_{SRA,k}$ is the tangent space for the kth product, $k = 1,2$. By the same argument, we have that $T_{SRA,k} = T_{SRA,k,1} \oplus \ldots \oplus T_{SRA,k,p}$, where $T_{SRA,k,j}$ is the tangent space for the jth component of the kth product in (5.4). We will now derive the tangent space $T_{SRA,k,j}$. Let $\mathcal{F}_1(j) = (A_2(j), \bar{A}(j-1), \bar{X}_A(j))$, and let $\mathcal{F}_2(j) = (\bar{A}(j-1), \bar{X}_A(j))$. Let $\alpha_k(j \mid \mathcal{F}_k(j)) = E(dA_k(j) \mid \mathcal{F}_k(j))$, $k = 1,2$. Then, the kth product, $k = 1,2$, in (5.4) can be represented as:

$$\prod_{j=1}^{p} \alpha_k(j \mid \mathcal{F}_k(j))^{dA_k(j)} \{1 - \alpha_k(j \mid \mathcal{F}(j))\}^{1-dA_k(j)}.$$

Note that

$$\alpha_k(j \mid \mathcal{F}_k(j)) = I(C_k \geq j, T_k > j)\lambda_k(j \mid \mathcal{F}_k(j)),$$

5.2. Mapping into Observed Data Estimating Functions 281

where $\lambda_k(j \mid \mathcal{F}_k(j)) = P(C_k = j \mid C_k \geq j, \mathcal{F}_k(j))$ is the conditional hazard of C_k, $k = 1, 2$.

Since $\alpha_k(j \mid \mathcal{F}_k(j))^{dA_k(j)}\{1 - \alpha_k(j \mid \mathcal{F}_k(j))\}^{1-dA_k(j)}$ is just a Bernoulli likelihood for the random variable $dA_k(j)$ with probability $\alpha_k(j \mid \mathcal{F}_k(j))$, it follows that the tangent space of $\alpha_k(j \mid \mathcal{F}_k(j))$ is the space of all functions of $(dA_k(j), \mathcal{F}_k(j))$ with conditional mean zero given $\mathcal{F}_k(j)$. Straightforward algebra shows that any such function V can be written as:

$$V(dA_k(j), \mathcal{F}_k(j)) - E(V \mid \mathcal{F}_k(j)) = \{V(1, \mathcal{F}_k(j)) - V(0, \mathcal{F}_k(j))\}dM_{G,k}(j), \tag{5.10}$$

where

$$\begin{aligned} dM_{G,k}(j) &= dA_k(j) - \alpha_k(j \mid \mathcal{F}_k(j)) \\ &= I(C_k = j) - \lambda_k(j \mid \mathcal{F}_k(j))I(C_k \geq j, T_k > j). \end{aligned}$$

Note that $I(C_k = j) = I(C_k = j, T_k > j)$.

Thus, the tangent space of $\alpha_k(j \mid \mathcal{F}_k(j))$ for a fixed j equals

$$T_{SRA,k,j} \equiv \overline{\{H(\mathcal{F}_k(j))\{dA_k(j) - \alpha_k(j \mid \mathcal{F}(j))\} : H\}},$$

where H ranges over all functions of $\mathcal{F}_k(j)$ for which the right-hand-side elements have finite variance. By factorization of the likelihood, we have

$$T_{SRA,k}(P_{F_X,G}) = T_{SRA,k,1} \oplus T_{SRA,k,2} \ldots \oplus T_{SRA,k,p}. \tag{5.11}$$

Equivalently,

$$T_{SRA,k}(P_{F_X,G}) = \overline{\left\{\sum_{j=1}^{p} H(j, \mathcal{F}_k(j))dM_{G,k}(j) : H\right\}}.$$

By representation (5.11), we have

$$\Pi(V \mid T_{SRA,k}) = \sum_{j=1}^{p} \Pi(V \mid T_{SRA,k,j}).$$

The projection $\Pi(V \mid T_{SRA,k,j})$ onto $T_{SRA,k,j}$ is obtained by first projecting on all functions of $(dA_k(j), \mathcal{F}_k(j))$ and subsequently subtracting its conditional expectation, given $\mathcal{F}_k(j)$:

$$E(V(Y) \mid dA_k(j), \mathcal{F}_k(j)) - E(E(V(D)(Y) \mid dA_k(j), \mathcal{F}_k(j)) \mid \mathcal{F}_k(j)).$$

By (5.10), this can be written as

$$\{E(V(Y) \mid dA_k(j) = 1, \mathcal{F}_k(j)) - E(V(Y) \mid dA_k(j) = 0, \mathcal{F}_k(j))\} dM_{G,k}(j),$$

so we can conclude that

$$\begin{aligned} \Pi(V(Y) \mid T_{SRA}(P_{F_X,G})) &= \sum_{k=1}^{2}\sum_{j=1}^{p} \{E(V(Y) \mid dA_k(j) = 1, \mathcal{F}_k(j)) \\ &\quad - E(V(Y) \mid dA_k(j) = 0, \mathcal{F}_k(j))\} dM_{G,k}(j). \end{aligned}$$

This completes the proof. □

5.2.5 Choosing the full data estimating function in MGLM

Consider the proposed estimating functions $IC(Y \mid Q, G, D_h(\cdot \mid \mu, \rho))$ defined as an projection of an initial estimating function $IC_0(Y \mid Q_0, G, D_h)$ onto the orthogonal complement of T_{SRA}. Suppose that the full data model is an m-variate generalized linear regression model $Z = g(X^* \mid \beta) + \epsilon$, where $E(K(\epsilon(\beta)) \mid X^*) = 0$, Z, ϵ are m-dimensional, and β is q-dimensional. For example, $T_j = g(X^* \mid \beta) + \epsilon_j$, $E(K(\epsilon_j) \mid X^*) = 0$, $j = 1, 2$, where X^* are baseline covariates. We assume that the covariates X^* are always observed. The full data estimating functions are $h(X^*)K(\epsilon)$, where $h(X^*)$ is a $q \times m$ bounded matrix function. It is of interest to provide a (closed-form) representation and estimate of the optimal choice h, which now might not necessarily correspond with the efficient influence curve as in Theorem 1.3 (due to the fact that we use a mapping $D \to IC(Y \mid Q, G, D)$ which is orthogonal to a *subspace* T_{SRA} of T_{CAR}). Application of theorem 2.11 teaches us that the optimal choice $h^*(X^*)_{q \times m}$ is given by

$$h^* = -E(d/d\beta IC(Y \mid K_\beta) \mid X^*)_{q \times m} E(IC(Y \mid K_\beta) IC(Y \mid K_\beta)^\top \mid X^*)^{-1},$$

where the latter factor is an inverse of an $m \times m$-matrix. Here $K_\beta(X) = K(\epsilon(\beta))$ and we used shorthand notation $IC(Y \mid K_\beta) = IC(Y \mid Q, Q, K_\beta)$. Thus, we now have a closed form representation of the optimal estimating function in our class of T_{SRA}-orthogonalized estimating functions based on multivariate right-censored data structures.

5.3 Bivariate Right-Censored Failure Time Data

In this section, we study locally efficient estimation with the classical bivariate right-censored data structure without any covariate process. This section is based on Quale, van der Laan, and Robins (2001).

5.3.1 Introduction

Marginal bivariate right-censored data arise when there are two time-to-event variables of interest (T_1, T_2) in which, for some observations, a process (independent of the event of interest) prevents us from observing the full time to event of one or both time variables. This process is represented by the censoring variables (C_1, C_2). Thus, in a bivariate right censored data set, we are seeing n i.i.d. copies of $Y = (\tilde{T}_1, \Delta_1, \tilde{T}_2, \Delta_2)$. Here $X = (T_1, T_2) \sim F$ (with corresponding bivariate survival function S) and $(C_1, C_2) \sim G$, where F and G are unspecified and (T_1, T_2) are independent of (C_1, C_2). Note that the distribution of $Y \sim P_{F,G}$ is indexed by F and G.

Let $\mu = \mu(F)$ be the parameter of interest. A typical parameter of interest is the survival function $\mu = S(t_1, t_2)$ at a given point (t_1, t_2).

We will consider estimation in three possible full data models. Below, we will review a large body of literature on estimation of F in the nonparametric full data model. In this case the full data model only has one estimating function for μ (e.g., $I(T_1 > t_1, T_2 > t_2) - \mu$ if $\mu = S(t_1, t_2)$). If one of the main purposes is to estimate a parameter that measures dependence between T_1 and T_2, then it might be sensible to assume a linear regression model such as $T_1 = \beta_0 + \beta_1 T_2 + \epsilon$, where $E(K(\epsilon) \mid T_2) = 0$ for a user-supplied monotone increasing function K. Now, β_1 is a parameter that measures the dependence of the location parameter identified by K of the conditional distribution of T_1, given T_2, on T_2. As possible choices of K, we recommend $I(\epsilon < 0) - p$ (p-quantile regression; e.g., $p = 0.5$ is the median regression), a smooth approximation of $I(\epsilon < 0) - 1/2$ (smooth median regression), or $K(\epsilon) = \min(\epsilon, \tau)$ for $\epsilon > 0$ and $K(\epsilon) = \max(\epsilon, -\tau)$ for $\epsilon < 0$ (truncated mean regression). In Section 2.2 of Chapter 2, we showed that the full data estimating functions are now $\{h(T_2)K(\epsilon(\beta)) : h\}$. Another possible full data structure model is the Cox proportional hazards model

$$\lambda_{T_1}(t \mid T_2)dt \equiv P(T_1 \in dt \mid T_1 \geq t, T_2) = \lambda_0(t)\exp(\beta_0 + \beta_1 T_2).$$

In Section 2.2 of Chapter 2 we showed that the full data estimating functions for β in this Cox proportional hazardsmodel are given by $\{\int\{h(t,T_2) - g(h)(t)\}dM(t) : h\}$, where $dM(t) = I(T_1 \in dt) - I(T_1 \geq t)\lambda_{T_1}(t \mid T_2)dt$ and

$$g(H)(t) = \frac{E\{h(t,T_2)I(T_1 \geq t)\exp(\beta_0 + \beta_1 T_2)\}}{E\{I(T_1 \geq t)\exp(\beta_0 + \beta_1 T_2)\}}.$$

In this model, β_1 measures the effect of T_2 on the hazard of the conditional distribution of T_1, given T_2.

There is no previous work on estimation of β in the latter two models. On the other hand, there are several existing nonparametric estimators of the bivariate survival function. Some prominent estimators include those of Dabrowska (1988), Prentice and Cai (1992a), Pruitt (1991), and van der Laan (1996a,b), among others. It is known that the NPMLE for continuous data is not consistent (Tsai, Leurgans, and Crowley, 1986). Thus, many of the existing bivariate estimators, including Dabrowska and Prentice-Cai, are explicit estimators based on representations of the bivariate survival function in terms of distribution functions of the data.

Pruitt (1991) proposed an estimator that is the solution of an ad hoc modification of the self-consistency equation. Pruitt's estimator tackles the nonuniqueness of the original self-consistency equation of the NPMLE by estimating conditional densities over the halflines implied by the singly censored observations. Van der Laan (1994b, 1996b) proves uniform consistency, $\sqrt{n}$-weak convergence, and validity of the bootstrap of Pruitt's estimator. However, this estimator is not asymptotically efficient,and its practical performance is not as strong as those of Dabrowska, Prentice–Cai, and van der Laan (van der Laan, 1997).

The Dabrowska and Prentice – Cai estimators have been shown to have good practical performance (Bakker, 1990; Prentice and Cai, 1992b; Pruitt, 1993, van der Laan, 1997) but are not, in general, nonparametrically efficient. Dabrowska's estimator is based on a clever representation of a multivariate survival function in terms of its conditional multivariate hazard measure. The Prentice–Cai estimator is related to Dabrowska's except that it also uses the Volterra structure suggested by Bickel (see Dabrowska, 1988). Also, as these estimators are based on smooth functionals of the data, results such as consistency, asymptotic normality, correctness of the bootstrap, and consistent estimation of the variance of the influence curve all hold by application of the functional delta method; see Gill (1992) and Gill, van der Laan, and Wellner (1995). In fact, both the Prentice–Cai and Dabrowska estimators are "locally" efficient in the sense that both are efficient at complete independence between T_1, T_2, C_1 and C_2 as proved in Gill, van der Laan, and Wellner (1995).

The "Sequence of Reductions NPMLE," or SOR-NPMLE, of van der Laan (1996a) makes use of the observation of Pruitt (1991) that the inconsistency of the NPMLE is due to the fact that singly censored observations imply halflines for T that do not contain any uncensored observations. To deal with this problem, van der Laan proposes to interval censor the singly censored observations by replacing the uncensored component, say T_{1i}, of the singly censored observations by the observation that T_{1i} lies in a small predetermined interval around T_{1i}. Van der Laan also proposes a further reduction based on the discretization of the C_i's to facilitate factorization of the joint likelihood into an F part and a G part to avoid having to estimate G. This estimator was shown to have good practical performance (van der Laan, 1997) in comparison with the Dabrowska, Prentice–Cai, and Pruitt estimators for small intervals around the uncensored components of singly censored observations. In van der Laan (1996a,b), it is shown that if the reduction of the data converges to zero slowly enough, then the SOR-NPMLE is asymptotically efficient.

As noted above, the Dabrowska, Prentice–Cai, and Pruitt estimators are not, in general, efficient estimators. As the SOR-NPMLE of van der Laan is "globally" efficient, a larger sample size may be necessary before its asymptotic properties take effect (this need for a larger sample size becomes more obvious when generalizing the estimator to higher dimensions). In addition, the SOR-NPMLE requires a choice of bandwidth.

Since the projection operator onto T_{CAR} does not exist in closed form, we use the representation $IC(\cdot \mid F, G, D) = A_F I_{F,G}^{-1}(D)$ (see Chapter 2) for the optimal mapping from full data estimating functions to observed data estimating functions, where $A_F(h)(Y) = E(h(Y) \mid X)$, $A_G^\top(V)(X) = E(V(Y) \mid X)$ is its adjoint and $I_{F,G} = A_F A_G^\top$ is the nonparametric information operator. We will assume

$$\overline{G}(T_1, T_2) > \delta > 0 \; F\text{-a.e.,} \tag{5.12}$$

which establishes the desired invertibility of the information operator and will make sure that the class of allowed full data structure functions $\mathcal{D}(\rho_1, G)$ contains all estimating functions of interest. However, we note that, by Theorem 1.7, our locally efficient doubly robust estimator, which uses user supplied estimators F_n and G_n of F and G, respectively, will still be CAN if F_n is consistent for the true F, even when assumption (5.12) is violated.

Artificial censoring: The condition (5.12) will be true if the distribution of (T_1, T_2) has compact support contained in a rectangle $[0, \tau_1] \times [0, \tau_2] \subset \mathbb{R}^2$ and $\bar{G}(\tau_1, \tau_2) > \delta > 0$. Consequently, as proposed in van der Laan (1996a,b), one can artificially censor the data so that this assumption holds in the following manner: given a (τ_1, τ_2) satisfying $\bar{G}(\tau_1, \tau_2) > 0$, if $\tilde{T}_j > \tau_j$, then set $\tilde{T}_j = \tau_j$ and $\Delta_j = 1$, $j = 1, 2$. The artificially censored data now follows a distribution $P_{F_\tau, G}$, where F_τ equals F on $[0, \tau_1) \times [0, \tau_2)$ and $F(\tau_1, \tau_2) = 1$ and $\bar{G}(\tau) > 0$, as required. This means that we can still estimate the bivariate distribution F on $[0, \tau_1) \times [0, \tau_2)$ with the artificially censored data structure. In practice, this means that we obtain more robust estimators of F on this rectangle.

Given user-supplied estimators F_n, G_n of F, G, $D_h \to IC(\cdot \mid F_n, G_n, D_h)$ is a mapping from full data estimating functions into observed data estimating functions. By the double robustness of $IC(Y \mid F, G, D)$ (Theorem 1.7), if either F_n or G_n (but not both) is inconsistent, then the resulting estimator μ_n will still be consistent and asymptotically normal. Thus, we are "protected" against the misspecification of the models chosen for either F or G (but not against misspecification of both). We propose to use a consistent nonparametric estimator (such as Dabrowska's) for G and a lower-dimensional (semiparametric or parametric) model for F. This has two beneficial properties: using a consistent estimator for G guarantees that the resulting estimator μ_n will be consistent and asymptotically normal, and our simulation studies indicate that using a lower-dimensional model for F (with Dabrowska for G) produces excellent practical performance (see Tables 5.3 and 5.6 later in this chapter). In addition, in many applications, one always observes (C_1, C_2) so that G can be well-estimated with the empirical distribution of (C_{1i}, C_{2i}), $i = 1, \ldots, n$.

Applying the mapping $IC(Y \mid F, G, D)$ to the full data structure estimating function $D(X) = I(T_1 > t_1, T_2 > t_2) - \mu$ yields a new class of nonparametric estimators of the bivariate survival function that is guaranteed to be consistent and asymptotically normal if either one of the user-supplied estimators F_n, G_n of F, G is consistent and is efficient in the nonparametric full data model if both estimators F_n, G_n are consistent. In the generalized linear regression, there is a whole class $\{h(T_2)K(\epsilon(\beta)) : h\}$ of full data estimating functions for β, and the optimal choice h_{opt} is defined as the solution of an integral equation in $h(T_2)$ provided in Chapter 2. Similarly, this is the case in the Cox proportional hazards model.

In the next subsection, we describe the locally efficient (LE) estimator for bivariate right-ensored data. In Subsections 5.3.3 and 5.3.4, we discuss implementation of the estimator for the three full data structure models in detail. In Subsection 5.3.5, we discuss the asymptotics of the estimator and construction of confidence intervals. In Subsection 5.3.6, we present an explicit theorem for the nonparametric full data structure model formally establishing the local efficiency of the estimator. In Subsection 5.3.7, we will present the results of a simulation study examining the performance of the LE estimator relative to Dabrowska's estimator, evaluating the amount of "protection" against misspecification of F or G that we get by using LE estimation and assessing the performance of estimated $(1 - \alpha)$ confidence intervals. Finally, in Subsection 5.3.8, we provide an application of the LE estimator on a data set from a twin study examining time to onset of appendicitis (Duffy, Martin, and Matthews, 1990).

5.3.2 Locally efficient estimation with bivariate right-censored data

Given any of the three full data models discussed above, let $\{D_h(\cdot \mid \mu) : h\}$ be the corresponding class of full data estimating functions for the parameter of interest μ. The optimal mapping from full data structure estimating functions to observed data estimating functions is

$$IC(Y|F, G, D) = A_F I_{F,G}^{-1}(D). \qquad (5.13)$$

Here, $A_F(\cdot) : L_0^2(F) \to L_0^2(P_{F,G})$ is the score operator for F and is defined as $E(\cdot \mid Y)$; $I_{F,G} : L_0^2(F) \to L_0^2(F)$ is the information operator and is defined as $A_G^T A_F$, where $A_G^T(\cdot) : L_0^2(P_{F,G}) \to L_0^2(F)$ is the transpose of the score operator for G and is defined as $E(\cdot \mid T_1, T_2)$. Thus IC can be seen as a mapping from a full data structure estimating function D to an observed data estimating function. In order for $I_{F,G}$ to be invertible, we need to impose the condition (5.12), which is $\overline{G}(T_1, T_2) > \delta > 0$, F-a.e. If F has compact support included in $[0, \tau_1] \times [0, \tau_2]$ with (τ_1, τ_2) and $P(C_1 > \tau_1, C_2 > \tau_2) > 0$, then condition (5.12) holds, and we showed in (5.12) how to artificially censor the data so that this assumption is true.

Given estimators F_n, G_n of F, G and a choice of full data estimating function D_{h_n}, we estimate μ with the solution of the estimating equation

$$0 = \sum_{i=1}^{n} IC(Y_i \mid F_n, G_n, D_{h_n}(\cdot \mid \mu)).$$

5.3. Bivariate Right-Censored Failure Time Data

Given an initial estimator μ_n^0, the corresponding one-step estimator of μ is given by

$$\mu_n^1 = \mu_n^0 + c_n^{-1} \frac{1}{n} \sum_{i=1}^n IC(Y_i \mid F_n, G_n, D_{h_n}(\cdot \mid \mu_n^0)), \qquad (5.14)$$

where $c_n = -d/d\mu 1/n \sum_i IC(Y_i \mid F_n, G_n, D_{h_n}(\cdot \mid \mu))|_{\mu=\mu_n^0}$. If $h_n = I_{F_n, G_n} I_{F_n, G_n}^{*-1}(D_{h_{eff,n}})$ estimates the optimal index h_{opt}, then $IC(Y_i \mid F_n, G_n, D_{h_n}(\cdot \mid \mu_n^0))$ is an estimate of the efficiency influence curve $IC(Y_i \mid F, G, D_{h_{opt}}(\cdot \mid \mu)) = A_F I_{F,G}^{*-1}(D_{h_{eff}})$. In particular, if the full data model is saturated and $\mu = S(t_1, t_2)$, then $D_{opt}(X \mid \mu) = I(T_1 > t_1, T_2 > t_2) - \mu$.

To understand what type of estimator F_n is needed, in the next paragraphs we will inspect the smoothness of $IC(Y \mid F, G, D)$ in F, G in more detail. We will conclude that one should use a discretized version of a *smooth* estimate $\tilde{F}_n$ of F with consistent densities, and one can use any discrete estimator G_n that consistently estimates G. This motivates us to consider parametric models for F and nonparametric models for G.

For a bivariate c.d.f., we define $F^1(t_1, t_2) = F(t_1, T_2) - F(t_1-, T_2)$ if $t_1 \to F(t_1, t_2)$ is discrete and $F^1(t_1, t_2) = d/dt_1 F(t_1, t_2)$ if $t_1 \to F(t_1, t_2)$ is absolute continuous with respect to Lebesgue measure. The score operator is given by

$$\begin{aligned}
A_F(s) &= E_F(s(T_1, T_2) \mid Y) \\
&= s(T_1, T_2) I(\Delta = (1,1)) \\
&\quad + \left\{ \frac{\int_{C_2}^\infty s(T_1, s_2) F^1(T_1, ds_2)}{\int_{C_2}^\infty F^1(T_1, ds_2)} \right\} I(\Delta = (1,0)) \\
&\quad + \left\{ \frac{\int_{C_1}^\infty s(s_1, T_2) F^2(ds_1, T_2)}{\int_{C_1}^\infty F^2(ds_1, T_2)} \right\} I(\Delta = (0,1)) \\
&\quad + \left\{ \frac{\int_{C_1}^\infty \int_{C_2}^\infty s(s_1, s_2) F(ds_1, ds_2)}{\int_{C_1}^\infty \int_{C_2}^\infty F(ds_1, ds_2)} \right\} I(\Delta = (0,0)).
\end{aligned}$$

Let $T = (T_1, T_2)$, $s = (s_1, s_2)$, $c = (c_1, c_2)$, $dc = (dc_1, dc_2)$, $ds = (ds_1, ds_2)$. The information operator $I_{F,G} = A_G^T A_F$ is given by

$$\begin{aligned}
I_{F,G}(s) &= A_G^T(A_F(s)) \\
&= E_G(A_F(s) \mid T_1, T_2) \\
&= \bar{G}(T_1, T_2) s(T_1, T_2) \\
&\quad - \frac{\int_0^{T_2} \left\{ \int_{c_2}^\infty s(T_1, s_2) F^1(T_1, ds_2) \right\} \bar{G}(T_1, dc_2)}{\int_{c_2}^\infty F^1(T_1, ds_2)} \\
&\quad - \frac{\int_0^{T_1} \left\{ \int_{c_1}^\infty s(s_1, T_2) F^2(ds_1, T_2) \right\} \bar{G}(dc_1, T_2)}{\int_{c_1}^\infty F^2(ds_1, T_2)}
\end{aligned}$$

$$+\frac{\int_0^T \{\int_c^\infty s(s_1,s_2) F(ds)\} G(dc)}{\int_c^\infty F(ds)}$$

$$= \overline{G}(T)s(T)$$
$$-\frac{\int_0^\infty \{\int_0^\infty I(c_2 \leq T_2, s_2 > c_2) s(T_1, s_2) F^1(T_1, ds_2)\} \bar{G}(T_1, dc_2)}{\int_{c_2}^\infty F^1(T_1, s_2) ds_2}$$
$$-\frac{\int_0^\infty \{\int_0^\infty I(c_1 \leq T_1, s_1 > c_1) s(s_1, T_2) F^2(ds_1, T_2)\} \bar{G}(dc_1, T_2))}{\int_{c_1}^\infty F^2(ds_1, T_2)}$$
$$+\frac{\int_0^\infty \{\int_0^\infty I(c_1 < T_1, s_1 > c_1) I(c_2 \leq T_2, s_2 > c_2) s(s) F(ds)\} G(dc)}{\int_c^\infty F(ds)}.$$

A straightforward application of Fubini's theorem gives us

$$I_{F,G}(s) = \overline{G}(T)s(T)$$
$$-\frac{\int_0^\infty \{\int_0^\infty I(c_2 \leq T_2, s_2 > c_2) s(T_1, s_2) \bar{G}(T_1, dc_2)\} F^1(T_1, ds_2)}{\int_{c_2}^\infty F^1(T_1, ds_2)}$$
$$-\frac{\int_0^\infty \{\int_0^\infty I(c_1 \leq T_1, s_1 > c_1) s(s_1, T_2) \bar{G}(dc_1, T_2)\} F^2(ds_1, T_2)}{\int_{c_1}^\infty F^2(ds_1, T_2)}$$
$$+\frac{\int_0^\infty \{\int_0^\infty I(c_1 \leq T_1, s_1 > c_1) I(c_2 \leq T_2, s_2 > c_2) s(s) G(dc)\} F(ds)}{\int_c^\infty F(ds)}.$$
(5.15)

In our estimate of $IC(Y \mid F, G, D)$, we substitute for F and G their discretized estimates (possibly on a fine grid) so that we only need to define the information operator and its inverse at discrete F and G. For example, the frailty estimator (Clayton and Cusick, 1985) F_n of F puts mass on the grid of uncensored values of Y_1 and Y_2. If there are m_1 unique uncensored values of Y_1 and m_2 unique uncensored values of Y_2, then the support is defined on an $m_1 \times m_2$ grid. Thus, the support of F_n can be represented by the $m_1 m_2$ dimensional vector $\tilde{t} = \{(t_{11}, t_{21}), \ldots, (t_{1m_1m_2}, t_{2m_1m_2})\}$, and thus our estimate of $I_{F,G}$ will be an $m_1 m_2 \times m_1 m_2$ matrix. An estimate of $F(dt_1, dt_2)$ can be obtained as follows

$$F_n(dt_1, dt_2) = F_n(t_1+\delta_1, t_2+\delta_2) - F_n(t_1, t_2+\delta_2) - F_n(t_1+\delta_1, t_2) + F_n(t_1, t_2).$$

Estimation of $G(dc_1, dc_2)$ is accomplished in a similar fashion.

For a discrete underlying distribution F, this discretization should provide a good estimate of the true $F(dt_1, dt_2)$, and thus the estimates of the information operator should approach the true $I_{F,G}$. If F is continuous, the grid defined by $\tilde{t}$ gets finer and finer with sample size, and F_n is a discretized version of an estimate $\tilde{F}$ of F for which $d/dx\tilde{F}$ consistently estimates d/dxF, then the estimated $I_{F_n,G}$ will converge to the true $I_{F,G}$. We refer the reader to van der Laan (1996a), in which a similar result is proved. Of course, as $m_1 m_2$ gets larger, it becomes more computationally expensive to calculate and invert the information operator (see Subsection 5.3.4). In practice, if the value $m_1 m_2$ becomes too large, it is also possible to discretize the data (e.g., round to fewer significant digits) so that the grid size $m_1 m_2$ is manageable. Both the simulation result in Table 5.11 later in this chapter and the data analysis verify that the estimator performs well for continuous data. We also note that $I_{F,G}$ is smooth enough in G so that a discrete estimator G_n that does not estimate a continuous density will still result in a consistent estimator I_{F,G_n} of $I_{F,G}$.

We now present a lemma that formalizes the expected property (see Theorem 2.1 and Lemma 1.9 and Section 2.4 of Chapter 2 about protection against misspecification of either F_n or G_n, but not both.

Lemma 5.1 *For any pair of measures P, P_1, we write $P \equiv P_1$ if dP/dP_1 and dP_1/dP are well-defined and have finite supremum norm. Let $\mathcal{F}$ be the set of bivariate failure time distributions with support included in $[0, \tau] \subset \mathbb{R}^2_{\geq 0}$. Let $\mathcal{G}$ be the set of bivariate censoring distributions G satisfying $\bar{G}(t_1, t_2) > \delta$ for some $\delta > 0$ for all $(t_1, t_2) \in [0, \tau] \subset \mathbb{R}^2_{\geq 0}$. For any $F_1 \in \mathcal{F}$ and $G_1 \in \mathcal{G}$, let $IC(Y \mid F_1, G_1, D)$ be defined as in (5.13). Then, given a $G_1 \in \mathcal{G}$, $E_{P_{F,G}}(IC(Y \mid F_1, G_1, D)) = E_F D(X)$ if either $F_1 = F$ and $G \ll G_1$ or $G_1 = G$ and $F_1 \equiv F$.*

We also have that, given $G_1 \in \mathcal{G}$, $E_{P_{F,G}} IC(Y \mid F_1, G_1, D) = E_F D(X)$ if either $F_1 = F$ and $G \ll G_1$ or $G_1 = G$ and F_1 is discrete. Finally, $E_G(IC(Y \mid F_1, G, D) \mid X) = D(X)$ F_X-a.e. at any $F_1 \in \mathcal{F}$ and $G \in \mathcal{G}$.

Proof. Let $(D[0, \tau], \|\cdot\|_\infty)$ be the Banach space consisting of real-valued functions defined on $[0, \tau]$ endowed with the supremum norm. Given a general F_1, we only know that, given a G_1 with $\bar{G}_1(T_1, T_2) > \delta > 0$, F-a.e., $I_{F_1, G_1} : L^2(F_1) \to L^2(F_1)$ is boundedly invertible as a Hilbert space operator, while if F_1 is discrete, then Gill, van der Laan, and Robins (2000) prove that $I_{F_1, G_1} : (D[0, \tau], \|\cdot\|_\infty) \to (D[0, \tau], \|\cdot\|_\infty)$ has a bounded inverse. Let us first consider the case where $G_1 = G$. By first taking the conditional expectation, given $X = (T_1, T_2)$, it follows that

$$E_{P_{F,G}} A_{F_1} (A_G^\top A_{F_1})^{-1}(D)(Y) = E_F D'(X),$$

where for general F_1, $D'(X) \equiv A_G^\top A_{F_1}(A_G^\top A_{F_1})^{-1}(D)$ equals $D(X)$ only in $L^2(F_1)$, and if F_1 is discrete, then $D'(X) = D(X)$ in $(D[0, \tau], \|\cdot\|_\infty)$. Thus, if $F_1 \equiv F$ or F_1 is discrete, then $E_{P_{F,G}} A_{F_1}(A_G^\top A_{F_1})^{-1}(D)(Y) = E_F D(X)$. This proves the unbiasedness for the case where $G_1 = G$.

Let us now consider the case where $F_1 = F$. Since $I_{F_X, G_1} : L^2_0(F_X) \to L^2_0(F_X)$ is 1-1 and onto under the condition $G_1 \in \mathcal{G}$, we can apply Theorem 1.7, which proves the result.
□

It should also be noted that the variance of $IC(Y \mid F, G, D_{h_{opt}}(\cdot \mid \mu))$ equals the information bound. In particular, if the full data model is

290   5. Multivariate Right-Censored Multivariate Data

nonparametric, $\mu = S(t_1, t_2)$, and $D(X) = I(T_1 > t_1, T_2 > t_2) - \mu$, then the variance of $IC(Y \mid F, G, D)$ equals the efficiency bound. This result allows us to calculate relative efficiency for any nonparametric bivariate estimator (see table 5.4 later in this chapter), which has not been available in the literature previously.

5.3.3 Implementation of the locally efficient estimator

To be specific, consider the case where $D(X) = I(T_1 > t_1, T_2 > t_2) - \mu$ so that the resulting estimator is a locally efficient estimator of $\mu(t_1, t_2) = S(t_1, t_2)$ in the nonparametric full data structure model. We use a consistent estimator such as Dabrowska's estimator for $\hat{\mu}_0$ in (5.14). In order to calculate the information operator, we must use estimators F_n and G_n to obtain $F_n(ds_1, ds_2)$, $G_n(dc_1, dc_2)$ as described in Subsection 5.3.2 for use in (5.15). Let $\tilde{t}$ represent the $m_1 m_2$ dimensional vector representing the discretization of the support of F described in Subsection 5.3.2. Let $\tilde{c} = \{(c_{11}, c_{21}), \ldots, (c_{1m_3}, c_{2m_3})\}$ be the set of points on which G_n puts mass. Then, the information operator will be an $m_1 m_2 \times m_1 m_2$ matrix, where the rows and columns are indexed by the values of $\tilde{t}$ (defined in Subsection 5.3.2).

Let $\widehat{I}^i_{F_n, G_n} = \widehat{I}_{F_n, G_n}(s)(t_{1i}, t_{2i})$, $t_\cdot = (t_{1\cdot}, t_{2\cdot})$, $dc_\cdot = (dc_{1\cdot}, dc_{2\cdot})$, $dt_\cdot = (dt_{1\cdot}, dt_{2\cdot})$, and $\overline{G}_n$ be the estimate of $\overline{G}$ obtained from G_n. The value of the information operator at the point (t_{1i}, t_{2i}) can be expressed as follows:

$$\widehat{I}^i_{F_n, G_n} = \overline{G}_n(t_{1i}, t_{2i}) s(t_{1i}, t_{2i})$$

$$+ \sum_{j:(t_{1i}, t_{2j}) \in \tilde{t}'} \left\{ \sum_{k=1}^{m_3} \frac{I(t_{2j} > c_{2k}, c_{2k} \leq t_{2i}) G_n([t_{1i}, \infty), dc_{2k})}{\sum_{l:(t_{1i}, t_{2l}) \in \tilde{t}} I(t_{2l} > c_{2k}) F_n(dt_{1i}, dt_{2l})} \right\}$$

$$\times s(t_{1i}, t_{2j}) F_n(dt_{1i}, dt_{2j})$$

$$+ \sum_{j:(t_{1j}, t_{2i}) \in \tilde{t}} \left\{ \sum_{k=1}^{m_3} \frac{I(t_{1j} > c_{1k}, c_{1k} \leq t_{1i}) G_n(dc_{1k}, [t_{2i}, \infty))}{\sum_{l:(t_{1l}, t_{2i}) \in \tilde{t}} I(t_{1l} > c_{1k}) F_n(dt_{1l}, dt_{2i})} \right\}$$

$$\times s(t_{1j}, t_{2i}) F_n(dt_{1j}, dt_{2i})$$

$$+ \sum_{j=1}^{m_1 m_2} \left\{ \sum_{k=1}^{m_3} \frac{I(t_j > c_k) I(c_k \leq t_i) G_n(dc_k)}{\sum_{l=1}^{m_1 m_2} I(t_l > c_k) F_n(dt_l)} \right\} s(t_j) F_n(dt_j).$$

Let $\Delta_i = (\Delta_{1i}, \Delta_{2i})$. The score estimator evaluated at Y_i may be estimated as follows:

$$\widehat{A}_{F_n}(s)(Y_i) = h(T_{1i}, T_{2i}) I(\Delta_i = (1, 1))$$

$$+ \sum_{j:(T_{1i}, t_{2j}) \in \tilde{t}} \left\{ \frac{I(t_{2j} > C_{2i}) s(T_{1i}, t_{2j}) F_n^1(T_{1i}, dt_{2j})}{\sum_{j:(T_{1i}, t_{2j}) \in \tilde{t}} I(t_{2j} > C_{2i}) F_n^1(T_{1i}, dt_{2j})} \right\} I(\Delta_i = (1, 0))$$

$$+ \sum_{j:(t_{1j},T_{2i})\in \tilde{t}} \left\{ \frac{I(t_{1j} > C_{1i})s(t_{1j},T_{2i})F_n^2(dt_{1j},T_{2i})}{\sum_{j:(t_{1j},T_{2i})\in \tilde{t}} I(t_{1j} > C_{1i})F_n^2(dt_{1j},T_{2i})} \right\} I(\Delta_i = (0,1))$$

$$+ \sum_{j=1}^{m_1 m_2} \left\{ \frac{I(t_j > C_i)h(t_j)F_n(dt_j)}{\sum_{j=1}^{m_1 m_2} I(t_j > C_i)F_n(dt_j)} \right\} I(\Delta_i = (0,0)).$$

Once we have $\widehat{A}_{F_n}$ and $\widehat{I}_{F_n,G_n}$, we can estimate the influence curve $IC(Y \mid F, G, \mu)$ by $IC(Y \mid F_n, G_n, D(\cdot \mid \widehat{\mu}_0)) = A_{F_n} I_{F_n,G_n}^{-}(D(\cdot \mid \widehat{\mu}_0))$, inverting the nonparametric information operator with standard matrix inversion or the algorithm (which avoids the inversion of high-dimensional matrices) in the next subsection. In the nonparametric full data model, there is only one choice for the full data estimating function, namely the efficient influence curve $S_{eff}^{*F} = D_{h_{eff}}$ for μ in the full data model.

Consider now the linear regression full data model $T_1 = \beta_0 + \beta_1 T_2 + \epsilon$, where $E(K(\epsilon) \mid T_2) = 0$ for a given K. If one is not concerned with optimal estimation, then one can select an ad hoc choice $D_h(X \mid \beta) = h(T_2)K(\epsilon(\beta))$ such as the efficient influence curve $S_{eff}^{*F} = D_{h_{eff}}$ for μ in the full data model as provided in Lemma 2.1 in Section 2.2 of Chapter 2. For the purpose of locally efficient estimation, we propose to use the following representation of the efficient influence curve (see Chapter 2)

$$IC(Y \mid F, G, D_{h_{opt}}) = A_F I_{F,G}^{*-1}(D_{h_{eff}}),$$

where

$$I_{F,G}^{*}(s) = \Pi(I_{F,G}(s) \mid \langle D_{h_{eff}} \rangle) + I_{F,G}(s) - \Pi(I_{F,G}(s) \mid T_{nuis}^{F,\perp})$$
$$\Pi(V \mid T_{nuis}^{F\perp}) = E(\{V(X) - E(V \mid T_2)\}K(\epsilon) \mid T_2)E(K(\epsilon)^2 \mid T_2)^{-1}K(\epsilon)$$
$$\Pi(V \mid \langle D_{h_{eff}} \rangle) = E(VD_{h_{eff}})E(D_{h_{eff}} D_{h_{eff}}^\top)^{-1} D_{h_{eff}}$$

for all $V(Y) \in L_0^2(P_{F,G})$. The last projection can be estimated trivially with empirical means. The projection operator onto $T_{nuis}^{F,\perp}$ can be estimated by substitution of an estimate F_n of the bivariate cumulative distribution function F. If one estimates F with a smooth parametric estimate F_n, then the conditional expectation of a function $V(T_1, T_2)$, given T_2, is obtained by integrating the density of F_n over T_1. Inversion of the information operator $I_{F,G}^{*}$ can be done by iteratively applying $I_{F,G}^{*}$ as shown in the next subsection. Thus, we conclude that we can estimate $I_{F,G}^{*-1}$ by substitution of a preferably smooth estimate F_n, an estimator G_n, a simple empirical covariance operator, and an estimate $h_n(T_2)K(\epsilon(\beta))$ of the full data efficient score $D_{h_{eff}}$.

Application of Theorem 2.4 and Theorem 2.5 in Chapter 2 shows that, under regularity conditions, the resulting estimator β_n will be efficient if both F_n and G_n are consistent and will remain consistent and asymptotically normally distributed if at least one of F_n and G_n is consistent.

Misspecification of h_n and the projection operator $\Pi(\cdot \mid T_{nuis}^{F,\perp})$ (as long as it maps into $\{h(T_2)K(\epsilon(\beta)) : h\}$) does not affect the consistency.

Locally efficient estimation in the multiplicative intensity full data model is described similarly with $\Pi(V \mid T_{nuis}^{F,\perp})$ now being the projection operator onto the orthogonal complement of the nuisance tangent space $T_{nuis}^{F,\perp} = \{\int (h - g(h))dM : h\}$ of the multiplicative intensity model for the full data structure $X = (T_1, T_2)$, as provided in Lemma 2.3.

5.3.4 Inversion of the information operator

In order to calculate $IC(Y \mid F_n, G_n, D)$, it is necessary to find a solution to the system of equations $\gamma = I_{F,G}^-(D)$. In addition, in order to calculate $IC(Y \mid F_n, G_n, \widehat{D}_{opt})$, one needs to find a solution to the system of equations $\gamma = I_{F,G}^{*-1}(D_{h_{eff}})$. The dimension of I_{F_n, G_n} is determined by the dimension m of the vector of points on which F_n puts mass and can be quite large, as mentioned in Subsection 5.3.3. In order to make this calculation computationally feasible, we used a result of van der Laan (1998) in which he developed an iterative algorithm for calculating γ. This algorithm requires km^2 steps for a constant k, and our implementation indicates that the constant k is quite small for reasonably large m.

In Chapter 2, we showed that

- if we have $\inf_{\|h\|_F=1, h \in T^F} \| A_F(h) \|_F > 0$, then $I_{F,G}^* : T^F(F) \to T^F(F)$ and $I_{F,G} : L_2^0(F) \to L_2^0(F)$ are 1-1.

- If there exists some $\delta > 0$ such that we have $\| A_F(h) \|_{P_{F,G}} \geq \delta$, then $I_{F,G} : L_2^0(F) \to L_2^0(F)$ and $I_{F,G}^* : T^F(F) \to T^F(F)$ are onto and have bounded inverse with operator norm smaller than or equal to $1/\delta^2$, and their inverses are given by

$$I_{F,G}^{-1} = \sum_{i=0}^{\infty} (I - I_{F,G})^i,$$

$$I_{F,G}^{*-1} = \sum_{i=0}^{\infty} (I - I_{F,G}^*)^i.$$

In addition, we proposed an iterative algorithm to calculate $\gamma = I_{F,G}^{*-}(D)$,

$$\gamma^{k+1} = D - (I - I_{F,G}^*)(\gamma^k),$$

where $\gamma^0 = D$ and iteration continued until $\| \gamma^{k+1} - \gamma^k \|_F < \epsilon$ for some $\epsilon > 0$ and similarly for $\gamma = I_{F,G}^{-1}(D)$.

In order to evaluate the practical performance of this algorithm in the context of the locally efficient estimation in the nonparametric bivariate right-censored data model, we recorded values of $\| \gamma^{k+1} - \gamma^k \|_{F_n}$ for each value of k over 100 simulated data sets (the data sets were generated with "low" dependency as described in Subsection 5.3.7). We chose $D = I(T_1 > t_1, T_2 > t_2) - S(t_1, t_2)$. The value of ϵ was chosen conservatively to be 1×10^{-7} to ensure accuracy in the calculation of γ, and for these simulated data sets, $m = 225$. The results may be seen in Figure 5.1 at the end of this chapter and indicate that the algorithm performs well. The values of $\| \gamma^{k+1} - \gamma^k \|_{F_n}$ appear to fall quickly after the first iteration, and the algorithm converges within 15 iterations for the time points chosen.

5.3.5 Asymptotic performance and confidence intervals

Consider the situation in which G_n is a consistent and efficient estimator of G according to the model that we have assumed on G. For example, G_n might be an efficient estimator of G under the assumption of a frailty model, G_n might be the SOR-NPMLE of van der Laan (1996a) under the nonparametric independence model (i.e., (C_1, C_2) is independent of (T_1, T_2)), or if (C_1, C_2) are always observed, one can estimate G with the empirical distribution of (C_{1i}, C_{2i}), $i = 1, \ldots, n$, in the nonparametric independence model. In addition, assume that F_n converges to some F_1 (in a strong sense so that f_n converges to f_1) not necessarily equal to the true F, which one expects to be the case if F_n is an estimate of F according to some guessed (semi)parametric model.

Our asymptotic Theorem 5.2 below proves that, under regularity conditions, $\widehat{\mu}$ is asymptotically linear with an influence curve

$$IC(Y) = IC(Y \mid F_1, G, D(\cdot \mid \mu)) - \Pi(IC(Y \mid F_1, G, D(\cdot \mid \mu)) \mid T_G), \quad (5.16)$$

where $T_G \subset L_0^2(P_{F,G})$ is the tangent space of G generated by all scores of the G part of the likelihood of Y, given by $L(G) = P(Y \mid (T_1, T_2))$, under the posed model for G. If $F_1 = F$, then $IC(Y \mid F_1, G, \mu)$ is orthogonal to T_{CAR} so that $IC(Y) = IC(Y \mid F, G, D(\cdot \mid \mu))$.

This shows that we can use $IC(Y \mid F_1, G, D(\cdot \mid \mu))$ as a conservative influence curve of our one-step estimator $\widehat{\mu}$, which is actually correct if our guessed model for F is correct (or if G is known so that T_G is empty). Thus, a conservative bound for the asymptotic variance of $\sqrt{n}(\widehat{\mu} - \mu)$ is given by, $\text{var}(IC(Y \mid F_1, G, D(\cdot \mid \mu)))$. Therefore, we may use our estimate $\widehat{IC}(Y) \equiv IC(Y \mid F_n, G_n, D)$ to obtain a 95% confidence interval for $\widehat{\mu}$ in the following way:

- Calculate $\widehat{\sigma}^2 = \frac{1}{n^2} \sum_{i=1}^n (\widehat{IC}(Y_i) - \overline{IC})^2$.

- CI $= (\widehat{\mu} - 1.96\widehat{\sigma}, \widehat{\mu} + 1.96\widehat{\sigma})$,

where

$$\overline{IC} = \frac{1}{n} \sum_{i=1}^n \widehat{IC}(Y_i).$$

If G_n is not an efficient estimator according to a model for G but is a good estimator such as Dabrowska's estimator, then we believe that this estimate of the limit variance and the corresponding confidence interval will still be a good practical choice. Our simulation study shows indeed the good practical performance of these confidence intervals for the case where G is estimated with Dabrowska's estimator.

Finally, we discuss some of the interesting implications of (5.16) for the nonparametric full data structure model. Firstly, $\widehat{\mu}$ becomes more efficient if one uses a more nonparametric model for G. Moreover, a fundamental result in Gill, van der Laan and Robins (1997) shows that if one only assumes coarsening at random on the conditional distribution of (C_1, C_2), given T_1, T_2 (and a nonparametric full data structure model), then any regular asymptotically linear estimator is efficient. This implies for the nonparametric full data model, under regularity conditions, that if one estimates G with a smoothed nonparametric maximum likelihood estimator such as the SOR-NPMLE of van der Laan (1996a), then $IC(Y \mid F^1, G, D(\cdot \mid \mu)) - \Pi(IC(Y \mid F^1, G, D(\cdot \mid \mu)) \mid T_G) = IC(Y \mid F, G, D(\cdot \mid \mu))$ for any F^1. In other words, in that case $\widehat{\mu}$ is efficient even when one guesses a wrong singleton $\{F^1\}$ as the model for F. By Lemma 1.8, we also have that if F is correct and $G_n \to G^1 \neq G$, then the estimating function $IC(Y \mid F, G^1, D(\cdot \mid \mu))$ is still orthogonal to T_{CAR} and is thus still the efficient influence curve. Thus, if one estimates F consistently, then $\widehat{\mu}$ is efficient even when one guesses a singleton $\{G^1\}$ as the model for G.

The practical performance of any estimator and, in particular, $\widehat{\mu}$, is a tradeoff between first- and second-order asymptotics. Although the first-order asymptotics suggest estimating F, G nonparametrically (or just G with a smoothed NPMLE), the fact is that such globally efficient estimators can suffer from large second-order terms. As described in Subsection 5.3.6, the influence curve depends on partial densities of F. Therefore, using a nonsmooth nonparametric estimator for F such as Dabrowska's is not appropriate. On the other hand, we want to be nonparametrically consistent in the model only assuming that (C_1, C_2) is independent of (T_1, T_2). To control the second-order terms of the estimator μ_n (i.e., to control the curse of dimensionality), and to still be nonparametrically consistent under the sole assumption that (C_1, C_2) is independent of (T_1, T_2), estimating G with Dabrowska's estimator or the empirical distribution if (C_1, C_2) is always observed, and guessing a low-dimensional model for F is a good strategy.

5.3.6 Asymptotics

In order to obtain a formal result with simple conditions, we will focus on the special case where the full data model is nonparametric and $D(X \mid \mu) = \kappa_{t_1,t_2}(T_1, T_2) - \mu$, where $\kappa_{t_1,t_2}(T_1, T_2) \equiv I(T_1 > t_1, T_2 > t_2)$. However, the

5.3. Bivariate Right-Censored Failure Time Data

results needed in our proof form a strong basis for an asymptotic theorem in the generalized linear regression and other full data structure models.

Let $IC(Y \mid F, G, \mu) \equiv IC(Y \mid F, G, D(\cdot \mid \mu))$. In this special case we present the one-step estimator as $\mu_n^1 = \mu_n^0 + 1/n \sum_i IC(Y_i \mid F_n, G_n, \mu_n^0)$, but we note that this actually reduces to:

$$\mu_n^1 = \frac{1}{n} \sum_{i=1}^n A_{F_n} I_{F_n, G_n}^{-1}(\kappa_{t_1, t_2}).$$

Thus μ_n^1 does not depend on the initial estimator. Since we advertised the one-step estimator μ_n^1 for which G_n is globally consistent, and F_n is locally consistent we are interested in applying Theorem 2.4 of Chapter 2, which assumes that G_n is estimated consistently. Theorem 2.4 and Lemma 5.1 directly translate into the following Theorem for our specific bivariate right-censored data structure.

For any pair of measures P, P_1, we write $P \equiv P_1$ if dP/dP_1 and dP_1/dP are well defined and have finite supremum norm. Let $\mathcal{F}$ be the set of bivariate failure time distributions with support included in $[0, \tau] \subset \mathbb{R}_{\geq 0}^2$. Let $\mathcal{G}$ be the set of bivariate censoring distributions satisfying that $\bar{G}(\tau) > \delta$ for some $\delta > 0$. For any $F_1 \in \mathcal{F}$ and $G_1 \in \mathcal{G}$, let $IC(Y \mid F_1, G_1, D)$ be defined as in (5.13). Application of Lemma 5.1 teaches us that $E_G(IC(Y \mid F_1, G, D(\cdot \mid \mu)) \mid X) = D(X \mid \mu)$ F_X-a.e. for all $F_1 \in \mathcal{F}$, which is a key condition of Theorem 2.4.

Theorem 5.2 *Let the full data model $\mathcal{M}^F$ for the distribution of $X = (T_1, T_2)$ be unspecified, and assume that the conditional distribution of (C_1, C_2), given X, satisfies CAR. Suppose that we observe n i.i.d. observations $Y_1, \ldots, Y_n$ of $Y = (\min(T_1, C_1), \Delta_1, \min(T_2, C_2), \Delta_2)$ or $Y = (C_1, C_2, \min(T_1, C_1), \min(T_2, C_2))$ (i.e., now the censoring times are observed as well). Let $P_{F,G}$ be the probability distribution of Y. We consider the one-step estimator μ_n^1 of $S(t_1, t_2)$:*

$$\mu_n^1 = \mu_n^0 + \frac{1}{n} \sum_{i=1}^n IC(Y_i \mid F_n, G_n, \mu_n^0).$$

Assume that F has compact support $[0, \tau]$ and $\bar{G}(\tau) > 0$. Assume that the limit F^1 specified in (ii) below is either discrete with support in $[0, \tau]$ or $F^1 \equiv F$. Then, by Lemma 5.1, $E_G(IC(Y \mid F^1, G, D) \mid X) = D(X)$ F_X-a.e.

Assume the following.

(i) $IC(\cdot \mid F_n, G_n, \mu_n^0)$ falls in a $P_{F_X, G}$-Donsker class with probability tending to 1.

(ii) $\| IC(\cdot \mid F_n, G_n, \mu_n^0) - IC(\cdot \mid F^1, G, \mu) \|_{P_{F_X, G}} \to 0$ in probability.

(iii) Define for a G_1

$$\Phi(G_1) = P_{F,G} IC(\cdot \mid F^1, G_1, \mu).$$

296   5. Multivariate Right-Censored Multivariate Data

Assume that

$$P_{F,G}\{IC(\cdot \mid F_n, G_n, \mu) - IC(\cdot \mid F_n, G, \mu)\} = \Phi(G_n) - \Phi(G) + o_P(1/\sqrt{n}).$$

If $IC(\cdot \mid F^1, G, \mu) = IC(\cdot \mid F, G, \mu)$, then μ_n^1 is asymptotically efficient. If also
(iv) $\Phi(G_n)$ is an asymptotically efficient estimator of $\Phi(G)$ for a CAR model containing the true G with tangent space $T_G(P_{F,G}) \subset T_{CAR}(P_{F,G})$, then μ_n^1 is a regular asymptotically linear estimator with influence curve given by

$$IC \equiv \Pi(IC(\cdot \mid F^1, G, \mu) \mid T_G^\perp(P_{F,G})),$$

where $\Pi(\cdot \mid T_G^\perp(P_{F,G}))$ is the projection operator on $T_G^\perp(P_{F,G})$ in the Hilbert space $L_0^2(P_{F,G})$.

Conditions (i) and (ii) of Theorem 2.4 require detailed understanding of the entropy of a class of functions containing $I_{F_n,G_n}^-(D)$ with probability tending to 1. Since the inverse of the information operator $I_{F,G}$ is, in general, only understood in an $L^2(F)$ sense, this is a hard task. However, in our proof of the next result we show that this inverse is well-understood in supremum norm and variation norm at a discrete F. This allows us to prove that our one-step estimator μ_n^1 using a discrete estimate F_n with support contained in a fixed set of (say) M points is consistent and asymptotically linear, and if F_n happens to be consistent, then it is also efficient. Our simulations suggest that μ_n^1 is also locally efficient if F_n is a discrete estimate of F according to an arbitrarily fine discrete approximation (depending on n) of a parametric or semiparametric smooth model. In other words, we are not claiming that our condition on F_n in Theorem 5.3 below is needed.

Theorem 5.3 *Let $Y = (C_1, C_2, \min(T_1, C_1), \min(T_2, C_2))$ include observing the censoring times. Assume that F has support contained in $[0, \tau] \subset \mathbb{R}_{\geq 0}^2$ and that $\bar{G}(\tau) > 0$. Let F_n be discrete with support contained in a fixed set of (say) M points in $[0, \tau]$, and assume $\| F_n - F^1 \|_\infty \to 0$ in probability for some discrete F^1 with $dF^1 > 0$ on each of the M-support points. Let G_n be the empirical distribution based on $(C_{1i}, C_{2i}), i = 1, \ldots, n$. Then, μ_n^1 is a regular asymptotically linear estimator with influence curve*

$$IC \equiv \Pi(IC(\cdot \mid F^1, G, D(\cdot \mid \mu)) \mid T_G^\perp(P_{F,G})),$$

where $T_G(P_{F,G}) = \overline{\{h(C_1, C_2) - E_G(h(C_1, C_2)) : h\}} \cap L_0^2(P_{F,G})$. In particular, if $F^1 = F$, then μ_n^1 is asymptotically efficient.

The projection operator is given by

$$\Pi(IC(\cdot \mid F^1, G, D(\cdot \mid \mu)) \mid T_G) = E(IC(Y \mid F^1, G, D(\cdot \mid \mu)) \mid C_1, C_2).$$

Proving conditions (i) and (ii) of Theorem 5.2 requires uniformly bounding the supremum and uniform sectional variation norm of $I_{F_n,G_n}^{-1}(D)$ for a given well-understood function D. The following important lemma establishes that the information operator in (F_n, G_n) is invertible w.r.t. the supremum norm and sectional variation norm uniformly in any of the possible realizations of (F_n, G_n) satisfying $\bar{G}_n(\tau) > \delta > 0$.

Lemma 5.2 *Let $\delta > 0$ and M points in $[0, \tau] \subset \mathbb{R}^2_{\geq 0}$ be given. Let $\mathcal{F}$ be a set of bivariate discrete distributions with support contained in these M points. Let $\mathcal{G}$ be a set of bivariate distributions all satisfying $\bar{G}(\tau) > \delta > 0$. Let $(D[0, \tau], \|\cdot\|_\infty)$ be the Banach space of bivariate real-valued cadlag functions on $[0, \tau]$ endowed with the supremum norm (see Neuhaus, 1971). We have that for any $F \in \mathcal{F}$ and $G \in \mathcal{G}$, $I_{F,G} : (D[0, \tau], \|\cdot\|_\infty) \to (D[0, \tau], \|\cdot\|_\infty)$ is invertible and*

$$\sup_{F \in \mathcal{F}, G \in \mathcal{G}} \sup_{h \in D[0,\tau], \|h\|_\infty = 1} \| I_{F,G}(h) \|_\infty < \infty.$$

Let $(D[0, \tau], \|\cdot\|_v)$ be the Banach space of bivariate real-valued cadlag functions on $[0, \tau]$ endowed with the uniform sectional variation norm

$$\| f \|_v = \max\left(\max_u \int | f(u, dv) |, \max_v \int | f(du, v) |, \int | f(du, dv) | \right).$$

We also have that for any $F \in \mathcal{F}$ and $G \in \mathcal{G}$, $I_{F,G} : (D[0, \tau], \|\cdot\|_v) \to (D[0, \tau], \|\cdot\|_v)$ is invertible and

$$\sup_{F \in \mathcal{F}, G \in \mathcal{G}} \sup_{h \in D[0,\tau], \|h\|_v = 1} \| I_{F,G}(h) \|_v < \infty.$$

Proof of Lemma 5.2. We will provide the supremum norm invertibility result and note that the variation norm invertibility result is proved similarly. A similar proof can be found in van der Laan (1996b) and van der Laan, and Gill (1999). We have $I_{F,G}(h)(X) = \bar{G}h(X) + K_{F,G}(h)(X)$, where $K_{F,G}$ is a linear operator involving a sum of three terms. These three terms integrate $s \to h(s, T_2)$, $s \to h(T_1, s)$ and $(s_1, s_2) \to h(s_1, s_2)$ w.r.t. $F(ds, \{T_2\})$, $F(\{T_1\}, ds)$, and $dF(s_1, s_2)$, respectively, over sets $[u, \infty)$, $[v, \infty)$, and $[u, \infty) \times [v, \infty)$, respectively, and subsequently integrate over u and v w.r.t. the sections of G and G itself. Therefore, $K_{F,G}$ is the composition of first calculating these three integrals with boundaries being the arguments of the function and subsequently integrating the integrals w.r.t. G. The first mapping only depends on the values of h at the support points of F, and it maps to step functions with jumps only at these support points. As a consequence, its range is M-dimensional (and it is bounded) so that this mapping is a compact operator on $(D[0, \tau], \|\cdot\|_\infty)$. Since the integral w.r.t. G maps compact sets to compact sets, it now follows that $K_{F,G} : (D[0, \tau], \|\cdot\|_\infty) \to (D[0, \tau], \|\cdot\|_\infty)$ is a compact operator.

Now, we note that $I_{F,G}/\bar{G}$ equals $h \to h + 1/\bar{G} K_{F,G}(h)$, which is thus an identity operator plus a compact operator since $\bar{G} > \delta > 0$. A well-known functional analysis result teaches us that if such an operator is 1–1, then it has a bounded inverse. We will now establish that $I_{F,G} : (D[0, \tau], \|\cdot\|_\infty) \to (D[0, \tau], \|\cdot\|_\infty)$ is 1–1. Assume that $\bar{G}(X)h(X) + K_{F,G}(h)(X) = 0$ for all $X \in [0, \tau]$. By the $L^2(F)$-invertibility of $I_{F,G}$, this implies that $h(x) = 0$ at each support point of F. Since $K_{F,G}(h)$ only integrates the values of h at the support points, this proves that $K_{F,G}(h)(X) = 0$ for all $X \in [0, \tau]$. Thus $\bar{G}(X)h(X) = 0$ for all $X \in [0, \tau]$, which proves that $h(X) = 0$ for all $X \in [0, \tau]$. This proves that $I_{F,G} : (D[0, \tau], \|\cdot\|_\infty) \to (D[0, \tau], \|\cdot\|_\infty)$ has a bounded inverse. Finally, it can be shown that the operator norm of the inverse $I_{F,G}^{-1}$ has to be bounded uniformly in $F \in \mathcal{F}$ and $G \in \mathcal{G}$ (see van der Laan (1996b) van der Laan, and Gill (1999) for the precise argument).

Proof of Theorem 5.3. Consider condition (i) of theorem 5.2. Firstly, we define the class of functions $\{(x, \delta) \to f(x, \delta) : f\}$, where $\delta \in \{0, 1\}^2$ and each of the four functions $x \to f(x, \delta)$ can vary over all functions in $D[0, \tau]$ with sectional variation norm $\|\cdot\|_v$ bounded by a fixed $M < \infty$. Norms are taken over $[0, \tau]$ only. This class of functions forms a Donsker class (see Gill, van der Laan, and Wellner; 1995, van der Laan, 1996a,b ; van der Laan, and Gill, 1999). Thus, it suffices to prove that $IC(\cdot \mid F_n, G_n, D)$ falls in this Donsker class with probability tending to 1. By assumption, we have that F_n is discrete on a fixed set of M points. By Lemma 5.2, this implies that $\| I_{F_n,G_n}^{-1}(D) \|_v < C < \infty$ for some $C < \infty$ uniformly in all F_n and all G_n with $\bar{G}_n(\tau) > \epsilon > 0$ for a fixed $\epsilon > 0$. Because $\bar{G}_n(\tau) \to \bar{G}(\tau)$ in probability, this proves that $I_{F_n,G_n}^{-1}(D)$ falls with probability tending to one in a $\|\cdot\|_v$ ball of functions in $(D[0, \tau], \|\cdot\|_v)$. Finally, note that $A_{F_n}(h)(x, \delta)$ equals $h(x)$ for $\delta = (1, 1)$ and (since F_n is discrete at M support points) the ranges of the three other terms are step functions at the M points. Given that f_n converges uniformly to f^1 and $f^1 > 0$ on each of the M points (by assumption), we also have that the denominators in the three censored terms of A_{F_n} are uniformly bounded away from zero. Now, it follows trivially that the uniform sectional variation norm of the functions $\{A_{F_n}(s)(\cdot, \delta) : \| s \|_v < C < \infty\}$, $\delta \in \{0, 1\}^2$, can be uniformly bounded, which proves condition (i) of Theorem 5.2.

In order to prove condition (ii) of Theorem 5.2, we note that

$$A_{F_n} I_{F_n,G_n}^{-}(D) - A_{F^1} I_{F^1,G}^{-1}(D) =$$
$$(A_{F_n} - A_{F^1}) I_{F^1,G}^{-1}(D) - A_{F_n} I_{F_n,G_n}^{-1} \{I_{F_n,G_n} - I_{F,G}\} I_{F^1,G}^{-1}(D). \quad (5.17)$$

Inspection of the information operator as a function of F makes clear that $IC(\cdot \mid F_n, G_n, D)$ depends on F_n through its density (due to the terms corresponding with the singly censored observations that contain partial densities F_1, F_2). On the other hand, integration by parts shows that it only depends on G_n through its c.d.f. Therefore, intuitively it is clear that consistent estimation of $IC(\cdot \mid F^1, G, D)$ requires an estimator F_n with consistent density f_n but just a consistent estimator G_n of the c.d.f. G. The proof works as follows. Let f_n, f^1 be the density of F_n, F^1 w.r.t. the counting measure on the M points. Because F_n is discrete, and $\| F_n - F^1 \|_\infty \to 0$, we have that f_n converges uniformly to f^1. Because

$\| f_n - f^1 \|_\infty \to 0$ and $I_{F^1,G}^{-1}(D)$ is uniformly bounded, by Lemma 5.2 we have that the first term on the right hand side of (5.17) converges uniformly to zero. Because $\| f_n - f^1 \|_\infty \to 0$ and $\| G_n - G \|_\infty \to 0$, it follows, by integration by parts, (see techniques in Gill, van der Laan, and Wellner (1995) and van der Laan (1996b)), that $(I_{F_n,G_n} - I_{F^1,G})(h)$ converges uniformly to zero for any uniformly bounded function h. By the fact that the operator norm of I_{F_n,G_n}^{-1} is uniformly bounded, this proves also that the second term in (5.17) converges uniformly to zero. This proves condition (ii) of Theorem 5.2.

Regarding condition (iii), we note that $\Phi(G_n) - \Phi(G) = P_{F,G_n-G}IC(\cdot \mid F^1, G_n, \mu)$. Thus condition (iii) requires showing $P_{F,G_n-G}IC(\cdot \mid F^1, G_n) - IC(\cdot \mid F_n, G_n) = o_P(1/\sqrt{n})$, where empirical process theory teaches us that $\| G_n - G \|_\infty = O_P(1/\sqrt{n})$. By integration by parts and the fact that $\| G_n - G \|_\infty = O_P(1/\sqrt{n})$, it follows that this holds if $\| f_n - f^1 \|_\infty \to 0$ in probability.

Finally, condition (iv) follows since the empirical c.d.f. G_n is an efficient estimator of G so that, in particular, $\Phi(G_n)$ is an efficient estimator of $\Phi(G)$. This proves all conditions of Theorem 5.2 and thus Theorem 5.3. □

5.3.7 Simulation methods and results for the nonparametric full data model

In this subsection we present the simulation results in Quale, van der Laan, and Robins (2001). In these simulation studies, we are interested in examining the performance in small samples of the nonparametric locally efficient estimator of $\mu = S(t_1, t_2)$ for a variety of combinations for the models for F and G, in particular the model that uses the Dabrowska estimator for G and a lower-dimensional model for F. The models used for F and G included the true distribution (representing small correctly specified parametric models), bivariate frailty models (representing semiparametric models), nonparametric models using Dabrowska's estimator, and a misspecification model (bivariate uniform distribution).

The simulation studies used a data-generation method in which the regularity condition (τ_1, τ_2) such that $P(T_1 > \tau_1, T_2 > \tau_2) = 0$, $P(C_1 > \tau_1, C_2 > \tau_2) = \delta$, where δ is bounded away from 0, is attained. We accomplish this by sampling T_1 from a truncated exponential distribution, namely

$$T_1 \sim U_1 \mid U_1 \leq \tau_1,$$

where U_1 is distributed as an exponential random variable with parameter λ_{t_1}. Then, we generate T_2 such that

$$T_2 \sim U_2 \mid U_2 \leq \tau_2,$$

where U_2 is distributed as an exponential random variable with parameter λ_{t_2}, and (T_1, T_2) are such that T_1 and T_2 are independent given an unobserved, gamma-distributed random variable Ω_t with variance α_t. (C_1, C_2)

are generated to have marginal exponential distributions with parameters λ_{c_1} and λ_{c_2}, respectively, and are independent given an unobserved gamma distributed random variable Ω_c with variance equal to α_c. τ_1 and τ_2 are chosen such that $\overline{G}(\tau_1, \tau_2) = \delta$, where δ is bounded away from zero. In these simulations, the value of δ was approximately 0.15. For computational feasibility and so that we could use the full grid of support points for F, for all but two simulations, the generated Y_1 and Y_2 were discretized so that the support of F was on $\{1, 2, \ldots 15\} \times \{1, 2, \ldots, 15\}$ and the support of G was $\{1, 2, \ldots\} \times \{1, 2, \ldots\}$. Two simulations were run in which the support of F was on the integers $\{1, 2, \ldots 40\} \times \{1, 2, \ldots, 40\}$ in order to verify that the locally efficient estimator works well in cases where the underlying F was less discrete. The amount of correlation between T_1 and T_2 was controlled by adjusting the α_t parameter, and the amount of censoring was controlled by the λ parameters. Further details for the data-generation method may be found in Quale, van der Laan, and Robins (2001).

In the simulation studies, we studied the small sample performance of the locally efficient estimator using a variety of models for F and G. Due to the data-generation scheme, using a bivariate frailty model would correspond to choosing semiparametric efficient estimators for F and G. Using the true distributions for F and G should give performance close to the efficiency bound and provide us with the best performance. Using Dabrowska's estimator for both F and G corresponds to the "globally" efficient estimator, as both F and G will be estimated consistently. However, as mentioned in Subsection 5.3.5, as Dabrowska's estimator is nonsmooth and highly nonparametric, it may not be the optimal choice for the estimator for F. Using a misspecification model ("guessing" a uniform distribution for F or G) should give us an indication of whether or not the locally efficient estimator is still consistent even if we "guess" wrong. The simulations were run with simulated data sets of size $n = 300$ over 625 iterations (except for the two continuous data simulations, in which the sample size was 100, so that the "grid size" defined by $m_1 m_2$ in Subsection 5.3.2 remained computationally feasible). Each simulation, aside from the first (described below), was run at two dependency levels, low ($\alpha_t = 0.5$, corresponding to a correlation between T_1 and T_2 of approximately 0.31) and high ($\alpha_t = 2$, corresponding to a correlation between T_1 and T_2 of approximately 0.72), and moderate censoring ($P(T_1 > C_1) = 0.30$).

In the first simulation, we generated data with heavy censoring on T_1 ($P(T_1 > C_1) = 0.65$), high correlation between T_1 and T_2 (0.72), and mild censoring on T_2 ($P(T_2 > C_2) = 0.30$). The frailty estimator was used for F, and Dabrowska's estimator was used for G. The results may be seen in Table 5.3. Here we see that the locally efficient estimator greatly outperforms Dabrowska's estimator, at points by almost a factor of 3. We see that the region where the LE estimator performs best is for the marginal distribution of T_1 ($t_2 = 0$). The marginal distribution of Dabrowska's estimator equals the Kaplan–Meier estimator based on $(\min(T_1, C_1), \Delta_1)$ and thus suffers heavily from the high amount of censoring. However, an efficient estimator tries to borrow information from T_2 when estimating the marginal distribution of T_1, which is in this simulation very beneficial since T_2 is almost always observed and T_1 and T_2 are strongly correlated.

We also ran two simulations in which we used the true distributions for F and G for the LE estimator at the dependency and censoring levels noted above and compared the result to Dabrowska's estimator (Table 5.4). If we use the true distributions for F and G, then the locally efficient estimator is asymptotically efficient so that the Monte Carlo variance should come close to achieving the efficiency bound. Thus, the ratios of mean squared error should be close to true relative efficiencies, which gives us a good measure of the performance of Dabrowska's estimator for this data-generating mechanism. As a result of the milder censoring, the results are not as dramatic as the previous simulation, but we see that the LE estimator outperforms Dabrowska's estimator.

In Tables 5.5 and 5.6, we see the result of the simulations for moderate censoring and two levels of dependence. In Table 5.5, we used the frailty estimator for both, and we see that the performance of the LE estimator is very good. However, in practice, we do not recommend using a lower dimensional model for both F and G, as that will not guarantee that S_n will be consistent. In table 5.6, we see that using Dabrowska's estimator for G does not result in a very large reduction in performance compared to the results in Table 5.5. Thus, using Dabrowska's estimator for G (or other consistent estimators of G) will guarantee that the LE estimator is always consistent, and gains performance relative to Dabrowska's estimator. Table 5.7 uses the Dabrowska estimator for both F and G and thus is a "globally" efficient estimator since both F and G are estimated consistently. However, the small sample performance is generally worse than Dabrowska's, underlining our statements that globally efficient estimators typically suffer from large second-order terms and also that Dabrowska's estimator being non-smooth and highly nonparametric, may be disadvantageous in estimation of partial densities of F.

Since we propose to use a lower-dimensional model for F for the LE estimator, there is the possibility that the model for F could be misspecified and not be consistent. Tables 5.8 and 5.9 are simulations that misspecify the distribution of F by "guessing" a uniform distribution for F. The results indicate that the estimator is still stable and the performance is still quite good relative to Dabrowska's estimator. A possible reason for this is that, for small samples, the second-order terms have more influence when you use a higher-dimensional model (e.g., frailty) than an extremely low-dimensional (uniform – zero unknown parameters) model. In Subsection 5.3.6, we proved that the first-order performance should actually deteriorate in the situation where we use the true distribution for G as opposed to estimating G, and a comparison of Table 5.9 (true G) and Table 5.8 (Dabrowska's estimator for G) shows that on the interior of the distribution, the model estimating G while misspecifying F indeed performs better. We believe that in the tails of the distributions the second-order terms generally dominate the first-order terms. Table 5.10 illustrates the "protection" property when G is misspecified. Although we propose to always use a consistent estimator for G in practice, these simulations indicate that indeed we are protected against misspecification of G.

The last set of simulations (Table 5.11) is for the case where the data are more "continuous"; namely, the support of F is on a 40 x 40 grid rather than a 15 x 15 grid as with the other simulations. For these simulations, both were run at a lower level of dependence, and one simulation estimated F with the frailty estimator and the true distribution for G, and the second simulation used the truth for both F and G, to validate that estimating an F that is less discrete gives an estimator that is still consistent and that $I_{F_n,G} \to I_{F,G}$. The results indicate that the locally efficient estimator performs well compared with Dabrowska's estimator that and the performance of the locally efficient estimator approaches the efficiency bound represented by the estimator using true F and true G.

Finally, Table 5.13 shows the estimated coverage probabilities of 95% confidence intervals constructed as described in subsection 5.3.5. Here we see that the confidence intervals provide estimates close to the ideal 0.95.

5.3.8 Data analysis: Twin age at appendectomy

To demonstrate the use of the LE estimator, we looked at a data set originally analyzed by Duffy, Martin, and Matthews (1990) of 1218 monozygotic female twins in which the outcome of interest was age (in years) at appendectomy. The data were obtained from a questionnaire sent in 1980 to twins over the age of 17 registered with the Australian National Health and Medical Research Council Twin Registry. Thus, if T_1 is the time to appendectomy of the first twin (where assignment of a twin to T_1 or T_2 was determined by birth order, where that information was available) and T_2 is the time to appendectomy of the second twin, then these time variables were censored by a common censoring variable C (i.e., $C_1 = C_2$). Specifically, the twin data can be represented by $Z_i = (Y_{1i}, Y_{2i}, \Delta_{1i}, \Delta_{2i}$, where $Y_{1i} = T_{1i} \wedge C_i$, $Y_{2i} = T_{2i} \wedge C_i$, $\Delta_{1i} = I(T_{1i} \leq C_i)$, and $\Delta_{2i} = I(T_{2i} \leq C_i)$, for $i = 1, \ldots, 1218$. To take advantage of this structure in the data, we estimated the distribution G of (C_1, C_2) using the well- known Kaplan–Meier estimator. Specifically, we created the variable $Z'_i = (Y'_i, \Delta'_i)$, where $Y'_i = \min(T_{1i}, T_{2i}, C_i)$ and $\Delta'_i = I(C \leq T_{1i} \wedge T_{2i})$, for $i = 1, \ldots, 1218$. Since $C_1 = C_2$, $P(C_1 > c_1, C_2 > c_2) = P(C > \max(c_1, c_2))$, and thus we can easily determine the estimate of the bivariate distribution of (C_1, C_2) from the univariate estimate of the distribution of C. To estimate the distribution of (T_1, T_2), we used the bivariate frailty estimator. There were 42 unique uncensored values of Y_1 and 41 unique uncensored values of Y_2; thus the set of support points $\tilde{t}$ (defined in subsection 5.3.2) had dimension 1722. The resulting estimate of the bivariate surface may be found in Figure 5.3.8.

We assessed the amount of dependence between T_1 and T_2 by utilizing two tests of independence developed by Quale and van der Laan (2000). The first tests the null hypotheses that the events $T_1 > t_{1i}$ and $T_2 > t_{2i}$ are independent for a given set of points $\mathbf{t} = \{(t_{1i}, t_{2i}), \ldots, (t_{1k}, t_{2k})\}$. This test involves looking at the difference between the locally efficient estimate of the bivariate survival function (no assumption of independence) and the bivariate product of the estimated marginals (which is correct under the assumption of independence) at the points $\mathbf{t}$. The distribution of this test statistic can be determined if one has an estimate of the influence curve. The second test tests the null hypothesis that all of the events mentioned above are independent, thus giving us an idea of the overall dependence of T_1 and T_2. We refer the reader to Quale and van der Laan (2000) for details. The results for the first test are given in Table 5.14 and indicate that the time to appendectomy appears to be more dependent the older the twins become. The second test resulted in a P-value less than 0.001 ($= P(\chi_{49} > 275.6)$ for χ_{49} a chi square random variable with 49 degrees of freedom), indicating that the time to appendectomy was related between the two twins (a result that Duffy, Martin, and Matthews (1990) found among the monozygotic female twins). Plots in Figure 5.3.8 of the conditional distributions $P(T_1 > t_1 \mid T_2 > t_2)$ versus the marginal distribution $P(T_1 > t_1)$ indicate this same pattern, as the curves diverge for larger values of t_2.

Also of interest is the question of whether or not the frailty was the correct model for S. To determine this, we looked at the difference between the locally efficient estimator and the estimator of S using the frailty estimator $(S_n(t_1, t_2) - \widehat{S}_{frail}(t_1, t_2))$. The results may be seen in Table 5.15, which tabulates the differences. The frailty estimator appears to be very close to the locally efficient estimator at all of the selected points (t_1, t_2), and indeed the frailty estimator lies within the 95% confidence interval for all of the selected points (t_1, t_2).

Remark

In this data set both failure times were subject to the same censoring variable. Thus this data structure corresponds with the univariate right-censored data structure $(C, \bar{X}_1(C), \bar{X}_2(C))$, where $X_k(t) = I(T_k \leq t)$, $k = 1, 2$, covered in chapter 3, where we developed a closed form locally efficient estimator. The generic locally efficient estimator used in this data analysis is thus asymptotically equivalent with this closed form locally efficient estimator.

Figure 5.1. Inverse algorithm performance. Plots of $\| \gamma^{k+1} - \gamma^k \|_F$ ("vector difference") versus iteration number k for $I_{F,G}$ calculated at 100 simulated data sets, for $\kappa(t_1,t_2) = I(T_1 > t_1, T_2 > t_2) - S(t_1,t_2)$, at points $\mathbf{t} = \{(2,2),(2,8),(8,2),(8,8)\}$, where $\dim(I_{F,G}) = 225$. The dotted line indicates ϵ, which was set at 1×10^{-7}.

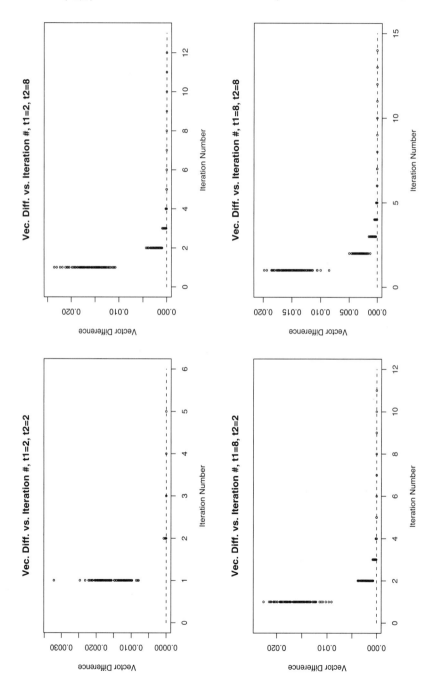

5.3. Bivariate Right-Censored Failure Time Data

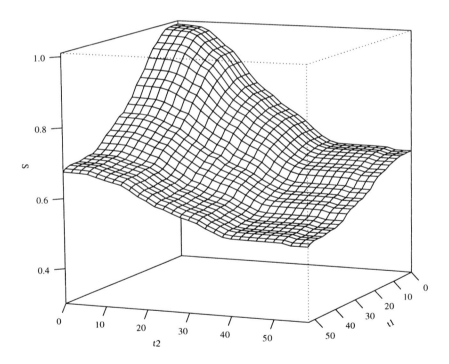

Figure 5.2. Estimated bivariate surface for twin appendectomy data, model for G: Kaplan Meier, model for F: bivariate frailty

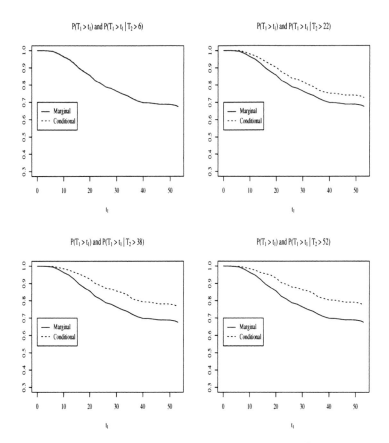

Figure 5.3. Conditional distributions ($P(T_1 > t_1 \mid T_2 > t_2)$) versus marginal distributions ($P(T_1 > t_1)$), twin data

Table 5.3. Heavy censoring on T_1 and high correlation; frailty F, Dabrowska G. MSE ratio for locally efficient estimator and Dabrowska's estimator ($\frac{MSE_{loc}}{MSE_{D_{ab}}}$) for a correlation between T_1 and T_2 of approximately 0.72. Simulations are for 300 subjects over 625 iterations, with $\lambda_{t_{1,2}} = 0.1$, $\lambda_{c_1} = 0.3$, and $\lambda_{c_2} = 0.08$, corresponding with $P(T_1 > C_1) = 0.65$ and $P(T_2 > C_2) = 0.30$.

	$t_2 = 0$	$t_2 = 1$	$t_2 = 2$	$t_2 = 4$	$t_2 = 6$	$t_2 = 8$	$t_2 = 10$
$t_1 = 0$	NA	1.03	1.02	1.00	0.98	0.96	0.95
$t_1 = 1$	1.13	0.99	0.95	0.93	0.93	0.92	0.93
$t_1 = 2$	1.10	0.94	0.92	0.90	0.91	0.89	0.91
$t_1 = 4$	0.93	0.88	0.88	0.89	0.89	0.88	0.89
$t_1 = 6$	0.76	0.77	0.80	0.87	0.87	0.87	0.86
$t_1 = 8$	0.58	0.60	0.65	0.74	0.75	0.75	0.73
$t_1 = 10$	0.34	0.36	0.38	0.44	0.49	0.50	0.52

5.3. Bivariate Right-Censored Failure Time Data   307

Table 5.4. Moderate censoring; low, high dependence; true F, true G. MSE ratio for estimates of S between the locally efficient estimator and Dabrowska's estimator ($\frac{MSE_{loc}}{MSE_{Dab}}$) for correlations between T_1 and T_2 of approximately 0.31 and 0.72. Simulations are for 300 subjects over 625 iterations, with $\lambda_{t_{1,2}} = 0.1$ and $\lambda_{c_{1,2}} = 0.08$, corresponding with $P(T_1 > C_1) = 0.30$ and $P(T_2 > C_2) = 0.30$.

	$t_2 = 1$	$t_2 = 2$	$t_2 = 4$	$t_2 = 6$	$t_2 = 8$	$t_2 = 10$
$t_1 = 1$	1.10,1.10	0.99,0.97	0.93,0.89	0.86,0.86	0.86,0.79	0.84,0.74
$t_1 = 2$	0.99,0.97	0.93,0.94	0.91,0.89	0.86,0.87	0.85,0.80	0.84,0.74
$t_1 = 4$	0.90,0.91	0.88,0.90	0.88,0.89	0.84,0.86	0.82,0.81	0.81,0.75
$t_1 = 6$	0.87,0.89	0.87,0.88	0.87,0.89	0.83,0.88	0.83,0.84	0.81,0.80
$t_1 = 8$	0.86,0.86	0.84,0.85	0.85,0.87	0.82,0.86	0.82,0.83	0.83,0.80
$t_1 = 10$	0.85,0.83	0.84,0.84	0.83,0.84	0.81,0.84	0.80,0.82	0.76,0.78

Table 5.5. Moderate censoring; low, high dependence; frailty F, frailty G. MSE ratio for estimates of S between the locally efficient estimator and Dabrowska's estimator ($\frac{MSE_{loc}}{MSE_{Dab}}$) for correlations between T_1 and T_2 of approximately 0.31 and 0.72. Simulations are for 300 subjects over 625 iterations, with $\lambda_{t_{1,2}} = 0.1$ and $\lambda_{c_{1,2}} = 0.08$, corresponding with $P(T_1 > C_1) = 0.30$ and $P(T_2 > C_2) = 0.30$.

	$t_2 = 1$	$t_2 = 2$	$t_2 = 4$	$t_2 = 6$	$t_2 = 8$	$t_2 = 10$
$t_1 = 1$	1.05,1.09	1.02,1.04	1.00,1.01	0.95,0.97	0.92,0.90	0.89,0.82
$t_1 = 2$	1.03,1.06	1.01,1.04	1.01,1.00	0.95,0.97	0.92,0.90	0.89,0.81
$t_1 = 4$	1.01,1.00	1.00,0.99	1.02,1.02	0.97,0.99	0.92,0.95	0.88,0.85
$t_1 = 6$	0.97,0.95	0.99,0.94	1.01,0.99	0.97,0.99	0.94,0.95	0.88,0.86
$t_1 = 8$	0.93,0.93	0.92,0.90	0.94,0.92	0.92,0.93	0.93,0.91	0.90,0.86
$t_1 = 10$	0.91,0.85	0.90,0.83	0.91,0.84	0.88,0.86	0.88,0.83	0.83,0.86

Table 5.6. Moderate censoring; low, high dependence; frailty F, Dabrowska G. MSE ratio for estimates of S between the locally efficient estimator and Dabrowska's estimator ($\frac{MSE_{loc}}{MSE_{Dab}}$) for correlations between T_1 and T_2 of approximately 0.31 and 0.72. Simulations are for 300 subjects over 625 iterations, with $\lambda_{t_{1,2}} = 0.1$ and $\lambda_{c_{1,2}} = 0.08$, corresponding to $P(T_1 > C_1) = 0.30$ and $P(T_2 > C_2) = 0.30$.

	$t_2 = 1$	$t_2 = 2$	$t_2 = 4$	$t_2 = 6$	$t_2 = 8$	$t_2 = 10$
$t_1 = 1$	1.03,1.03	1.01,1.02	1.00,0.99	0.99,0.96	0.96,0.91	0.93,0.83
$t_1 = 2$	1.02,1.02	1.01,1.01	1.00,0.99	0.99,0.97	0.96,0.91	0.93,0.84
$t_1 = 4$	1.00,0.98	1.00,0.99	1.01,0.99	0.98,0.96	0.97,0.92	0.93,0.86
$t_1 = 6$	0.97,0.97	0.98,0.97	0.99,0.97	0.98,0.97	0.97,0.93	0.93,0.89
$t_1 = 8$	0.96,0.92	0.96,0.93	0.95,0.94	0.95,0.94	0.95,0.92	0.91,0.89
$t_1 = 10$	0.93,0.87	0.93,0.88	0.92,0.88	0.90,0.90	0.90,0.88	0.87,0.86

Table 5.7. Moderate censoring; low, high dependence; Dabrowska F, Dabrowska G. MSE ratio for estimates of S between the locally efficient estimator and Dabrowska's estimator ($\frac{MSE_{loc}}{MSE_{D_{ab}}}$) for correlations between T_1 and T_2 of approximately 0.31 and 0.72. Simulations are for 300 subjects over 625 iterations, with $\lambda_{t_{1,2}} = 0.1$ and $\lambda_{c_{1,2}} = 0.08$, corresponding to $P(T_1 > C_1) = 0.30$ and $P(T_2 > C_2) = 0.30$.

	$t_1 = 1$	$t_1 = 2$	$t_1 = 4$	$t_1 = 6$	$t_1 = 8$	$t_1 = 10$
$t_2 = 1$	1.03,1.05	1.02,1.04	1.03,1.03	1.01,1.01	1.02,1.01	1.08,1.04
$t_2 = 2$	1.03,1.02	1.02,1.02	1.02,1.01	1.01,1.00	1.03,1.00	1.11,1.03
$t_2 = 4$	1.03,0.99	1.01,1.00	1.04,1.03	1.01,1.01	1.04,0.99	1.12,0.98
$t_2 = 6$	1.04,1.00	1.04,1.02	1.05,1.02	1.01,1.00	1.05,1.00	1.13,1.01
$t_2 = 8$	1.10,0.97	1.09,0.99	1.07,1.00	1.05,1.02	1.05,0.97	1.16,0.97
$t_2 = 10$	1.17,1.10	1.20,1.06	1.14,1.06	1.11,1.06	1.07,0.97	1.27,0.90

Table 5.8. Moderate censoring; low, high dependence; misspecification (Uniform) F, Dabrowska G. MSE ratio for estimates of S between the locally efficient estimator and Dabrowska's estimator ($\frac{MSE_{loc}}{MSE_{D_{ab}}}$) for correlations between T_1 and T_2 of approximately 0.31 and 0.72. Simulations are for 300 subjects over 625 iterations, with $\lambda_{t_{1,2}} = 0.1$ and $\lambda_{c_{1,2}} = 0.08$, corresponding to $P(T_1 > C_1) = 0.30$ and $P(T_2 > C_2) = 0.30$.

	$t_2 = 1$	$t_2 = 2$	$t_2 = 4$	$t_2 = 6$	$t_2 = 8$	$t_2 = 10$
$t_1 = 1$	1.01,1.01	1.00,0.99	0.97,0.97	0.94,0.94	0.90,0.91	0.85,0.86
$t_1 = 2$	1.00,0.99	0.99,0.99	0.97,0.97	0.94,0.94	0.90,0.90	0.85,0.86
$t_1 = 4$	0.97,0.97	0.97,0.97	0.96,0.96	0.94,0.95	0.91,0.90	0.85,0.85
$t_1 = 6$	0.94,0.94	0.94,0.94	0.93,0.94	0.92,0.94	0.90,0.91	0.86,0.86
$t_1 = 8$	0.91,0.91	0.91,0.91	0.91,0.91	0.91,0.92	0.89,0.91	0.86,0.86
$t_1 = 10$	0.87,0.88	0.86,0.87	0.86,0.87	0.84,0.88	0.82,0.86	0.80,0.84

Table 5.9. Moderate censoring; low, high dependence; misspecification (Uniform) F, true G. MSE ratio for estimates of S between the locally efficient estimator and Dabrowska's estimator ($\frac{MSE_{loc}}{MSE_{D_{ab}}}$) for correlations between T_1 and T_2 of approximately 0.31 and 0.72. Simulations are for 300 subjects over 625 iterations, with $\lambda_{t_{1,2}} = 0.1$ and $\lambda_{c_{1,2}} = 0.08$, corresponding to $P(T_1 > C_1) = 0.30$ and $P(T_2 > C_2) = 0.30$.

	$t_1 = 1$	$t_1 = 2$	$t_1 = 4$	$t_1 = 6$	$t_1 = 8$	$t_1 = 10$
$t_2 = 1$	1.03,1.03	0.93,0.94	0.89,0.89	0.89,0.89	0.89,0.90	0.88,0.89
$t_2 = 2$	0.94,0.94	0.91,0.92	0.88,0.89	0.88,0.88	0.87,0.87	0.86,0.86
$t_2 = 4$	0.89,0.88	0.90,0.88	0.88,0.88	0.86,0.87	0.85,0.86	0.84,0.85
$t_2 = 6$	0.90,0.89	0.89,0.87	0.86,0.86	0.85,0.88	0.82,0.86	0.80,0.87
$t_2 = 8$	0.91,0.90	0.90,0.87	0.85,0.86	0.83,0.88	0.82,0.88	0.80,0.88
$t_2 = 10$	0.95,0.95	0.93,0.92	0.89,0.88	0.86,0.88	0.80,0.91	0.81,0.94

5.3. Bivariate Right-Censored Failure Time Data

Table 5.10. Moderate censoring; low, high dependence; frailty F, misspecification (Uniform) G. MSE ratio for estimates of S between the locally efficient estimator and Dabrowska's estimator ($\frac{MSE_{loc}}{MSE_{Dab}}$) for correlations between T_1 and T_2 of approximately 0.31 and 0.72. Simulations are for 300 subjects over 625 iterations, with $\lambda_{t_{1,2}} = 0.1$ and $\lambda_{c_{1,2}} = 0.08$, corresponding to $P(T_1 > C_1) = 0.30$ and $P(T_2 > C_2) = 0.30$.

	$t_2 = 1$	$t_2 = 2$	$t_2 = 4$	$t_2 = 6$	$t_2 = 8$	$t_2 = 10$
$t_1 = 1$	1.08,1.08	1.07,1.06	1.06,1.02	1.00,0.97	0.95,0.91	0.92,0.87
$t_1 = 2$	1.07,1.05	1.06,1.05	1.06,1.01	1.01,0.97	0.96,0.92	0.92,0.86
$t_1 = 4$	1.04,1.00	1.04,1.00	1.05,1.03	1.01,0.98	0.97,0.96	0.93,0.90
$t_1 = 6$	0.97,0.94	0.98,0.94	1.00,0.99	0.99,0.98	0.99,0.96	0.97,0.92
$t_1 = 8$	0.94,0.91	0.94,0.90	0.93,0.93	0.95,0.94	0.97,0.93	0.97,0.91
$t_1 = 10$	0.93,0.87	0.93,0.86	0.91,0.88	0.91,0.90	0.93,0.90	0.95,0.92

Table 5.11. Moderate censoring; low, high dependence, support for F on $\{1, 2, \ldots, 40\} \times \{1, 2, \ldots, 40\}$. MSE ratio for estimates of S between the locally efficient estimator (frailty F, true G and true F, true$G$) and Dabrowska's estimator ($\frac{MSE_{loc}}{MSE_{dab}}$) for a correlation between T_1 and T_2 of approximately 0.31. Simulations are for 300 subjects over 625 iterations, with $\lambda_{t_{1,2}} = 0.0333$ and $\lambda_{c_{1,2}} = 0.03$, corresponding to $P(T_1 > C_1) = 0.34$ and $P(T_2 > C_2) = 0.34$.

	$t_2 = 1$	$t_2 = 2$	$t_2 = 4$	$t_2 = 6$	$t_2 = 8$	$t_2 = 10$
$t_1 = 1$	1.00,1.06	0.98,0.98	0.98,0.97	0.97,0.96	0.95,0.92	0.94,0.94
$t_1 = 2$	0.98,0.99	0.98,0.97	0.99,0.97	0.98,0.96	0.97,0.93	0.94,0.93
$t_1 = 4$	0.97,0.95	0.97,0.94	0.98,0.94	0.98,0.95	0.99,0.95	0.97,0.97
$t_1 = 6$	0.97,0.95	0.96,0.92	0.96,0.92	0.98,0.96	0.98,0.92	0.93,0.90
$t_1 = 8$	0.95,0.91	0.95,0.91	0.96,0.91	0.96,0.92	0.98,0.94	0.95,0.94
$t_1 = 10$	0.93,0.89	0.93,0.89	0.94,0.89	0.94,0.91	0.88,0.87	0.84,0.85

Table 5.12. Moderate censoring; low, high dependence; continuous data; frailty F, Dabrowska G. MSE ratio for estimates of S between the locally efficient estimator and Dabrowska's estimator ($\frac{MSE_{loc}}{MSE_{Dab}}$) for correlations between T_1 and T_2 of approximately 0.31 and 0.72. Simulations are for 100 subjects over 625 iterations, with $\lambda_{t_{1,2}} = 0.1$ and $\lambda_{c_{1,2}} = 0.08$, corresponding to $P(T_1 > C_1) = 0.30$ and $P(T_2 > C_2) = 0.30$.

	$t_2 = 1$	$t_2 = 2$	$t_2 = 4$	$t_2 = 6$	$t_2 = 8$	$t_2 = 10$
$t_1 = 1$	1.01,1.02	1.01,1.03	0.99,0.99	0.97,0.97	0.95,0.95	0.92,0.93
$t_1 = 2$	1.01,1.01	1.02,1.01	1.00,1.01	0.96,0.99	0.95,0.97	0.91,0.94
$t_1 = 4$	1.00,1.00	1.00,1.01	1.00,1.00	0.96,1.00	0.96,0.98	0.90,0.96
$t_1 = 6$	1.00,0.97	1.00,0.97	0.99,0.99	0.98,1.00	0.93,0.97	0.85,0.91
$t_1 = 8$	0.99,0.98	0.99,0.97	0.99,0.97	0.98,0.96	0.92,0.95	0.81,0.85
$t_1 = 10$	1.00,0.98	1.00,0.99	0.99,0.96	0.92,0.95	0.85,0.95	0.74,0.82

Table 5.13. Empirical coverage probabilities for estimated 95% confidence intervals for the locally efficient estimator; moderate censoring; low, high dependence; frailty F, Dabrowska G. Results for correlations between T_1 and T_2 of approximately 0.31 and 0.72. Simulations are for 300 subjects over 625 iterations, with $\lambda_{t_{1,2}} = 0.1$ and $\lambda_{c_{1,2}} = 0.08$, corresponding to $P(T_1 > C_1) = 0.30$ and $P(T_2 > C_2) = 0.30$.

	$t_2 = 1$	$t_2 = 2$	$t_2 = 4$	$t_2 = 6$	$t_2 = 8$	$t_2 = 10$
$t_1 = 1$	0.92,0.91	0.92,0.92	0.92,0.94	0.92,0.92	0.90,0.91	0.92,0.92
$t_1 = 2$	0.90,0.90	0.90,0.92	0.90,0.91	0.90,0.90	0.90,0.91	0.90,0.90
$t_1 = 4$	0.91,0.91	0.91,0.92	0.91,0.91	0.92,0.93	0.91,0.91	0.92,0.90
$t_1 = 6$	0.89,0.91	0.91,0.90	0.89,0.92	0.90,0.90	0.90,0.92	0.89,0.92
$t_1 = 8$	0.91,0.93	0.91,0.94	0.91,0.93	0.91,0.95	0.92,0.94	0.92,0.93
$t_1 = 10$	0.91,0.94	0.92,0.93	0.90,0.94	0.91,0.92	0.91,0.92	0.91,0.94

Table 5.14. Pointwise tests of independence for twin data.

	$t_1 = 6$	$t_1 = 12$	$t_1 = 20$	$t_1 = 28$	$t_1 = 36$	$t_1 = 44$	$t_1 = 52$
$t_2 = 6$	0.298	0.083	0.022	0.032	0.072	0.11	0.11
$t_2 = 12$	0.179	<0.001	<0.001	<0.001	<0.001	<0.001	<0.001
$t_2 = 20$	0.345	<0.001	<0.001	<0.001	<0.001	<0.001	<0.001
$t_2 = 28$	0.604	<0.001	<0.001	<0.001	<0.001	<0.001	<0.001
$t_2 = 36$	0.402	<0.001	<0.001	<0.001	<0.001	<0.001	<0.001
$t_2 = 44$	0.319	<0.001	<0.001	<0.001	<0.001	<0.001	<0.001
$t_2 = 52$	0.307	<0.001	<0.001	<0.001	<0.001	<0.001	<0.001

Table 5.15. Difference between the locally efficient estimate of the bivariate distribution and the bivariate frailty estimate for twin data $(S_n - \widehat{S}_{frailty})$.

	$t_1 = 4$	$t_1 = 12$	$t_1 = 20$	$t_1 = 28$	$t_1 = 36$	$t_1 = 44$	$t_1 = 52$
$t_2 = 4$	-0.0003	-0.006	-0.015	-0.015	-0.026	-0.025	-0.021
$t_2 = 12$	0.004	0.002	-0.008	-0.007	-0.021	-0.020	-0.017
$t_2 = 20$	0.004	0.004	0.003	-0.004	-0.011	-0.011	-0.008
$t_2 = 28$	0.001	-0.002	-0.002	-0.006	-0.013	-0.015	-0.012
$t_2 = 36$	0.006	0.001	-0.008	-0.012	-0.017	-0.019	-0.017
$t_2 = 44$	0.001	-0.002	-0.009	-0.015	-0.020	-0.023	-0.021
$t_2 = 52$	-0.004	-0.007	-0.014	-0.021	-0.027	-0.030	-0.027

6
Unified Approach for Causal Inference and Censored Data

6.1 General Model and Method of Estimation

Let $A(t)$ represent a time-dependent action process as observed on a randomly sampled subject. A general example can be $A(t) = (A_1(t), A_2(t), A_3(t), A_4(t))$, where $A_1(t) = I(C \leq t)$ jumps to 1 when the subject is right-censored, $A_2(t)$ is a counting process that jumps when the subject is monitored, $A_3(t)$ indicates which of the covariates are measured at time t, and $A_4(t)$ denotes the treatment that the subject receives at time t. In other words, $A(t)$ can denote both censoring/missingness and treatment actions. Let $\mathcal{A}$ be the set of possible sample paths of $A(\cdot)$. For technical reasons and simplicity, we will assume that $A(t)$ only changes values at given time points $t = 1, 2, \ldots, p$ and that $\mathcal{A}$ is finite. We note that this does not diminish the practical applicability of the methods presented in this chapter since one can approximate a continuous action process with an arbitrarily fine discrete approximation. In addition, we will present the formulas in such a way that they can be applied to continuous data as well, although we do not present regularity conditions and proofs.

We will denote the sample paths $A(1), \ldots, A(p)$ with A or $\bar{A}$. For each possible action regime $a = (a(t) : t)$, we define $X_a(t)$ as the data that one would observe on the subject if, possibly contrary to the fact, the subject had been assigned action regime a. We assume that $X_{\bar{a}}(t) = X_{\bar{a}(t-)}(t)$ (i.e., the action-specific outcome X_a at time t is only affected by actions before time t). One refers to $X_a = (X_a(t) : t)$ as an action-specific counterfactual. The baseline covariates are included in $X_a(1) = X(1)$. The observed data on a randomly selected subject are given by

$$Y = (A, X_A) = (A(1), \ldots, A(p), X_A(1), \ldots, X_A(p)).$$

Alternatively, one can represent this data structure by the ordered sequence

$$Y = (X(1), A(1), X_{A(1)}(2), A(2), \ldots, X_{\bar{A}(p-1)}(p), A(p)).$$

One defines $X_{\bar{A}(j-1)}(j)$ such that it becomes a constant equal to its final value after the time point at which no more data is collected on the subject (e.g., the minimum of time till right-censoring and time till death). We will also denote $X_{\bar{A}(j-1)}(j)$ with $X(j)$ so that one can also denote the observed data structure with $(X(1), A(1), \ldots, X(p), A(p))$.

Note that this data structure is a censored (i.e., coarsened) data structure of the full data $X = (X_a : a)$ whose a-specific components are X_a, where A represents the generalized censoring variable.

Let the distribution F_X of X be modeled by some full data model $\mathcal{M}^F$. We assume that the conditional distribution of A, given X, satisfies the sequential randomization assumption (SRA):

$$g(\bar{A} \mid X) = \prod_t g(A(t) \mid \bar{A}(t-), X) = \prod_t g(A(t) \mid \bar{A}(t-), \bar{X}_A(t)). \quad (6.1)$$

Note that SRA implies CAR. By CAR, the likelihood of Y is given by

$$dP_{F_X, G}(Y) = \prod_{j=1}^p \left\{ dP(X(j) \mid \bar{A}(j-1), \bar{X}(j-1)) \right\} g(\bar{A} \mid X). \quad (6.2)$$

The factor in set braces is the F_X-part of the likelihood of Y.

Since we assumed that $A(t)$ is discrete, the product integral in (6.1) becomes a finite product. In general, for continuous $A(t)$, one needs to assume that the product integral is appropriately defined. Typically, $A(t)$ consists of counting processes. If $A(t)$ is a vector of continuous counting processes, then one defines (6.1) as the partial likelihood, which is formally defined in Andersen, Borgan, Gill, and Keiding (1993). This partial likelihood assumption (6.1) is the continuous analog of the sequential randomization assumption on a discrete action mechanism in longitudinal studies.

We pose a model $g_\eta(A(t) \mid \bar{A}(t-), \bar{X}_A(t))$ for $g(A(t) \mid \bar{A}(t-), \bar{X}_A(t))$ and estimate the unknown parameter η by maximum likelihood:

$$\eta_n = \max{}_\eta^{-1} \prod_{i=1}^n \prod_t g_\eta(A_i(t) \mid \bar{A}_i(t-), \bar{X}_{i, A_i}(t)).$$

If $A(t) = (A_1(t), \ldots, A_k(t))$ is multivariate, then one can further factorize the multivariate probability $g(A(t) \mid \bar{A}(t-), \bar{X}_A(t))$. For example, if $A(t) = (A_1(t), A_2(t))$, then $g(A(t) \mid \bar{A}(t-), \bar{X}_A(t)) = g(A_1(t) \mid$

$A_2(t), \bar{A}(t-), \bar{X}_A(t))g(A_2(t) \mid \bar{A}(t-), \bar{X}_A(t))$, so in this case we have

$$g(\bar{A} \mid X) = \prod_{j=1}^{p} g(A(j) \mid \bar{A}(j-1), X)$$
$$= \prod_{j=1}^{p} g(A_1(j) \mid \mathcal{F}_1(j)) \prod_{j=1}^{p} g(A_2(j) \mid \mathcal{F}_2(j)), \quad (6.3)$$

where $\mathcal{F}_1(j) \equiv (A_2(j), \bar{A}(j-1), \bar{X}_A(j))$ and $\mathcal{F}_2(j) \equiv (\bar{A}(j-1), \bar{X}_A(j))$ are two observable histories. Since the different univariate conditional probabilities denote different mechanisms (e.g., a treatment mechanism, a monitoring mechanism, or a censoring mechanism), it is natural to model them separately. In that case, the corresponding maximum likelihood estimators maximize separate partial likelihoods.

This framework of representing the observed data and modeling the action (censoring/treatment) mechanism imitates the formal framework for doing causal inference (Robins, 1992, 1994, 1998a,b,c, 1999), in which case $A(t)$ is a treatment process. It has been our experience that this way of representing the observed data and modeling is very useful both for censored data structures and for mixtures of censored and causal inference data structures. It provides a unified framework for deriving a class of estimating functions and corresponding highly efficient estimators. We applied this approach in chapter 5 to obtain highly efficient estimators for the multivariate right-censored data structure on time-dependent processes, which is an example of a pure censored data structure.

The corresponding general approach for deriving a class of estimating functions is as follows. Let $D \to IC_0(Y \mid Q_0, G, D)$ be an initial mapping from full data estimating functions $D_h(X \mid \mu, \rho)$ into observed data estimating functions for μ with nuisance parameters G and $Q_0(F_X, G)$ that satisfies for a non empty set of full data functions $\mathcal{D}(\rho_1(F_X), G)$: for all $G \in \mathcal{G}$, $F_X \in \mathcal{M}^F$ $E_G(IC_0(Y \mid Q_0, G, D) \mid X) = D(X)$ F_X-a.e. for all possible Q_0 and $D \in \mathcal{D}(\rho_1(F_X), G)$. Convenient choices $IC_0(Y \mid G, D)$ in the form of an "inverse of probability of action weighted" mapping are often available. We refer the reader to Section 2.3 and Subsection 3.3.1 of Chapter 3 for the reparametrization of this restricted class of full data structure estimating functions $\{D_h(\cdot \mid \mu, \rho) : h \in \mathcal{H}^F(\mu, \rho, \rho_1, G)\}$, where the index set $\mathcal{H}^F(\mu, \rho, \rho_1, G) \subset \mathcal{H}^F$ is such that these full data structure estimating functions are elements of $\mathcal{D}(\rho_1, G)$, to $\{D_h^r(\cdot \mid \mu, \rho') : h \in \mathcal{H}^F\}$ by incorporating the extra nuisance parameters ρ_1 and G (needed to map any $h \in \mathcal{H}^F$ into $\mathcal{H}^F(\mu, \rho, \rho_1, G)$) in the nuisance parameter of D_h^r. This reparametrization is specified in (2.14) and, for notational convenience, we denote this reparametrized class of full data structure estimating functions with $\{D_h(\cdot \mid \mu, \rho) : h \in \mathcal{H}^F\}$ again, where ρ now includes the old ρ, ρ_1, and G. We showed this reparametrization in action in a right-censored data example covered in Examples 2.3, 2.4 and 2.5 in Chapter 2. We refer the reader to these examples.

The general theory of Chapter 2 teaches us that one should try to make an initial mapping $D_h \to IC_0(Y \mid D_h)$ from full data estimating functions D_h to observed data estimating functions orthogonal to a subspace of $T_{CAR} = \{v(A, X_A) : E(V(A, X_A) \mid X) = 0\} \cap L_0^2(P_{F_X,G})$ and preferably to T_{CAR} itself. Let T_{SRA} be the tangent space of G under the sole assumption SRA (6.1). It follows immediately that $T_{SRA} \subset T_{CAR}$. Robins, Rotnitzky, and Scharfstein (1999) prove that under the following non-identifiable assumption CAR and SRA are equivalent.

Assumption of CAR-SRA Equivalence: Given action regimes a and a^* let u^* be the smallest time u for which $a(u) \neq a^*(u)$. Then for all a and a^*, $(\overline{X}_a(t), \overline{X}_{a^*}(t); t > u^*)$ has a non-degenerate joint distribution given $\overline{X}_a(u^*-)$.

This assumption essentially says you cannot know with certainty the effect on an outcome at time t of a treatment history $\overline{a}(t-)$ on a particular subject from knowledge of the effect of a treatment history $\overline{a}^*(t-)$ on the same subject unless the treatment histories are identical. The practical import of this result is that when our model $\mathcal{M}^F$ for the law of X contains distributions that satisfy the assumption of CAR-SRA Equivalence, then imposing CAR implies the same model $\mathcal{M}(CAR)$ for the observable data Y as does imposing SRA.

Robins, Rotnitzky, and Scharfstein (1999) show that the assumption of CAR-SRA Equivalence holds when A denotes a pure treatment action, a common right censoring time, a single monitoring time as with current status data, or any combination of the three. However it will not hold if A denotes a multivariate censoring process or an interval censoring process. To be specific, in Chapter 5 we have $A(t) = (A_1(t) = I(C_1 \leq t), A_2(t) = I(C_2 \leq t))$ and $X_{a_1,a_2} = (X_{1,a_1}, X_{2,a_2})$ (i.e., C_2 has no effect on the first component of X_a, and C_1 has no effect on the second component of X_a). The assumption fails because if two actions $a = (a_1.a_2)$ and a^* agree in their first component a_1 but differ in their second component after time u^*, then $X_{a_1,a_2}(t)$ and $X_{a_1^*,a_2^*}(t)$ have a degenerate distribution fot $t > u$ since the two vectors $X_{a_1,a_2}(t)$ and $X_{a_1^*,a_2^*}(t)$ have identical first components $X_{1,a_1}(t)$. In this case, we will typically have that SRA is a significantly stronger assumption than CAR, (i.e., $T_{CAR} \not\subset T_{SRA}$) and that the projection operator onto T_{CAR} does not exist in closed form. Additionally, if the data structure is high-dimensional, this implies that orthogonalizing IC_0 w.r.t. T_{CAR} is not computationally practical.

We can still improve efficiency and obtain the double robustness property of our estimating function $IC_0(Y \mid Q_0, G, D_h(\cdot \mid \mu, \rho))$ within a practical framework by orthogonalizing IC_0 w.r.t. T_{SRA}. Thus, we define the new estimating function $IC(Y \mid Q_0, Q, G, D_h(\cdot \mid \mu, \rho))$ given by

$$IC_0(Y \mid Q_0, G, D_h(\cdot \mid \mu, \rho)) - IC_{SRA}(Y \mid Q, G),$$

where $IC_{SRA}(Y \mid Q, G)$ is a well-defined function on $\mathcal{Y} \times \mathcal{Q} \times \mathcal{G}$ so that $IC_{SRA}(Y \mid Q(F_X, G), G)$ equals

$$\Pi(IC_0(Y \mid Q_0(F_X, G), G, D_h(\cdot \mid \mu(F_X), \rho(F_X, G))) \mid T_{SRA}) \text{ in } L_0^2(P_{F_X, G}).$$

Suppose that $A = (A_1, A_2)$. Theorem 1.1 provides the following representation of this projection $\Pi(IC_0 \mid T_{SRA})$:

$$\sum_{k=1}^{2}\sum_{t=1}^{p} E(IC_0(Y) \mid A_k(t), \mathcal{F}_k(t)) - E(IC_0(Y) \mid A_k(t-1), \mathcal{F}_k(t)), \quad (6.4)$$

where $\mathcal{F}_1(t) = (A_2(t), \bar{A}(t-), \bar{X}_A(t))$ and $\mathcal{F}_2(t) = (\bar{A}(t-), \bar{X}_A(t))$.
We have

$$E(IC_0(Y) \mid A_k(t-1), \mathcal{F}_k(t)) = E(Q_k(A_k(t), \mathcal{F}_k(t)) \mid \mathcal{F}_k(t)),$$

where

$$Q_k(F_X, G)(A_k(t), \mathcal{F}_k(t)) \equiv E(IC_0(Y) \mid A_k(t), \mathcal{F}_k(t)), \ k = 1, 2.$$

Thus, the projection $\Pi(IC_0 \mid T_{SRA})$ can be represented as

$$IC_{SRA}(Y \mid Q_1, Q_2, G) \equiv \sum_{k=1}^{2}\sum_{t} Q(F_X, G)(A_k(t), \mathcal{F}_k(t))$$

$$- \sum_{k=1}^{2}\sum_{t}\sum_{\delta} Q_k(F_X, G)(\delta, \mathcal{F}_k(t)) P(A_k(t) = \delta \mid \mathcal{F}_k(t)),$$

where δ ranges over the possible outcomes of $A_k(t)$. Let $Q = (Q_0, Q_1, Q_2)$ so that we can denote the proposed estimating function with $IC(Y \mid Q, G, D) = IC_0(Y \mid Q_0, G, D) - IC_{SRA}(Y \mid (Q_1, Q_2), G)$.

Given a possibly data adaptive choice h_n for the full data estimating function $D_{h_n}(\cdot \mid \mu, \rho)$, estimates G_n, Q_n, ρ_n we would estimate μ by solving

$$0 = \sum_{i=1}^{n} IC(Y_i \mid Q_n, G_n, D_{h_n}(\cdot \mid \mu, \rho_n)).$$

In absolute generality, we can estimate the conditional expectations $E(IC_0(Y) \mid A_k(t) = \delta, \mathcal{F}_k(t))$ (semi)parametrically by regressing an estimate of $IC_0(Y)$ onto t and covariates extracted from the past $(A_k(t), \mathcal{F}_k(t))$. Here, we assume a model $E(IC_0(Y) \mid A_k(t), \mathcal{F}_k(t)) = g_t(W(t) \mid \beta)$. It is often the case that $g_t(W(t) \mid \beta)$ is known for t larger than a certain endpoint (often random) τ. In that case, each subject contributes observations $(t = j, A_k(j), \mathcal{F}_k(j)), j = 1, \ldots, \tau \leq p$. Another method would be to regress an estimate of $IC_0(Y)$ onto covariates extracted from $\mathcal{F}_k(t)$ among observations with $A_k(t) = \delta$ and subsequently smooth all of these t-specific regression estimates over t, taking into account the variance of each them (e.g., by weighting them by 1 over the number of observations used to fit the regression).

In order to obtain a doubly robust estimator of μ, one needs to estimate $Q = Q(F_X, G)$ with a substitution estimator $Q(F_n, G_n)$. We proposed a general maximum likelihood estimation method in Section 1.6, where the conditional expectations under P_{F_n,G_n} are evaluated by Monte-Carlo simulation. We presented the likelihood $dP_{F_X,G}(Y)$ in (6.2).

Let $\tilde{IC}_{SRA}$ denote the limit of the estimator $\hat{IC}_{SRA}$ as $n \to \infty$. Then, as in Chapter 2, we consider the minor modification $IC_0 - c^*_{nu}\tilde{IC}_{SRA}$ of IC, where $c^*_{nu} = \langle IC_0, \tilde{IC}_{SRA}^\top\rangle\langle \tilde{IC}_{SRA}, \tilde{IC}_{SRA}^\top\rangle^{-1}$ so that $c^*_{nu}\tilde{IC}_{SRA} = \Pi(IC_0 \mid \langle \tilde{IC}_{SRA}\rangle)$ is the projection of IC_0 onto the space spanned by $\tilde{IC}_{SRA}$, which guarantees that μ_n is asymptotically linear with an influence curve that is more efficient than $IC_0(Y)$. Thus, by setting IC_0 equal to the influence curve of an initial estimator μ_n^0, the resulting estimate μ_n will be guaranteed to be more efficient than μ_n^0, even when Q_n is heavily misspecified. Note that c^*_{nu} can be estimated with empirical covariance matrix of $\widehat{IC}_0 = (\widehat{IC}_0(Y_1), \ldots, \widehat{IC}_0(Y_n))$, $\widehat{IC}_{SRA} = (\widehat{IC}_{SRA}(Y_1), \ldots, \widehat{IC}_{SRA}(Y_n))$. Recall that the estimate $c^*_{nu,n}$ approximates 1 if $\widehat{IC}_{SRA}$ approximates $IC_{SRA} = \Pi(IC_0 \mid T_{SRA})$. Therefore $c^*_{nu,n}$ can also be used to select a good fit Q_n.

Let $IC(Y \mid \mu) = IC(Y \mid Q, G, c_{nu}, D_h(\cdot \mid \mu, \rho))$ denote the limit of $\widehat{IC}(Y \mid \mu) \equiv IC(Y \mid Q_n, G_n, D_{h_n}(\cdot \mid \mu, \rho_n))$ for $n \to \infty$. Wald-type confidence intervals for μ are directly available if we assume that the model for G is correctly specified. Let $T_G \subset T_{SRA}$ be the observed data tangent space of G under this model. In that case, application of Theorem 2.4 of Chapter 2 teaches us that, under the specified regularity conditions of Theorem 2.4, μ_n is asymptotically linear with influence curve $-c^{-1}\{IC(Y \mid \mu) - \Pi(IC \mid T_G)\}$, where $c = d/d\mu P_{F_X,G}IC(Y \mid \mu) = d/d\mu P_{F_X,G}IC_0(Y \mid \mu)$. Thus a conservative confidence band for μ can be based on the following conservative estimate of the covariance matrix of the normal limit distribution of $\sqrt{n}(\mu_n - \mu)$,

$$\hat{\Sigma} = c_n^{-1}\frac{1}{n}\sum_{i=1}^n \widehat{IC}(Y_i)\widehat{IC}(Y_i)^\top c_n^{-1\top},$$

where c_n is the empirical estimate of the derivative matrix c.

The following lemma can be used to calculate the actual projection $\Pi(IC \mid T_G)$ of IC onto the tangent space T_G of the action mechanism, if $A(t)$ is a counting process and modelled with a multiplicative intensity model. The proof of this lemma is completely analogue to the proof of Lemma 3.2 in Section 3.3.

Lemma 6.1 *For each action regime $a(\cdot) = (a(t) : t = 1, \ldots, p) \in \mathcal{A}$, we define an action specific time-dependent process $X_a(\cdot)$. Suppose $X_a(t) = X_{\bar{a}(t-)}(t)$, $t = 1, \ldots, p+1$. Let $X = (X_a : a \in \mathcal{A})$ be the full-data structure and let $Y = (A, X_A)$ be the observed data structure, where $A = (A(1), \ldots, A(p))$ and $X_A = (X_A(1), \ldots, X_A(p+1))$. Suppose that*

6.1. General Model and Method of Estimation

$A(t)$ is counting process. Assume SRA:

$$P(dA(j) = 1 \mid \bar{A}(j-1), X) = P(dA(j) = 1 \mid \bar{A}(j-1), \bar{X}_A(j)),$$

$j = 1, \ldots, p$. We consider the special case where $A(t)$ is discrete on a fine grid (i.e., p is large) so that a multiplicative intensity model $\alpha_A(t_j) = E(dA(t_j) \mid \mathcal{F}(t_j)) = Y_A(t_j)\lambda_{0A}(t_j)\exp(\beta_A W(t_j))$, $j = 1, \ldots, k$, is appropriate: note that the $\alpha_A(t_j)$ are now conditional probabilities.

The conditional distribution $g(\bar{A} \mid X)$ equals the partial likelihood of $A(\cdot)$ w.r.t. observed history $\mathcal{F}(t) = (\bar{A}(t-), \bar{X}_A(t))$ for the discrete multiplicative intensity model $\alpha_A(t) \equiv E(dA(t) \mid \mathcal{F}(t)) = Y_A(t)\lambda_{0A}(t)\exp(\beta_A W(t))dt$,

$$g(\bar{A} \mid X) = \prod_{t=1}^{p} \alpha_A(t)^{dA(t)}(1 - \alpha_A(t)dt)^{1-dA(t)}.$$

Let $dM_G(t) \equiv dA(t) - \alpha_A(t)dt$. The score for the regression parameter β_A is given by

$$S_{\beta_A} = \int W(t)dM_G(t).$$

The tangent space $T_{\Lambda_{0A}}$ is given by

$$T_{\Lambda_{0A}} = \overline{\left\{\int g(t)dM_G(t) : g\right\}}.$$

We have

$$\Pi\left(\int H(t, \mathcal{F}(t))dM_G(t) \mid T_{\Lambda_{0A}}\right) = \int g(H)(t)dM_G(t) \quad (6.5)$$

$$\equiv \int \frac{E\{H(t,\mathcal{F}(t))Y_A(t)\exp(\beta_A W(t))\}}{E\{Y_A(t)\exp(\beta_A W(t))\}}dM_G(t).$$

Thus, the efficient score of β_A is given by

$$\begin{aligned}S^*_{\beta_A} &= S_{\beta_A} - \Pi(S_{\beta_A} \mid T_{\Lambda_{0A}}) \\ &= \int \left\{W(t) - \frac{E\{W(t)Y_A(t)\exp(\beta_A W(t))\}}{E\{Y_A(t)\exp(\beta_A W(t))\}}\right\}dM_G(t)\end{aligned}$$

and

$$T_{\Lambda_{0A},\beta_A}(P_{F_X,G}) = \langle S^*_{\beta_A}\rangle \oplus \overline{\left\{\int g(t)dM_G(t) : g\right\}}. \quad (6.6)$$

Given any function $V(Y) \in L^2(P_{F_X,G})$, we have $\Pi(V \mid T_{SRA}) = \int H_V(t, \mathcal{F}(t))dM_G(t)$, where $H_V(t, \mathcal{F}(t)) = H_{V,1}(t, \mathcal{F}(t)) - H_{V,2}(t, \mathcal{F}(t))$ with $H_{V,1} = E(V(Y) \mid dA(t) = 1, \mathcal{F}(t))$ and $H_{V,2} = E(V(Y) \mid dA(t) = 0, \mathcal{F}(t))$. Thus, given any function $V(Y)$, we have

$$\Pi(V \mid T_{\Lambda_{0A}}) = \int g(H_V)(t)dM_G(t).$$

Thus, given any function $V(Y)$, we have that $\Pi(V \mid T_{\Lambda_{0A},\beta_A})$ is given by

$$E(VS_{\beta_A}^{*\top})E(S_{\beta_A}^* S_{\beta_A}^{*\top})^{-1}S_{\beta_A}^* + \int \{g(H_{V,1}) - g(H_{V,2})\}(t)dM_G(t). \quad (6.7)$$

If one uses an estimator $Q_n = Q(F_n, G_n)$ separately estimating F_X and G components of $Q(F_X, G)$, then, under the regularity conditions of Theorem 2.5, μ_n will be asymptotically linear in model $\mathcal{M}$. In this case, we propose to use the bootstrap to estimate the variability of the estimator μ_n.

Organization In Sections 6.2, 6.3 and 6.4, we apply this general methodology to estimate the causal effect as defined by marginal structural models of a time-dependent (and time-independent) treatment in a longitudinal study with no censoring and with right-censoring (i.e., $A(t)$ includes treatment and right-censoring). In section 6.4, we also present a data analysis to illustrate these methods. In section 6.5, we consider estimation of the causal regression parameters in a marginal structural nested model and estimation of dynamic treatment-regime-specific survival functions. In this section, we also provide a small simulation for dynamic treatment regimes in point treatment study. Section 6.6 applies the methodology to estimate an effect of exposure on an outcome through a regression in a longitudinal study with right-censoring when the exposure process is only measured on a subsample of the subjects (i.e., $A(t)$ includes right-censoring and missingness indicators). Finally, in Section 6.7 we consider estimation in a longitudinal study in which subjects are randomly monitored and right censored, resulting in right censored interval censored data on time-variables of interest (i.e., $A(t)$ includes monitoring and right-censoring). Estimation in each of these problems is challenging, and no literature on the last two estimation problems is available, but the general methodology presented in this section provides high-quality estimation procedures.

6.2 Causal Inference with Marginal Structural Models

Let $A(t)$ represent a time-dependent treatment process that potentially changes value at a finite prespecified set of points $t = 1, \ldots, p$. Let $\mathcal{A}$ be the set of possible sample paths of A, where we assume that $\mathcal{A}$ is finite. For each possible treatment regime a, we define $X_a(t)$ as the data that one would observe on the subject if, possibly contrary to the fact, the subject had followed treatment regime a. It is natural to assume that $X_a(t) = X_{\bar{a}(t-)}$ (i.e., the counterfactual outcome at time t is not affected by treatment given after time t). One refers to $X_a = (X_a(t) : t = 1, \ldots, p+1)$ as a (counter)factual. Suppose that $X_a = (Z_a, L_a)$ consists of an outcome process Z_a and covariate process L_a. The baseline covariates are included

in $L_a(1) = L(1)$. The observed data structure is given by
$$Y = (A, X_A) = (A, Z_A, L_A).$$
Respecting the ordering in which the data is colelcted, we can also represent this as
$$(Z(1), L(1), A(1), \ldots, Z_A(p), L_A(p), A(p), Z_A(p+1), L_A(p+1)).$$
The observed data structure can be viewed as a censored data structure $Y = \Phi(A, X) \equiv (A, X_A)$ on the full data $X = (X_a : a \in \mathcal{A})$. The general methodology presented in Section 6.1 can be used to construct locally efficient estimators of parameters in causal inference models.

Robins (1998b, 1999) introduces a class of full data models that are called marginal structural models (MSM). These are models for the marginal distribution of X_a of X for a fixed a for each a, typically describing models for a conditional distribution of a treatment specific outcome Y_a within levels of (i.e. conditional on) covariates V. An example of an MSM is the marginal structural generalized linear regression model of a counterfactual outcome of interest on baseline covariates. Let Y_a^* be a counterfactual outcome of interest such as $Y_a(\tau)$ at an endpoint τ; then, such a model would be of the form
$$Y_a^* = m(a, V \mid \beta) + \epsilon_a, \text{ where } E(\epsilon_a \mid V) = 0. \tag{6.8}$$
V is a vector of baseline covariates included in $L_A(1) = L(1)$, and $m(a, V \mid \beta)$ is a specified function of a, V, β. For example, we could consider a linear regression model:
$$Y_a^* = \beta_0 + \beta_1 \text{cum}(a) + \beta_2 V + \epsilon_a,$$
where cum(a) is a summary measure of the cumulative history $\bar{a}(\tau)$.

Our tasks are 1) to find the orthogonal complement of nuisance tangent space in the full data model and corresponding set of full data estimating functions and 2) to find $IC_0(Y \mid G, D)$ and $\Pi(IC_0(Y \mid G, D) \mid T_{SRA})$ and thereby a mapping $D \rightarrow IC_0(Y \mid G, D) - \Pi(IC_0(Y \mid, G, D) \mid T_{SRA})$ from full data estimating functions into observed data estimating functions. To be concrete, we will assume the full data model (6.8), although our results generalize immediately to any marginal structural model such as the marginal structural Cox proportional hazards model $\lambda_{T_a}(t \mid V) = \lambda_0(t) \exp(\beta_0 a + \beta V)$ for the hazard of a treatment specific survival time T_a, given V.

Recall that the full data structure is $X = (X_a : a)$. Marginal structural models $\mathcal{M}^F$ assume a model for the marginal random variable X_a for each a. Thus $\mathcal{M}^F = \cap_a \mathcal{M}_a^F$, where $\mathcal{M}_a^F$ only assumes the restriction on the distribution of X_a. For example, in the model above we have $\mathcal{M}_a^F = \{F_X : E(Y_a^* \mid V) = m(a, V \mid \beta)\}$. Let $T_{nuis,a}^{F,\perp}$ be the orthogonal complement of $\mu = \beta$ in model $\mathcal{M}_a^F$. In Section 2.2 of Chapter 2, we proved for the multivariate generalized linear regression model that $T_{nuis,a}^{F,\perp} = \{h(V)\epsilon_a(\beta) : h\}$.

Since the orthogonal complement of an intersection is the sum of the orthogonal complements, $T_{nuis}^{F,\perp} \supset \{\sum_{a\in\mathcal{A}} h(a,V)\epsilon_a(\beta) : h\}$, where we typically have equality. Thus, the set of full data estimating functions of interest is given by

$$\left\{D_h(X \mid \beta) = \sum_{a\in\mathcal{A}} h(a,V)\epsilon_a(\beta) : h\right\}.$$

Under our assumption that A is discrete, CAR is equivalent with $g(a \mid X) = b(a, X_a)$ for some function b. Since $g(\bar{A} \mid X) = \prod_t g(A(t) \mid \bar{A}(t-), X)$ a natural way to impose CAR is to assume SRA (6.1), $g(A(t) \mid \bar{A}(t), X) = g(A(t) \mid \bar{A}(t-), \bar{X}_A(t))$ (SRA). In words, for all t the conditional distribution of $A(t)$, given $X, \bar{A}(t-)$, equals the conditional distribution of $A(t)$, given $\bar{A}(t-)$ and the observed part $\bar{X}_A(t)$ of X. As described above, Robins, Rotnitzky, and Scharfstein (1999) show under certain conditions, CAR and SRA are equivalent and thus generate the same tangent space. Given a MSM, Robins (1999) also describes assumptions that are weaker than SRA but generate the same model for the observed data and thus the same tangent space as under SRA. An example of such a weaker assumption for the MSM model (6.8) is the SRA for Y_a^* only

$$Y_a^* \text{ II } A(t) \mid \bar{A}(t-1), \bar{X}(t) \text{ for all } a \text{ and } t. \tag{6.9}$$

Define

$$IC_0(Y \mid G, D_h) = \frac{h(A,V)\epsilon(\beta)}{g(\bar{A} \mid X)},$$

where $\epsilon(\beta) = \epsilon_A(\beta)$. By SRA, we have that $g(\bar{A} \mid X)$ is only a function of $Y = (A, X_A)$ and thus that $D_h \to IC_0(Y \mid G, D_h)$ indeed maps a full data estimating function into an observed data estimating function. If

$$\max_{a\in\mathcal{A}} \left|\frac{h(a,V)\epsilon_a(\beta)}{g(a \mid X)}\right| < \infty \; F_X\text{-a.e}, \tag{6.10}$$

where $\mathcal{A}$ is the support of the marginal distribution of A, then

$$E(IC_0(Y \mid G, D_h) \mid X) = \sum_{a\in\mathcal{A}} h(a,V)\epsilon_a(\beta) = D_h(X) \; F_X\text{-a.e.}$$

A fundamental condition in our asymptotics Theorem 2.4 for this estimator μ_n^0 of μ is that $\mathcal{D}(\rho_1(F_X), G)$ is non empty, where $\mathcal{D}(\rho_1(F_X), G)$ is defined as the set of full data structure estimating functions for which $E_G(IC_0(Y \mid G, D) \mid X) = D(X) \; F_X$-a.e. Clearly (6.10) guarantees that $\mathcal{D}(\rho_1(F_X), G)$ is non-empty. In other words, we need that h_n and G are such that (6.10) holds. The condition on the support

$$\{a(t) : g(a(t) \mid \bar{A}(t-) = \bar{a}(t-), \bar{X}_A(t)) > 0\} \text{ is non-random} \tag{6.11}$$

for all t, or equivalently,

$$g(a(t) \mid \bar{A}(t-1) = \bar{a}(t-1), \bar{X}_A(t)) > 0 \text{ for all possible } a(t), F_X\text{-a.e.},$$

(given a $\bar{a}(t-1)$) guarantees that each possible full data structure estimating function is an element of the set $\mathcal{D}(\rho_1(F_X), G)$ (see 2.13)). This condition is needed to have nonparametric identifiability of $E[Y_a^* \mid V]$ for all a. It says that, at any point in time t, each *possible* treatment $a(t)$ among subjects with a treatment past $\bar{a}(t-)$ needs to have a chance of being selected, whatever the observed $\bar{X}(t)$ might be. If the assumption (6.11) does not hold in a particular application of interest, then $\mathcal{D}(\rho_1(F_X), G)$ may still be non-empty and β may still be identifiable. We then effectively restrict h_n by making the membership requirement $D_{h_n}(\cdot \mid \mu(F_X), \rho(F_X, G)) \in \mathcal{D}(\rho_1(F_X), G)$ an additional parameter of the full data estimating function in the manner described in Section 6.1.

In our particular case, this comes down to making h a function of the denominator $g(\bar{A} \mid X)$ in such a way that, if the denominator $g(\bar{a} \mid x) = 0$ for a possible x, then $h(\bar{a}, V) = 0$. Clearly, this might not always be possible, which means that $\mathcal{D}(\rho_1, G)$ is empty (i.e., our particular parameter of interest is simply not estimable from the data based on this choice of IC_0).

Given an estimate of g, one can estimate β by solving

$$0 = \frac{1}{n} \sum_{i=1}^n \frac{h(A_i, V_i)\epsilon_i(\beta)}{g_n(\bar{A}_i \mid X_i)}.$$

We refer to this estimator as the "inverse probability of treatment weighted" (IPTW) estimator. The observed data likelihood for g is given by $\prod_j g(A(j) \mid \bar{A}(j-), \bar{X}_A(j))$, which can be modeled by modeling the conditional distribution of $A(j)$, given the past, for each j separately, or one can use time j as a covariate and assume common parameters for each $g(A(j) \mid \bar{A}(j-), \bar{X}_A(j))$, $j = 1, \ldots, p$. If $A(j)$ is discrete, then a multinomial logistic regression model extracting covariates from the past is appropriate (see Brookhart, and van der Laan, 2002a, Robins, Hernan, and Brumback, 2000, for a discussion and application of this model). Let $\mathcal{G}$ be the model for g.

Consider a restricted treatment model $\mathcal{G}^* = \{g \in \mathcal{G} : g(A(j) \mid \bar{A}(j-), \bar{X}_A(j)) = g(A(j) \mid \bar{A}(j-), V)\}$ assuming sequential randomization w.r.t. $\bar{A}(j-), V$. Since $g(\bar{A} \mid X) = \prod_j g(A(j) \mid \bar{A}(j-), \bar{X}_A(j))$, under this restricted model we have $g(\bar{A} \mid X) = g(\bar{A} \mid V)$. Consequently, $m(A, V \mid \beta) = E(Y^* \mid A, V)$ is a regression of Y^* onto A, V. Thus, Lemma 2.1 teaches us that, if the true treatment mechanism is an element of $\mathcal{G}^*$ and the additional covariates beyond V are non-informative, that is, $\bar{X}_A(\tau - 1) \perp Y_A(\tau) \mid V, \bar{A}(\tau - 1)$, then the optimal estimating function for β is given by:

$$\frac{\frac{d}{d\beta} m(A, V \mid \beta)}{E(\epsilon(\beta)^2 \mid A, V)} \epsilon(\beta). \tag{6.12}$$

For any g in our posed model $\mathcal{G}$ for the treatment mechanism, let $g^* = g^*(g)$ be a projection of g onto $\mathcal{G}^*$ in some sense. For example, the Kullback–Leibner projection of g onto $\mathcal{G}^*$ corresponds with maximum likelihood estimation of G as above for $\mathcal{G}$, but now restricted to model $\mathcal{G}^*$. If we set

$$h^*_{opt}(A,V) = g^*(\bar{A} \mid X) \frac{\frac{d}{d\beta} m(A, V \mid \beta)}{E(\epsilon(\beta)^2 \mid A, V)}, \qquad (6.13)$$

then $IC_0(Y \mid G, D_{h^*_{opt}})$ reduces to (6.12) if the true treatment mechanism happens to be an element of $\mathcal{G}^*$. Let h_n be an estimator of this locally optimal direction h^*_{opt}. Then, the IPTW estimator β_n is CAN if the treatment mechanism $g(\bar{A} \mid X)$ is modeled correctly. This estimator has the attractive property that it is easy to compute (one just applies standard regression software, but one assigns a weight to each subject) and, by theorem 2.3, it always improves on the naive estimator assuming that there is no confounding beyond the variables that one has adjusted for in the regression.

The set of all observed data estimating functions can be represented as $\{IC(Y \mid Q, G, D_h) = IC_0(Y \mid G, D_h) - IC_{SRA}(Y \mid Q, G) : h \in \mathcal{H}^F\}$, where the projection term is defined in (6.4). Theorem 1.2 provides us with the projection on the tangent space T_{SRA}. This gives us the observed data estimating functions $IC(Y \mid Q, G, D_h)$ given by

$$\frac{h(\bar{A}, V)\epsilon_{\bar{A}}(\beta)}{g(\bar{A} \mid X)} - \sum_{k=1}^{2} \sum_{j} \{E(IC_0(Y) \mid A_k(j), \mathcal{F}_k(j)) - E(IC_0(Y) \mid \mathcal{F}_k(j))\},$$

where we used the shorthand notation $IC_0(Y) = IC_0(Y \mid G, D_h)$.

In Bryan, Yu, and van der Laan (2002) we implemented the IPTW-estimator specified above corresponding with the estimating function $IC_0(Y \mid G, D_{h^*_{opt}})$ and the one-step estimator corresponding with the estimating function $IC(Y \mid \beta)$ involving the projection of IC_0 onto T_{SRA}. Here we estimated Q by regressing observations $\hat{IC}_0(Y_i)$ onto covariates extracted from $A_k(j), \mathcal{F}_k(j)$. We used these estimators to estimate the causal effect of initiation time of a treatment on the hazard of survival under a particular marginal structural linear logistic regression model with four parameters; given a subject has not failed yet, the probability of failure in the upcoming interval is given by

$$logit(P(Y_{\bar{a}}(k) = 1 \mid Y_{\bar{a}}(k-1) = 0) = \alpha_0 + ((1-a(k))t_k + a(k)t^*)\alpha_1$$
$$+ a(k)\alpha_2 + a(k)(t_k - t^*)\alpha_3.$$

Here t^* denotes the time-point at which treatment is initiated and $A(k) = I(t^* \geq k)$ is the indicator for being on treatment. Below, we report the relative efficiency of the IPTW, the one-step estimator, and the naive regression estimator. Here α_2 actually measures the immediate treatment effect. It is of interest to see that the one-step estimator is four times as efficient as the IPTW estimator, which shows that the one-step estimator

6.2. Causal Inference with Marginal Structural Models

can truly dramatically improve on an initial estimator in these causal inference models. For details, we refer the reader to Bryan, Yu, and van der Laan (2002).

	α_0	α_1	α_2	α_3
One-step w.r.t. IPTW	0.8841	0.8420	0.2656	0.5047
IPTW w.r.t unweighted	0.5217	0.7814	0.2455	0.7867

Regarding estimation of $Q(F_X, G)$, in Section 6.4, we present a plug-in estimator $Q(F_n, G_n)$ of $Q(F_X, G)$ separately estimating the F_X and G components, which yields a doubly robust estimator β_n of β. We already discussed the doubly robust estimation method based on maximum likelihood estimation as presented in Section 1.6. If A is time-independent, then the nuisance parameter Q is a simple function of a regression $E(\epsilon \mid A, W)$ and $g(A \mid W)$, so that doubly robust estimators are easy to compute, as shown in Section 6.3).

If the treatment process only changes value at random monitoring times among a given discrete set of potential monitoring times, then the following model for $g(\bar{A} \mid X)$ is appropriate. Let $N(t)$ be a counting process jumping at the times t at which $A(t)$ changes value. In the model above $N(t)$ was deterministic with jumps at $j = 1, \ldots, p$. Let $\mathcal{F}(t) = (\bar{A}(t-), \bar{X}_A(t))$, which thus excludes observing $dN(t)$. Let $\alpha(t \mid \mathcal{F}(t)) = E(dN(t) \mid \mathcal{F}(t))$ be the intensity of $N(t)$ w.r.t. $\mathcal{F}(t)$. Let $\mathcal{F}_1(t) = (N(t), A_2(t), \mathcal{F}(t))$ and $\mathcal{F}_2(t) = (N(t), \mathcal{F}(t))$. Consider the model

$$g(A \mid X) = \prod_{\{t: dN(t)=1\}} g(A_1(t) \mid \mathcal{F}_1(t)) \prod_{\{t: dN(t)=1\}} g(A_2(t) \mid \mathcal{F}_2(t))$$

$$\times \prod_t \alpha(t \mid \mathcal{F}(t))^{dN(t)} (1 - \alpha(t \mid \mathcal{F}(t)))^{1-dN(t)},$$

where the third product is the partial likelihood for the intensity α as defined formally in Andersen, Borgan, Gill, and Keiding (1993). Thus, in this case, $g(\bar{A} \mid X)$ has an additional parameter α, but the first two products are analogous to the parametrization (6.3) for discrete A.

By factorization of $g(\bar{A} \mid X)$, the following theorem is the natural extension of Theorem 1.2. Since we do not want to claim to have considered the technical issues involved for a continuous counting process, we state the theorem for the case where $N(t)$ is discrete (i.e., it only jumps at prespecified grid points). However the theorem is expressed in such a way that it may immediately be applied to data in continuous time. This theorem is based on an analogous theorem in Robins (1999).

Theorem 6.1 *Consider the causal inference data structure* $Y = (A, X_A) \sim P_{F_X, G}$. *Let* $N(t)$ *be a counting process jumping at the times* t *at which* $A(t)$ *changes value, and assume that* $A(t)$ *can only change value at prespecified grid points* $t_1 < \ldots < t_p$. *Let* $\mathcal{F}(t) = (\bar{A}(t-), \bar{X}_A(t))$, which thus excludes observing $dN(t)$. Let $\alpha(t \mid \mathcal{F}(t)) = E(dN(t) \mid \mathcal{F}(t))$. Let $\mathcal{F}_1(t) = (N(t), A_2(t), \mathcal{F}(t))$ and $\mathcal{F}_2(t) = (N(t), \mathcal{F}(t))$. We assume the following model for the conditional probability distribution of A, given X:

$$g(A \mid X) = \prod_{\{t:dN(t)=1\}} g(A_1(t) \mid \mathcal{F}_1(t)) \prod_{\{t:dN(t)=1\}} g(A_2(t) \mid \mathcal{F}_2(t))$$

$$\times \prod_t \alpha(t \mid \mathcal{F}(t))^{dN(t)} (1 - \alpha(t \mid \mathcal{F}(t)))^{1-dN(t)}.$$

Let $\mathcal{G}(SRA)$ be the set of such conditional distributions and let $T_{SRA}(P_{F_X,G})$ be the corresponding observed data tangent space of G. We have that

$$T_{SRA} = \overline{\left\{ \sum_{k=1}^{2} \int \{V(A_k(t), \mathcal{F}_k(t)) - E(V \mid \mathcal{F}_k(t))\} dN(t) : V \right\}}$$

$$\oplus \overline{\left\{ \int H(u, \mathcal{F}(u)) dM_\alpha(u) : H \right\}}.$$

In addition, for any function $V \in L_0^2(P_{F_X,G})$ the projection $\Pi(V \mid T_{SRA})$ is given by

$$\sum_{k=1}^{2} \int \{E(V(Y) \mid A_k(u), \mathcal{F}_k(u)) - E(V(Y) \mid \mathcal{F}_k(u))\} dN(u)$$

$$+ \int H_V(u, \mathcal{F}(u)) dM_\alpha(u),$$

where

$$H_V(u, \mathcal{F}(u)) = E(V \mid \mathcal{F}(u), dN(u) = 1) - E(V \mid \mathcal{F}(u), dN(u) = 0)$$

and $dM_\alpha(t) \equiv dN(t) - \alpha(t \mid \mathcal{F}(t))$.

This provides us with a formula for $IC_{SRA}(Y \mid Q(F_X, G), G, D) = \Pi(IC_0(D) \mid T_{SRA})$ for this type of model for the treatment mechanism, and thereby corresponding estimates.

6.2.1 Closed Form Formula for the Inverse of the Nonparametric Information Operator in Causal Inference Models.

It follows from Theorem 2.7 in Chapter 2 that to construct an efficient estimator of the parameters of a MSM we need to be able to invert the nonparametric information operator $\mathbf{I}_{F_X} = A_G^\top A_{F_X}$ where $A_{F_X}(\cdot) = E_{F_X}(\cdot \mid Y)$, $A_G^\top(\cdot) = E_G(\cdot \mid X)$ with $Y = (A, X_A)$ and $X = (X_a, a \in \mathcal{A})$.

Suppose that the Assumption of CAR-SRA Equivalence holds. Then Gill and Robins (2001) prove that the stronger assumption

$$\overline{X}_a \coprod \overline{X}_{a^*} \mid \overline{X}_a(u^*-) \text{ for all } a, a^* \tag{6.14}$$

6.2. Causal Inference with Marginal Structural Models

places no restriction on the law of the observed data Y even when sequential randomization and a MSM are imposed. Here we recall that u^* is the smallest time u for which $a(u) \neq a^*(u)$. Now, by Theorem 2.7, the efficient score for μ in the model $\mathcal{M}(CAR)$ for the observed data Y can be represented as $A_{F_X} \mathbf{I}_{F_X,G}^{-1} D_{opt}$ when, as we shall assume, there exists D_{opt} in the orthogonal complement $T_{nuis}^{F,\perp}(F_X)$ to the full data nuisance tangent space satisfying $\Pi\left[I^{-1}(D_{opt})\,|\,T_{nuis}^{F,\perp}(F_X)\right] = S_{eff}^{*F}(\cdot \mid F_X)$. Now, as discussed above, we can always assume that X satisfies (6.14) without changing our model for Y and thus without affecting the efficient score. Now, any $D = d(X)$ in the range of $\mathbf{I}$ can clearly be written as $\int b(a, X_a)\,d\mu(a)$ for some $b(a, X_a)$, where $\mu(\cdot)$ is a carrying measure. With $X_a = \overline{X}_a(p+1) = (X_a(1), ..., X_a(p+1))$ and $a = (a(1), ..., a(p))$, Robins (1999) proved by explicit calculation that under assumption (6.14 and CAR

$$\mathbf{I}_{F_X,G}^{-1}\left[\int b(a, X_a)\,d\mu(a)\right] =$$

$$\int d\mu(\overline{a})\,\{g[\overline{a}(p)\mid X_a]\}^{-1} E_{F_X}\left[b(a, X_a)\mid \overline{X}_a(p+1)\right]$$

$$- \sum_{m=2}^{p+1} \frac{E_{F_X}\left[b(a, X_a)\mid \overline{X}_a(m-1)\right]}{g[\overline{a}(m-1)\mid X_a]}\,\{1 - g[a(m-1)\mid \overline{a}(m-2), X_a]\}.$$

Robins (1999) uses this explicit formula for the inverse of the nonparametric information operator to calculate the efficient score for a MSM with a time-independent treatment. We now give an alternative representation of the latter formula for $\mathbf{I}_{F_X,G}^{-1}$ that allows immediate generalization to continuous time action mechanisms. Let $\alpha(t\mid \overline{a}(t-), X_a) = pr\left(A(t) \neq \overline{A}(t-)\mid \overline{A}(t-) = \overline{a}(t-), X_a\right)$ which we referred to as $\alpha(t\mid \mathcal{F}(t))$ in Theorem 6.1. Then, under CAR and equation (6.14,

$$\mathbf{I}_{F_X,G}^{-1}\left[\int b(a, X_a)\,d\mu(a)\right]$$

$$= \int d\mu(\overline{a})\,\left\{\{g[\overline{a}(p)\mid X_a]\}^{-1} E_{F_X}\left[b(a, X_a)\mid \overline{X}_a(p+1)\right]\right\}$$

$$- \sum_{t=1}^{p} \alpha(t\mid \overline{a}(t-), X_a)\, E_{F_X}\left[b(a, X_a)\mid \overline{X}_a(t)\right] \left(\prod_{u=1}^{t}\{1 - \alpha(u\mid \overline{a}(u-), X_a)\}\right)^{-1}$$

$$+ \sum_{\{t;a(t)\neq a(t-)\}} g(a(t)\mid \overline{a}(t-), a(t) \neq a(t-), X_a)\, E_{F_X}\left[b(a, X_a)\mid \overline{X}_a(t)\right] \times$$

$$\left.\left(\prod_{u=1}^{t}\{1 - \alpha(u\mid \overline{a}(u-), X_a)\}\right)^{-1}\right\}$$

To apply this formula to a treatment process with a continuous intensity, we redefine $\sum_{t=1}^{p}$ as the integral between 1 and $p+1$ w.r.t. the Lebesgue measure, $\alpha\left(t|\overline{a}\left(t-\right),X_a\right) = \lim_{dt \to 0} pr\left(A\left(t+dt\right) \neq A\left(t-\right) | \overline{A}\left(t-\right) = \overline{a}\left(t-\right), X_a\right)/dt$ and condition on $\overline{X}_a\left(t-\right)$ rather than $\overline{X}_a\left(t\right)$.

6.3 Double Robustness in Point Treatment MSM

Let A be a treatment variable that is time-independent and $\mathcal{A}$ its set of possible outcomes. Let $(Z_a : a \in \mathcal{A})$ be a vector-random variable whose components are the treatment-specific outcomes. Suppose now that we observe on each subject a treatment variable A, an outcome $Z = Z_A$, and baseline covariates W,

$$Y = (W, A, Z = Z_A),$$

where W are the observed baseline covariates. The full data structure is $X = ((Z_a : a), W)$, with the collection of treatment-specific outcomes Z_a and the baseline covariates W, while the observed data structure Y is a simple function of X and the treatment (i.e., censoring) variable A. Consider as the full data structure model a marginal structural generalized linear regression model

$$Z_a = m(a, V \mid \beta) + \epsilon_a, \text{ where } E(\epsilon_a \mid V) = 0. \tag{6.15}$$

$V \subset W$ is a baseline covariate included in W and $m(a, V \mid \beta)$ is a specified function of a, V, β. For example, we could consider a linear regression model

$$Z_a = \beta_0 + \beta_1 a + \beta_2 V + \epsilon_a.$$

The randomization assumption on the treatment mechanism $g(a \mid X)$ is stated as

$$g(a \mid X) \equiv P(A = a \mid X) = P(A = a \mid W) \equiv g(a \mid W).$$

The observed data likelihood for g is given by $\prod_{i=1}^{n} g(A_i \mid W_i)$, which can be modeled with a logistic regression or multinomial logistic regression model. Let $\mathcal{G}$ be the model for g.

The set of full data estimating functions is given by

$$\left\{ D_h(X \mid \beta) = \sum_{a \in \mathcal{A}} h(a, V) \epsilon_a(\beta) : h \right\}.$$

Define

$$IC_0(Y \mid G, D_h) = \frac{h(A, V)\epsilon(\beta)}{g(A \mid X)},$$

where $\epsilon(\beta) = \epsilon_A(\beta)$. By the randomization assumption, we have that $g(A \mid X)$ is only a function of A, W and thus that $D_h \to IC_0(Y \mid G, D_h)$ indeed maps a full data estimating function into an observed data estimating function. If $\max_{a \in \mathcal{A}} h(a, V)/g(a \mid W) < \infty$ F_W-a.e., then

$$E(IC_0(Y \mid G, D_h) \mid X) = \sum_{a \in \mathcal{A}} h(a, V)\epsilon_a(\beta) = D_h(X) \ F_X\text{-a.e.}$$

Given an estimate of g, one can estimate β by solving an IPTW estimating function:

$$0 = \frac{1}{n}\sum_{i=1}^{n} \frac{h(A_i, V_i)\epsilon_i(\beta)}{g_n(A_i \mid X_i)}.$$

Consider a restricted treatment model $\mathcal{G}^* = \{g \in \mathcal{G} : g(a \mid W) = g(a \mid V)\}$ assuming randomization w.r.t. V. Under this restricted model, we have that $m(A, V \mid \beta) = E(Z \mid A, V)$ is a regression of Z onto A, V. Thus, Lemma 2.1 teaches us that, if W and Z are conditionally independent, given V, A, then the optimal estimating function for β is given by

$$\frac{\frac{d}{d\beta}m(A, V \mid \beta)}{E(\epsilon(\beta)^2 \mid A, V)}\epsilon(\beta). \tag{6.16}$$

For any g in our posed model $\mathcal{G}$ for the treatment mechanism, let $g^* = g^*(g)$, an element in $\mathcal{G}^*$ in some sense close to g (e.g., one estimates g^* with maximum likelihood estimation for $\mathcal{G}$ but now restricted to model $\mathcal{G}^*$). If we set

$$h^*_{opt}(A, V) = g^*(\bar{A} \mid X)\frac{\frac{d}{d\beta}m(A, V \mid \beta)}{E(\epsilon(\beta)^2 \mid A, V)},$$

then $IC_0(Y \mid G, D_{h^*_{opt}})$ reduces to (6.16) if the true treatment mechanism happens to be an element of $\mathcal{G}^*$. Let h_n be an estimator of this locally optimal direction h^*_{opt}. Then, the IPTW estimator β_n is CAN if the treatment mechanism $g(\bar{A} \mid X)$ is modeled correctly. This estimator has the attractive property that it is easy to compute and it improves on the naive regression estimator that works under the assumption that there is no confounding beyond the variables that one has adjusted for in the regression.

As in Section 6.1, the set of all observed data estimating functions can be represented as $\{IC(Y \mid Q, G, D_h) = IC_0(Y \mid G, D_h) - IC_{RA}(Y \mid Q, G) : h\}$, where $IC_{RA}(\cdot \mid Q(F_X, G), G) = \Pi(IC_0(Y \mid G, D_h) \mid T_{RA})$ in $L^2_0(P_{F_X,G})$ and T_{RA} is the tangent space under the randomization assumption on $g(A \mid X)$. We have

$$T_{RA} = \overline{\{h(A, W) - E(h(A, W) \mid W) : h\}}.$$

Thus, the projection of a function $U \in L^2_0(P_{F_X,G})$ of the observed data Y onto T_{RA} is given by

$$\Pi(U \mid T_{RA}) = E(U \mid A, W) - E(U \mid W).$$

328   6. Unified Approach for Causal Inference and Censored Data

To calculate the projection of IC_0 onto T_{RA}, we note that

$$E(h(A,V)\epsilon(\beta)/g(A\mid X)\mid A,W) = h(A,V)/g(A\mid X)E(\epsilon(\beta)\mid A,W)$$
$$E(h(A,V)\epsilon(\beta)/g(A\mid X)\mid W) = \sum_a h(a,V)E(\epsilon(\beta)\mid A=a,W).$$

Thus, the set of all observed data estimating functions orthogonal to T_{RA} indexed by h is given by

$$IC(Y\mid Q,g,D_h(\cdot\mid\beta)) = \frac{h(A,V)\epsilon_A(\beta)}{g(\bar{A}\mid X)} - \frac{h(A,V)}{g(A\mid X)}E(\epsilon(\beta)\mid A,W)$$
$$+ \sum_a h(a,V)E(\epsilon(\beta)\mid A=a,W).$$

Here $Q(F_X)(A,W) \equiv E(\epsilon(\beta)\mid A,W)$ and $g(A\mid X)$ are the nuisance parameters of this estimating function for β. We have the following double robustness result for this class of estimating functions.

Lemma 6.2 *If $h(A,V)/g^1(A\mid W)$ is a uniformly bounded random variable, then*

$$E_{F_X,G}IC(Y\mid Q(F_X),g^1,D_h(\cdot\mid\beta)) = 0.$$

If $\max_{a\in\mathcal{A}} h(a,V)/g(a\mid W) < \infty$ F_W-a.e., then

$$E_{F_X,G}IC(Y\mid Q^1,g,D_h(\cdot\mid\beta)) = 0 \text{ for all uniformly bounded } Q^1.$$

As the estimator of β, we propose the solution β_n of the estimating equation

$$0 = \sum_{i=1}^n IC(Y_i\mid Q_n,g_n,D_{h_n}(\cdot\mid\beta)),$$

where Q_n is an estimator of the regression $E(\epsilon(\beta_n^0)\mid A,W)$ of $\epsilon(\beta_n^0)$ on A,W according to some regression model $\mathcal{Q}$, and g_n, h_n are defined above as the estimator of the treatment mechanism and a locally optimal direction, respectively. Due to the double protection of the estimating equation, under the regularity conditions of Theorem 2.5, this estimator β_n will be CAN if either $\mathcal{G}$ or the regression model $\mathcal{Q}$ are correctly specified.

It is of interest to compare this doubly robust estimator with an alternative method studied in Neugebauer, van der Laan (2002), which builds on the approach followed by most epidemiologists and biostatisticians involving estimation of $E(Y\mid A,W)$ by carrying out a linear regression adjusting for all confounders W. Firstly, we note that the regression method $E(Y\mid A,W)$ is answering a question driven by the actual confounders coming up in the data set, instead of answering a preposed question. The relationship of this to the concepts of "treatment interaction" and 'effect modification' in epidemiology is discussed by Robins, Hernán, and Brumback (2000). To describe the estimator studied in Neugebauer, van der Laan (2002), we note that $E(Y_a\mid V) = E(E(Y\mid A=a,W)\mid V)$. Define

$Y_a(W) \equiv E(Y \mid A = a, W)$. Let $\hat{E}(Y \mid A, W)$ be an estimate of this regression according to some regression model, and let $\hat{Y}_a(W) = \hat{E}(Y \mid A = a, W)$ be the evaluation of this regression at $A = a$ and W. Since $E(Y_a(W) \mid V) = m(a, V \mid \beta)$, one can now regres for each a, $\hat{Y}_a(W)$ on V, and thereby obtain an estimate of β. The latter estimation problem is a standard repeated measures regression model, where each subject contributes multiple outcomes $Y_a(W)$, $a \in \mathcal{A}$, and the regression of outcome $Y_a(W)$ on V is given by $m(a, V \mid \beta)$. Lemma 2.1 provides us with the class of estimating functions and the optimal estimating function. Let $\mathcal{A}$ be discrete with m possible values. The class of estimating functions is given by $h(V)\vec{\epsilon}(\beta)$, where $h(V)$ is a $k \times m$-matrix function, and $\vec{\epsilon}(\beta) = (\epsilon_a(\beta) : a \in \mathcal{A})$. A simple estimator β_n^* of β is thus given by fitting a regression of an outcome Z on covariates A, V, assuming the regression model $E(Z \mid A, V) = m(A, V \mid \beta)$, with the pooled sample in which each subject contributes m lines of data $(\hat{Y}_a(W), V, A = a)$, $a \in \mathcal{A}$.

Note that estimation of $Q(F_X)$ is equivalent with estimating the regression $E(Y \mid A, W)$. Suppose that we use the same model for $E(Y \mid A, W)$ as the one used in the estimator β_n^* described in the previous paragraph. If the model for $E(Y \mid A, W)$ is wrong, then β_n^* is inconsistent, while the doubly robust estimator β_n will still be consistent if the treatment mechanism $g(A \mid W)$ is correctly estimated. On the other hand, if $E(Y \mid A, W)$ is correctly modeled, then both estimators β_n and β_n^* are consistent. This shows that β_n is truly a more nonparametric estimator than the estimator β_n^*. Notice that, by Lemma 6.2, if $E(Y \mid A, W)$ is consistently estimated, then β_n is even consistent if $g(A = a \mid W) = 0$ for some treatment values a, while the IPTW estimator is now inconsistent. The practical impact of this result is highlighted in a forthcoming paper by Neugebauer and van der Laan (2002). We proved this robustness against the identifiability condition on g in Section 1.6, Theorems 1.6 and 1.7.

6.4 Marginal Structural Model with Right-Censoring

For each possible treatment regime $a_1 = (a_1(t) : t = 1, \ldots, p)$ for an random treatment regime A_1, we define a counterfactual random variable $X_{a_1} = (X_{a_1}(t) : t)$, where $X_{a_1}(t) = (Y_{a_1}(t), L_{a_1}(t))$, Y_{a_1} is a time-dependent outcome process, and L_{a_1} is a time-dependent covariate process. Let $\mathcal{A}_1$ be the support of A_1. It is assumed that $X_{a_1}(t)$ only depends on a_1 through $(a_1(s) : s < t)$. Let time be discrete at $j = 1, \ldots, p+1$. The full data structure is $X = (X_{a_1} : a_1)$.

Suppose now that the data can be right censored by C. We define the observed data by

$$Y = (C, \bar{X}_{A_1}(C), \bar{A}_1(C)).$$

In other words, we observe the treatment-specific process X_{A_1} corresponding with the treatment that the subject actually received up until the follow-up time C. Let $A_2(t) = I(C \leq t)$ be a process that jumps at the censoring time C.

Let $a_2 = \bar{a}_2$ be a potential sample path for A_2; that is, a_2 is a function of time whose initial value equals 0 and jumps to 1 at some time $j = 1, ..., p$ or at ∞ (corresponding to no censoring) and remains at 1 after jumping. Let $c(a_2)$ be the time that a_2 jumps to 1 so $C = c(A_2)$. Define $X_{a_1, a_2}(t) = X_{a_1}(\min\{t, c(a_2)\})$ so $X_{a_1}(t)$ is $X_{a_1, a_2}(t)$ for a_2 that jumps at ∞. Finally, redefine $X = (X_{a_1, a_2} : a_1, a_2)$

The observed data can be written as $Y = (A, X_A)$, where $A(t) = (A_1(\min(C, t)), A_2(t))$ and $X_A(t) = X_{A_1}(\min(C, t))$, $A = (A(1), ..., A(p))$, and $X_A = (X_A(1), ..., X_A(p+1))$. This means that we can apply the general methodology described in Section 6.1. To describe the likelihood of the data (so that one can apply, in particular, the general double robust estimation methodology of Section 1.6), we use the following ordering of the data

$$(X(1), A(1), ..., X_{\bar{A}(p-1)}(p), A(p), X_{\bar{A}(p)}(p+1)),$$

where $A(j) = (A_1(\min(j, C)), A_2(j))$, $j = 1, ..., p$.

Let us first assume a concrete marginal structural model. For that purpose, let $Y_{a_1}(t) = I(T_{a_1} \leq t)$, where T_{a_1} is a treatment-specific survival time. If $X_{a_1} = \bar{X}_{a_1}(T_{a_1})$, then we define $C = \infty$ if $C \geq T = T_{\bar{A}_1}$ so that C is always observed. Suppose that one is interested in estimation of the causal effect of the treatment regime a_1 on the survival time, adjusted for some baseline covariates V. In that case, one might want to assume a model for the intensity of the counting process $Y_{a_1}(t)$ w.r.t. to history $\bar{Y}_{a_1}(t), V$,

$$E(dY_{a_1}(t) \mid \bar{Y}_{a_1}(t), V) = I(T_{a_1} \geq t)\lambda_{a_1}(t \mid V, \beta), \qquad (6.17)$$

where

$$\lambda_{a_1}(t \mid V, \beta) \equiv P(Y_{a_1}(t) = 1 \mid Y_{a_1}(t-1) = 0, V)$$

denotes the treatment specific hazard of failing at time t. Since we assumed that time is discrete, a natural model is the logistic regression model,

$$P(Y_{a_1}(j) = 1 \mid Y_{a_1}(j-1) = 0, V) = m(j, \bar{a}_1(j-1), V \mid \beta)$$
$$\equiv \frac{1}{1 + \exp(\beta_0 + \beta_1 j + \beta_2 \text{sum}(\bar{a}_1(j-1)) + \beta_3 V)},$$

where $\text{sum}(\bar{a}_1(j-1))$ is some known summary measure of the treatment past $\bar{a}_1(j-1)$. The goal is now to estimate the causal parameter β.

The orthogonal complement of the nuisance tangent space in the full data model assuming (6.17) for a given a_1 is given by

$$\left\{ \sum_{j=1}^{T_{a_1}} h(j, V) dM_{a_1, \beta}(j) : h \right\},$$

where
$$dM_{a_1,\beta}(j) = I(T_{a_1} = j) - I(T_{a_1} \geq j)\lambda_{a_1}(j \mid V, \beta).$$
Thus
$$T_{nuis}^{F,\perp}(F_X) \supset \overline{\left\{ D_h(X \mid \beta) \equiv \sum_{a_1 \in \mathcal{A}_1} \sum_{j=1}^{T_{a_1}} h(j, \bar{a}_1(j), V) dM_{a_1,\beta}(j) : h \right\}},$$

and, under regularity conditions, one will have equality. This implies the class of full data structure estimating functions.

The sequential randomization assumption states that for all $j \in \{1, \ldots, p\}$

$$g(A(j) \mid \bar{A}(j-1), X) = g(A(j) \mid \bar{A}(j-1), \bar{X}_A(j)). \tag{6.18}$$

At an $A = (A_1, A_2)$ with $A_2(t) = I(C \leq t)$, we have

$$g(\bar{A} \mid X) = \prod_{j=1}^{C} g(A(j) \mid \bar{A}(j-1), X) \tag{6.19}$$

$$= \prod_{j=1}^{C} g_1(A_1(j) \mid A_2(j), \bar{A}(j-1), \bar{X}_A(j)) \prod_{j=1}^{C} g_2(A_2(j) \mid \bar{A}(j-1), \bar{X}_A(j)).$$

Let $\mathcal{F}_1(j) = (A_2(j), \bar{A}(j-1), \bar{X}_A(j))$ and $\mathcal{F}_2(j) = (\bar{A}(j-1), \bar{X}_A(j))$ so that

$$g(A(j) \mid \bar{A}(j-1), X) = g_1(A_1(j) \mid \mathcal{F}_1(j)) g_2(A_2(j) \mid \mathcal{F}_2(j)).$$

The first product in (6.19) represents the treatment mechanism, while the second product represents the censoring mechanism. Note that the products are over j from 1 till the minimum of C and the time $T-1$ till (say) death or another time at which data collection on a subjects stops. After $\min(C, T-1)$, both $A_2(j)$ and $A_1(j)$ become degenerate so that the corresponding factors in (6.19) equal 1 and do thus not contribute to the product. By the same argument, the summations defining projections onto the tangent space T_{SRA} as provided below only run till $\min(C, T-1)$ as well.

We will need to assume models for both mechanisms. Let g_{1,γ_1} be a parametrization of the treatment mechanism. If treatment can only change value at a subset $\mathcal{S}$ of $\{1, \ldots, p\}$, then the model should respect this constraint on the treatment mechanism: that is, $g_1(A_1(j) \mid \mathcal{F}_1(j)) = 0$ for $j \notin \mathcal{S}$.

In addition, we assume a model for the intensity $\alpha_{\gamma_2}(j \mid \mathcal{F}_2(j)) = E(dA_2(j) \mid \mathcal{F}_2(j)) = I(C \geq j) E(dA_2(j) \mid \mathcal{F}_2(j), C \geq j)$. If $X_{a_1} = \bar{X}(T_{a_1})$, then we have $E(dA_2(j) \mid \mathcal{F}_2(j)) = I(C \geq j, T \geq j+1) E(dA_2(j) \mid \mathcal{F}_2(j), C \geq j, T \geq j+1)$. For example, we could assume a logistic regression model

$$\alpha_{\gamma_2}(j \mid \mathcal{F}_2(j)) = \frac{1}{1 + \exp(m(j, W(j) \mid \gamma_2))}, \tag{6.20}$$

where $W(j)$ are functions of the observed past $\mathcal{F}_2(j)$. By factorization of the likelihood $P_{F_X, G}(dy)$ in F_X and G parts, the maximum likelihood of $\gamma = (\gamma_1, \gamma_2)$ is defined by

$$\gamma_n = \max_\gamma{}^{-1} \prod_{i=1}^{n} \prod_{j=1}^{\min(C_i, T_i-1)} g_{1,\gamma_1}(A_{1i}(j) \mid \mathcal{F}_{1,i}(j)) g_{2,\gamma_2}(A_{2i}(j) \mid \mathcal{F}_{2,i}(j)).$$

If the models for g_1 and g_2 have no common parameters, then

$$\gamma_{1n} = \max_{\gamma_1}{}^{-1} \prod_{i=1}^{n} \prod_{j=1}^{\min(C_i, T_i-1)} g_{1,\gamma_1}(A_{1i}(j) \mid \mathcal{F}_{1,i}(j))$$

and

$$\gamma_{2n} = \max_{\gamma_2}{}^{-1} \prod_{i=1}^{n} \prod_{j=1}^{\min(C_i, T_i-1)} \alpha_{\gamma_2}(j \mid \mathcal{F}_{2i}(j))^{dA_2(j)} \{1 - \alpha_{\gamma_2}(j \mid \mathcal{F}_{2i}(j))\}^{1-dA_2(j)}.$$

If we assume the logistic regression model (6.20), then γ_{2n} can be obtained by applying the S-plus function GLM() with logit link to the pooled sample $(A_{ki}(j), j, W_i(j))$, $i = 1, \ldots, n$, $j = 1, \ldots, \min(C_i, T_i-1)$, treating this data as i.i.d. observations of a Bernoulli random variable A_k with covariates time t and W. We will denote the posed models for g_1 and g_2 with $\mathcal{G}_1$ and $\mathcal{G}_2$, respectively.

We define the following inverse weighted mapping from the full data to the observed data estimating functions:

$$IC_0(Y \mid G, D_h) \equiv \left\{ \sum_{j=1}^{T} h(j, \bar{A}_1(j), V) dM_{\bar{A}_1, \beta}(j) \right\} \frac{I(C \geq T)}{g(\bar{A}_1, \bar{A}_2(T-1) = 0 \mid X)}. \tag{6.21}$$

Under the assumption that $\{a_1(j) : P(A_1(j) = a_1(j) \mid \bar{A}_2(j) = 0, \bar{A}_1(j-1) = \bar{a}_1(j-1), \bar{X}_{A_1}(j)) > 0\}$ is non-random (i.e., this support does not depend on $\bar{X}_{A_1}(j)$) and, $\{a_2(j) : P(A_2(j) = a_2(j) \mid \bar{A}_2(j-1) = 0, \bar{A}_1(j-1) = \bar{a}_1(j-1), \bar{X}_{A_1}(j)) > 0\}$ is non-random, then for a given $D_h(X) = \sum_{a_1 \in \mathcal{A}_1} D_{h_{a_1}}(X_{a_1})$, we have $E(IC_0(Y \mid G, D_h) \mid X) = D_h(X)$ F_X-a.e. It is often possible to weaken this assumption, as discussed in the previous sections. Alternatively, we could use inverse weighting within the summation:

$$IC_0(Y \mid G, D_h)(Y) \equiv \sum_{j=1}^{T} h(j, \bar{A}_1(j), V) dM_{\bar{A}_1, \beta}(j) \frac{I(C \geq j)}{g(\bar{A}_1(j), \bar{A}_2(j-1) = 0 \mid X)}. \tag{6.22}$$

To orthogonalize IC_0, we must find the projection of $IC_0(Y)$ onto $T_{SRA} = T_{CAR}$ by applying Theorem 1.2. Firstly, by factorization of $g(\bar{A} \mid X)$ into a treatment mechanism and censoring mechanism, we have

$$T_{SRA}(P_{F_X, G}) = T_{SRA,1}(P_{F_X, G}) \oplus T_{SRA,2}(P_{F_X, G}),$$

6.4. Marginal Structural Model with Right-Censoring

where

$$T_{SRA,1} = \overline{\left\{ \sum_j V(A_1(j), \mathcal{F}_1(j)) - E(V \mid \mathcal{F}_1(j)) : V \right\}}$$

and

$$T_{SRA,2} = \overline{\left\{ \sum_j V(A_2(j), \mathcal{F}_2(j)) - E(V \mid \mathcal{F}_2(j)) : V \right\}}$$

$$= \overline{\left\{ \sum_j \{V(1, \mathcal{F}_2(j)) - V(0, \mathcal{F}_2(j))\} dM_2(j) : V \right\}}$$

$$= \overline{\left\{ \sum_j H(j, \mathcal{F}_2(j)) dM_2(j) : H \right\}}.$$

Here

$$dM_2(j) = dA_2(j) - E(dA_2(j) \mid \mathcal{F}_2(j)) = dA_2(j) - \alpha_2(j \mid \mathcal{F}_2(j)).$$

The projection of any function $V(Y) \in L^2(P_{F_X,G})$ onto $T_{SRA,1}(P_{F_X,G})$ is given by:

$$\Pi(V \mid T_{SRA,1}) = \sum_{j=1}^{C} E(V \mid A_1(j), \mathcal{F}_1(j)) - E(V \mid \mathcal{F}_1(j)).$$

The projection of any function $V(Y) \in L^2(P_{F_X,G})$ onto $T_{SRA,2}$ is given by

$$\sum_{j=1}^{C} \{E(V \mid dA_2(j) = 1, \mathcal{F}_2(j)) - E(V \mid dA_2(j) = 0, \mathcal{F}_2(j))\} dM_2(j).$$

Substitution of $V = IC_0(Y \mid G, D_h)$ given by (6.21) yields

$$\Pi(IC_0 \mid T_{SRA}) = \sum_{j=1}^{C} E(IC_0(Y) \mid A_1(j), \mathcal{F}_1(j))$$

$$- \sum_{j=1}^{C} \sum_{a_1(j)} E(IC_0(Y) \mid a_1(j), \mathcal{F}_1(j)) g_1(a_1(j) \mid \mathcal{F}_1(j))$$

$$- \sum_{j=1}^{C} E(IC_0(Y) \mid C > j, \mathcal{F}_2(j)) dM_2(j)$$

$$\equiv IC_{SRA}(Y \mid Q, G),$$

where we define $Q_1(j, \mathcal{F}_1(j)) = E(IC_0(Y) \mid A_1(j), \mathcal{F}_1(j))$, $Q_2(j, \mathcal{F}_2(j)) = E(IC_0(Y) \mid C > j, \mathcal{F}_2(j))$ and let $Q = (Q_1, Q_2)$ denote both of these parameters. We can now define the desired mapping from full data estimating functions to observed data estimating functions for β indexed by nuisance parameters Q and G:

$$IC(Y \mid Q, G, D_h) = IC_0(Y \mid G, D_h(\cdot \mid \beta)) - IC_{SRA}(Y \mid Q, G).$$

It is of interest to note that $IC(Y \mid Q, G, D_h)$ is the same for IC_0 that uses within summation inverse weighting as IC_0 that uses inverse weighting outside the summation.

Given estimators Q_{1n}, Q_{2n}, G_n and a possibly data-dependent index h_n, we estimate β by solving the estimating equation

$$0 = \frac{1}{n} \sum_{i=1}^{n} IC(Y_i \mid Q_n, G_n, D_{h_n}(\cdot \mid \beta)).$$

Estimation of Q_{kn} can be carried out by regressing $IC_0(Y \mid G_n, D_{h_n}(\cdot \mid \beta_n^0))$ onto time j and covariates extracted from the past $\mathcal{F}_k(j)$, $k = 1, 2$, as discussed in section 6.1. To obtain a doubly robust estimator of μ, one can estimate the F_X and G part of the likelihood of the observed data with maximum likelihood estimation and evaluate the conditional expectations under the estimated distribution P_{F_n, G_n} of the data with Monte Carlo simulation. The latter method is described in detail in Section 1.6.

A sensible choice for $h(j, \bar{A}_1(j), V)$ in (6.22) is given by:

$$h(j, \bar{A}_1(j), V) = g^*(\bar{A}_1(j), \bar{A}_2(j-1) \mid V) \frac{d/d\beta \lambda_{A_1}(j \mid V, \beta)}{\lambda_{A_1}(j \mid V, \beta)(1 - \lambda_{A_1}(j \mid V, \beta))},$$

where g^* is the action mechanism assuming, possibly contrary to the fact, sequential randomization of $A_1(j), A_2(j)$ w.r.t. the treatment past, censoring past, and V. This g^* is estimated by fitting the same models as assumed for the true action mechanism, but where we now exclude all variables of the past beyond $\bar{A}(j)$ and V. Implementation of the corresponding inverse probability of action weighted estimator corresponds with fitting the logistic regression model

$$E(Y(j) \mid \bar{Y}(j-1), \bar{A}_1(j-1), V) = I(Y(j-1) = 0) m(j, \bar{A}_1(j-1), V),$$

with standard logistic regression software, applying it to a pooled sample in which each subject contributes multiple observations, where one assigns to each subject's j-specific observation a weight

$$W(j) = I(C \geq j) \frac{g^*(\bar{A}_1(j), \bar{A}_2(j-1) \mid V)}{g(\bar{A}_1(j), \bar{A}_2(j-1) \mid X)}.$$

6.4.1 Doubly robust estimators in marginal structural models with right-censoring

We have that $Q(F_X, G)$ is a simple function of $E_{P_{F_X, G}}(IC_0(Y) \mid \mathcal{F}(t))$ for particular observable histories $\mathcal{F}(t)$. In Section 1.6, we proposed to estimate the data generating distribution $P_{F_X, G}$ of the observed data with

6.4. Marginal Structural Model with Right-Censoring

maximum likelihood estimation according to models $\mathcal{G}$ and $\mathcal{M}^{F,w}$, separately estimating the G and F_X part of this likelihood, and subsequently, evaluate the conditional expectation under this maximum likelihood estimator P_{F_n,G_n} with Monte-Carlo simulation. In this section, we provide non-likelihood methods only requiring estimation of regressions. The next theorems provide a representation of $E(IC_0(Y) \mid \mathcal{F}(t))$ in terms of F_X parameters and G, where each F_X parameter is simply a regression of an observed random variable that does not depend on G or G_n on an observed past. Estimation each of these regressions according to user-supplied regression models plus our usual estimator G_n of G yields an estimator Q_n of $Q(F_X, G)$. Since each regression is separately modeled, the resulting estimator Q_n of $Q(F_X, G)$ cannot necessarily be represented as $Q(F_n, G_n)$ for some full data structure distribution F_n, since the functional form of the user-supplied time t-specific regression models might be incompatible with any joint distribution. Thus this approach does not correspond with posing a proper working model for F_X. Nonetheless, this estimator Q_n estimates the F_X and G components in the $Q(F_X, G)$ separately and therefore exploits the protection property $E_{F_X,G} IC(Y \mid Q(F_X, G_1), G_1, D)) = 0$ for all $G_1 \in \mathcal{G}(CAR)$. Thus from a practical perspective, if one does a good job in modeling the regressions defining the F_X-parameters, then the estimator μ_n will be robust against misspecification of the model for G in the sense that the bias of the estimator of μ will be small even if the user-supplied regression models are incompatible. We refer to Robins (2000) and Robins and Rotnitzky (2001) for a general discussion on such generalized doubly robust estimators. The formulas presented in this subsection generalize those in Robins (2000) and Tchetgen, and Robins (2002).

We have seen that most full data structure models allow either an IPAW mapping, IC_0, that involves weighting by the inverse of the probability of the complete action regime, as in (6.21), or that it involves weighting by the inverse of the probability of the action regime up until time t at each time point t, as in (6.22). The next theorem covers the first case.

Theorem 6.2 *For each possible treatment regime $a_1 = (a_1(t) : t)$, we define a counterfactual random variable $X_{a_1} = (X_{a_1}(t) : t)$, where $X_{a_1}(t) = (R_{a_1}(t) = I(T_{a_1} \leq t), L_{a_1}(t))$ and T_{a_1} is a treatment-specific stopping time (e.g., death) for this process X_{a_1}. Thus $X_{a_1}(t) = X_{a_1}(\min(t, T_{a_1}))$. It is assumed that $X_{a_1}(t)$ only depends on a_1 through $(a_1(s) : s < t)$. The treatment-specific full data structure is defined by $\bar{X}_{a_1}(T_{a_1})$. The full data structure is $X = (X_{a_1} : a_1)$. Let C be a right-censoring time and let $A_2(t) = I(C \leq t)$. Define $A(t) = (A_1(\min(C, t)), A_2(t))$. We define the observed data by:*

$$Y = (\bar{A}(T), \bar{X}_{A_1}(\min(T, C))).$$

In other words, we observe the treatment-specific process X_{A_1} corresponding with the treatment that the subject actually received up until the minimum of the follow-up time C and T_{A_1}. Assume that all processes are discrete in the sense that they are discrete-valued and only change at time points labeled by $1,\ldots,p$. Assume that the conditional density $g(\bar{A} \mid X)$ of $\bar{A}$, given X, satisfies the sequential randomization assumption

$$g(\bar{A} \mid X) = \prod_{j=1}^{p} g(A(j) \mid \bar{A}(j-1), \bar{X}_A(j)).$$

Assume that $g(\bar{a} \mid X) > 0$ F_X-a.e. for all $\bar{a}$ in the support of the marginal distribution of $\bar{A}$.

Let $\mathcal{F}(t) = (\bar{A}_2(t-1), \bar{A}_1(\min(t,C,T)), \bar{X}_{A_1}(\min(t,C)))$. For notational simplicity, let $Z(t) \equiv (\bar{A}_1(\min(t,T)), \bar{X}_{A_1}(t))$ so that $\mathcal{F}(t) = (\bar{A}_2(t-1), \bar{Z}(\min(t,C)))$.

For any function $D(\bar{A}_1, \bar{X}_{A_1}, T) = D_1(\bar{A}_1(T), \bar{X}_{A_1}(T))$ (for some function D_1), consider

$$IC_0(Y \mid G, D) = \frac{I(\bar{A}_2(T-1) = 0)}{g(\bar{A}_1(T), \bar{A}_2(T-1) \mid X)} D(\bar{A}_1, \bar{X}_{A_1}, T).$$

(Note that $C = T$, still implies that we observe $\bar{X}_{A_1}(T)$.) We have (here, $dR(u) = I(T=u)$)

$$E(IC_0(Y) \mid \mathcal{F}(t)) = \frac{I(\bar{A}_2(T-1) = 0)}{g(\bar{A}_1(T), \bar{A}_2(T-1) \mid X)} I(T \leq t) D(\bar{A}_1, \bar{X}_{A_1}, T)$$
$$+ \int_{\{u:u>t\}} E\left(\frac{I(\bar{A}_2(u-1) = 0)}{g(\bar{A}_1(u), \bar{A}_2(u-1) \mid X)} D(\bar{A}_1, \bar{X}_{A_1}, u) dR(u) \mid \mathcal{F}(t) \right).$$

Define

$$g(u,t) \equiv E\left(\frac{I(\bar{A}_2(u-1) = 0)}{g(\bar{A}_1(u), \bar{A}_2(u-1) \mid X)} D(\bar{A}_1, \bar{X}_{A_1}, u) dR(u) \mid \mathcal{F}(t) \right).$$

We have for $u > t$

$$g(u, t = j) = \frac{I(\bar{A}_2(j-1) = 0)}{g(\bar{A}_1(j), \bar{A}_2(j-1) \mid X)} (\phi_j \circ \ldots \circ \phi_{u-1}) \{D(\bar{A}_1, \bar{X}_{A_1}, u) dR(u)\},$$

where for any random variable B

$$\phi_j(B) \equiv E\left(\sum_{a_1(j+1)} B I(A_1(j+1) = a_1(j+1)) \mid \bar{A}_2(j) = 0, \bar{A}_1(j), \bar{X}_{A_1}(j) \right).$$

The proof of the theorem is a direct consequence of the following lemma.

Lemma 6.3 *Consider the setting and definitions of Theorem 3.1. Let $u \in \{1,\ldots,p\}$ be given. If $E(B \mid \mathcal{F}(u)) = \frac{I(\bar{A}_2(u-1)=0)}{g(\bar{A}_1(u), \bar{A}_2(u-1)\mid X)} D_u(\bar{Z}(u))$ for some function D_u of $\bar{Z}(u)$, then $E(B \mid \mathcal{F}(u-1)) =$*

6.4. Marginal Structural Model with Right-Censoring

$\frac{I(\bar{A}_2(u-2)=0)}{g(\bar{A}_1(u-1),\bar{A}_2(u-2)|X)}D_{u-1}(\bar{Z}(u-1))$, where $D_{u-1}(\bar{Z}(u-1))$ is given by

$$E\left(\sum_{a_1(u)} D_u(\bar{Z}(u))I(A_1(u)=a_1(u)) \mid \bar{A}_2(u-1)=0, \bar{Z}(u-1)\right).$$

Thus, iteration of this result shows that for any $j \in \{1, \ldots, u-1\}$

$$E(B \mid \mathcal{F}(j)) = \frac{I(\bar{A}_2(j-1)=0)}{g(\bar{A}_1(j),\bar{A}_2(j-1) \mid X)} D_j(\bar{Z}(j)),$$

where

$$D_j(\bar{Z}(j)) = \phi_j \circ \ldots \circ \phi_{u-1}(D_u).$$

Proof. For notational convenience, let $w(u) = \frac{I(\bar{A}_2(u-1)=0)}{g(\bar{A}_1(u),\bar{A}_2(u-1)|X)}$, and we redefine $D = D_u(\bar{Z}(u))$, $X(j) = X_{A_1}(\min(j,C))$, $A_1(j) = A_1(\min(j,C))$, and $Z(j) = Z(\min(j,C))$ (i.e., the latter processes are truncated at C). Thus we can now represent $\mathcal{F}(u)$ as $(\bar{Z}(u), \bar{A}_2(u-1))$. Let $w_1(u) = 1/\prod_{j=1}^{u} g(A_1(j) \mid \bar{A}_1(j-1), \bar{X}(j), \bar{A}_2(j-1))$ and $w_2(u) = I(\bar{A}_2(u) = 0)/\prod_{j=1}^{u} g(A_2(j) \mid \bar{Z}(j), \bar{A}_2(j-1))$, and note that $w(u) = w_1(u) * w_2(u-1)$.

By assumption, we have $E(B \mid \mathcal{F}(u)) = w_1(u)w_2(u-1)D$. By $E(B \mid \mathcal{F}(u-1)) = E(E(B \mid \mathcal{F}(u)) \mid \mathcal{F}(u-1))$, it follows that

$$E(B \mid \mathcal{F}(u-1)) = E\left(w(u)D \mid \bar{A}_2(u-2), \bar{Z}(u-1)\right).$$

By first conditioning on $\bar{A}_2(u-1), \bar{Z}(u-1)$, and noticing that $w_2(u-1)$ is only a function of $\bar{A}_2(u-1)$ and $\bar{Z}(u-1)$, it follows that the last expression equals:

$$E\left(w_2(u-1)E\left(D*w_1(u) \mid \bar{A}_2(u-1)=0, \bar{Z}(u-1)\right) \mid \bar{A}_2(u-2), \bar{Z}(u-1)\right).$$

Integrating w.r.t. $A_2(u-1)$ yields now:

$$w_2(u-2)E\left(E\left(D*w_1(u) \mid \bar{A}_2(u-1)=0, \bar{Z}(u-1)\right) \mid \bar{A}_2(u-2), \bar{Z}(u-1)\right),$$

which thus equals

$$w_2(u-2)E\left(D*w_1(u) \mid \bar{A}_2(u-2)=0, \bar{Z}(u-1)\right).$$

By first conditioning on $(\bar{A}_2(u-1), \bar{A}_1(u-1), \bar{X}_{A_1}(\min(u,C))$ in the conditional expectation, so that we only integrate w.r.t. $A_1(u)$, we obtain

$$w_2(u-2)E\left(\sum_{a_1} I(A_1(u)=a_1)D*w_1(u-1) \mid \bar{A}_2(u-2)=0, \bar{Z}(u-1)\right).$$

Since $w_1(u-1)$ is only a function of $\bar{A}_2(u-2), \bar{Z}(u-1)$, and $w_1(u-1)w_2(u-2) = w(u-1)$, we obtain as final expression

$$w(u-1)E\left(\sum_{a_1} I(A_1(u)=a_1)D \mid \bar{A}_2(u-2)=0, \bar{Z}(u-1)\right).$$

By SRA, we can replace $\bar{A}_2(u-2)$ by $\bar{A}_2(u-1)$. This proves the lemma. □

Theorem 6.3 *Consider the setting of Theorem 6.2. For any function $D(\bar{A}_1, \bar{X}_{A_1}, T) = D_1(\bar{A}_1(T), \bar{X}_{A_1}(T))$ (for some function D_1), consider*

$$IC_0(Y \mid G, D) = \sum_{u \leq T} \frac{I(\bar{A}_2(u-1) = 0)}{g(\bar{A}_1(u), \bar{A}_2(u-1) \mid X)} D(\bar{A}_1, \bar{X}_{A_1}, u).$$

We have

$$E(IC_0(Y) \mid \mathcal{F}(t)) = \sum_{\{u:u \leq t\}} \frac{I(\bar{A}_2(u-1) = 0)}{g(\bar{A}_1(u), \bar{A}_2(u-1) \mid X)} I(T \geq u) D(\bar{A}_1, \bar{X}_{A_1}, u)$$

$$+ \sum_{\{u:u > t\}} E\left(\frac{I(\bar{A}_2(u-1) = 0)}{g(\bar{A}_1(u), \bar{A}_2(u-1) \mid X)} I(T \geq u) D(\bar{A}_1, \bar{X}_{A_1}, u) \mid \mathcal{F}(t)\right).$$

Define for $u > t$

$$g(u, t) \equiv E\left(\frac{I(\bar{A}_2(u-1) = 0)}{g(\bar{A}_1(u), \bar{A}_2(u-1) \mid X)} I(T \geq u) D(\bar{A}_1, \bar{X}_{A_1}, u) \mid \mathcal{F}(t)\right).$$

We have for $u > t$

$$g(u, t = j) = \frac{I(\bar{A}_2(j-1) = 0)}{g(\bar{A}_1(j), \bar{A}_2(j-1) \mid X)} (\phi_j \circ \ldots \circ \phi_{u-1}\{D_1\}),$$

where

$$D_1 \equiv D(\bar{A}_1, \bar{X}_{A_1}, u) I(T \geq u).$$

This theorem follows directly from Lemma 6.3.

Estimation of each of the components ϕ_j, $j < u - 1$, in the recursive representation of $g(u, t)$ only involves regressions of observed outcomes (after having estimated ϕ_i, $i > j$) on covariates extracted from $\bar{Z}(j)$ among subjects with $C \geq j + 1$. The conditional expectations w.r.t. the indicator $I(T \geq u)$ can be transformed into an intensity of $dR(t)$ w.r.t. to an observed past, which can be estimated with partial likelihood estimation, as discussed in Subsection 3.5.4.

6.4.2 Data Analysis: SPARCS

In this subsection, we analyze data using the longitudinal logistic marginal structural model for the hazard of survival (6.17). We will first introduce the data set and the variables that we choose for the analysis.

The data are from the SPARCS (Study of Physical Performance and Age Related Changes in Sonomans) project. SPARCS is a community-based longitudinal study of physical activity and fitness in people ≥ 55 years of age who live in the city and environs of Sonoma, California.

Data for this analysis are based on the home evaluation component from the first three evaluations of the females of the cohort (May 1993–Dec.

6.4. Marginal Structural Model with Right-Censoring 339

1994, Sep.,1995–Nov., 1996, and June 1998–Oct.1999). At baseline, there are 1197 subjects, of which 155 subjects develop a cardiovascular condition during the study, 181 subjects die before the end of the study, 58 subjects drop out before the end of the study, and the remaining 959 subjects are censored at the end of the study.

The goal of the study is to estimate the causal effect of activity score ($GSM\_ORD(t)$) on mortality. The activity score is discretized into four values $\{1, 2, 3, 4\}$ representing low to vigorous exercise. Let $A_1(t) \equiv I(GSM\_ORD(t) \geq 3)$ be the indicator of engaging in moderate or vigorous levels of activity at time t since entry in the study. Here, $A_1(t)$ represents the time-dependent treatment variable.

We use the following time-independent covariates: "Age" is the age at first (baseline) interview, "Decline" is an indicator of a dramatic drop in activity 5 and 10 years prior to baseline interview, "Habitual" is mutually exclusive indicators of consistent vigorous levels of activity in the past, and "Team" is an indicator of whether the individual participated in high school sports. The time-dependent covariates are given by "Cardiovascular", is an indicator that jumps to 1 (and stays 1) if someone develops a cardiovascular condition, "Other health", is an indicator of having been told by a doctor to have one of a number of conditions spanning a number of diseases, "self-perception of health", is a four-level categorical variable with values excellent, good, fair, poor, "NRB" is a clinical measure of performing everyday tasks that is computed as a weighted average over a number of tasks weighted by the level of difficulty of each of the tasks, "Body Mass Index" (BMI); and "Ex-smoking", is an indicator of being a current smoker. Notice that these factors are considered predictive of future activity score and survival and are therefore time-dependent confounders of the treatment. The detailed descriptions of these variables can be found in Tager, Haight, Hollenberg, and Satariano.(2000).

For a given treatment regime $a_1(\cdot)$, let $X_{a_1}(\cdot)$ represent the time-dependent treatment-specific counterfactual process that includes time-independent covariates W and the time-dependent covariates $L_{a_1}(\cdot)$. Let τ be the time between entry and end of study, which is considered a completely independent random variable in our analysis. This type of censoring does not need to be addressed in any special way since we can make it part of the counterfactual processes $X_{a_1}(t) \equiv X_{a_1}(\min(t, \tau))$ of interest without changing the meaning of the causal parameters in our marginal structural model for the hazard of survival time T_{a_1}. Let C be the drop-out time of a subject (i.e., some subjects drop out before the end of the study τ) The observed data can be represented as

$$Y = (C, \bar{X}_{A_1}(C), \bar{A}_1(C)). \tag{6.23}$$

Preprocessing of the data

To simplify the problem, we assume that the evaluations are made every 2.5 years even though the actual value ranges between 2 and 3 years. To use the discrete causal model described in this section, we discretize the data by 6 months. For example, a follow up time of 58 months will be transformed to 9. Thus, there are five time points between two evaluations of a subject. Recall that the activity score and the covariate processes are subject to change only at each evaluation time ($t = 0, 5, 10$).

Marginal structural models

We consider two marginal structural logistic regression models, for the hazard of survival. In the first model we adjust for $V = (Card, Age)$.
Model 1:

$$\begin{aligned}
P(Y_{\bar{a}_1}(j) = 1 | \bar{Y}_{\bar{a}_1}(j-1) = 0, V) &= I(\bar{Y}_{\bar{a}_1}(j) \text{ is at risk of jump}) \times \\
&\quad \text{logit}^{-1}(\beta_0 + \beta_1 a_1(j) + \beta_2 j + \beta_3 Age + \\
&\quad \beta_4 Card + \beta_5 Age \times a_1(j) + \\
&\quad \beta_6 Age \times j + \beta_7 Card \times a_1(j) + \\
&\quad \beta_8 Card \times j + \beta_9 Age \times Card).
\end{aligned}$$

Here $Y_{\bar{a}_1}(j) = I(T_{\bar{a}_1} \leq j)$, $I(\bar{Y}_{\bar{a}_1}(j)$ is at risk of jump$) = I(\min(C, T_{\bar{a}_1}) \geq j, j < \tau)$ and $Card$ is the baseline measurement of cardiovascular condition (cardiovascular variable in the first round). In the second model, we do not adjust for baseline covariates.
Model 2:

$$\begin{aligned}
P(Y_{\bar{a}_1}(j) = 1 | \bar{Y}_{\bar{a}_1}(j-1) = 0) &= I(\bar{Y}_{\bar{a}_1}(j) \text{ is at risk of jump}) \times \\
&\quad \text{logit}^{-1}(\beta_0 + \beta_1 a_1(j) + \beta_2 j).
\end{aligned}$$

We assume that the probability of the treatment conditional on the past treatment and past covariate history follows a logistic regression model

$$\begin{aligned}
\lambda_j(\gamma) &= P(A_1(j) = 1 | \bar{A}_1(j-1), \bar{X}(j)) \\
&\equiv \text{logit}^{-1}(\gamma_0 + \gamma_1 A_1(j-1) + \gamma_2 j + \gamma_3^\top L(j) + \gamma_4^\top W),
\end{aligned}$$

where $L(j)$ represents the time-dependent covariates mentioned above and W represents the baseline covariates. Let $\hat{\gamma}$ be the maximum partial likelihood estimator (MLE) of γ; that is, $\hat{\gamma}$ maximizes the partial likelihood,

$$\begin{aligned}
L(\gamma) &= \Pi_i L_i(\gamma) \\
&\equiv \Pi_i \Pi_j \lambda_{ji}(\gamma)^{A_{1i}(j)} (1 - \lambda_{ji}(\gamma))^{1 - A_{1i}(j)},
\end{aligned}$$

which can be computed using standard software (e.g., glm() in S-plus).

6.4. Marginal Structural Model with Right-Censoring

Let $A_2(\cdot) \equiv I(C \leq \cdot)$. We assume that the intensity model for the dropout process is

$$E(dA_2(j)|\bar{A}_2(j), \bar{X}(j)) = \pi_j(\gamma^*), \qquad (6.24)$$

where

$$\pi_j(\gamma^*) = \text{logit}^{-1}\left(\gamma_0^* + \gamma_1^* A_1(j) + \gamma_2 j + \gamma_3^{*\top} L(j) + \gamma_4^{*\top} W\right).$$

Let $\widehat{\gamma}^*$ be the partial maximum likelihood estimator (MLE) of γ^* maximizing:

$$\begin{aligned} L(\gamma^*) &= \Pi_i L_i(\gamma^*) \\ &= \Pi_i \Pi_j \pi_{ji}(\gamma^*)^{A_2(j)} (1 - \pi_{ji}(\gamma^*))^{1-A_2(j)}. \end{aligned}$$

Results

The following table records the estimates of β based on the naive method, IPTW, and the one-step Newton-Raphson for solving the T_{SRA}-orthogonalized IPTW-estimating function. Estimated standard errors for the one-step and IPTW estimators are reported in parentheses.

	Naive	IPTW	One-Step
$\widehat{\beta}_0$	-12.5435	-13.2424 (1.4244)	-12.9429 (1.3994)
$\widehat{\beta}_1$	0.6861	1.1873 (1.4727)	0.8018 (1.4274)
$\widehat{\beta}_2$	-0.1163	-0.0618 (0.1553)	-0.0825 (0.1517)
$\widehat{\beta}_3$	0.1048	0.1132 (0.0179)	0.1091 (0.0176)
$\widehat{\beta}_4$	4.8012	4.2989 (1.6576)	4.4791 (1.5922)
$\widehat{\beta}_5$	-0.0202	-0.0263 (0.0192)	-0.0204 (0.0185)
$\widehat{\beta}_6$	0.0025	0.0017 (0.0020)	0.0019 (0.0019)
$\widehat{\beta}_7$	0.4386	0.6898 (0.3672)	0.6885 (0.3502)
$\widehat{\beta}_8$	0.0101	0.0191 (0.0400)	0.0179 (0.0391)
$\widehat{\beta}_9$	-0.0535	-0.0488 (0.0204)	-0.0509 (0.0195)

The coefficient of $A_1(j)$ is $\beta_{Mod} \equiv \beta_1 + \beta_5 Age + \beta_7 Card$, which is estimated by $\widehat{\beta}_{Mod} = \widehat{\beta}_1 + \widehat{\beta}_5 Age + \widehat{\beta}_7 Card$. The estimated covariance matrix of $\widehat{\beta}$ provides us with an estimate of the standard error of $\widehat{\beta}_{Mod}$. The following table records the estimates of β_{Mod} for the subjects with age between 60 and 80 years based on the naive, IPTW, and one-step estimators. The standard errors are reported in parentheses.

		60	65	70	75	80
Card=0	Naive	-0.52	-0.62	-0.72	-0.82	-0.92
	IPTW	-0.38	-0.51	-0.65	-0.78	-0.91
		(0.37)	(0.30)	(0.25)	(0.22)	(0.23)
	One-Step	-0.42	-0.52	-0.62	-0.73	-0.83
		(0.36)	(0.29)	(0.24)	(0.21)	(0.22)
Card=1	Naive	-0.08	-0.18	-0.28	-0.38	-0.49
	IPTW	0.30	0.17	0.0390	-0.09	-0.22
		(0.40)	(0.34)	(0.30)	(0.29)	(0.30)
	One-Step	0.26	0.16	0.05	-0.04	-0.14
		(0.38)	(0.32)	(0.28)	(0.27)	(0.29)

Notice that these results suggest that, among people without a heart condition at baseline, high levels of activity have a positive causal effect on survival, and the effect becomes larger with baseline age. However, among people with a heart condition at baseline, high levels of activity have no significant effect on survival.

Below, we report the parameter estimates $\widehat{\gamma}$ and $\widehat{\gamma}^*$ for the treatment and censoring mechanism.

	Treatment	Censoring
(Intercept)	3.3247 (0.7239)	-8.4037 (1.8283)
k	-0.1557 (0.0221)	0.0711 (0.0333)
$A_1(k)$	—	0.0281 (0.2790)
$A_1(k-1)$	2.2622 (0.1113)	—
Age	-0.0472 (0.0070)	0.0246 (0.0174)
Habitual	0.2046 (0.1116)	-0.1524 (0.2777)
Team	0.1750 (0.1127)	-0.1524 (0.2777)
Decline	-0.3075 (0.1171)	-0.1382 (0.3057)
BMI	-0.0169 (0.0108)	0.0083 (0.0278)
NRB	0.5662 (0.2470)	0.7564 (0.6777)
Cardiovascular	0.2418 (0.1577)	-0.5955 (0.4450)
Other health	0.1737 (0.1213)	-0.4503 (0.3107)
Perception of health	-0.3094 (0.1525)	0.4342 (0.3832)
Current smoking	-0.5319 (0.2044)	-0.1533 (0.5790)
Ex-smoking	0.1496 (0.1124)	0.2043 (0.2760)

We also computed a slight alternative p_n^* of the projection constant $c_{nu,n}^*$. Let p_n^* be the empirical estimate of the correlation matrix p^* between $IC_0 -$

IC_{SRA} and IC_{SRA}. This empirical correlation matrix ($\times 10^4$) is given by

$$\begin{pmatrix} 96 & -5 & -101 & -69 & 15 & 7 & 77 & -16 & -4 & -13 \\ -9 & 0 & 10 & 7 & -1 & -1 & -7 & 2 & 0 & 1 \\ -75 & 4 & 80 & 54 & -12 & -6 & -61 & 12 & 3 & 10 \\ -68 & 3 & 72 & 49 & -10 & -5 & -55 & 11 & 3 & 9 \\ 20 & -1 & -21 & -14 & 3 & 2 & 16 & -3 & -1 & -3 \\ 14 & -1 & -15 & -10 & 2 & 1 & 12 & -2 & -1 & -2 \\ 56 & -3 & -60 & -41 & 9 & 4 & 45 & -9 & -2 & -8 \\ -24 & 1 & 25 & 17 & -4 & -2 & -19 & 4 & 1 & 3 \\ -5 & 0 & 5 & 3 & -1 & 0 & -4 & 1 & 0 & 1 \\ -19 & 1 & 20 & 14 & -3 & -1 & -15 & 3 & 1 & 3 \end{pmatrix}.$$

This indicates that we have succeeded well in estimating the projection IC_{SRA}.

The estimates of β for Model 2 are reported in the following table. Again, the estimated standard errors are reported in parentheses.

	Naive	InvWght	OneStep
$\widehat{\beta_0}$	-4.4552	-4.8602 (0.1855)	-4.8532 (0.1782)
$\widehat{\beta_1}$	-1.0833	-0.4594 (0.1846)	-0.4448 (0.1684)
$\widehat{\beta_2}$	0.0755	0.0798 (0.0201)	0.0758 (0.0196)

We refer to Bryan, Yu, van der Laan (2002) for further details on this data analysis.

6.4.3 A simulation for estimators of a treatment-specific survival function

In this subsection we construct a locally efficient estimator of the treatment-specific distribution function $\mu = P(T_{a_1} \leq t)$ if treatment $A_1(t) = A_1(0)$ is time-independent and discrete-valued and the full data model is chosen to be nonparametric. We can represent the observed data by $Y = (A_1, \tilde{T}_{A_1} = \min(T_{A_1}, C), \bar{W}_{A_1}(\tilde{T}_{A_1}))$, where A_1 is the treatment, C is the right-censoring time, T_{a_1} is the treatment-specific survival time, and $W_{a_1}(t)$ is the treatment-specific covariate process. Rhus, the only difference with the above is that the full data model is saturated so that the full data estimating function is $D_{opt}(X \mid \mu) = I(T_{a_1(0)} \leq t) - \mu$ and that $A_1(t) = A_1(0)$. This is carried out in Hubbard, van der Laan, and Robins (1999). The efficient influence curve $IC(Y \mid Q, G, D_{opt}) = IC_0(Y \mid G, D_{opt}) - IC_{SRA}(Y \mid Q, G)$ can be represented as

$$IC^*(Y) = \frac{I(A_1 = a_1)}{g_1(A_1 \mid W(0))} \frac{I(T \leq t)\Delta}{\bar{G}_2(T \mid X, A_1)} \qquad (6.25)$$
$$+ \frac{I(A_1 = a_1)}{g_1(A_1 \mid W(0))} \int F(t \mid \bar{W}(u), A_1, \tilde{T} > u) \frac{dM_{G_2,a_1}(u)}{\bar{G}_2(u \mid X, A_1)}$$

$$-\frac{I(A_1 = a_1) - g_1(a_1 \mid W(0))}{g_1(a_1 \mid W(0))} F(t \mid W(0), A_1 = a_1) - \mu,$$

where $W(0)$ represents all baseline covariates, $W(t)$ represents the observed covariate process

$$g_1(a_1 \mid W(0)) = P(A_1 = a_1 \mid W(0)),$$
$$\bar{G}_2(u \mid X, A_1 = a_1) = P(C \geq u \mid A_1 = a_1, X),$$

and $dM_{G_2,a_1}(u)$ is given by

$$I(A_1 = a_1) \left\{ I(C \in du, \Delta = 0) - I(\tilde{T} \geq u) \frac{dG_2(u \mid X, A_1 = a_1)}{\bar{G}_2(u \mid X, A_1 = a_1)} \right\}.$$

Here we let Q represent the parameters $(F(t \mid \bar{W}(u), A_1, \tilde{T} > u), F(t \mid W(0), A_1 = a_1))$. Let IC^{**} be defined by the same expression (6.25) defining IC^*, but excluding the final term $-\mu$. Thus $IC^* = IC^{**} - \mu$. Notice that, given estimators g_{1n} of the treatment assignment, G_{2n} of the censoring mechanism G_2 and an estimator Q_n of $Q(F_X)$, the locally efficient estimator solving $0 = \sum_i (\hat{IC}^*(Y_i \mid \mu))$ is given by:

$$\mu_n = \frac{1}{n} \sum_{i=1}^{n} \hat{IC}^{**}(Y_i).$$

We will refer to this estimator in the next simulation study as the one-step estimator because it also corresponds with the first step of the Newton-Raphson algorithm for solving the estimating equation $0 = \sum_i (\hat{IC}^*(Y_i \mid \mu))$. Below, we will report a summary of the simulation study carried out in Hubbard, van der Laan, and Robins (1999).

Two relevant treatments

Firstly, we present two simulations that examine the performance of our one-step estimator when one is interested in the marginal treatment survival curve and two or more treatments exist. The first simulation examines the performance when treatment assignment and the failure time are marginally dependent, but these random variables are conditionally independent given the covariate. In this case, the simple Kaplan–Meier estimator performed on each treatment group is inconsistent, so the advantage of the locally efficient one-step estimator is a reduction in bias. In the second simulation, treatment assignment is done completely at random, but there exists a binary covariate (W) that strongly predicts failure. In this case, the performance of the one-step estimator should be superior to that of the Kaplan–Meier estimator by reducing the variance of estimation. The reduction in variance occurs by accounting for the non-uniform distribution of W within each subsample defined by the treatment group. In this way, the one-step estimator reduces the bias conditional on realized chance association between W and treatment. Although the Kaplan–Meier

6.4. Marginal Structural Model with Right-Censoring

estimator is consistent for repeated experiments under this scenario, it can be significantly biased in any realized sample if by bad luck the potential confounder W is unevenly distributed among the treatment groups (Robins and Morgenstern, 1987).

For both simulations, we use the two families of data-generating models:

$$F(t \mid W, A_1) = \frac{1}{1 + \exp(-(\beta_0^T + \beta_1^T t + \beta_2^T W + \beta_3^T A_1))}, \quad (6.26)$$

$$G_2(c \mid W, A_1) = \frac{1}{1 + \exp(-(-10 + c))},$$

where $W \in (0, 1)$ with equal probability and treatment $A_1 \in (0, 1)$. The β's and $P(A_1 = 1 \mid W = w)$ vary with the simulation. In the first simulation, we simply use the known values of G, $F(t \mid W, S)$ and the propensity score $P(A_1 = 1 \mid W)$ when calculating our estimators. In the second simulation, we again use the known values of G_2 and $F(t \mid W, A_1)$, but we estimate $P(A_1 \mid W)$ even though treatment assignment and W are independent. Our one-step estimator should improve over the estimator that uses the known values of the propensity score.

Simulation 1. For this simulation

$$\begin{align}
(\beta_0^T, \beta_1^T, \beta_2^T, \beta_3^T) &= (-10, 1, 5, -5), \\
P(A_1 = 1 \mid W = 1) &= 0.90, \\
P(A_1 = 1 \mid W = 0) &= 0.10.
\end{align}$$

Thus, those subjects with $W = 1$ have a shorter mean survival time than those with $W = 0$. If $W = 1$, however, then the subject has a much higher probability of receiving treatment ($A_1 = 1$) relative to those subjects with $W = 0$. Furthermore, those with treatment have a higher mean survival than controls ($A_1 = 0$). Thus, W confounds the relationship of treatment and survival because the treatment group will contain differentially more subjects with shorter survival times. This will result in an overestimation of $F_{A_1=1}(t)$ and underestimation of $F_{A_1=0}(t)$ by the stratified Kaplan–Meier estimator. However, the one-step estimator should successfully adjust for the confounding of assignment and treatment effect that occurs through W.

Instead of reporting the results of repeated iterations, we present the graphical results of a single iteration (Figure 6.1). As one can see, the Kaplan–Meier estimator performed on the two subsamples ($A_1 = 0$ and $A_1 = 1$) provides a biased estimate of the marginal treatment distribution. As anticipated, the Kaplan–Meier estimator underestimates the treatment survival distribution and overestimates the control distribution. However, the locally efficient one-step estimator consistently estimates both distributions.

Simulation 2. For this simulation,

$$(\beta_0^T, \beta_1^T, \beta_2^T, \beta_3^T) = (-30, 3, 15, -15),$$

346   6. Unified Approach for Causal Inference and Censored Data

Figure 6.1. Estimates of the distribution function under non random assignment for simulation 1. □ = truth, + = one-step, and △ = Kaplan–Meier.

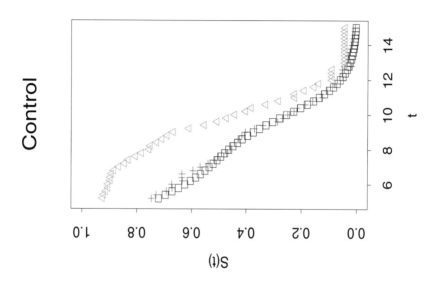

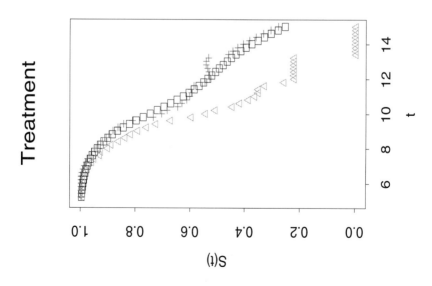

$$P(A_1 = 1 \mid W = 1) = 0.50,$$
$$P(A_1 = 1 \mid W = 0) = 0.50.$$

In this case, assignment is done completely at random; however, W has such a strong effect on survival that nonuniform distribution of W among the subjects in the two treatment groups can have a strong confounding effect (i.e., conditional bias) in the sample. Thus, we should gain over the Kaplan–Meier estimates by modeling $P(A_1 \mid W)$.

The graphical results of four iterations of simulation 2 are shown in Figure 6.2. Because for this simulation the Kaplan–Meier estimates of the treatment distributions are consistent (treatment assignment was done completely at random), these estimates do not depart from the true distributions as dramatically as in simulation 1. However, by estimating the propensity score, the one-step estimator provides an estimate of the treatment survival distribution that is closer, on average, to the true distribution than the Kaplan–Meier estimator. Note that the improvement over the Kaplan–Meier estimator in this circumstance will be a function of how strongly W affects survival. In this case, W significantly affects the mean survival, so small discrepancies in the distribution of W between subsamples defined by treatment group ($A_1 = 0$ and $A_1 = 1$) will result in confounding by W within any *realized* sample. Thus, one can substantially improve efficiency relative to the Kaplan–Meier estimator by modeling the propensity score. See Robins and Morgenstern (1987) for further discussion of the relationship between unconditional efficiency and conditional bias given an ancillary or approximate ancillary statistic.

6.5 Structural Nested Model with Right-Censoring

For each possible treatment regime $a_1 = (a_1(t) : t = 1, \ldots, K)$, we define a counterfactual random variable $X_{a_1} = (X_{a_1}(t) : t)$, where $X_{a_1}(t) = (Y_{a_1}(t), L_{a_1}(t))$, Y_{a_1} is a time-dependent outcome process, and L_{a_1} is a time-dependent covariate process. It is assumed that $X_{a_1}(t)$ only depends on a_1 through $\bar{a}_1(t-) = (a_1(s) : s < t)$. Let time be discrete at $j = 1, \ldots, K$.

Dynamic treatment regimes. Since we will also be concerned with estimating dynamic treatment regime specific distributions, we will include dynamic treatment regime specific processes X_d in our full-data structure as well. A V-specific dynamic treatment regime is a deterministic rule for assigning treatment at time j, where the rule is a function of a V-history $\bar{V}(j) = (V(1), \ldots, V(j))$ collected in the study. Let $d = (d_1, d_2, \ldots, d_K)$ be a dynamic treatment regime, where $d_j(\cdot)$ is a function of $\bar{V}(j)$. Let X_d be the dynamic treatment regime specific counterfactual random variable. The full data structure is $X = (X_d : d)$, where d ranges over the set of V-specific dynamic treatment regimes including all static treatment

348   6. Unified Approach for Causal Inference and Censored Data

Figure 6.2. Estimates of the distribution function under random assignment for simulation 2. □ = truth, + = one-step, and △ = Kaplan–Meier.

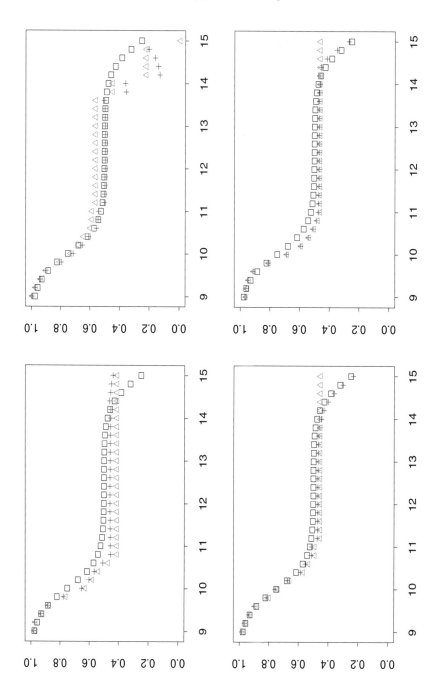

6.5. Structural Nested Model with Right-Censoring

regimes $a_1(\cdot)$. Again, it is assumed that $X_d(t)$ only depends on d through $\bar{d}_{t-1} \equiv (d_1, \ldots, d_{t-1})$.

Let C be a right-censoring time. We define the observed data by

$$Y = (C, \bar{X}_{A_1}(C), \bar{A}_1(C)).$$

In other words, we observe the treatment-specific process X_{A_1} corresponding with the treatment that the subject actually received up until the follow-up time C.

Let $A_2(t) = I(C \leq t)$ be a process that jumps at the censoring time C. Let $a_2 = \bar{a}_2$ be a potential sample path for A_2, that is, a_2 is a function of time whose initial value equals 0 and jumps to 1 at some time $j = 1, \ldots, p$ or at ∞ (corresponding to no censoring) and remains at 1 after jumping. Let $c(a_2)$ be the time that a_2 jumps to 1 so $C = c(A_2)$. Define $X_{a_1,a_2}(t) = X_{a_1}(\min\{t, c(a_2)\})$ so $X_{a_1}(t)$ is $X_{a_1,a_2}(t)$ for a_2 that jumps at ∞. Finally, redefine $X = (X_{a_1,a_2} : a_1, a_2)$

Then we can define the observed data as $Y = (A, X_A)$, where $A = (\bar{A}_1(C), A_2)$. This means that we can apply the general methodology described in Section 6.1.

The sequential randomization assumption states that for all $j \in \{1, \ldots, K\}$

$$g(A(j) \mid \bar{A}(j-1), X) = g(A(j) \mid \bar{A}(j-1), \bar{X}_A(j)).$$

At an $A = (A_1, A_2)$ with $A_2(t) = I(C \leq t)$, we have

$$g(\bar{A} \mid X) = \prod_{j=1}^{C} g(A(j) \mid \bar{A}(j-1), X) \quad (6.27)$$

$$= \prod_{j=1}^{C} g_1(A_1(j) \mid A_2(j), \bar{A}(j-1), \bar{X}_A(j)) \prod_{j=1}^{C} g_2(A_2(j) \mid \bar{A}(j-1), \bar{X}_A(j)).$$

Let $\mathcal{F}_1(j) = (A_2(j), \bar{A}(j-1), \bar{X}_A(j))$ and $\mathcal{F}_2(j) = (\bar{A}(j-1), \bar{X}_A(j))$ so that

$$g(A(j) \mid \bar{A}(j-1), X) = g_1(A_1(j) \mid \mathcal{F}_1(j)) g_2(A_2(j) \mid \mathcal{F}_2(j)).$$

The first product in (6.27) represents the treatment mechanism, while the second product represents the censoring mechanism. For modelling and estimating both mechanisms we refer to the presentation and setting of the previous section. Let $\mathcal{G}$ denote the model for the action mechanism $g(\bar{A} \mid X)$.

Marginal structural nested full data model. The following model can be applied to any continuous outcome. To be specific, we will assume that $Y_{a_1}(t) = I(T_{a_1} \geq t)$, where T_{a_1} is the treatment-regime-specific survival time. We assume that the treatment specific survival times T_{a_1} are continuous. A quantile–quantile function $\gamma(t)$ linking two continuous distributions F_1, F_2 is defined by $\gamma(t) = F_1^{-1} F_2(t)$. It maps a p-th quantile $q_{2,p}$ of F_2

into the pth $q_{1,p}$ quantile of F_1; that is, if $X_j \sim F_j$, $j = 1, 2$, then

$$P(X_1 \leq F_1^{-1} F_2(q_{2,p})) = F_2(q_{2,p}) = p$$

so that $q_{1,p} = F_1^{-1} F_2(q_{2,p})$. In particular, it can be used to map a random variable X_2 with distribution F_2 into a random variable $F_1^{-1} F_2(X_2)$ with distribution F_1. Note that a quantile–quantile function is a monotone increasing function from $F_1^{-1}(0)$ at 0 to $F_1^{-1}(1)$ at ∞.

A marginal structural nested model is a model for the quantile–quantile function $F_1^{-1} F_2$ of two conditional treatment-specific survival times only differing in the treatment regime at time point m, where both have treatment set equal to zero after time m. Let $\bar{V}(m) \subset \bar{X}(m)$ be a subset of the complete process $(\bar{Y}(m), \bar{L}(m))$. These two conditional distributions are given by

$$F_{(\bar{a}_1(m-1),0)}(\cdot \mid \bar{v}_{\bar{a}_1}(m)) \equiv P(T_{\bar{a}_1(m-1),0} \leq \cdot \mid \bar{v}_{\bar{a}_1}(m)),$$
$$F_{\bar{a}_m,0}(\cdot \mid \bar{v}_{\bar{a}_1}(m)) \equiv P(T_{\bar{a}_1(m),0} \leq \cdot \mid \bar{v}_{\bar{a}_1}(m)).$$

Now, we define γ_m, $m = 1, \ldots, K$, as the quantile–quantile function corresponding with these choices F_1, F_2, respectively:

$$\gamma_m(t \mid \bar{v}(m), \bar{a}_1(m)) = F_{(\bar{a}_1(m-1),0)}^{-1}(F_{\bar{a}_m,0}(\cdot \mid \bar{v}_{\bar{a}_1}(m)) \mid \bar{v}_{\bar{a}_1}(m)). \quad (6.28)$$

Since γ_m measures the effect of a final treatment action $a_1(m)$ at time m on survival, this quantile–quantile function is called a blip function. We will assume that $\gamma_m(t \mid \bar{v}(m), \bar{a}_1(m))$ is parametrized by an unknown finite dimensional parameter ψ. We will here assume that $\bar{V}(m)$ includes $\bar{Y}(m)$. A possible model for γ_m is, for $t > t_m$

$$\gamma_\psi(t \mid \bar{v}(m), \bar{a}_1(m)) = t + \delta_m(t) \{a_1(m) \{\psi_1 + \psi_2 a_1(m-1) + \psi_3 w(m)\}\},$$

and $\gamma_\psi(t \mid \bar{v}(m), \bar{a}_1(m)) = t$ for $t \leq t_m$, where $w(m)$ is a function of $\bar{v}(m)$, $\delta_m(t) = \min(t, t_{m+1}) - t_m$, and $a_1(m)$ is a treatment assigned over a time interval $(t_m, t_{m+1}]$. Alternatively, $\gamma_\psi(t \mid \bar{v}(m), \bar{a}_1(m))$ equals for $t > t_m$

$$t + \delta_m(t) \{\exp(a_1(m)\{\psi_1 + \psi_2 a_1(m-1) + \psi_3 w(m)\}) - 1\}.$$

and it equals t for $t \leq t_m$. This class of models, as introduced in van der Laan, Murphy, and and Robins (2002) generalizes the structural nested failure time model of Robins which assumes $V = X$ (i.e., in a structural nested failure time model, the quantile–quantile function conditions on all treatment confounders). This generalization is important if one is concerned with estimating the effect of dynamic treatment regimes that are only functions of a (e.g., small) subset $V \subset L$. These models can also be used for continuous outcomes that are not survival times, such as measurements made at an endpoint τ.

Analyzing dynamic treatment regimes. Let T_d be the dynamic treatment-regime-specific survival time, and let F_d be its marginal distribution function: $F_d(t) = P(T_d \leq t)$. Marginal structural nested models

6.5. Structural Nested Model with Right-Censoring

are particularly effective in modeling and estimating a dynamic treatment-regime-specific distribution function F_d, as we will now show (see also Robins' work on structural nested models and van der Laan, Murphy, and Robins, 2002). Specifically, let

$$H = h(T \mid \bar{V}(K), \bar{A}_1(K)) \equiv \gamma_1 \circ \ldots \circ \gamma_{K-1} \circ \gamma_K(T), \quad (6.29)$$

where we used the shorthand notation $\gamma_m(\cdot) = \gamma_m(\cdot \mid \bar{V}(m), \bar{A}_1(m))$, $m = 1, \ldots, K$. Thus, we evaluate the quantile–quantile functions γ_m at the observed histories $\bar{V}(m), \bar{A}_1(m)$. By the aforementioned property of a quantile–quantile function, $h(T_{\bar{a}_1} \mid \bar{V}_{\bar{a}_1}(K), \bar{a}_1(K))$ is a random variable with the same marginal distribution as the population distribution F_0 of survival T_0 had all treatment been witheld:

$$h(T_{\bar{a}_1} \mid \bar{V}_{\bar{a}_1}(K), \bar{a}_1(K)) \sim F_0 \text{ for all } \bar{a}_1.$$

Application of this operator $h(\cdot)$ (6.29) is often referred to as "blipping down".

Let γ_m^{-1} denote the inverse of γ_m, $m = 1, \ldots, K$. Given a V-specific dynamic treatment-regime d, consider the function

$$h^{-1}(s \mid \bar{V}(k), d) = \gamma_{k,d}^{-1} \circ \gamma_{k-1,d}^{-1} \cdots \circ \gamma_{1,d}^{-1}(s), \quad (6.30)$$

where we used the shorthand notation $\gamma_{m,d}^{-1}(\cdot) = \gamma_m^{-1}(\cdot \mid \bar{V}(m), \bar{A}_1(m) = \bar{d}_m(\bar{V}(m)))$, $m = 1, \ldots, K$. Here, we also used the notation $\bar{d}_m = (d_1, \ldots, d_m)$ as a function of $\bar{V}(m)$ for the treatment assigned by the rule d up to and including time m. Thus for the failure time models given above, at the first m such that $\gamma_m^{-1}(u)$ is less than $m + 1$, we would have $h^{-1}(u \mid \bar{V}(k), d) = \gamma_m^{-1}(u)$.

Again, by the mentioned property of the quantile–quantile function, Robins (1997) shows that, under the local rank preservation assumption that $\gamma_m(T_{\bar{a}_1(m),0} \mid \bar{V}_{\bar{a}_1(m),0}) = T_{\bar{a}_1(m),0}$ with probability 1,

$$h^{-1}(T_0 \mid \bar{V}_d(K), d) = T_d \text{ with probability 1.}$$

Here it is assumed that T_d has compact support $[0, K]$ for some $K < \infty$. One refers to applying the operator h^{-1} as "blipping up". As a consequence, under local rank preservation, Robins (1997, 1998c) shows that we have

$$1 - F_{\bar{d}}(t) = \int I(h^{-1}(T_0 \mid \bar{V}(int(t)), d) > t) \prod_{m=1}^{int(t)} dF_{\bar{d}}(V(m) \mid \bar{V}(m-1), T_0) dF_0(T_0).$$
$$(6.31)$$

Here $int(t)$ is the largest integer value less than t.

Robins (1997, 1998c) proceeds now as follows. Suppose that we can express, under local rank preservation and SRA, these treatment specific distributions of $(\bar{V}_d, T_0)$ in terms of observed data distributions. Then the resulting formula for $1 - F_{\bar{d}}(t)$ in terms of the observed data distribution will also hold without the local rank preservations, because, even under SRA, local rank preservation is an assumption that cannot be identified from the data. Thus, consistent estimation of a dynamic treatment-regime-specific survival function requires constructing consistent estimates of ψ, F_0, and $F_{\bar{V}_d}(\cdot \mid T_0)$ under local rank preservation and the SRA. Then, substitution of these estimates in the formula (6.31) results now in a consistent estimate of $F_{\bar{d}}(t)$, under SRA even without local rank preservation.

Specifically, it follows, by the G-computation formula, that were the sequential randomization assumption to hold given data on $V = \bar{V}$ (i.e., were equation (6.27 to hold with $\bar{V}_A(j) = \bar{V}(j)$ replacing $\bar{X}_A(j)$) the distribution of T_d would be represented in terms of observed data distributions as follows:

$$1 - F_{\bar{d}}(t) = \int I(h^{-1}(H \mid \bar{V}(int(t)), d) > t) dF(H, \bar{V}(t)), \qquad (6.32)$$

where $dF(H, \bar{V}(t))$ is

$$\prod_{m=1}^{int(t)} dF(V(m) \mid T > m, \bar{V}(m-1), \bar{A}(m-1) = \bar{d}_{m-1}(\bar{V}(m-1)), H) dF_0(H).$$

Here, the product is taken to be zero if any of the conditioning events cannot occur (i.e., have density 0).

One could evaluate this latter integral with the following Monte Carlo simulation: 1) simulate H from its distribution (which is the same distribution as that of T_0) and then simulate V_m from $f(\cdot \mid \bar{V}(m-1), H, \bar{A}(m-1) = \bar{d}_{m-1}(\bar{V}(m-1)))$ for $m = 1, ..., K$.

In the next subsection, we will first derive a class of estimating functions for ψ and, subsequently, we will discuss estimation of F_0 and the law of T_d when sequential randomization does not hold given data on $\bar{V}$ but only given the full data $\bar{X}$.

Since the G-computation formula for dynamic treatment regimes is such a fundamental building block for causal inference methods we provide here its simplest version, which is easy to prove. We refer to Robins (1997, 1998c) for details, and to Gill, Robins (2001), and Yu, van der Laan (2002) for its extensions to the continuous case. Other references of interest are Robins, Rotnitzky, and Scharfstein (1999), Robins (1986).

Theorem 6.4 *(G-computation formula, Robins, 1986, 1997)* Consider the setting above, where the full-data structure $X = (X_d : d)$ is a collection of V-specific dynamic treatment-regime-specific random variables, and the observed data structure is $Y = (\bar{A}(p), \bar{X}_A(p + 1))$, where $\bar{A}(t) = (A(1), ..., A(t))$, $\bar{X}_A(t) = (X_A(1), ..., X_A(t))$. Assume that the treatment mechanism satisfies SRA: that is, $g(A(t) \mid \bar{A}(t-1), X) = g(A(t) \mid \bar{A}(t-1), \bar{X}_A(t))$, $t = 1, ..., p$. In addition, assume that all random variables $X_a(t)$ are discrete valued. Given a dynamic treatment regime $d(\cdot)$, consider the formula:

$$f_d(x) = \prod_{j=1}^{p+1} f(X(j) \mid \bar{X}(j-1), \bar{A}(j-1) = \bar{d}_j(\bar{V}(j-1))),$$

where $f(\cdot \mid \bar{X}(j-1), \bar{A}(j-1))$ is the conditional probability of $X(j)$, given $\bar{X}(j-1), \bar{A}(j-1)$, $j = 1, \ldots, p+1$.

We have

$$P(X_d = x) = f_d(x).$$

This result provides us with an alternative method for estimation of $F_d(t) = P(T_d \leq t)$ which involves 1) assuming a model for the conditional distributions of $X(j)$, given the observed past $\bar{X}(j-1), \bar{A}(j-1)$ (i.e., the F_X-part of the likelihood), 2) maximum likelihood estimation of the F_X-part of the likelihood, and 3) evaluation of the G-computation formula for $F_d(t)$ by Monte-Carlo simulation. However, the alternative approach discussed below based on a marginal structural nested model and its corresponding representation (6.31) of $F_d(t)$ has a particular appeal since testing $H_0 : \psi = 0$ provides a test for no effect of V-specific dynamic treatment regimes, where the α-level of the test carries the same robustness against misspecification of nuisance parameters (of α) as our doubly robust estimator of α (i.e., it relies on correct specification of either the F_X-part or the G-part of the observed data likelihood).

6.5.1 The orthogonal complement of a nuisance tangent space in a structural nested model without censoring

Let $\mathcal{G}^* \subset \mathcal{G}$ be the restricted model consisting of all action mechanisms in $\mathcal{G}$ of the form (6.27) satisfying $g_2(A_2(j) = 0 \mid \mathcal{F}_2(j)) = 1$ for all $j \leq T$ (i.e., there is no censoring) and $g_1(A_1(j) \mid \bar{X}(j), \bar{A}_1(j-1)) = g_1(A_1(j) \mid \bar{V}(j), \bar{A}_1(j-1))$. Treatment is sequentially randomized w.r.t. $\bar{V}$ as well as $X = \bar{X}$ in the sense that $g_1(A_1(j) \mid X, \bar{A}_1(j-1)) = g_1(A_1(j) \mid \bar{V}(j), \bar{A}_1(j-1))$. Note that the observed data model for the reduced data structure $(\bar{Y}_{A_1}, \bar{V}_{A_1}, \bar{A}_1)$ implied by the marginal structural full data structure model and $\mathcal{G}^*$ is the structural nested failure time model as in Robins et al. (1992), Robins (1993b, 1998a). Robins (1993b, 1998a) proves the following result.

Lemma 6.4 (*Structural nested model*) *Consider the reduced uncensored data $Y_r \equiv (\bar{Y}_{A_1} = T_{A_1}, \bar{V}_{A_1}, \bar{A}_1)$ in the structural nested model $\mathcal{M}(G^*)$ with $G^* \in \mathcal{G}^*$ known (i.e., censoring is absent and the SRA w.r.t. $\bar{V}$ holds). Suppose that the regularity conditions needed to have the density of Y_r w.r.t. a dominating measure (using the transformation theorem for $(T, \bar{V}, \bar{A}_1) \to (H(\psi), \bar{V}, \bar{A}_1))$ are given by*

$$f(Y_r) = \frac{dH(\psi)}{dT} f_0(H(\psi)) \prod_{m=1}^{int(T)} f(V(m) \mid \bar{V}(m-1), \bar{A}_1(m-1), H(\psi))$$

$$\times g^*(A(m) \mid \bar{A}(m-1), \bar{V}(m)), \tag{6.33}$$

where we note that $\bar{V}(m-1)$ includes the event $T > m$. hold. Here

$$H(\psi) = h(T \mid \bar{V}(K), \bar{A}_1(K), \psi),$$

and f_0 is the density of T_0.

The orthogonal complement $T_{nuis,r}^\perp$ of the nuisance tangent space of ψ is given by

$$\overline{\left\{ \sum_{m=1}^{int(T)} h(\mathcal{F}_m) - E_{G^*}(h(\mathcal{F}_m) \mid \bar{V}(m), \bar{A}_1(m-1), H(\psi)) : h \right\}}, \tag{6.34}$$

where $\mathcal{F}_m \equiv (\bar{V}(m), \bar{A}_1(m), H)$, and $H = H(\psi_0)$ with ψ_0 the true value of ψ.

The projection operator on this space is given as follows. For $D(H, \bar{A}_1(K), \bar{V}(K)) \in L_0^2(P_{F_X,G})$, we have

$$\Pi(D \mid T_{nuis,r}^\perp) = \sum_{m=1}^{int(T)} E(D \mid \bar{V}(m), \bar{A}_1(m), H) - E(D \mid \bar{V}(m), \bar{A}_1(m-1), H).$$

Let

$$S_\psi(Y_r) = \frac{d}{d\psi} \log \left(d/dT H(\psi) \prod_{m=1}^{int(T)} f(V(m) \mid \bar{V}(m-1), \bar{A}_1(m-1), H(\psi)) \right)$$

be the score of ψ (note that $\bar{V}(m-1)$ includes $T > m$). The efficient score is thus given by

$$\Pi(S_\psi \mid T_{nuis,r}^\perp) = \sum_{m=1}^{int(T)} E(S_\psi \mid \mathcal{F}_m) - E(S_\psi \mid \bar{V}(m), \bar{A}_1(m-1), H).$$

Consider now the model $\mathcal{M}(\mathcal{G}^*)$ for the distribution of Y_r. Let

$$T_{SRA}^* = \overline{\left\{ \sum_{m=1}^{int(T)} h(\bar{A}(m), \bar{V}(m)) - E_{G^*}(h \mid \bar{A}(m-1), \bar{V}(m)) : h \right\}}$$

be the tangent space of G in this model. We have that the orthogonal complement of the nuisance tangent space in this model is given by:

$$T_{nuis,r}^\perp(\mathcal{M}(\mathcal{G}^*)) = T_{nuis,r}^\perp - \Pi(T_{nuis,r}^\perp \mid T_{SRA}^*)$$

(i.e., subtract from each element in $T_{nuis,r}^\perp$ its projection on T_{SRA}^* and take the closure of the linear span of all of these elements).

6.5. Structural Nested Model with Right-Censoring

We have for $D(H, \bar{A}_1(int(T)), \bar{V}(int(T))) \in L_0^2(P_{F_X,G})$

$$\Pi(D \mid T^{\perp}_{nuis,r}(\mathcal{M}(\mathcal{G}^*))) =$$
$$\sum_{m=1}^{int(T)} D_m - \{E(D_m \mid \bar{A}_1(m), \bar{V}(m)) - E(D_m \mid \bar{A}_1(m-1), \bar{V}(m))\},$$

where

$$D_m = E(D \mid \bar{V}(m), \bar{A}_1(m), H) - E(D \mid \bar{V}(m), \bar{A}_1(m-1), H).$$

This gives us also a representation of $T^{\perp}_{nuis,r}(\mathcal{M}(\mathcal{G}^*))$:

$$T^{\perp}_{nuis,r}(\mathcal{G}^*) = \left\{ \sum_{m=1}^{int(T)} h(\bar{V}(m), \bar{A}_1(m), H) - E(h \mid \bar{V}(m), \bar{A}_1(m)) : h \right\}$$
$$- \left\{ \sum_{m=1}^{int(T)} E(h \mid \bar{V}(m), \bar{A}_1(m-1), H). - E(h \mid \bar{V}(m), \bar{A}_1(m-1)) : h \right\} \quad (6.35)$$

We give here a proof that is easy to understand and provides further insight in the structural nested model.

Proof. Let $A(m) = A_1(m)$ in this proof. We take the likelihood (6.33) as the starting point. Firstly, consider the nonparametric likelihood

$$f_0(H) \prod_{m=1}^{K} f(V(m) \mid \bar{A}(m-1), \bar{V}(m-1), H) f(A(m) \mid \bar{A}(m-1), \bar{V}(m), H),$$

where $H = H(\psi)$. Recall $\bar{V}(m)$ includes $\bar{Y}(m)$, where $Y(m) = I(T \leq m)$. The products run from $m = 1, \ldots, int(T)$ because the conditional distributions are degenerate for $m \geq T$: i.e. after time T the processes stay constant. If we put no constraints on any of these conditional distributions, then this is a completely nonparametric model for the distribution of $(H(\psi), \bar{V}(T), \bar{A}(T))$. It is of interest to note that our model likelihood (6.33) differs from the nonparametric likelihood only by imposing the constraints

$$f(A(m) \mid \bar{A}(m-1), \bar{V}(m), H(\psi)) = f(A(m) \mid \bar{A}(m-1), \bar{V}(m)),$$

$m = 1, \ldots, int(T)$, which gives us a sense of where our information for ψ comes from: one needs to choose ψ so that $H(\psi)$ is independent of $A(m)$ given the past $\bar{A}(m-1), \bar{V}(m)$. The tangent space for the nonparametric likelihood is $L_0^2(P_{F_X,G^*})$, and it is the orthogonal sum (by factorization of the likelihood) of the tangent spaces corresponding with the $2K+1$ factors

$$L_0^2(P_{F_X,G}) = H_0 \oplus \sum_{m=1}^{K} H_{1m} \oplus \sum_{m=1}^{K} H_{2m},$$

where

$$H_0 = L_0^2(F_0),$$
$$H_{1m} = \{h(\bar{V}(m), \bar{A}(m-1), H) - E(h \mid \bar{V}(m-1), \bar{A}(m-1), H) : h\},$$
$$H_{2m} = \{h(\bar{V}(m), \bar{A}(m), H) - E(h \mid \bar{V}(m), \bar{A}(m-1), H) : h\}.$$

Here we note that these functions equal zero for $m > int(T)$. Given a $D \in L_0^2(P_{F_X,G})$, we have a corresponding decomposition $D = D_0 + \sum_m D_{1m} + \sum_m D_{2m}$, where these projections on the subspaces H_0, H_{1m}, H_{2m} are given by:

$$D_0 = \Pi(D \mid H_0) = E(D \mid H),$$
$$D_{1m} = \Pi(D \mid H_{1m})$$
$$= E(D \mid \bar{V}(m), \bar{A}(m-1), H) - E(D \mid \bar{V}(m-1), \bar{A}(m-1), H),$$
$$D_{2m} = \Pi(D \mid H_{2m})$$
$$= E(D \mid \bar{V}(m), \bar{A}(m), H) - E(D \mid \bar{V}(m), \bar{A}(m-1), H).$$

From the likelihood (6.33), it follows that the nuisance tangent space $T_{nuis,r}(G^*)$ for G^* known and the nuisance tangent space $T_{nuis,r}(\mathcal{G}^*)$ for G^* unknown are given by

$$T_{nuis,r}(G^*) = H_0 \oplus \sum_{m=1}^{K} H_{1m},$$
$$T_{nuis,r}(\mathcal{G}^*) = H_0 \oplus \sum_{m=1}^{K} H_{1m} \oplus \sum_{m=1}^{K} H_{2m}^*,$$

where

$$H_{2m}^* \equiv \{h(\bar{V}(m), \bar{A}(m)) - E(h \mid \bar{V}(m), \bar{A}(m-1)) : h\} \subset H_{2m}$$

are subspaces of H_{2m}, $m = 1, \ldots, K$. It follows now that

$$D - \Pi(D \mid T_{nuis,r}(G^*)) = D_0 + \sum_m D_{1m} + \sum_m D_{2m} - \left(D_0 + \sum_{m=1}^{K} D_{1m}\right)$$
$$= \sum_m D_{2m},$$

which proves all statements about the model with G^* known. Similarly,

$$D - \Pi(D \mid T_{nuis,r}(\mathcal{G}^*)) = D_0 + \sum_{m=1} D_{1m} + \sum_{m=1} D_{2m}$$
$$- \left(D_0 + \sum_{m=1} D_{1m} + \sum_{m=1} \Pi(D_{2m} \mid H_{2m}^*)\right)$$
$$= \sum_{m=1}^{int(T)} D_{2m} - (E(D_{2m} \mid \bar{A}(m), \bar{V}(m)) - E(D_{2m} \mid \bar{A}(m-1), \bar{V}(m))),$$

which proves the last statement. □

The class of estimating functions (6.34) indexed by h provides the class of all estimating functions, including the optimal estimating function, for model $\mathcal{M}(\mathcal{G}^*)$. The optimal choice is obtained by setting h equal to

$$h^*_{opt,m} = E\left(S_\psi(\bar{V}, \bar{A}_1) \mid \bar{V}(m), \bar{A}_1(m), H(\psi)\right). \tag{6.36}$$

The class of estimating functions (6.35) indexed by h is orthogonalized w.r.t. T_{SRA}, where T_{SRA} denotes the tangent space of the treatment mechanism under the assumption of SRA for the reduced uncensored data Y_r. Notice that these orthogonalized estimation functions are a subset of (6.34). Due to the orthogonality, the estimating functions in (6.35) are doubly robust in the sense that they are unbiased if either the treatment mechanism G^* is correctly specified or the conditional expectations over $H(\psi)$, given observed pasts, are consistently estimated. Consequently, these estimating functions for ψ can be used to construct doubly robust estimators based on the reduced uncensored data. For example, the choice $h(H, \bar{A}_1(m), \bar{V}(m)) = A_1(m)H$ yields the estimating function

$$\sum_{m=1}^{int(T)} \{H - E(H \mid \bar{A}_1(m), \bar{V}(m))\}\{A_1(m) - E_{G^*}(A_1(m) \mid \bar{A}_1(m-1), \bar{V}(m))\},$$

where $E(H(\psi) \mid \bar{A}_1(m), \bar{V}(m)) = E(H(\psi) \mid \bar{A}_1(m-1), \bar{V}(m))$ at the true parameter value ψ. Note that indeed this estimating function for ψ based on the reduced data remains unbiased if only one of the two nuisance parameters $E(H(\Psi) \mid \bar{A}(m-1), \bar{V}(m))$ and G^* is misspecified. It is trivial to see, by conditioning on $\bar{A}_1(m), \bar{V}(m)$, that the estimating function is unbiased if $E(H(\Psi) \mid \bar{A}(m-1), \bar{V}(m))$ is correctly specified. At correctly specified G^*, first condition on $\bar{A}_1(m), \bar{V}(m)$ and then notice that $E(H(\psi) \mid \bar{A}_1(m), \bar{V}(m))$ does not depend on $A_1(m)$.

6.5.2 A class of estimating functions for the marginal structural nested model

We will derive a class of estimating functions in our model $\mathcal{M}(\mathcal{G})$ in terms of $T^\perp_{nuis,r}$. Given $g \in \mathcal{G}$, let $g^*(g)$ be an element in $\mathcal{G}^*$ close to g in some sense. In Subsection 2.3.4 in Chapter 2, we introduced the general method (2.22) of inverse weighting a class of estimating functions whose conditional expectation w.r.t. a special censoring mechanism G^* maps into $T^{F,\perp}_{nuis}(F_X)$ (i.e., these might be estimating functions developed under a restricted censoring model). Applying this method to the class of estimating functions $T^\perp_{nuis,r}$ developed under SRA w.r.t. the collapsed data, yields the following mapping into observed data estimating functions $IC_0(Y \mid G, \psi, h)$:

$$\left\{ \sum_{m=1}^{int(T)} h(\mathcal{F}_m) - E_{G^*}(h(\mathcal{F}_m) \mid \bar{V}(m), \bar{A}_1(m-1), H) \right\} W. \tag{6.37}$$

Here $\mathcal{F}_m \equiv (H, \bar{A}_1(m), \bar{V}(m))$, and

$$\begin{aligned}
W &= W(G) \\
&\equiv \frac{g^*(\bar{A}_1, \bar{A}_2 = 0 \mid X)}{g(\bar{A}_1, \bar{A}_2 = 0 \mid X)} \\
&= I(C \geq T) \frac{\prod_{j=1}^{\min(C,T-1)} g_1^*(A_1(j) \mid A_2(j), \bar{A}(j-1), \bar{V}(j))}{\prod_{j=1}^{\min(C,T-1)} g_1(A_1(j) \mid \mathcal{F}_1(j)) g_2(A_2(j) = 0 \mid \mathcal{F}_2(j))},
\end{aligned}$$

is the Radon–Nykodym derivative of G^* w.r.t. G.

If we make the strong identifiability assumption that $\max_{\bar{a}_1} g^*(\bar{a}_1, \bar{A}_2 = 0 \mid X)/g(\bar{a}_1, \bar{A}_2 = 0 \mid X) < \infty$ F_X-a.e., then we have $h \to E_G(IC_0(Y \mid G, \psi, h) \mid X)$ maps into $E(T_{nuis,r}^{\perp} \mid X) \subset T_{nuis}^{F,\perp}(F_X)$ for all indices h. Because $T_{nuis,r}^{\perp}$ is the orthogonal complement of the nuisance tangent space in the structural nested model for the collapsed data, one expects to have

$$E(T_{nuis,r}^{\perp} \mid X) = T_{nuis}^{F,\perp}(F_X). \tag{6.38}$$

If (6.38) holds, then application of Theorem 1.3 teaches us that the orthogonal complement of the nuisance tangent space in the observed data model $\mathcal{M}(CAR)$ can be represented as $\{IC_0(\cdot \mid G, h) - \Pi(IC_0 \mid T_{CAR}) : h\}$, where T_{CAR} equals T_{SRA} for this particular data structure. This onto conjecture (6.38) is shown to hold in van der Laan, Murphy, Robins (2002).

It therefore remains to find the projection onto T_{SRA} for our observed data structure. By simply applying Theorem 1.2, we derived the projection of $IC_0(Y)$ onto $T_{SRA} = T_{CAR}$ in the previous example

$$\begin{aligned}
\Pi(IC_0 \mid T_{SRA}) &= \sum_{j=1}^{C} E(IC_0(Y) \mid A_1(j), \mathcal{F}_1(j)) \\
&\quad - \sum_{j=1}^{C} \sum_{a_1(j)} E(IC_0(Y) \mid a_1(j), \mathcal{F}_1(j)) g_1(a_1(j) \mid \mathcal{F}_1(j)) \\
&\quad - \sum_{j=1}^{C} E(IC_0(Y) \mid C > j, \mathcal{F}_2(j)) dM_2(j) \\
&\equiv IC_{SRA}(Y \mid Q, G),
\end{aligned}$$

where we define $Q_1(j, \mathcal{F}_1(j)) = E(IC_0(Y) \mid A_1(j), \mathcal{F}_1(j))$, $Q_2(j, \mathcal{F}_2(j)) = E(IC_0(Y) \mid C > j, \mathcal{F}_2(j))$, and let $Q = (Q_1, Q_2)$ denote both of these parameters. We can now define the desired optimal mapping into observed data estimating functions for ψ indexed by nuisance parameters Q and G:

$$IC(Y \mid Q, G, \psi, h) = IC_0(Y \mid G, \psi, h) - IC_{SRA}(Y \mid Q, G).$$

We propose to set h_n equal to an estimator of h_{opt}^* (6.36). The score S_ψ can be estimated by assuming parametric models for the conditional covariate distributions, and h_{opt}^* can be estimated by regressing this estimated score on covariates extracted from the past and time j. In order to deal with the right-censoring, we can apply inverse probability of censoring weighting, provided $Pr[C \geq T \mid X] \geq 0$ with probability 1. This latter condition will fail when there is administrative censoring by end of follow up before all individuals have died. In that case, one wants to treat the processes up till artificial censoring as full data structure and use the "artificial censoring" methods as described in Robins (1992) to modify the estimating functions so that they still identify the parameter of interest ψ.

6.5.3 Analyzing dynamic treatment regimes

In the following, we would replace ψ by an estimator ψ_n as proposed above. We wish to compute by **Monte Carlo** simulation $F_{\bar{d}}(t)$ using the formula (6.32). Firstly, we note that this formula (6.32) equals the F_X-parameter $1 - F_{\bar{d}}(t)$ under the data generating distribution $P_{F_X, G^*} \in \mathcal{M}(\mathcal{G}^*)$ in the structural nested model $\mathcal{M}(\mathcal{G}^*)$ for the reduced data structure $Y_r \equiv (\bar{Y}_{A_1}, \bar{V}_{A_1}, \bar{A}_1)$ (where P_{F_X, G^*} is defined by replacing the G-part of the true data generating distribution $dP_{F_X, G}$ by a G^* which is only a function of V, and assuming SRA w.r.t. V, but leaving the full-data distribution F_X unchanged). Thus we need to estimate

$$\prod_{m=1}^{int(T)} dF(V(m) \mid T > m, \bar{V}(m-1), \bar{A}(m-1) = \bar{d}_m(\bar{V}(m-1)), H(\psi_0)),$$

where $dF(\cdot \mid \cdot)$ denotes the conditional distribution of $V(j)$, given the past and $H(\psi_0)$, corresponding to the distribution P_{F_X, G^*}. For the purpose of clarity, let us first consider the case where there is no censoring. If one assumes a parametric model $dF_\theta(V(m) \mid \bar{V}(m-1), \bar{A}(m-1), H(\psi))$ for this conditional probability, then the score functions w.r.t. θ corresponding with the likelihood $\prod_i dF_\theta(V_i(m) \mid T_i > m, \bar{V}_i(m-1), \bar{A}_i(m-1), H(\psi))$ are unbiased estimating functions for θ under P_{F_X, G^*}. As shown above (see (6.37)), multiplying these scores with the inverse probability of treatment weights $W(G) = dG(Y \mid X)/dG^*(Y \mid X)$ now results in unbiased observed data estimating functions for θ under the true data generating distribution $P_{F_X, G}$. In other words, one can estimate θ with standard maximum likelihood methods by assigning weights W_i to each subject i, $i = 1, \ldots, n$.

Similarly, $(I(H(\psi) \leq t) - F_0(t))W(G)$ is an unbiased estimating function for $F_0(t)$ in model $\mathcal{M}(\mathcal{G})$. Finally, to deal with the right-censoring, one needs to inverse weight by $I(C_i > k)/\widehat{P}(C > k \mid X)$ (i.e., the probability of being uncensored), as in Chapter 3. For a simulation study and data analysis of a longitudinal study using these estimates of dynamic treatment-regime specific survival functions see Aiyou, and van der Laan (2002).

6.5.4 Simulation for dynamic regimes in point treatment studies

Dynamic treatment regimes already have nice applications in point treatment studies, where one is interested in determining the optimal way of assigning treatment at baseline based on some pretreatment variables. Suppose that we observe on each randomly sampled subject a treatment A, a survival time T, and pretreatment covariates (V, L). Our data consist of n i.i.d. observations (A_i, V_i, L_i, T_i), $i = 1, \ldots, n$. The full data structure $X = ((T_a, a), V, L)$ is the vector of treatment-specific survival times and the baseline covariates V, L, while the observed data structure (A, V, L, T_A) is a missing data structure on this full data structure. We assume that A is randomized w.r.t. V, L: $P(A = a \mid X) = P(A = a \mid V, L)$. Consider as the full data model the structural nested model that assumes that

$$T_0 = h(T_a, V, L) \equiv T_a \exp\{a(\psi_1 + \psi_2 * V + \psi_3 * L)\} \text{ in distribution.}$$

(Note that $H(\psi) = h(T, V, L)$.) This corresponds with the following model for the quantile-quantile function $F_{T_0}(F_{T_a}^{-1}(\cdot \mid V, L) \mid V, L)$,

$$\gamma_j(t \mid V, L, a) = t + (\min(t, t_{j+1}) - t_j) \times \\ (\exp(a\{\psi_1 + \psi_2 * V + \psi_3 * L\} - 1)),$$

where $t_1, \ldots, t_K$ is a fine partition of $[0, \infty)$. We could have assumed a marginal structural nested model by only including V in the blip function and thus $h(cdot)$, which would be an appropriate model if one is only concerned with estimating dynamic treatment regimes that are based only on V.

In this subsection, we will simulate data from the model above and estimate (ψ_1, ψ_2, ψ_3) and five treatment-specific survival curves of T_d corresponding with dynamic treatment regimes $d(V, L)$ that are functions of V and L. We will consider the treatment regimes always control, always treatment, $A = 1$ iff $V > 0$ and $L > 5$, $A = 1$ iff $f(V, L) < 0$, and $A = 1$ iff $f(V, L) > 0$, where $f(V, L)$ is the linear form in the blip function with ψ replaced by its estimator ψ_n. Notice that the fourth dynamic treatment regime is an optimal treatment regime, given the model. The fact that the optimal dynamic treatment regime is defined by the blip function is a particularly nice fact for dynamic treatment regimes for point treatments.

We simulate from this structural nested model as follows. Let T_0 follow an exponential distribution with mean λ, where we set $\lambda = 5$. Suppose that (V, L), given T_0, follows a bivariate normal distribution with mean vector (μ_V, μ_L), where $\mu_V = \alpha_{11} + \alpha_{12} T_0$ and $\mu_L = \alpha_{21} + \alpha_{22} T_0$. We set $\alpha = [-0.1, 5; 0.01, 0.01]$. The covariance matrix is defined by the three parameters $(\sigma_v, \sigma_L, \rho)$, which are set equal to $(1, 5, 0.5)$. Subsequently, we draw the treatment variable $A \in \{0, 1\}$ from a Bernoulli distribution with

$$\text{logit} Pr(A = 1 \mid V, L, T_0) = \beta_0 + \beta_1 V + \beta_2 L,$$

where $\beta = [-0.1, 0.1, 0.1]$. Finally, the observed survival time T is decided by the blip-up operator defined by

$$T_0 = \int_0^T \exp\{A(\psi_1 + \psi_2 v + \psi_3 L)\},$$

where $\psi = [-0.3, 0.2, 0.1]$.

Our estimating function corresponds with the index $h(\bar{A}(m), \bar{V}(m), H(\psi)) = A(m)H(\psi)$. We assume correctly a logistic regression model for $P(A = 1 \mid V, L)$, and we assume a normal distribution for $P(V \mid L, T_0)$ and $P(L \mid T_0)$ with mean linear in the conditioning covariates, which we estimate with linear regression. The five true survival curves are given in Figure 6.3. As we see, it is indeed the case that the dynamic treatment regime $A = 1$ iff $f(V, L) < 0$ is the best, but the differences are not dramatic. It is of interest to see if one can still distinguish these survival curves based on data.

For sample size $n = 500$, our estimate of ψ is given by $\hat{\psi} = (-0.35, 0.20, 0.12)$, and our estimated standard errors are $SE(\hat{\psi}) = (0.14, 0.09, 0.02)$. The estimated survival curves of the five different regimes are given in Figure 6.4. We see that the estimated survival curves are close to the true survival curves and are, in particular, ordered correctly.

Figure 6.3. Estimated survival curves in simulation of Structural Nested model I on one point-time regime, where $f(v, L) = \hat{\psi}_1 + \hat{\psi}_2 v + \hat{\psi}_3 L$, and sample size=500.

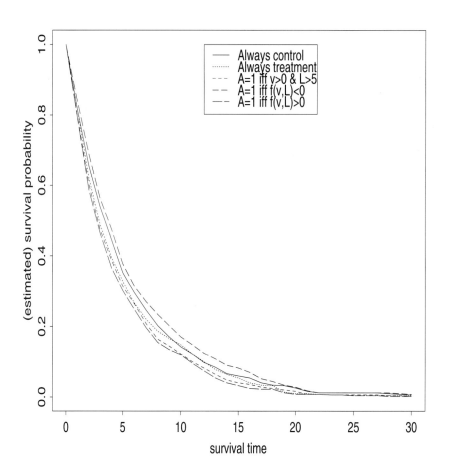

6.6 Right-Censoring with Missingness.

Let $X(t) = (Z(t), E(t), E^*(t), V(t), V^*(t))$, where $Z(t)$ represents an outcome process (such as lung function at time t), $E(t)$ represents true exposure such as personally monitored air pollution, $E^*(t)$ represents a surrogate for this true exposure, such as air pollution exposure calculated from measurements at fixed central monitoring stations in the area, $V(t)$ are covariates that one wants to adjust for when estimating the effect of true exposure on the outcome, and $V^*(t)$ includes other measured covariates. Let T be some endpoint, either fixed or random, and let the full data be $X = \bar{X}(T)$.

Figure 6.4. true survival curves in simulation of structural nested model I on one point-time regime, where $f(v, L) = \psi_1 + \psi_2 v + \psi_3 L$ and sample size=500.

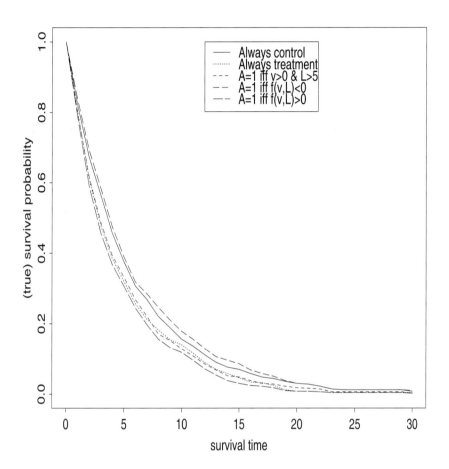

In this example, we consider the situation where the true exposure E is only measured on a subset of the subjects and, as usual, there is also right-censoring. Let ξ be the indicator that the process E is not observed, and let C be the follow-up time of the subject, where $C = \infty$ if $C > T$. Let $X^-(t) = (Z(t), E^*(t), V(t), V^*(t))$. The observed data structure is $Y = (C, \xi, \xi \bar{X}^-(C) + (1-\xi)\bar{X}(C))$.

Given a full data model $\mathcal{M}^F$, let μ be a full data parameter of interest, and let $\{D_h(X \mid \mu, \rho) : h\}$ be a class of full data estimating functions. For example, if time is discrete at $j = 1, \ldots, T$, T being fixed, then the full data model could be the multivariate regression model

$$E(Z_j \mid X^*) = m_j(X^* \mid \beta),$$

where $X^*(t) = (E(t), V(t))$ and $m_j(X^* \mid \beta) = m_j(\bar{X}^*(j) \mid \beta)$ only depends on X^* through $\bar{X}^*(j)$, $j = 1, \ldots, T$. In this case, the full data estimating functions are $\{h(X^*)\epsilon(\beta) : h\}$, where $\epsilon(\beta) = Z - m(X^* \mid \beta)$. If Z_j is a discrete variable, then one could assume a multinomial logistic regression model for $P(Z_j = m \mid \bar{X}^*(j))$ and model the effect of time $t = j$ parametrically. In this case the likelihood for the full data model is a product over time of these multinomial probabilities so that (as in the previous example) the full data estimating functions are sums over time j of unbiased j-specific estimating functions.

Let $A(0) = \xi$ and $A(t) = I(C \leq t)$; then, the censoring process is completely identified by $A = (A(t) : t)$ so that the observed data are a function of X and A. Let $\mathcal{F}(t) = (\bar{A}(t-), \bar{X}_{\bar{A}}(t))$, and let $W = X(0)$ be the baseline covariates measured on each subject. We will assume SRA (i.e., $A(t)$ is independent of X, given $\mathcal{F}(t)$). In that case we have that the conditional density of $\bar{A}$, given X, is given by the partial likelihood of $A(t)$ w.r.t. history $\mathcal{F}(t)$,

$$\begin{aligned}
g(\bar{A} \mid X) &= P(A(0) = 1 \mid W)^{A(0)} \{1 - P(A(0) = 1 \mid W)\}^{1-A(0)} \\
&\quad \times \prod_{t>0} E(dA(t) \mid \mathcal{F}(t))^{dA(t)} \{1 - E(dA(t) \mid \mathcal{F}(t))\}^{1-dA(t)} \\
&= \left\{ \prod_{t>0} \alpha_1(dt)^{dA(t)} \{1 - \alpha_1(dt)\}^{1-dA(t)} \right\}^{A(0)} \\
&\quad \times \left\{ \prod_{t>0} \alpha_0(dt)^{dA(t)} \{1 - \alpha_0(dt)\}^{1-dA(t)} \right\}^{1-A(0)},
\end{aligned}$$

where

$$\begin{aligned}
\alpha_1(dt) &= E(dA(t) \mid A(0) = 1, \bar{X}^-(t)) = I(C \geq t)\Lambda_1(dt \mid \bar{X}^-(t)), \\
\alpha_0(dt) &= E(dA(t) \mid A(0) = 0, \bar{X}(t)) = I(C \geq t)\Lambda_0(dt \mid \bar{X}(t)).
\end{aligned}$$

Here $\Lambda_1(dt \mid \bar{X}^-(t)) = P(C \in dt \mid C \geq t, A(0) = 1, \bar{X}^-(t))$ and $\Lambda_0(dt \mid \bar{X}(t)) = P(C \in dt \mid C \geq t, A(0) = 0, \bar{X}(t))$.

Since SRA implies CAR, we have that the density of Y factorizes in an F_X and a G part, with the G part being $g(\bar{A} \mid X)$. As mentioned in Section 1, the maximum likelihood estimator can be obtained with standard S-plus functions Coxph() (Cox proportional hazards) or Glm() (logistic regression). The observed data tangent space T_{SRA} generated by the parameter $g(\bar{A} \mid X)$ when only assuming SRA is the space of scores spanned by the scores $\frac{d}{d\epsilon} \log(g_\epsilon(A \mid X))$ of all possible one-dimensional submodels $g_\epsilon(A \mid X)$. It is straightforward to show

$$\begin{aligned}
T_{SRA} &= \overline{\{V(A(0), W) - E(V(A(0), W) \mid W) : V\}} \\
&\oplus \overline{\left\{ \int H(t, \mathcal{F}(t)) dM_C(t) : H \right\}},
\end{aligned}$$

where $dM_C(t) = dA(t) - E(dA(t) \mid \mathcal{F}(t))$. The projection $\Pi(V \mid T_{SRA})$ of a function V onto T_{SRA} is given by

$$\{E(V \mid A(0) = 1, W) - E(V \mid A(0) = 0, W)\}(A(0) - P(A(0) = 1 \mid W))$$
$$+ \int \{E(V \mid C = t, \mathcal{F}(t)) - E(V \mid C > t, \mathcal{F}(t))\} dM_C(t).$$

Given a full data estimating function $D_h(X \mid \mu, \rho)$ for μ, we can define an IPCW observed data estimating function by

$$IC_0(Y \mid G, D_h) = D_h(X \mid \mu, \rho) \frac{I(C > T, A(0) = 0)}{\bar{G}_0(T \mid X)},$$

where

$$\begin{aligned}
\bar{G}_0(c \mid X) &\equiv P(C > c, A(0) = 0 \mid X) \\
&= P(\bar{A}(c) = 0 \mid X) \\
&= P(A(0) = 0 \mid W) \prod_{t \leq c} P(A(t) = 0 \mid A(0) = 1, \mathcal{F}(t)) \\
&= (1 - \Pi(W)) \exp\left(-\int_0^c \alpha_0(dt)\right).
\end{aligned}$$

Thus, an estimate of the intensities α_0, α_1 provides us, in particular, with an estimate of this denominator.

For this choice of IPCW-mapping $IC_0(Y) = IC_0(Y \mid G, D)$, the projection of IC_0 onto T_{SRA} is given by

$$\begin{aligned}
IC_{SRA} &= -E(IC_0(Y) \mid A(0) = 0, W)\{A(0) - P(A(0) = 1 \mid W)\} \\
&\quad - \int E(IC_0(Y) \mid C > t, \mathcal{F}(t)) dM_C(t).
\end{aligned}$$

Thus G-orthogonalized IPCW estimating functions are given by

$$\begin{aligned}
IC(Y \mid Q, G, D_h) &= IC_0(Y \mid G, D) + E(IC_0(Y \mid G, D) \mid A(0) = 0, W) \\
&\quad + \int E(IC_0(Y \mid G, D) \mid C > t, A(0) = 0, \mathcal{F}(t)) dM_C(t),
\end{aligned}$$

where $Q = Q(F_X, G)$ has components Q_0, Q_1 defined by

$$\begin{aligned}
Q_0(W) &\equiv E(IC_0(Y \mid G, D) \mid A(0) = 0, W \\
&= \frac{1}{1 - \Pi(W)} E(D(X) \mid W) \\
Q_1(t, \mathcal{F}(t)) &\equiv E(IC_0(Y \mid G, D) \mid C > t, A(0) = 0, \mathcal{F}(t)) \\
&= \frac{1}{\bar{G}_0(t \mid X)} E(D(X) \mid \bar{X}(t)).
\end{aligned}$$

Given a full data index h_n, we can use $IC(Y \mid Q, G, D_{h_n}(\cdot \mid \mu, \rho))$ as an estimation function for μ with nuisance parameters Q, G, ρ, just as in our previous examples.

6.7 Interval Censored Data

Consider a study in which an event time T is of interest. Suppose that the event is not directly observable and that its status can only be observed at random monitoring times. Let $L(t)$ be a covariate process, and assume that this covariate process is also only measured at the random monitoring times. Let $X^*(t)$ be a process that is observed from the start of the study until a fixed (e.g., every subject is followed up for 5 years) or random (such as death) endpoint τ, where $I(\tau \leq t)$ is a component of $X^*(t)$. Thus $X^*(t)$ contains directly observable events such as death that are therefore not subject to interval censoring. Let $X^*(0)$ represent the baseline covariates. If we define $R(t) = I(T \leq t)$, then the full data process is $X(t) \equiv (R(t), L(t), X^*(t))$, and the full data structure is $X = \bar{X}(\tau)$. We redefine $X(t) = X(\min(t,\tau))$ to indicate that the process stops changing after time τ.

Define $A(t) = \sum_{j=1}^{M} I(C_j \leq t)$ as a process that jumps at each monitoring time, where we set $C_j = \infty$ if $C_j > \tau$. The observed data structure is

$$Y = (\bar{X}^*(\tau), C_1, X(C_1), \ldots, C_M, X(C_M)).$$

For any given realization $A = a$ with jump points $c_1 < \ldots < c_M$, we define X_a as $(X(c_1), \ldots, X(c_M))$. The observed data can then be represented as

$$Y = (\bar{A}, X_{\bar{A}}), \tag{6.39}$$

which means that we can apply the methodology presented in Section 6.1 of this chapter. At the end of this section, we will show how one can straightforwardly extend this data structure to also allow for informative right-censoring (e.g., τ is the minimum of the end of the study and an informative dropout time), but for clarity we will first only focus on the missingness due to a random monitoring scheme $(C_1, \ldots, C_M)$.

The distribution of Y is indexed by the full data distribution F_X and the conditional distribution of $\bar{A}$, given X. Let $\mathcal{M}^F$ be a full data model, and let $\mu = \mu(F_X)$ be the parameter of interest. For example, the full data model might be nonparametric and $\mu = \int r(t)\{1 - F(t)\}dt$. Other examples are $\log(T) = \beta Z + \epsilon$, where $E(K(\epsilon(\beta)) \mid Z) = 0$ for some given monotone function K, and the Cox proportional hazards model $\lambda_{T|Z}(t \mid Z) = \lambda_0(t)\exp(\beta Z)$. For each of these models, the class of full data estimating functions is known and given in Section 2.2 of Chapter 2. Let $\{D_h(T, Z \mid \mu) : h\}$ denote this set of full data estimating functions for μ, where we assume $D_h(T, Z) = D_h(\min(T, \tau), Z)$.

Let $\mathcal{F}(t) = (\bar{A}(t-), \bar{X}_A(t))$ represent the history observed at time t. We model $g(A \mid X)$ with the partial likelihood of A w.r.t. history $\mathcal{F}(t)$,

$$g(\bar{A} \mid X) = \prod_t \lambda_A(t \mid X)^{\Delta A(t)} \prod_t (1 - \lambda_A(t \mid X))^{1-\Delta A(t)}, \tag{6.40}$$

where

$$\lambda_A(t \mid X) = E(dA(t) \mid \mathcal{F}(t))$$

is the intensity of A w.r.t. $\mathcal{F}(t)$, which can be defined for continuous $A(t)$ and discrete $A(t)$ that only jump at prespecified points $t_1, \ldots, t_K$. The partial likelihood assumption (6.40) is the continuous analog of SRA on a discrete action mechanism in longitudinal studies. As explained previously, the partial likelihood assumption is stronger than assuming CAR. We denote the t-specific term in the product integral with $g(A(t) \mid \bar{A}(t), X)$ so that $g(\bar{A} \mid X) = \prod_t g(A(t) \mid \bar{A}(t), X)$.

If $A(t)$ is continuous, then we can assume a multiplicative intensity model

$$\lambda_A(t \mid X) = Y^*(t)\lambda_0(t)\exp(\beta W(t)),$$

where $Y^*(t) = I(A(t)$ is at risk of jumping$)$ and $W(t)$ are functions of the observed past $\mathcal{F}(t)$. For discrete $A(t)$, a logistic regression model $Y^*(t)/(1 + \exp(\beta_0(t) + \beta_1 W(t)))$ can be assumed. These models can be fit with maximum likelihood estimation using standard software, as noted in Section 6.1.

We will assume that $\lambda_A(t \mid X) > 0$ on each $t \in [a, \tau]$ with $D'(t, Z) > 0$ F_X-a.e., where a is the left point of the support of $\lambda_A(t \mid X)$. This left support point a is allowed to depend on the always observed covariates $\bar{X}^*(\tau)$. Thus, it is sufficient if subjects are always at risk of being monitored up to the endpoint τ, but if one assumes a smooth-median or truncated mean regression model $\log(T) = \beta Z + \epsilon$ so that $D'(t, Z)$ will be equal to zero outside a sub nterval of $[a, \tau]$, then one does not necessarily need to monitor the whole support of T (see also Section 4.4 in Chapter 4). We will now propose the initial mapping $D_h \to IC_0(Y \mid G, D_h)$ into observed data estimating functions

$$IC_0(Y \mid G, D) \equiv \sum_{j=1}^{M} \frac{D'(C_j, Z)(1 - \Delta_j)}{\lambda_A(C_j \mid X)} + D(a, Z), \qquad (6.41)$$

where $D'(t, Z) = d/dt D(t/Z)$ if A is continuous. If $A(t)$ is a counting process that can only jump at fixed time points $t_0, t_1, \ldots$, then one should replace $D'(t_k, Z)$ by $D(t_{k+1}, Z) - D(t_k, Z)$. Since IC_0 only sums up monitoring times $C_j < T < \tau$, it only involves a summation over observed monitoring times. By SRA, we also have that $\lambda_A(C_j \mid X)$ depends on X and $\bar{A}(C_j-)$ only through the observed history $\mathcal{F}(C_j)$. Thus, it follows that IC_0 is indeed a function of the observed data Y.

We will now prove that this mapping indeed satisfies $E(IC_0(Y \mid G, D) \mid X) = D(X)$. Consider the case where A is a continuous process. One can imitate the proof for the case where A is discrete and $D'(C, Z) = 0$ between the support points of A. We have $A(t) = \sum_{j=1}^{M} A_j(t)$, where $A_j(t) \equiv I(C_j \leq t)$. Let $\lambda_{A,j}(t \mid X)$ be the intensity of $A_j(t)$ w.r.t. $\mathcal{F}(t)$ so that $\lambda_A(t \mid X) =$

$\sum_{j=1}^{M} \lambda_{A,j}(t \mid X)$. It now follows that

$$
\begin{aligned}
E(IC_0(Y \mid G, D) \mid X) &= \sum_{j=1}^{M} \int_0^T D'(t, Z) \frac{\lambda_{A,j}(t \mid X)}{\lambda_A(t \mid X)} I(\lambda_A(t) > 0) dt \\
&\quad + D(a, Z) \\
&= \int_0^T D'(t, Z) I(\lambda_A(t) > 0) dt + D(a, Z) \\
&= \int_a^{\min(b,T)} D'(t, Z) dt + D(a, Z) \\
&= D(\min(b, T), Z) = D(T, Z). \qquad (6.42)
\end{aligned}
$$

To orthogonalize this initial class of observed data estimating functions, we note that $\Pi(IC_0(Y) \mid T_{SRA})$ is given by

$$\int \{E(IC_0(Y) \mid dA(t) = 1, \mathcal{F}(t)) - E(IC_0(Y) \mid dA(t) = 0, \mathcal{F}(t))\} dM_A(t),$$

and $dM_A(t) = dA(t) - \lambda_A(t \mid X)$. This defines now the $\mathcal{G}(SRA)$-orthogonalized class of estimating functions $IC(Y \mid Q, G, D_h(\cdot \mid \mu, \rho))$, where the additional nuisance parameter Q is given by $Q(t, \mathcal{F}(t)) \equiv E(IC_0(Y \mid G, D) \mid A(t), \mathcal{F}(t))$. One can estimate β with the solution of the corresponding estimating equation $0 = \sum_i IC(Y_i \mid Q_n, G_n, D_h(\cdot \mid \mu, \rho_n))$, where Q can be directly estimated by regressing an estimate of $IC_0(Y \mid G, D)$ onto time t, $A(t)$ (or equivalently $dA(t)$) and functions of the past $\mathcal{F}(t)$. Given an estimate of this regression, one obtains an estimate of $E(IC_0(Y \mid G, D) \mid dA(t) = 1, \mathcal{F}(t))$ and $E(IC_0(Y \mid G, D) \mid dA(t) = 0, \mathcal{F}(t))$ by evaluating it at $t, dA(t) = 1, \mathcal{F}(t)$ and $t, dA(t) = 0, \mathcal{F}(t)$, respectively.

6.7.1 Interval censoring and right-censoring combined

We will now extend this methodology for interval censored data to also allow for right-censoring. Let C^* be a right-censoring time at which subjects drop out of the study, where we set $C^* = \infty$ if $C^* > \tau$. Let $A_m(t) = \sum_{j=1}^{M} I(C_j \leq t)$ be the monitoring process, and recall the representation (6.39) $Y = (A_m, X_{\bar{A}_m})$ of the interval censored data structure above which corresponded with observing $\bar{Y}(t) \equiv (\bar{A}_m(t), \bar{X}_{A_m}(t))$ over time $t \in [0, \tau]$. The right censored interval censored data structure can be represented as

$$Y_c \equiv (C^*, \bar{Y}(C^*)) = (C^*, \bar{A}_m(C^*), \bar{X}_{\bar{A}_m}(C^*)).$$

Let $A_c(t) = I(C^* \leq t)$ and $A(t) = (A_c(t), A_m(\min(t, C^*)))$ be the joint action process including right-censoring and monitoring actions; then, we can represent Y again as $Y = (A, X_A)$, where $\bar{X}_A(t) = \bar{X}_{\bar{A}_m}(\min(t, C^*))$. Thus, the distribution of Y is indexed by the full data distribution F_X and the conditional distribution of $\bar{A}$, given X. Let $\mathcal{M}^F$ be a full data model, and let $\mu = \mu(F_X)$ be the parameter of interest. Let $\{D_h(T, Z \mid \mu) : h\}$ denote the set of full data estimating functions for μ, where we assume $D_h(T, Z) = D_h(\min(T, \tau), Z)$.

Let $\mathcal{F}_c(t) \equiv (\bar{A}(t-), \bar{X}_A(t))$ and $\mathcal{F}_m(t) \equiv (A_c(t), \bar{A}(t-), \bar{X}_A(t))$. We model $g(\bar{A} \mid X)$ with the partial likelihood of A,

$$g(\bar{A} \mid X) = \prod_t \left[\lambda_c(t \mid \mathcal{F}_c(t))^{dA_c(t)}\{1 - \lambda_c(t \mid \mathcal{F}_c(t))\}^{1-dA_c(t)}\right.$$

$$\times \prod_t \left[\lambda_m(t \mid \mathcal{F}_m(t))^{dA_m(t)} \prod_t \{1 - \lambda_m(t \mid \mathcal{F}_m)\}^{1-dA_m(t)},\right.$$

where

$$\lambda_m(t \mid \mathcal{F}_m(t)) = E(dA_m(t) \mid \mathcal{F}_m(t))$$

is the intensity of A_m w.r.t. $\mathcal{F}_m(t)$ and

$$\lambda_c(t \mid \mathcal{F}_c(t)) = E(dA_c(t) \mid \mathcal{F}_c(t))$$

is the intensity of A_c w.r.t. $\mathcal{F}_c(t)$. Both intensities can be defined for continuous $A(t)$ and discrete $A(t)$, which can only jump at prespecified points $t_1, \ldots, t_K$. We denote the t-specific term in the product integral with $g(A(t) \mid \bar{A}(t-), X)$ so that $g(\bar{A} \mid X) = \prod_t g(A(t) \mid \bar{A}(t-), X)$.

Above, we already discussed modeling and estimating λ_m. If $A_c(t)$ is continuous, then we can assume a multiplicative intensity model

$$\lambda_c(t \mid \mathcal{F}_c(t)) = I(C \geq t, \tau \geq t)\lambda_0(t) \exp(\beta W(t)).$$

For discrete $A_c(t)$, we can assume a logistic regression model. These models can be fit by maximum likelihood estimation using standard software, as noted in Section 6.1.

We adapt (6.41) by inverse weighting with the probability of censoring

$$IC_0(Y \mid G, D) \equiv \left\{\sum_{j=1}^{M} \frac{D'(C_j, Z)(1 - \Delta_j)}{\lambda_A(C_j \mid X)} + D(a, Z)\right\} \frac{I(C^* > \tau)}{\bar{G}_c(\tau \mid \mathcal{F}_c(\tau))},$$

where

$$\bar{G}_c(\tau \mid \mathcal{F}_c(\tau)) \equiv \prod_{t \in [0,\tau]} (1 - \Lambda_c(dt \mid \mathcal{F}_c(t)))$$

and Λ_c is the cumulative intensity corresponding with λ_c. Alternative inverse weighting schemes (e.g., within the summation) as provided in Chapter 3 are also available. If $A(t)$ is a counting process that can only jump at fixed time points $t_0, t_1, \ldots$, then one should replace $D'(t_k, Z)$ by $D(t_k, Z) - D(t_{k-1}, Z)$. As above, it follows that IC_0 is indeed a function of the observed data Y. We now also need to assume, in addition to the assumptions made on λ_m in the previous subsection, that $\bar{G}_c(\tau \mid \mathcal{F}_c(\tau)) > \delta >$

0 F_X-a.e. By first conditioning on $(X, \bar{A}_m)$ and subsequently imitating the proof (6.42) above, it follows that indeed $E(IC_0(Y \mid G, D) \mid X) = D(X)$.

We can now use $IC(Y \mid Q, G, D) \equiv IC_0(Y \mid G, D) - \Pi(IC_0(Y \mid G, D) \mid T_{SRA})$, possibly extended with the projection constant, as mapping from full data estimating functions to observed data estimating functions, where

$$\Pi(IC_0 \mid T_{SRA}) = -\int \{E(IC_0(Y) \mid C^* > t, \mathcal{F}_c(t))\} \, dM_c(t)$$
$$+ \int E(IC_0(Y) \mid dA_m(t) = 1, \mathcal{F}_m(t)) dM_m(t)$$
$$- \int E(IC_0(Y) \mid dA_m(t) = 0, \mathcal{F}_m(t)) dM_m(t),$$

$dM_c(t) = dA_c(t) - \Lambda_c(dt \mid \mathcal{F}_c(t))$, and $dM_m(t) = dA_m(t) - \Lambda_m(dt \mid \mathcal{F}_m)$. Proposals for estimation of these regressions defining the unknown parameter Q are provided in Section 6.1.

For another approach to interval censored data in longitudinal studies, see van der Laan (2000).

References

Andersen, P.K., and Gill, R.D. (1982), Cox's regression for counting processes: A large sample study. *Annals of Statistics*, **10**(4): 1100–1120.

Andersen, P.K., Borgan, O., Gill, R.D., and Keiding, N. (1993), *Statistical Models Based on Counting Processes*, Springer, New York.

Andrews, C., van der Laan, M.J., and Robins, J.M. (2002), Locally efficient estimation of regression parameters using current status data, revised for publication in *Journal of the American Statistical Association*.

Bacchetti, P. (1996), Reporting delays of deaths with AIDS in the United States, *Journal of Acquired Immune Deficiency Syndromes and Human Retrovirology*, **13**, 363–367.

Bakker, D.M. (1990), Two nonparametric estimators of the survival function of bivariate right-censored observations, Report BS-R9035, Centre for Mathematics and Computer Science, Amsterdam.

Bang, H, and Tsiatis, A.A. (2002), Median regression with censored medical cost data, *Biometrics*, **58**, 643–650.

Barlow, R.E., Bartholomew, D.J., Bremner, J.M., and Brunk, H.D. (1972), *Statistical Inference under Order Restrictions*, John Wiley, New York.

Bickel, P.J. (1982), On adaptive estimation, *Annals of Statistics*, **10**, 647–671.

Bickel, P.J., Klaassen, A.J., Ritov, Y. and Wellner, J.A. (1993), *Efficient and adaptive inference in semi-parametric models*, Johns Hopkins University Press, Baltimore.

Breiman, L. and Friedman, J.H. and Olshen, R.A. and Stone, C.J. (1984), *Classification and Regression Trees*, Wadsworth, Belmont.

Brillinger, D.R. (1983), A generalized linear model with Gaussian regressor variables. *A Festschrift for Erich L. Lehmann*, 97–114.

Brookhart, A., and van der Laan, M.J. (2002a), An event history model for welfare transition data, Technical report, University of California, Berkeley.

Brookhart, A., van der Laan, M.J. (2002b), A semiparametric model selection criterian: Applications to causal inference models. Technical report, Division of Biostatistics, University of California, Berkeley, to be submitted.

Bryan, J., Yu, Z., and van der Laan, M.J. (2002), Analysis of longitudinal marginal structural models, Technical report, Division of Biostatistics, University of California, Berkeley, to be submitted.

Burke, M.D. (1988), Estimation of a bivariate survival function under random censorship, *Biometrika* **75**, 379–382.

Campbell, G., and Földes, A. (1982), Large-sample properties of nonparametric bivariate estimators with censored data, in: *Nonparametric Statistical Inference*, B.V. Gnedenko, M.L. Puri, and I. Vincze (Eds.), North-Holland, Amsterdam, pp. 103–122.

Chamberlain, G. (1987), Asymptotic efficiency in estimation with conditional moment restrictions, *Journal of Econometrics*, **34**, 305–324.

Chen, A., and van der Laan, M.J. (2002), Estimation of dynamic treatment regimes with marginal structural nested failure time models, manuscript in process, University of California, Berkeley.

Clayton, D.G. (1978), A model for association in bivariate life tables and its application in epidemiological studies of a familial tendency in chronic disease incidence, *Biometrika*, **65**, 141–151.

Clayton, D.G. (1991), A Monte Carlo method for Bayesian inference in frailty models, *Biometrics*, **47**, 467–485.

Clayton, D.G., and Cuzick, J. (1985), Multivariate generalizations of the proportional hazards model (with discussion), *Journal of the Royal Statistical Society, Series B,* **148**, 82–117.

Colford, J.M., Sega, M., Tabnak, F., Chen, M., Sun, R., and Tager, I., (1997), Temporal trends and factors associated with survival after *Pneumocystis carinii* pneumonia in California, 1983–1992, *American Journal of Epidemiology*, **146**, 115–127.

Costigan, T. and Klein, J. (1993), Multivariate survival analysis based on frailty models, in : *Advances in Reliability*, A. Basu (Ed.) North-Holland, New York, pp.43–58.

Cox, D.R., Fitzpatrick, R., Gore, E., Spiegelhalter, D.J., and Jones, D.R. (1992), Quality-of-life assessment: Can we keep it simple?, *Journal of the Royal Statistical Society, A* **155**, 353–393.

Dabrowska, D.M. (1988), Kaplan–Meier estimate on the plane, *Annals of Statististics*, **16**, 1475–1489.

Dabrowska, D.M. (1989), Kaplan–Meier estimate on the plane: Weak convergence, LIL, and the bootstrap, *Journal of Multivariate Analysis*, **29**, 308–325.

Datta, S., Satten, G.A., and Datta, S. (2000), Nonparametric estimation for the three-stage irreversible illness-death model, *Biometrics*, **56**, 841–848.

Davis, R.B., and Anderson, J.R. (1989), Exponential survival trees, *Statistics in Medicine*, **8**, 947–961.

Dempster, A.P., Laird, N.M., and Rubin, D.B. (1977), Maximum likelihood from incomplete data via the EM-algorithm, *Journal of the Royal Statistical Society*, **39**, 1–38.

Diamond, I.D., McDonald, J.W., and Shah, I.H. (1986), Proportional hazards models for current status data: Application to the study of differentials in age at weaning in Pakistan, *Demography* **23**, 607–620.

Diamond, I.D., and McDonald, J.W. (1991), The analysis of current status data, in *Demographic Applications of Event History Analysis*, J. Trussell, R. Hankinson, and J. Tilton (Eds.), Oxford University Press, Oxford.

Diggle, P.J., Liang, K.-Y.,and Zeger, S.L. (1994), *Analysis of Longitudinal Data*, Oxford Statistical Science Series, Oxford Science Publications, Oxford.

Dinse, G.E. and Lagakos, S.W. (1982), Nonparametric estimation of lifetime and disease onset distributions from incomplete observations, *Biometrics*, **38**, 921–932.

Dominici, and Zeger, S.L. (2001), Smooth quantile ration estimation, submitted for publication.

Duffy, D.L., Martin, N.G., and Matthews, J.D. (1990), Appendectomy in Australian twins, *American Journal of Human Genetics*, **47**, 590–592.

Duan, N., Li, K-C (1987), Distribution-free and link-free estimation for the sample selection model, *J. Econometrics*, **35**, 25–35.

Duan, N., Li, K-C (1991), Slicing regression: A link-free regression method, *Annals of Statistics*, **19**, 505–530.

Efron, B. (1967), The two sample problem with censored data, *Proceedings of the 5th. Berkeley Symposium on Mathematical Statistics and Probability*, University of California Press, Berkeley, pp. 830–853.

Efron, B. , (1990), More efficient bootstrap computations, *Journal of the American Statistical Association*, **85**, 79–89.

Efron, B., and Tibshirani, R.J. (1993), *An Introduction to the Bootstrap*, Chapman and Hall, London.

Eisenberg, J.N.S., Wade, T.J., Hubbard, A., Abrams, D.I., Leiser, R.J., Charles, S., Vu, M., Saha, S., Wright, C.C., Levy, D.A., Jensen, P., and Colford, J.M. (2002), Association between water treatment methods and diarrhea in HIV positive individuals, accepted for publication in Journal of Epidemiology and Infection.

Friedman, J.H. (1984), A variable span smoother, Technical report, Department of Statistics, Stanford University, Stanford, CA.

Friedman, J.H. (1991), Multivariate adaptive regression splines, *Annals of Statistics* **19** (1), 1–67.

van de Geer, S. (1994), Asymptotic normality in mixture models, preprint, University of Leiden, the Netherlands.

Gelber, R.D., Gelman, R.S. and Goldhirsch, A. (1989), A quality of life oriented endpoint for comparing therapies, *Biometrics*, **45**, 781–795.

Gelber, R.D., Goldhirsch, A., and Cavalli, F. (1991), Quality of life adjusted evaluation of a randomized trial comparing adjuvant therapies for operable breast cancer (for the international breast cancer study group), *Annals of Internal Medicine*, **114**, 621–628.

Gelber, R.D., Lenderking, W.R., Cotton D.J., Cole, B.F., Fischl, M., Goldhirsch, A., and Testa, M.A. (1992), Quality-of-life evaluation in a clinical trial of zidovudine therapy in patients with mildly symptomatic HIV infection, *Annals of Internal Medicine*, **116**, 961–966.

Gelber, R.D., Cole, B.F., Gelber, S., and Goldhirsch, A. (1995), Comparing treatments using quality-adjusted survival: The Q-TWIST Method, *American Statistician*, **49**, 161–169.

Genest, C., and MacKay, R. J. (1986), The joy of copulas: Bivariate distributions with given marginals, *American Statistician*, **40**, 280–283.

Genest, C., and Rivest, L.P. (1993), Statistical inference procedures for bivariate Archimedean copulas, *Journal of the American Statistical Association*, **88**, 1034–1043.

Gill, R.D. (1983), Large sample behaviour of the product-limit estimator on the whole line, *Annals of statistics*, **11**, 49–58.

Gill, R.D. (1984), Understanding Cox's regression model: A martingale approach, *Journal of the American Statistical Association*, **79**(386), 441–447.

Gill, R.D. (1989), Non-and semi-parametric maximum likelihood estimators and the von mises method (Part 1), *Scandinavian Journal of Statistics*, **16**, 97–128.

Gill, R.D. (1992), Multivariate survival analysis, *Theory of Probability and Its Applications* (English Translation), **37**, 18–31 and 284–301.

Gill, R.D. (1993), Lectures on survival analysis, in: D. Bakry, R.D. Gill, and S. Molchanov, École d'Été de Probabilités de Saint Flour XXII-1992, P. Bernard Ed.; Lecture Notes in Mathematics, Springer, Berlin.

Gill, R.D., and Johansen, S. (1990), A survey of product integration with a view towards application in survival analysis, *Annals of Statistics*, **18**, 1501–1555.

Gill, R.D., van der Laan, M.J., and Robins, J.M. (1997), Coarsening at random: Characterizations, conjectures and counter-examples, in: *Proceedings of the First Seattle Symposium in Biostatistics*, 1995, D.Y. Lin and T.R. Fleming (eds), Lecture Notes in Statistics, Springer, New York, pp. 255–294.

Gill, R.D., van der Laan, M.J., and Robins, J.M. (2000), *Locally efficient estimation with censored data and high-dimensional covariate processes*, Technical report No. 85, Division of Biostatistics, University of California, Berkeley.

Gill, R.D., van der Laan, M.J., and Wellner, J.A. (1995), Inefficient estimators of the bivariate survival function for three models, *Annales de l'Institut Henri Poincaré*, **31**, 545–597.

Gill, R.D., and Robins, J.M. (2001), Causal inference for complex longitudinal data: the continuous case, *Annals of Statistics*, **29**, 1785–1811

Gill, R.D., and van der Vaart, A.W. (1993), Non- and semi-parametric maximum likelihood estimators and the von Mises method (part 2), *Scandinavian Journal of Statistics***20**, 271–288.

Giné, E., and Zinn, J. (1990). Bootstrapping general empirical measures. *Annals of Probability*, **18**, 851–869.

Glasziou, P.P., Simes, R.J., and Gelber, R.D. (1990), Quality adjusted survival analysis, *Statistics in Medicine*, **9**, 1259–1276.

Goldhirsch, A., Gelber, R.D., Simes, R.J., Glasziou, P.P., and Coates, A. (1989), Costs and benefits of adjuvant therapy in breast cancer: A quality adjusted survival analysis, *Journal of Clinical Onconlogy*, **7**, 36–44.

Gordon, L., and Olshen, R.A. (1985), Tree-structured survival analysis, *Cancer Treatment Reports*, **69**, 1065–1069.

Green, P.J. and Silverman, B.W. (1994), *Nonparametric Regression and Generalized Linear Models: A Roughness Penalty Approach*, Chapman and Hall, London

Groeneboom, P. (1991), Nonparametric maximum likelihood estimators for interval censoring and deconvolution, Technical report No. 378, Department of Statistics, Stanford University, Stanford, CA.

Groeneboom, P., and Wellner, J.A. (1992), *Information Bounds and Nonparametric Maximum Likelihood estimation*, Birkhäuser, Boston.

Härdle, W. (1993), *Applied Nonparametric Regression*, Econometric Society Monographs, Cambridge University Press, Cambridge, U.K.

Hansen, L.P. (1982), Large sample properties of generalized method of moments estimators, *Econometrica*, **50**, 1029–1054.

Hastie, T.J., and Tibshirani, R.J. (1990a), *Generalized Additive Models*, Chapman and Hall, London.

Hastie, T.J. and Tibshirani, R.J. (1990b), Exploring the nature of covariate effects in the proportional hazards model, *Biometrics*, **46** (4), 1005–1016.

Heitjan, D.F. (1993), Ignorability and coarse data: Some biomedical examples, *Biometrics,* **49**, 1099–1109.

Heitjan, D.F., and Rubin, D.B. (1991), Ignorability and coarse data, *Annals of statistics*, **19**, 2244–2253.

Henneman, T, and van der Laan, M.J. (2002), Marginal structural models in point treatment studies, Technical report, Division of Biostatistics, University of California, Berkeley.

Hernan, M., Brumback, B., and Robins, J.M. (2000), Marginal structural models to estimate the causal effect of zidovudine on the survival of HIV-positive men, *Epidemiology*, **11**(5), 561–570.

Hougaard, P. (1986), A class of multivariate failure time distributions, *Biometrika*, **73**(3), 671–678.

Hougaard, P. (1987), Modeling multivariate survival, *Scandinavian Journal of Statistics*, **14**, 291–304.

Hu, P.H., and Tsiatis, A.A. (1996), Estimating the survival function when ascertainment of vital status is subject to delay, *Biometrika*, **83**, 371–380.

Huang, J., and Wellner, J.A. (1995), Asymptotic normality of the NPMLE of linear functionals for interval censored data, case I, *Statistica Neerlandica*, **49**, 153–163.

Huang, J. (1996), Efficient estimation for the proportional hazards model with interval censoring, *Annals of Statistics*, **24**, 540–568.

Hubbard, A.E., van der Laan, M.J., and Robins, J.M. (1999), Nonparametric locally efficient estimation of the treatment specific survival distribution with right censored data and covariates in observational studies, in: *Statistical Models in Epidemiology: The Environment and Clinical Trials*, E. Halloran, D. and Berry, (Eds.) Springer-Verlag, New York pp. 135–178.

Hubbard, A.E., van der Laan, M.J., Enaroria, W.,and Colford, J. (2000), Nonparametric survival estimation when death is reported with delay, *Lifetime Data Models*, **6**, 237–250.

Ichida, J.M., Wassell, J.T., and Keller, M.D. (1993), Evaluation of protocol change in burn-care management using the Cox proportional hazards model with time-dependent covariates, *Statistics in Medicine*, 12, 301-310.

Jacobsen, M., and Keiding, N. (1995), Coarsening at random in general sample spaces and random censoring in continuous time, *Annals of Statistics*, **23**, 774–786.

Jewell, N.P., Malani, H.M., and Vittinghoff, E. (1994), Nonparametric estimation for a form of doubly censored data with application to two problems in AIDS, *Journal of the American Statistical Association*, **89**, 7–18.

Jewell, N.P., and Shiboski, S.C. (1990), Statistical analysis of HIV infectivity based on partner studies, *Biometrics*, **46**, 1133–1150.

Joe, H. (1993), Parametric families of multivariate distributions with given marginals, *Journal of Multivariate Analysis,* **46**, 262–282.

Kalbfleish, J.D., and Prentice, R.L. (1980), *The Statistical Analysis of Failure Time Data,* Wiley Series in Probability and Mathematical statistics, Wiley, NewYork.

Kaplan, E.L., and Meier, P. (1958), Nonparametric estimation from incomplete observations. *Journal of the American Statistical Association,* **53**, 457–481.

Keiding, N. (1991), Age-specific incidence and prevalence (with discussion), *Journal of the Royal Statistical Society Series A,* **154**, 371–412.

Keles, S., van der Laan, M.J (2002), Survival prediction with sieves and cross-validation, to be submitted for publication in *Bernoulli.*

Keles, S., van der Laan, M.J., and Robins, J.M. (2002), Estimation of the bivariate survival function in the presence of time dependent covariates, submitted for publication as chapter in the Volume *Survival Analysis,* edited by Professor C.R. Rao and Professor N. Balakrishnan in the book series *Handbook of Statistics.*

Kiefer, J., and Wolfowitz, J. (1956), Consistency of the maximum likelihood estimator in the presence of infinitely many incidental parameters, *Annals of Statistics,* **27**, 887–906.

Klaassen, C.A.J. (1987), Consistent estimation of the influence function of locally asymptotically linear estimators, *Annals of Statistics,* **15**, 1548–1562.

Klein, J. (1992), Semiparametric estimation of random effects using the Cox model based on the EM algorithm, *Biometrics,* **48**, 795–806.

Klein, J.P., and Moeschberger, M.L. (1997), *Survival Analysis: Techniques for Censored and Truncated Data,* Springer, New York.

Kodell, R.L., Shaw, G.W., and Johnson, A.M. (1982), Nonparametric joint estimators for disease resistance and survival functions in survival/sacrifice experiments, *Biometrics,* **38**, 43–58.

Kooperberg, C. and Stone, C.J. and Truong, Y.K. (1995), Hazard regression, Journal of the American Statistical Association, **90** (429), 78–94.

Korn, E.L. (1993), On estimating the distribution function for quality of life in cancer clinical trials, *Biometrika,* **80**, 535–542.

van der Laan, M.J. (1990), Analysis of Dabrowska's estimator of the bivariate survival function, Masters thesis, Utrecht University, The Netherlands.

van der Laan, M.J. (1994), Modified EM-equations-estimator of the bivariate survival function, *Mathematical Methods of Statistics,* **3**, 213–243.

van der Laan, M.J. (1997), Nonparametric estimators of the bivariate survival function under random censoring, *Statistica Neerlandica,* **51**(2) 178–200.

van der Laan, M.J. (1996a), Efficient estimator of the bivariate survival function and repairing NPMLE, *Annals of statistics*, **24**, 596–627.

van der Laan, M.J. (1996b), *Efficient and inefficient estimation in semiparametric models*, C.W.I. Tract 114, Centre of Computer Science and Mathematics, Amsterdam, The Netherlands.

van der Laan, M.J. (1998), Identity for NPMLE in censored data models, *Lifetime Data Models*, **4**, 83–102.

van der Laan, M.J. (2000), Estimation with interval censored data in longitudinal studies. Technical report, University of California, Berkeley.

van der Laan, M.J., and Andrews, C. (2000), The NPMLE in a class of doubly censored current status data models with applications to AIDS partner studies, *Biometrika*, **87**(1), 61–71.

van der Laan, M.J., Bickel, P.J., and Jewell, N.P. (1997), Singly and doubly censored current status data, estimation, asymptotics and regression, *Scandinavian Journal of statistics*, **24**, 289–308.

van der Laan, M.J., Dominici, F., and Zeger, S.L. (2002), Locally efficient estimation of the quantile-quantile function in a two-sample problem, manuscript in process.

van der Laan, M.J., and Gill, R.D. (1999), Efficiency of NPMLE in nonparametric missing data models, *Mathematical Methods of Statistics*, **8**(2), 251–276.

van der Laan, M.J., and Hubbard A. (1997), Estimation with interval censored data and covariates, *Lifetime Data Models*, **3**, 77–91.

van der Laan, M.J., and Hubbard, A. (1998), Locally efficient estimation of the survival distribution with right-censored data and covariates when collection of the data is delayed, *Biometrika*, **85**, 771–783.

van der Laan, M.J., and Hubbard, A. (1999), Locally efficient estimation of the quality adjusted lifetime distribution with right censored data and covariates, *Biometrics*, **55**, 530–536.

van der Laan, M.J., Hubbard, A.E., and Robins, J.M. (2002), Locally efficient estimation of a multivariate survival function in longitudinal studies, *Journal of the American Statistical Association*, **97**, 494–508.

van der Laan, M.J., Murphy, S.A., and Robins, J.M. (2002), Analyzing dynamic regimes using marginal structural nested mean models, to be submitted.

van der Laan, M.J., and Jewell, N.P. (2002), Current status and right-censored data structures when observing a marker at the censoring time, to appear in *Annals of Statistics*.

van der Laan, M.J., Jewell, N.P., and Peterson, D.R. (1997), Efficient estimation of the lifetime and disease onset distribution, *Biometrika*, **84**, 539–554.

van der Laan, M.J, and McKeague, I. (1997), Efficient estimation from right-censored Data when failure idicators are Missing at Random. *Annals of Statistics*, **26**, 164–182.

van der Laan, M.J., and Robins, J.M. (1998), Locally efficient estimation with current status data and time-dependent covariates. *Journal of the American Statistical Association*, **93** (442), 693–701.

van der Laan, M.J., and van der Vaart, A.W. (2002), Estimating a survival distribution with current status data and high-dimensional covariates, submitted to Annals of Statistics.

van der Laan, M.J., and Yu, Z (2001), Comments on the millennium paper "Inference for semiparametric models: Some questions and an answer," by P.J. Bickel and J. Kwon, in the millennium series of Statistica Sinica, 910–917.

Lapidus, G., Braddock, M., Schwartz, R., Banco, L., and Jacobs, L. (1994), Accuracy of fatal motorcycle-injury reporting on death certificates, *Accident Analysis and Prevention*, **26**, 535–542.

Lawless, J.F. (1995), The analysis of recurrent events for multiple subjects, *Applied Statistics Journal of the Royal Statistical Society Series C*, **44**(4), 487–498.

Lawless, J.F., and Nadeau, C. (1995), Some simple robust methods for the analysis of recurrent events, *Technometrics*, **37**(2), 158–168.

Lawless, J.F., Nadeau, C., and Cook, R.J. (1997), Analysis of mean and rate functions for recurrent events, In *Proceedings of the First Seattle Symposium in Biostatistics*, Lecture Notes in Statistics volume 123, Springer, New York, pp. 37–49.

Leblanc, M., and Crowley, J. (1992), Relative risk trees for censored data, *Biometrics*, **48**, 411–425.

Lin, D.Y., Robins, J.M., and Wei, L.J. (1996), Comparing two failure time distributions in the presence of dependent censoring, *Biometrika*, **83**, 381–393.

Lin, D.Y., Sun, W., and Ying, Z. (1999), Nonparametric estimation of the gap time distribution for Serial events with censored data, *Biometrika*, **86**, 59–70.

Lin, D.Y., Wei, L.J., Yang, I., Ying, Z. (2000), Semiparametric regression for the mean and rate functions of recurrent events, *Journal of the Royal Statistical Society series B - Statistical Methodology*, **62**(PT4): 711–730.

Lipsitz, S.R., Ibrahim, J.G., and Zhao, L.P. (1999), A weighted estimating equation for missing covariate data with properties similar to maximum likelihood, *Journal of the American Statistical Association*, **94**, 1147–1160.

Little, R.J.A., and Rubin, D.B. (1987), *Statistical Analysis with Missing Data*, Wiley, New York.

Lo, S.-H. (1991), Estimating a survival function with incomplete cause-of-death data, *Journal of Multivariate Analysis*, **39**, 217–235.

Luenberger, D.G (1969), *Optimization by Vector Space Methods*, John Wiley and Sons, New York.

Mark, S.D., and Robins, J.M. (1993), Estimating the causal effect of smoking cessation in the presence of confounding factors using a rank preserving structural failure time model, *Statistics in Medicine*, **12**, 1605–1628.

McCullagh, P., and Nelder, J.A. (1990), *Generalized Linear Models*, second edition, Monographs on Statistics and Applied Probability, Chapman and Hall, London.

Molinaro, A., van der Laan, M.J., and Dudoit, S. (2002), Prediction of survival with regression trees and cross-validation, to be submitted.

Morrison D. , (1990), *Multivariate Statistical Methods*, third edition, McGraw-Hill Publishing Co., San Francisco.

Murphy, S.A., van der Laan, M.J., and Robins, J.M. (2001), *Marginal mean models for dynamic treatment regimes*, Journal of the American Statistical Association, **96**, 1410–1424.

Neuhaus, G. (1971), On weak convergence of stochastic processes with multidimensional time parameter, *Annals of Mathematics and Statistics* **42**, 1285–1295.

Neugebauer, R., and van der Laan, M.J. (2002), Why prefering doubly robust estimation? Application to point treatment marginal structural models, submitted for publication in *Journal of Statistical Planning and Inference*.

Newey, W.K. (1990), Semiparametric efficiency bounds. *Journal of Applied Econometrics*, **5**, 99–135.

Newey, W.K., and McFadden, D. (1994), Large sample estimation and hypothesis testing, *Handbook of Econometrics*, **4**, McFadden, D., and Engle, R. (Eds.), Amsterdam, North-Holland, 2113–2245.

Oakes, D. (1989), Bivariate survival models Iinduced by frailties, *Journal of the American Statistical Association*, 84, 487–493.

Padian, N., Marquis, L., Francis, D.P., Anderson, R.E., Rutherford, G.W. , O'Malley, P.M., and Winkelstein, W. (1987), Male-to-female transmission of Human Immunodeficiency Virus, *Journal of the American Medical Association*, **258**, 788–790.

Padian, N., Shiboski, S.C., Glass, S.O., and Vittinghoff, E. (1997), Heterosexual transmission of HIV in northern California: Results from a ten year study, *American Journal of Epidemiology*, **146**, 350–357.

Pavlic, M., and van der Laan, M.J. (2002), Fitting mixtures with unspecified number of components using cross-validation, Special issue on Mixtures of *Computational Statistics and Data Analysis*, to appear.

Pavlic, M., van der Laan, M.J., and Buttler, S. (2001), Recurrent events analysis in the presence of time dependent covariates and dependent censoring, revised for publication in *Journal of the Royal Statistical Society*.

Pearl, J. (1995), Causal diagrams for empirical research, *Biometrika*, **82**, 669–710.

Pearl, J., and Robins, J.M. (1995), Probabilistic evaluation of sequential plans from causal models with hidden variables, In P. Besnard and S. Hanks (Eds.), *Uncertainty in Artificial Intelligence*, **11**, 444–453, San Frnacisco, Morgan Kaufman.

Pearl, J. (2000), *Models, Reasoning and Inference*, Cambridge University Press, Cambridge, United Kingdom.

Pepe, M.S., and Cai, J. (1993), Some graphical displays and marginal regression analysis for recurrent failure times and time-dependent covariates, *Journal of the American Statistical Association*, **88**(423), 811–820.

Portier, C.J. (1986), Estimating the tumor onset distribution in animal carcinogenesis experiments, *Biometrika*, **73**, 371–378.

Portier, C.J., and Dinse, A. (1987), Semiparametric analysis of tumor incidence rates in survival/sacrifice experiments, *Biometrics*, **43**, 107–114.

Prentice, R.L., and Cai, J. (1992a), Covariance and survivor function estimation using censored multivariate failure time data, *Biometrika*, **79**, 495–512.

Prentice, R.L., and Cai, J. (1992b), Marginal and conditional models for the analysis of multivariate failure time data, J.P. Klein, and P.K. Goel (Eds.) in: *Survival Analysis State of the Art*, Kluwer, Dordrecht.

Pruitt, R.C. (1991), Strong consistency of self-consistent estimators: general theory and an application to bivariate survival analysis, Technical Report no. 543, University of Minnesota, Minneapolis.

Pruitt, R.C. (1993), Small sample comparisons of six bivariate survival curve estimators, *Journal of Statistics and Computer simulation*, **45**, 147–167.

Quale, C.M., and van der Laan, M.J. (2000), Inference with bivariate truncated data, *Lifetime Data Analysis*, **6**(4), 391–408.

Quale, C.M., van der Laan, M.J., and Robins, J.M. (2002), Locally efficient estimation with bivariate right censored data, revised for publication in Journal of the American Statistical Association.

Rabinowitz, D. and Jewell, N.P. (1996), Regression with doubly censored current status data, *Journal of the Royal Statstical Society B*, **58**, 541–550.

Rabinowitz, D., Tsiatis, A., and Aragon, A. (1995), Regression with interval-censored data, *Biometrika*, **82**, 501–513.

Ritov, Y., and Wellner, J.A. (1988), Censoring, martingales, and the Cox model, *Contemporary Mathematics*, **80**, 191–219.

Robins, J.M. (1986), A new approach to causal inference in mortality studies with sustained exposure periods - Application to control of the healthy worker survivor effect, *Mathematical Modelling*, **7**, 1393–1512, with 1987 Errata in *Computers and Mathematics with Applications*, **14**, 917–921, 1987 Addendum to A new approach to causal inference in mortality studies with sustained exposure periods

- Application to control of the healthy worker survivor effect, *Computers and Mathematics with Applications*, **14**, 923–945; and 1987 Errata to "Addendum to a new approach to causal inference in mortality studies with sustained exposure periods - Application to control of the healthy worker survivor effect," *Computers and Mathematics with Applications*, **18**, 477.

Robins, J.M. (1987), A graphical approach to the identification and estimation of causal parameters in mortality studies with sustained exposure periods, *Journal of Chronic Disease*, (40, Supplement), **2**. 139s-161s.

Robins, J.M. (1989a), The analysis of randomized and non-randomized AIDS treatment trials using a new approach to causal inference in longitudinal studies, in: *Health Service Research Methodology: A Focus on AIDS*, L. Sechrest, H. Freeman, and A. Mulley (Eds.), U.S. Public Health Service, National Center for Health Services Research, pp. Washington, DC, 113–159.

Robins, J.M. (1989b), The control of confounding by intermediate variables., *Statistics in Medicine*, **8**, 679–701.

Robins, J.M. (1992), Estimation of the time-dependent accelerated failure time model in the presence of confounding factors, *Biometrika*, **79**, 321–334.

Robins, J.M. (1993a), Information recovery and bias adjustment in proportional hazards regression analysis of randomized trials using surrogate markers, *Proceedings of the Biopharmaceutical section, American Statistical Association*, American Statistical Association, Alexandria, VA, pp. 24–33.

Robins, J.M. (1993b), Analytic methods for estimating HIV treatment and cofactor effects, *Methodological Issues of AIDS Mental Health Research*, Eds: Ostrow D.G., Kessler R., New York: Plenum Publishing, 213–290. Reproduced with permission of Plenum Publishing.

Robins, J.M. (1994), Correcting for non-compliance in randomized trials using structural nested mean models, *Communications in Statistics*, **23**, 2379–2412.

Robins, J.M. (1995a,b), An analytic method for randomized trials with informative censoring, Parts 1 and 2 *Lifetime Data Analysis* **1**, 241–254 and 417–434.

Robins, J.M. (1996), Locally efficient median regression with random censoring and surrogate markers, in: *Lifetime Data: Models in Reliability and Survival Analysis*, N.P. Jewell, A.C. Kimber, M.-L. Ting Lee, and G.A. Whitmore (Editors), 263–274, Kluwer Academic Publishers, Dordrecht, the Netherlands.

Robins, J.M. (1997), Causal inference from complex longitudinal data, Latent Variable Modeling and Applications to Causality.*Lecture Notes in Statistics*, **120**, M. Berkane (Editor), New York, Springer Verlag, 69–117.

Robins, J.M. (1998a). Correction for non-compliance in equivalence trials, *Statistics in Medicine*, **17**, 269–302.

Robins, J.M. (1998). Marginal Structural Models versus Structural Nested Models as Tools for Causal Inference. In: AAAI Technical Report Series; Spring 1998 Symposium on Prospects for a Common Sense Theory of Causation. Stanford, CA, March 1998 (to appear).

Robins, J.M. (1998b). Marginal structural models, in: 1997 *Proceedings of the American Statistical Association*, American Statistical Association, Alexandria, VA, pp. 1–10.

Robins, J.M. (1998c). Structural nested failure time models, in: Survival Analysis, P.K. Andersen and N. Keiding (Section Eds.), *The Encyclopedia of Biostatistics*, P. Armitage and T. Colton, (Eds.), Chichester, U.K., John Wiley and Sons, pp. 4372–4389.

Robins, J.M. (1999), Marginal structural models versus structural nested models as tools for causal inference. in: *Statistical Models in Epidemiology: The Environment and Clinical Trials*, M.E. Halloran and D. Berry (Eds.), IMA Volume 116, Springer-Verlag, New York, pp. 95-134.

Robins, J.M. (2000), Robust estimation in sequentially ignorable missing data and causal inference models, *Proceedings of the American Statistical Association.*, American Statistical Association, Alexandria, VA.

Robins, J.M., and Finkelstein, D. (2000), Correcting for noncompliance and dependent censoring in an AIDS clinical trial with inverse probability of censoring weighted (IPCW) log-rank tests, *Biometrics*, **56**, 779–788.

Robins, J.M., Blevins D., Ritter G., and Wulfsohn M. (1992), G-estimation of the effect of prophylaxis therapy for pneumocystis carinii pneumonia on the survival of AIDS patients, *Epidemiology*, **3**, 319–336. Please see also the following link for the Errata to the article: Errata to G-estimation of the effect of prophylaxis therapy for pneumocystis carinii pneumonia on the survival of AIDS patients, *Epidemiology*, **4**, 189, Reproduced with permission of the publisher, Lippincott, Williams and Wilkins.

Robins, J.M., and Gill, R.D. (1997), Non-response models for the analysis of non-monotone ignorable missing data, *Statistics in Medicine*, **16**, 39–56.

Robins, J.M., and Greenland S. (1994), Adjusting for differential rates of PCP prophylaxis in high- versus low-dose AZT treatment arms in an AIDS randomized trial, *Journal of the American Statistical Association*, **89**, 737–749.

Robins, J.M., Hernan, M., and Brumback, B. (2000), Marginal structural models and causal inference in epidemiology, *Epidemiology*, **11** 5), 550–560.

Robins, J.M., Hsieh, F-S., and Newey, W. (1995), Semiparametric efficient estimation of a conditional density with missing or mismeasured covariates, *Journal of the Royal Statistical Society B*, **57**, 409–424.

Robins, J.M., Mark S.D., and Newey, W.K. (1992), Estimating exposure effects by modeling the expectation of exposure conditional on confounders. *Biometrics*, **48**, 479–495.

Robins, J.M., and Morgenstern, H. (1987), The foundations of confounding in epidemiology. *Computers and Mathematics with Applications*, **14**, 869–916.

Robins, J.M., and Ritov, Y. (1997), Toward a curse of dimensionality appropriate (CODA) asymptotic theory for semi-parametric models, *Statistics in Medicine*, **16**, 285–319.

Robins, J.M., and Rotnitzky, A. (1992), Recovery of information and adjustment for dependent censoring using surrogate markers, *Aids Epidemiology, Methodological Issues*, Birkhäuser, Boston.

Robins, J.M., and Rotnitzky, A. (1995), Semiparametric efficiency in multivariate regression models with missing data, *Journal of the American Statistical Association*, **90**, 122–129.

Robins, J.M., and Rotnitzky, A. (2001), Comments on the millennium paper "Inference for semiparametric models: Some questions and an answer," by P.J. Bickel and J. Kwon, in the *millennium series of Statistica Sinica*, 920–936.

Robins, J.M., Rotnitzky, A. and, van der Laan, M.J. (1999), Discussion of "On Profile Likelihood" by S.A. Murphy and A.W. van der Vaart, *Journal of the American Statistical Association* **95**, 477–482.

Robins, J.M., Rotnitzky, A. and Scharfstein, D. (1999), Sensitivity analysis for selection bias and unmeasured confounding in missing data and causal inference models. In: *Statistical Models in Epidemiology: The Environment and Clinical Trials*, Halloran, M.E. and Berry, D., (eds.), IMA **116**, New York, Springer-Verlag, 1-92.

Robins, J.M., Rotnitzky, A., and Zhao L.P. (1994), Estimation of regression coefficients when some regressors are not always observed, *Journal of the American Statistical Association*, **89**, 846–866.

Robins, J.M., Rotnitzky, A., and Zhao, L-P. (1995), Analysis of semiparametric regression models for repeated outcomes in the presence of missing data, *Journal of the American Statistical Association*, **90**, 106–121.

Robins, J.M., and Tsiatis A. (1991), Correcting for non-compliance in randomized trials using rank-preserving structural failure time models, *Communications in Statistics*, **20**, 2609–2631.

Robins, J.M., and Wang, N. (1998), Discussion on the papers by Forster and Smith and Clayton et al., *Journal of the Royal Statistical Society B*, **60** (Part 1), 91–93.

Rosenbaum, P.R. (1984), Conditional permutation tests and the propensity score in observational studies, *Journal of the American Statistical Association*, **79**, 565–574.

Rosenbaum, P.R. (1987), Model-based direct adjustment, *Journal of the American Statistical Association*, **82**, 387–394.

Rosenbaum, P.R. (1988), Permutation tests for matched pairs with adjustments for covariates, *Applied Statistics*, **37**, 401–411.

Rosenbaum, P.R., and Rubin, D.B. (1983), The central role of the propensity score in observational studies for causal effects, *Biometrika*, **70**, 41–55.

Rosenbaum, P.R., and Rubin, D.B. (1984), Reducing bias in observational studies using subclassification on the propensity score, *Journal of the American Statistical Association*, **79**, 516–524.

Rosenbaum, P.R., and Rubin, D.B. (1985), Constructing a control group using multivariate matched sampling methods that incorporate the propensity score, *Journal of the American Statistical Association*, **39**, 33–38.

Rossini, A.J., and Tsiatis, A.A. (1996), A semiparametric proportional odds regression model for the analysis of current status data, *Journal of the American Statistical Association*, **91**(N434), 713–721.

Rotnitzky, A., and Robins, J.M. (1995a), Semi-parametric estimation of models for means and covariances in the presence of missing data, *Scandinavian Journal of Statistics*, **22**, 323–333.

Rotnitzky, A., and Robins, J.M. (1995b), Semiparametric regression estimation in the presence of dependent censoring, *Biometrika*, **82**, 805–820.

Rotnitzky, A., and Robins, J.M. (1997), Analysis of semiparametric regression models with non-ignorable non-response, *Statistics in Medicine*, **16**, 81–102.

Rotnitzky, A., Robins, J.M., and Scharfstein, D. (1998), Semiparametric regression for repeated outcomes with nonignorable nonresponse, Journal of the American Statistical Association, **93** (444), 1321–1339.

Rubin, D. B. (1976). Inference and missing data. *Biometrika* **63** 581–590.

Rubin, D.B. (1978), Bayesian inference for causal effects: The role of randomization, *Annals of Statistics*, **6**, 34–58.

Scharfstein, D.O., Robins, J.M., and van der Laan, M.J. (2002), Locally efficient estimation in the bivariate location shift model, to be submitted.

Ruud, P.A. (1983), Sufficient conditions for the consistency of maximum likelihood estimation despite misspecification of distribution in multinomial discrete choice models, *Econometrica*, **51**, 225–228.

Ruud, P.A. (1986), Consistent estimation of limited dependent variable models despite misspecification of distribution. *J. Econometrics*, **32**, 157–187.

Scharfstein, D.O., Rotnitzky, A., and Robins, J.M. (1999), Adjusting for non-ignorable drop out using semiparametric non-response models, *Journal of the American Statistical Association*, **94**, 1096–1120.

Scharfstein, D.O., Rotnitzky, A., and Robins, J.M. (1999b), Comments and rejoinder. *Journal of the American Statistical Association*, **94** (448), 1121–1146.

Segal, M.R. (1988), Regression trees for censored data, *Biometrics*, **44** (1), 35–47.

Shen, X. (2000), Linear regression with current status data, *Journal of the American Statistical Association*, **95** 451, 842–852.

Shiboski, S.C., and Jewell, N.P. (1992), Statistical analysis of the time dependence of HIV infectivity based on partner study data, *Journal of the American Statistical Association*, **87**, 360–372.

Small, C.G., and McLeish, D.L. (1994), *Hilbert Space Methods in Probability and Statistical Inference*, John Wiley and Sons, New York.

Strawderman, R.L. (2000), Estimating the mean of an increasing stochastic process at censored stopping time, *Journal of the American Statistical Association*, 95, 1192–1208.

Sun, J. and Kalbfleish, D. (1993), The analysis of current status data on point processes, *Journal of the American Statistical Association*, **88**, 1449–1454.

Tager, I., Haight, T., Hollenberg, A., and Satariano, B. (2000), *Physical Functioning and Mortality in Elderly Females*, unpublished manual, School of Public Health, University of California, Berkeley.

Tchetgen, E and Robins, J.M. (2002), Doubly robust estimation of the marginal structural proportional hazards model, submitted for publication.

Tsai, W-Y., Leurgans, S., and Crowley, J. (1986), Nonparametric estimation of a bivariate survival function in the presence of censoring, *Annals of Statistics*, **14**, 1351–1365.

Turnbull, B.W. (1976), The empirical distribution with arbitrarily grouped censored and truncated data, *Journal of the Royal statistical Society*, B **38**, 290–295.

Turnbull, B.W. and Mitchell, T.J. (1984), Nonparametric estimation of the distribution of time to onset for specific diseases in survival/sacrifice experiments, *Biometrics*, **40**, 41–50.

van der Vaart, A.W. (1988), *Statistical Estimation in Large Parameter Spaces*, CWI Tract, Centre for Mathematics and Computer Science, Amsterdam.

van der Vaart, A.W. (1991), On differentiable functionals, *Annals of Statistics*, **19**, 178–204.

van der Vaart, A.W. (1998), *Asymptotic Statistics*, Cambridge series in Statistical and probabilistic Mathematics, Cambridge University Press, Cambridge, U.K.

van der Vaart, A.W. (2001), On a theorem by James Robins, Technical report, Free University, Amsterdam, The Netherlands.

Wellner, J.A. (1982), Asymptotic optimality of the product limit estimator, *Annals of Statistics* **10**, 595–602.

van der Vaart, A.W. and Wellner, J.A. (1996), *Weak Convergence and Empirical Processes*, Springer-Verlag, New York.

Wang, W., and Wells, M.T. (1998), Nonparametric estimation of successive duration times under dependent censoring, *Biometrika*, **85**, 561–572.

Zhao, H., and Tsiatis, A.A. (1997), A consistent estimator for the distribution of quality adjusted survival time, *Biometrika*, **84**, 339–348.

Yu, Z., van der Laan, M.J. (2002), A Monte-Carlo simulation method for doubly robust estimation in longitudinal studies, to be submitted.

Yu, Z., van der Laan, M.J. (2002), Construction of counterfactuals and the G-computation formula, to be submitted to Annals of Statistics.

Author Index

Andersen, P.K., 13, 39, 109, 173, 175, 177, 185, 187, 192, 199, 221, 235, 270, 312, 323
Anderson, J.R., 224
Andrews, C., 247, 250, 252, 255
Aragon, A., 250

Bacchetti, P., 179
Bakker, D.M., 284
Barlow, R.E., 247
Bartholomew, D.J., 247
Bickel, P.J., 9, 18, 20, 61, 103, 145, 247
Borgan, O., 13, 39, 109, 173, 175, 177, 187, 192, 199, 221, 235, 270, 270, 323
Breiman, L., 224
Bremner, J.M., 247
Brookhart, A., 50, 321
Brumback, B., 49, 55
Brunk, H.D., 247
Bryan, J., 11, 322
Burke, M.D., 182
Buttler, S., 185

Cai, J., 182, 191, 283, 284
Campbell, G., 182
Cavalli, F., 179
Chen, M., 180
Clayton, D.G., 183, 209, 288
Coates, A., 179
Cole, B.F., 179
Colford, J.M., 180
Cook, R.J., 191
Costigan, T, 183, 209
Cotton, D.J., 179
Cox, D.R., 179
Crowley, J., 182, 224, 283
Cuzick, J., 183, 209, 288

Dabrowska, D.M., 129, 182, 273, 283
Davis, R.B., 224
Dempster, A.P., 26
Diamond, I.D., 246
Diggle, P.J., 13, 17
Dinse, G.E., 246, 263
Duan, N., 13
Dudoit, S., 225
Duffy, D.L., 286, 302, 303

Efron, B., 145, 182
Enaroria, W., 180

Finkelstein, D., 177, 216
Fischl, M., 179
Fitzpatrick, R., 179
Földes, A., 182
Friedman, J., 224

van de Geer, S., 247
Gelber, R.D., 179
Gelber, S., 178
Gelman, R.S., 179
Genest, C., 209
Gill, R.D., 13, 185, 13, 39, 109, 173, 175, 177, 187, 192, 199, 221, 235, 270,

270, 312, 323, 185, 28, 64, 145, 223, 182, 284, 222, 192, 24, 30, 32, 182, 294, 129, 222, 182, 273, 284, 298, 299, 289
Glass, S.O., 261
Glasziou, P.P., 179
Goldhirsch, A., 179
Gordon, L., 224
Gore, E., 179
Green, P.J., 13
Greenland, S., 11
Groeneboom, P., 247

Hastie, T.J., 13
Heitjan, D.F., 24
Henneman, T., 11
Hernan, M., 49, 55
Hougaard, P., 183, 209
Hsieh, F.-S., 10
Hu, P.H., 180
Huang, J., 247, 250
Hubbard, A.E., 11, 177, 179, 180, 181, 183, 210, 214, 343

Ibrahim, J.G., 13
Ichida, J.M., 214

Jacobsen, M., 24
Jewell, N.P., 234, 236, 246, 261, 263. Joe, H., 209
Johansen, S., 192
Johnson, A.M., 263
Jones, D.R., 179

Kalbfleish, D., 173, 246
Kaplan, E. L., 28
Keiding, N., 13, 24, 39, 109, 173, 175, 177, 187, 192, 199, 221, 235, 246, 270, 312, 323
Keles, S., 270
Keller, M.D., 214
Kiefer, J., 45
Klaassen, A.J., 9, 18, 20, 32, 61, 103, 145
Klein, J., 183, 209, 214
Kodell, R.L., 263
Kooperberg, C., 224
Korn, E.L., 179

van der Laan, M.J., 11, 11, 94, 94, 247, 250, 252, 255, 50, 321, 322, 323, 24, 30, 32, 182, 294, 129, 222, 182, 273, 284, 298, 299, 177, 343, 180, 270, 129, 273, 218, 284, 284, 284, 292, 182, 283, 284, 289, 293, 298, 222, 283, 284, 297, 298, 165, 292, 247, 297, 298, 289, 181, 179, 183, 214, 210, 128, 234, 236, 263, 247, 254, 128, 185, 303, 126, 300, 270, 370
Lagakos, S.W., 263
Lawless, J.F., 191
Leblanc, M., 224
Lenderking, W.R., 179
Leurgans, S., 182, 283
Liang, K.-Y., 13, 17
Lipsitz, S.R., 13
Little, R.J.A., 13, 26
Lin, D.Y., 182 , 191, 191, 212

MacKay, R.J., 209
Malani, H.M., 247
Mark, S.D., 13, 11
Martin, N.G., 286, 302, 303
Matthews, J.D., 286, 302, 303
McCullagh, P., 13
McDonald, J.W., 246
Meier, P., 28
Mitchell, T.J., 263
Moeschberger, M.L., 214
Molinaro, A., 225
Morrison, D., 256
Murphy, S.A., 128

Nadeau, C., 191
Nelder, J.A., 13
Neugebauer, R., 13
Neuhaus, G., 297
Newey, W.K., 9, 11

Oakes, D., 183, 209
Olshen, R.A., 224

Padian, N., 261
Pavlic, M., 10, 94, 185

Pearl, J., 13
Pepe, M.S., 191
Peterson, D.R., 263
Portier, C.J., 246
Prentice, R.L., 173, 182, 283, 284
Pruitt, R.C., 284, 284

Quale, C.M., 126, 270, 300, 303

Rabinowitz, D., 250
Ritov, Y., 9, 18, 20, 32, 61, 103, 145, 185, 247
Rivest, L.P., 209
Robins, J.M., 10, 247, 250 252, 255, 24, 30, 32, 182, 294, 55, 177, 343, 180, 270, 289, 183, 214, 210, 128, 247, 254, 11, 128, 126, 300, 270, 11, 11, 11, 10, 177, 265, 11, 10, 11, 49, 11, 11, 49, 50, 11, 50, 177, 216, 11, 49, 11, 32, 247, 9, 32, 177, 182, 204, 265, 10, 10, 10, 46, 10, 11, 10, 10
Rosenbaum, P.R., 11
Rossini, A.J., 250
Rotnitzky, A., 9, 10, 32, 46, 177, 182, 204, 265
Rubin, D.B., 13, 11, 24, 26
Ruud, P.A., 13

Sega, M., 180
Segal, M., 224
Scharfstein, D., 13
Shah, I.H., 246
Shaw, G.W., 263
Shen, X., 250
Shiboski, S.C., 246, 261
Silverman, B.W., 13
Simes, R.J., 179
Spiegelhalter, D.J., 179
Stone, C., 224, 224
Sun, J., 246
Sun, R., 180
Sun, W., 182, 212

Tabnak, F., 180
Tager, I., 180
Testa, M.A., 179
Tibshirani, R.J., 13
Truong, Y.K., 224

Tsai, W.-Y., 182, 283
Tsiatis, A.A., 11, 179, 180, 250
Turnbull, B.W., 182, 263

van der Vaart, A.W., 9, 14, 145, 150, 152, 221, 223
Vittinghoff, E., 247, 261

Wang, N., 10
Wang, W., 182
Wassell, J.T., 214
Wellner, J.A., 9, 18, 20, 61, 103, 145, 129, 222, 182, 273, 284, 298, 299, 247, 247, 185, 28, 145, 150, 152, 221
Wei, L.J., 191, 191
Wells, M.T., 182
Wolfowitz, J., 45

Yang, I., 191, 191
Ying, Z., 182, 191, 191, 212
Yu, Z., 11, 322
Zeger, S.L., 13, 17
Zhao, H., 179
Zhao L.P., 10, 46

Subject Index

AIDS-partner study, 260
action process, 312
asymptotically linear, 19, 30

bivariate right-censored data (see also multivariate right-censored data), 76, 216, 267, 282
bootstrap, 145
burn victim data, 214

canonical gradient, 57, 61, 154
causal effect/marginal structural model, 48, 318, 330
causal effect/structural nested model/marginal structural nested model, 347
causal inference, 313, 318, 330
cause-specific censoring, 175
cause-specific monitoring, 234
censoring/missingness, 17
coarsening at random, 24, 25, 28, 173, 233
competing risk/failure time data, 232
convex parameter, 69, 135
copula models, 209
Cox proportional hazards model, 173
cross-sectional data, 232
cross-validation, selection of nuisance parameter models, 94
current status data, 121, 156, 246, 263

curse of dimensionality, 28

double protection against misspecification, 42, 135
doubly robust estimator, 81, 256

efficient estimator, 61
efficient influence curve/function, 32, 44, 154
efficient score, 20
estimating function, 41, 55, 62, 111
estimating equation, 140, 141,

factorization of density/likelihood, 26
frailty models, 209, 299
full data estimating functions, 103

gradient, 57

ignoring information on censoring mechanism, 135
influence curve/function, 19, 30
information operator (see also nonparametric information operator), 121, 164
interval censored data, 365, 368
inverse probability of censoring weighted estimator, 33, 36, 121, 183
IPTW estimator, 50, 322

kernel smoothing, 234

locally efficient estimation, 21, 41, 286, 334
logistic regression, 173, 269

mapping into observed data estimating functions, 125, 128, 131, 137
marginal structural model, 127, 318, 330
maximum likelihood estimator, 28, 199, 200
missing covariate, 16, 157
missingness, 362
mixture models, 71.
monotone censored data, 172
multinomial logistic regression model, 200
multivariate current status data, 233
multivariate failure time regression model, 208
multivariate generalized regression model, 16, 105, 205, 206, 245
multivariate right-censored data, 126, 129, 143, 181, 266, 273
multiplicative intensity model, 107, 184, 199, 270

nuisance tangent space, 19, 56

Subject Index

Newton–Raphson algorithm, 107
nonparametric information operator, 204, 288

observed data model, 40, 103
one-step estimator, 44, 141, 252, 295
optimal estimating function, 20, 44, 50, 154, 205, 206, 245
orthogonal complement of nuisance tangent space, 19, 32, 35, 55, 64, 105, 132
orthogonalizing estimating functions, 131

partial likelihood, 39, 270, 312
pathwise derivative, 57
prediction of survival, 224
proportional rate models, 190
protection against misspecification of convex parameter, 69, 135
protection of estimating functions (see also double protection): 69

quality adjusted survival, 177

regression with current status data, 247
repeated measures, 16
reporting delay, 179
right-censored data, 17, 25, 28, 32, 132, 136, 330, 362, 368

scores, 19, 41
score operator, 121
sequential randomization assumption, 48, 268, 312

tangent space, 33, 56
treatment-specific survival, 343

Example Index

Bivariate location shift model for failure time data, 76.
Current status data with time-dependent covariates, 121, 156
Current status data on a counting process with a surrogate process, 233
Cross-sectional data on competing failure times, 232, 242, 243
(Optimal) IPTW mapping, 163.
Marginal right-censored data, 136
Mixtures (semiparametric models, locally efficient estimation), 71.
Multivariate current status data with a covariate process up until the monitoring time, 233
Multivariate generalized linear regression, 113
Multivariate right-censored data structure with time-dependent covariates, 126, 129, 267, 273, 267.
Marginal structural model, 48,127
Repeated measures data with missing covariate, 16, 29, 33, 45, 157
Repeated measures data with right-censoring, 17, 30, 47
Right-censored data with time-dependent covariate process, 115, 125, 132
Right-censored data with time-independent covariates, 28, 32, 116, 117, 119.
Structural nested model: 347
Tangent space examples: 56, 56, 58, 60, 63

Springer Series in Statistics (continued from p. ii)

Knottnerus: Sample Survey Theory: Some Pythagorean Perspectives.
Kotz/Johnson (Eds.): Breakthroughs in Statistics Volume I.
Kotz/Johnson (Eds.): Breakthroughs in Statistics Volume II.
Kotz/Johnson (Eds.): Breakthroughs in Statistics Volume III.
Küchler/Sørensen: Exponential Families of Stochastic Processes.
Le Cam: Asymptotic Methods in Statistical Decision Theory.
Le Cam/Yang: Asymptotics in Statistics: Some Basic Concepts, 2nd edition.
Liu: Monte Carlo Strategies in Scientific Computing.
Longford: Models for Uncertainty in Educational Testing.
Mielke/Berry: Permutation Methods: A Distance Function Approach.
Pan/Fang: Growth Curve Models and Statistical Diagnostics.
Parzen/Tanabe/Kitagawa: Selected Papers of Hirotugu Akaike.
Politis/Romano/Wolf: Subsampling.
Ramsay/Silverman: Applied Functional Data Analysis: Methods and Case Studies.
Ramsay/Silverman: Functional Data Analysis.
Rao/Toutenburg: Linear Models: Least Squares and Alternatives.
Reinsel: Elements of Multivariate Time Series Analysis, 2nd edition.
Rosenbaum: Observational Studies, 2nd edition.
Rosenblatt: Gaussian and Non-Gaussian Linear Time Series and Random Fields.
Särndal/Swensson/Wretman: Model Assisted Survey Sampling.
Schervish: Theory of Statistics.
Shao/Tu: The Jackknife and Bootstrap.
Simonoff: Smoothing Methods in Statistics.
Singpurwalla and Wilson: Statistical Methods in Software Engineering:
    Reliability and Risk.
Small: The Statistical Theory of Shape.
Sprott: Statistical Inference in Science.
Stein: Interpolation of Spatial Data: Some Theory for Kriging.
Taniguchi/Kakizawa: Asymptotic Theory of Statistical Inference for Time Series.
Tanner: Tools for Statistical Inference: Methods for the Exploration of Posterior
    Distributions and Likelihood Functions, 3rd edition.
van der Laan: Unified Methods for Censored Longitudinal Data and Causality.
van der Vaart/Wellner: Weak Convergence and Empirical Processes: With
    Applications to Statistics.
Verbeke/Molenberghs: Linear Mixed Models for Longitudinal Data.
Weerahandi: Exact Statistical Methods for Data Analysis.
West/Harrison: Bayesian Forecasting and Dynamic Models, 2nd edition.

ALSO AVAILABLE FROM SPRINGER!

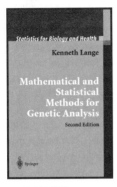
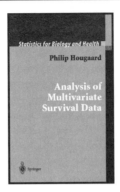
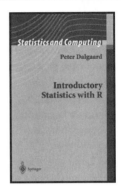

KENNETH LANGE
MATHEMATICAL AND STATISTICAL METHODS FOR GENETIC ANALYSIS
Second Edition

Mathematical, statistical, and computational principles relevant to genetic analysis are developed hand in hand with applications to population genetics, gene mapping, risk prediction, testing of epidemiological hypotheses, molecular evolution, and DNA sequence analysis.

This second edition expands the original edition by over 100 pages and includes new material on DNA sequence analysis, diffusion processes, binding domain identification, Bayesian estimation of haplotype frequencies, case-control association studies, the gamete competition model, QTL mapping and factor analysis and, the Lander-Green-Kruglyak algorithm of pedigree analysis.

2002/384 PAGES/HARDCOVER/ISBN 0-387-95389-2
STATISTICS FOR BIOLOGY AND HEALTH

PHILIP HOUGAARD
ANALYSIS OF MULTIVARIATE SURVIVAL DATA

Survival data or more general time-to-event data occurs in many areas, including medicine, biology, engineering, economics, and demography, but previously standard methods have required that all time variables are univariate and independent. This book extends the field by allowing for multivariate times. Applications where such data appear are survival of twins, survival of married couples and families, time to failure of right and left kidney for diabetic patients, life history data with time to outbreak of disease, complications and death, recurrent episodes of diseases and cross-over studies with time responses.

2000/480 PP./HARDCOVER/ISBN 0-387-98873-4
STATISTICS FOR BIOLOGY AND HEALTH

PETER DALGAARD
INTRODUCTORY STATISTICS WITH R

This book provides an elementary-level introduction to R, targeting both non-statistician scientists in various fields and students of statistics.

The main mode of presentation is via code examples with liberal commenting of the code and the output, from the computational as well as the statistical viewpoint. Brief sections introduce the statistical methods before they are used. A supplementary R package can be downloaded and contains the data sets. All examples are directly runnable and all graphics in the text are generated from the examples.

The statistical methodology covered includes statistical standard distributions, one- and two-sample tests with continuous data, regression analysis, one- and two-way analysis of variance, regression analysis, analysis of tabular data, and sample size calculations.

2002/288 PP./SOFTCOVER/ISBN 0-387-95475-9
STATISTICS AND COMPUTING

To Order or for Information:

In the Americas: **CALL:** 1-800-SPRINGER or **FAX:** (201) 348-4505 • **WRITE:** Springer-Verlag New York, Inc., Dept. S449, PO Box 2485, Secaucus, NJ 07096-2485 • **VISIT:** Your local technical bookstore
• **E-MAIL:** orders@springer-ny.com

Outside the Americas: **CALL:** +49/30/8/27 87-3 73
• +49/30/8 27 87-0 • **FAX:** +49/30 8 27 87 301
• **WRITE:** Springer-Verlag, P.O. Box 140201, D-14302 Berlin, Germany • **E-MAIL:** orders@springer.de

PROMOTION: S449

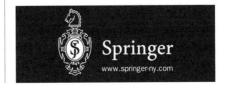